About the Author

Danny Wedding, PhD, MPH, retired from the University of Missouri School of Medicine to become the Associate Dean for Management and International Programs at the California School of Professional Psychology, Alliant International University, San Francisco. In this role, he had oversight responsibility for psychology graduate programs in Hong Kong, Tokyo, and Mexico City. He subsequently chaired the Department of Behavioral Science and Neuroscience for the American University of Antigua School of Medicine and served in a variety of roles for the American University of the Caribbean in Sint Maarten. Danny is a retired navy captain who was a Robert Wood Johnson Health Policy Fellow, working in the Senate, and an APA Congressional Science Fellow, working in the House of Representatives. He is the former editor of *PsycCRITIQUES: Contemporary Psychology – APA Review of Books*, the senior editor for Hogrefe's book series on *Advances in Psychotherapy: Evidence-Based Practice*, and the coauthor of *Positive Psychology at the Movies: Using Films to Build Virtues and Character Strengths.* Danny's best-known book is *Current Psychotherapies,* now in its 11th edition. He lives in West Linn, Oregon, where he continues to write and lecture on the portrayal of mental illness in contemporary cinema.

Movies and Mental Illness

Using Films to Understand Psychopathology

5th edition

Danny Wedding

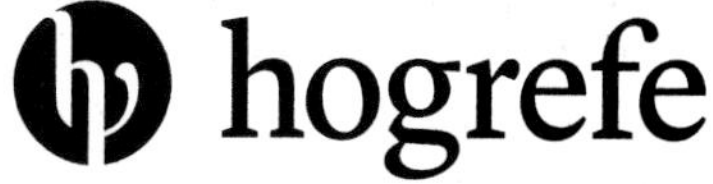

Library of Congress Cataloging in Publication information for the print version of this book is available via the Library of Congress Marc Database under the Library of Congress Control Number 2023945581

Library and Archives Canada Cataloguing in Publication

Title: Movies and mental illness : using films to understand psychopathology / Danny Wedding.
Names: Wedding, Danny, author.
Description: 5th edition. | Includes bibliographical references and index.
Identifiers: Canadiana (print) 20230537707 | Canadiana (ebook) 20230537715 | ISBN 9780889375536 (softcover) | ISBN 9781616765538 (PDF) | ISBN 9781613345535 (EPUB)
Subjects: LCSH: Psychology, Pathological—Study and teaching—Audio-visual aids. | LCSH: Mental illness in motion pictures. | LCSH: Mental illness.
Classification: LCC RC459 .W43 2023 | DDC 616.89—dc23

www.hogrefe.com

PUBLISHING OFFICES

USA:	Hogrefe Publishing Corporation, 44 Merrimac Street, Suite 207, Newburyport, MA 01950 Phone (978) 255 3700; E-mail customersupport@hogrefe.com
EUROPE:	Hogrefe Publishing GmbH, Merkelstr. 3, 37085 Göttingen, Germany Phone +49 551 99950 0, Fax +49 551 99950 111; E-mail publishing@hogrefe.com

SALES & DISTRIBUTION

USA:	Hogrefe Publishing, Customer Services Department, 30 Amberwood Parkway, Ashland, OH 44805 Phone (800) 228 3749, Fax (419) 281 6883; E-mail customersupport@hogrefe.com
UK:	Hogrefe Publishing, c/o Marston Book Services Ltd., 160 Eastern Ave., Milton Park, Abingdon, OX14 4SB Phone +44 1235 465577, Fax +44 1235 465556; E-mail direct.orders@marston.co.uk
EUROPE:	Hogrefe Publishing, Merkelstr. 3, 37085 Göttingen, Germany Phone +49 551 99950 0, Fax +49 551 99950 111; E-mail publishing@hogrefe.com

OTHER OFFICES

CANADA:	Hogrefe Publishing Corporation, 82 Laird Drive, East York, Ontario M4G 3V1
SWITZERLAND:	Hogrefe Publishing, Länggass-Strasse 76, 3012 Bern

Printed and bound in the USA

ISBN 978-0-88937-553-6 (print) • ISBN 978-1-61676-553-8 (PDF) • ISBN 978-1-61334-553-5 (EPUB)
https://doi.org/10.1027/00553-000

Dedication

For Ryan Niemiec and Mary Ann Boyd

Two wonderful colleagues who walked beside me on this long and fascinating journey ...

Acknowledgments

I am constantly writing about and discussing movies, and there are numerous friends and colleagues to acknowledge. Many of the new film entries included in each new edition of *Movies and Mental Illness* grew out of discussions with these individuals, especially those who are mental health professionals interested in the fascinating ways in which psychopathology is portrayed in film.

Rob Dimbleby, my Hogrefe editor, is an extraordinary publisher, a true visionary, and a valued friend. I appreciate his enthusiasm for publishing an expanded and enhanced fifth edition.

I am also grateful to Mary Ann Boyd and Ryan Niemiec, cherished colleagues and friends, who served as coauthors of the first four editions of *Movies and Mental Illness.* This edition is dedicated to the two of them. Their ideas and writing are found on almost every page, but I remain solely responsible for any errors.

Many people provided specific feedback or suggestions relating to the psychopathology or movie portions of the book. These comments helped me make solid improvements in this edition. Thanks go to my colleagues in two divisions of the American Psychological Association: The Society for Media Psychology and Technology, and the Society for the Psychology of Aesthetics, Creativity, and the Arts. The members of these two divisions made multiple recommendations for films we have included in this new edition.

I benefited from hundreds of discussions about films with my oldest son, Joshua Wedding, and my peripatetic younger son, Jeremiah Wedding (whose decision to major in film studies was no doubt influenced by my habit of watching two or three movies each week). Kayley Harrington, Kristine Harrington, and Thomas Harrington also made numerous useful suggestions, along with their respective partners, Aaron Bach, Laurie Dukart, and Krystle Bartholomew.

I also benefited from numerous films discussed with my wonderful wife, Karen Harrington; she shares my passion for films (but not always my passion for films dealing with depression, pathology, and suicide). Karen's mother, Dorothea (Dody) Schwaiger, also helped with this edition – in part by walking away from several films after 15 minutes, helping Danny know when films were too confusing, provocative, or disturbing for the typical viewer (e.g., *Bone Tomahawk, The Snowtown Murders*, and *We Need to Talk About Kevin*).

Dr. Kimberly Kirkland arranged for me to spend the fall semester, 2022, in Sint Maarten (the Dutch side of the island) where I served for one semester as interim Associate Dean for student affairs for the American University of the Caribbean (AUC), a medical school where I have taught off and on for 20 years. I worked *very* hard, but my evenings and weekends were free (and lonely). This provided time to see dozens of films, and I was able to finalize this book while on the island.

Ms. Mounia Hanzazi, an AUC librarian, was also tremendously helpful in ensuring I had access to primary source material while away from my usual libraries and librarians.

This book has opened some incredible speaking opportunities. Drs. Moira Nakousi and Daniel Soto arranged for me to present talks on *Movies and Mental Illness* in Santiago, Chile; Dr. Catherine Sun invited me to keynote a conference in counseling psychology in Hong Kong; Dr. Saths Cooper invited me to present on the topic at the International Congress of Psychology in Cape Town, South Africa; Prof. Paul Crawford arranged for me to present at an International Health Humanities conference sponsored by the University of Nottingham; and I was able to present on the topic of bipolar disorders and cinema at the 12th International Review of Bipolar Disorders in Nice, France. The Nice talk coincided with the by-invitation-only

Cannes Film Festival (*Festival de Cannes*), and I was able to use a flyer for *Movies and Mental Illness* to establish my credentials as a serious scholar and a writer with a genuine interest in films.

Finally, I want to thank the seven individuals who translated earlier editions of *Movies and Mental Illness* into Spanish, Korean, Turkish, Japanese, German, Italian, and Polish.

I appreciate the feedback from my colleagues, friends, family, as well as the many readers who have taken time to share suggestions and opinions. I hope you will let me know when you come across a great film that should be discussed in the next edition.

Contents

Foreword to the Fifth Edition

When Dr. Wedding asked me to write this foreword, I experienced the full range of what I guess are pretty predictable emotions. Rather than naming the rather embarrassing first iteration of my feelings, I'll ask you instead to picture my 5-foot 6-inch frame walking through the majestic woods of New Hampshire with a puffed-up chest and a spring to my step. I've written about movies for much of my career, and *Movies and Mental Illness* is the altar on which every mental health professional who writes about film has felt compelled to leave an offering. Dr. Wedding's book is a masterpiece. Nobody else has come even close to the scholarship, creativity, and almost impossible inclusiveness that await you in this fifth edition. As a result of this high, it took me longer than I'd care to admit to actually put pen to paper. Instead, I imagined over and over again that I had already written what would be the most celebrated essay in the history of the world that endeavors to discuss film and psychology. This, I recognized, was the Walter Mitty stage of writing. I was Danny Kaye in 1947 or Ben Stiller in 2013. The same Walter in both films, and both films perfectly capturing my state of mind. That's the magic of movies.

But next came anxiety and fear. After all, if I have placed this book on the altar, then it is, by definition, beyond description. Imagine trying to write an introduction to something for which your admiration has come close to worship. It is akin to describing something awesome, something that is in its essence uncapturable. The magic of movies struck again. This time nearly suffocating me in one of those groovy space suits in *2001: A Space Odyssey*. I was dumbstruck as I watched the planet Jupiter grow large and ominous, and my writing was delayed despite the pesky fact that the clock refused to stop ticking.

Like a delirious pinball, I ricocheted from one film to the next, looking to rescue myself from the paralysis of my task. I settled on the warnings of Captain Picard in *Star Trek: Generations*. Chatting with Commander Riker, Picard contemplates the passage of time. "Someone once told me that time was a predator that stalked us all our lives," he muses. And to be honest, I was awfully close to being captured and devoured by time's most pernicious weapon – that monster we call procrastination. But then I remembered that Picard, ever the optimist, turned the metaphor of predatory time on its head. "I rather believe that time is a companion," he tells us. "What we leave behind is not as important as how we lived." If we are talking about how we live, then it is here that I must confess that I have lived my life with and through the movies. My father took me to see *2001: A Space Odyssey* when it came back to the theaters in the mid-1970s. I have been enamored of Star Trek from the moment I had the capacity to turn on the television set by myself. Onscreen stories are inextricably tied to who and to what I am.

As I thought more about this foreword, I borrowed from the sense of responsibility and challenge that virtually every story about the intoxication of exploration has at some point unfailingly depicted. This assignment would not become the *game over* moment from *Aliens* that has come to exemplify giving up. This assignment would be my invitation to discover and to be amazed. My paralytic fear became Caliban's resolve in *The Tempest*. "Sometimes a thousand twangling instruments will hum about mine ears," he says. Rather than eschewing the island that made him, he embraces and celebrates the magic of his predicament. To me, Caliban's thousand instruments are the countless movies that have enriched my life. As if to prove my point, I noted that *The Tempest* has enjoyed more than five different movies adaptations, and I adore every one of them. If the deformed Caliban can look upon his island with wonder, then I can certainly write this foreword with the same spirit of discovery and awe.

By now you'll sense that the biggest impediment to my celebrating *Movies and Mental Illness* wasn't time, or grandiosity, or even my lingering fear of abject failure. The impediment was the subject itself. To borrow again from Shakespeare, the "past is prologue." I have never not loved movies. As such, I lose all sense of time when I thumb through this book. Wedding so seamlessly mixes the nuanced world of psychiatry with the nuanced world of movies that every time I sat down to write this essay, I would read a chapter or two, and then I was off to the cinema yet again. The wonder of our modern world is the immense and immediate accessibility of film. All you need is a laptop or a theater and a willingness to pay a few bucks. Because of this book, I discovered gems like *The Boy Who Could Fly*, revisited long forgotten favorites like *Birdy*, and soared through the clouds with the giddy and increasingly dangerous teens in *Chronicle*. In other words, every time I opened this book, I risked getting lost in at least three movies, each well over an hour long. I therefore feel this foreword ought to contain at least some form of warning. *Movies and Mental Illness* is that gift that at the same time becomes the best kind of trap. Hours will collapse as you read. You will turn to YouTube to search for the most obscure but illuminating movie clips. You will scan your local library for the DVD of that film that is no longer streaming. If you live in a rural setting as I do, you'll drive hours to see that one film that just happens to be playing at that funky arthouse cinema nestled like a shrine on Main Street in some small New England town.

The real impediment to this foreword is knowing when to stop reading and to start writing. For a psychiatrist, this book is like the table of luscious food in *Pan's Labyrinth*, but without the terror of the Pale Man to stop you from eating. Without the Pale Man's menace, you have infinitely more freedom than the girl in Guillermo Del Toro's haunting film. You can take more than just a grape. But with a feast like this at your fingertips, how in the world does one begin?

I suppose it is best to start with what is perhaps already obvious. Since humans have been humans, we've told stories. We had movies way before we had movie projectors. Homer describes each scene of *The Odyssey* as if he were intimately familiar with the local cinema in ancient Athens.

> But Odysseus aimed and shot Antinous square in the throat
> and the point went stabbing clean through the soft neck and out –
> and off to the side he pitched, the cup dropped from his grasp
> as the shaft sank home, and the man's lifeblood came spurting
> out his nostrils –
> thick red jets –
> a sudden thrust of his foot –
> he kicked away the table –
> food showered across the floor,
> the bread and meats soaked in a swirl of bloody filth.
>
> (Book 22, *Slaughter in the Hall*, translated by Robert Fagles)

My goodness, this could have been written by Quentin Tarantino! The magic of stories rests in their iterative dialectic. We hear or we watch the same tales again and again, and yet when these stories are done well, they feel as fresh as the break of day. Thank goodness for the endless creativity of humanity.

But there is another constant with which this introduction must reckon. The variety of stories that we tell is matched only by the variety of madness that we suffer. Depression, mania, psychosis ... these illnesses have been described for thousands of years. Say what you want about the flawed *Diagnostic and Statistical Manual of Mental Disorders*, 5th edition (DSM-5). I will maintain that some form of the DSM was written long before the American Psychiatric Association (APA) claimed this catalogue as its own. Pathological states of mind have always been integral to our stories. In fact, I would go so far as to say that pathological states of mind are the *essence* of our stories. If you'll accept this supposition, then it stands to reason that movies themselves are perhaps our best and most accessible modalities toward understanding representations of mental illness. They are also among the most jarring means through which we can observe the many ways that these illnesses and their treatments can be dangerously represented. Is *One Flew Over the Cuckoo's Nest* (1975) a warning against the cultural entanglement of the conforming lens of psychiatric diagnosis, or a celebration of the uncrushable potency of human individualism? The answer, I'd argue, is both. Not surprisingly, this iconic film is mentioned more than 20 times in *Movies and Mental Illness*.

What makes *Movies and Mental Illness* so special is that it goes beyond simply cataloguing the mental states that occur in movies. Wedding writes that *Cuckoo's Nest* shows us the dangers inherent in the powers given to psychiatric hospitals, and at the same time compares it with the 1948 film, *The Snake Pit*. He notes that the risk of inhumane treatment for psychiatrically ill individuals exists whether the person being treated is feigning the illness, as in *Cuckoo's Nest*, or quite authentically suffering from a psychiatric syndrome, as in *The Snake Pit*. These nuggets of truth are the golden bits of wisdom that rest within the pages that follow.

Stories are incredibly powerful, and stories told on the screen are perhaps the most powerful of all. Movies invite us and envelope us. They challenge us and they rescue us. There are hundreds of movies mentioned in *Movies and Mental Illness*, each one a different story, and each one a variation on the same familiar theme. After all, a good movie is nuanced and fresh and, simultaneously, recognizable and familiar. This book works because the same can be said of psychiatric illness. Each person suffering from mental illness is overwhelmingly different and relentlessly familiar. We know people who suffer. We *are* people who suffer. The thread that ties us to movies is the thread that ties us to each other, and that is the thread of common experience. As we sit currently in the midst of an epidemic of mental suffering, the thread of psychological anguish is an all too common experience. This is hardly a newsflash, but we must keep this in mind as we read this book. Movies represent a potent arm in our arsenal toward fighting the stigma against mental illness. Movies can also help us to find new ways to understand and to treat psychiatric syndromes.

In *Spiderman*, Uncle Ben tells Peter Parker, "With great power comes great responsibility." That's what this book gives its readers: Power and responsibility. And to prove my point, it is worth remembering that this very sentiment was expressed in stories well before there were movie screens. In the first century BC, the fable of *The Sword of Damocles* tells us that Damocles becomes terrified when he is allowed by King Dionysius to occupy the throne for even a day. The responsibility of this power overwhelms him, and he gladly steps away from his brief stint as king. As with all good stories, this warning surfaces again and again throughout the millions of stories we've told each other since the beginning of time. From Damocles to Spiderman, we see through stories the responsibility we carry, and it is in this spirit that I ask you to enjoy this book. Read the following pages carefully, and watch the movies that you discover thoughtfully. If you teach about mental illness, this book should never leave your desk. If you are a clinician treating mental illness, this book should be among your most cherished guides. And if you suffer yourself, then let this book be your salve.

We are all in this together. We are all, all of us, teachers and clinicians and patients. Fortunately for all of us, this amazing book is written for whatever hat we happen to be wearing at the time that we begin to read.

Steven Schlozman, MD
Chief of Child Psychiatry
University of Vermont

Preface

Drama is life with the dull bits cut out.

Alfred Hitchcock

I wrote *Movies and Mental Illness* because of my conviction that films are a powerful medium for teaching students (in psychology, social work, medicine, nursing, and counseling), engaging patients, and educating the public about the fascinating world of psychopathology. In addition, I wrote the book because I genuinely love watching and talking about movies. While the title is *Movies and Mental Illness*, this book also addresses serious problems that do not reflect mental illness per se, including neurodevelopmental disorders, physical or sexual abuse, and violence.

The first edition of *Movies and Mental Illness* grew out of a series of lunchtime conversations between a psychiatric nurse (Mary Ann Boyd) and me. Inevitably, these conversations included some discussion of recent films we had seen, and whether we thought the portrayal of whatever illness was depicted was accurate. The notes grew into a series of index cards, and the index cards eventually became the first edition. Later, a gifted young psychologist and cinephile named Ryan Niemiec joined the team. Mary Ann and Ryan have both moved on to other projects, but I have persisted in watching hundreds of new films and adding some discussion of almost all of them to this edition.

There are numerous changes made to each new edition, in part because dozens of excellent films have been released over the 8 years or so between editions that need to be included in any book that purports to be both contemporary and comprehensive. Over a hundred recent films have been added to Appendix 6 that illustrate psychopathology. Although it is impossible to list every film depicting every disorder, the book identifies and discusses the most important films that illustrate or involve psychopathology. The reader will find a significant number of these new films discussed in the relevant chapters.

Films are remarkable pedagogical tools, and my students have always appreciated the time I have taken to collect and organize video clips to use in the classroom. For example, I believe watching Michael Haneke's *Amour* captures the pathos associated with caregiving with raw emotion and a vivid power that can never be had by simply reading about neuropathology.

One way to approach *Movies and Mental Illness* is to simply start with Appendix 6 and a highlighter, identifying interesting films, and then seeing what I have to say about them in the book.

I have updated the list of favorite films in each category ("Author Picks"). Mary Ann Boyd and Ryan Niemiec helped me identify these films. We did not always agree about which films were most important for readers to see, but we negotiated and debated each list and eventually selected around 10 films for each chapter that balanced artistic merit and clinical relevance. This addition is in response to the frequent requests for our recommendations for movies that can be used to help train mental health professionals and students from various health professionals.

I relied heavily on Rotten Tomatoes and the Internet Movie Database (IMDb) to refresh my memory on films that I had viewed years ago, or to get a second opinion regarding ratings for films.

I have continued to expand the sections on international films in each chapter. Often these films are more powerful and accurate than anything filmmakers in the United States have produced. I hope this will entice readers to watch more foreign language films; this is an especially interesting and rewarding way to learn about other cultures. In addition, watching foreign language films using Language Learning with Netflix (LLN) makes acquisition of a new language relatively easy and almost fun.

In discussing psychopathology, I occasionally reveal endings or surprise twists to films, and this may spoil these films for some readers. I apologize in advance if this occurs.

The book was originally designed to supplement core texts in abnormal psychology; if the book is being used in this way, the relevant core chapters in the primary text should be read before reviewing the corresponding chapter in *Movies and Mental Illness.* Professors using the text to teach psychopathology can download supplemental material (see Notes on Supplementary Materials at the end of the book for instructions on how to obtain them) including questions that can be assigned to students to answer before coming to class. In addition, each appendix is available to download and share with students.

I will occasionally present detailed and specific information about mental illness, but these facts are almost incidental to the discussion of the films themselves, and I have tried to avoid redundancy with the many fine textbooks that already explain psychopathology in considerable detail. I assume the reader will look up unfamiliar terms or discuss them in class, and I have not always defined each new term.

I am a clinical psychologist and a college professor, and I've found that the judicious use of films dramatically increases students' and clients' understanding of abnormal behavior. For example, when lecturing about alcoholism, I sometimes supplement my lectures with a "demonstration" of delirium tremens using *The Lost Weekend* to illustrate withdrawal, and Denzel Washington's character in *Flight* to illustrate tolerance. Before a lecture on bipolar disorder, I ask my students to watch *Touched With Fire* or *Silver Linings Playbook.* All four films provide intensity that simply cannot be captured by a classroom lecture or on the printed page. Likewise, when working with a client going through a divorce who becomes incensed over the behavior of their spouse, I might recommend watching *Kramer vs. Kramer* or *The Squid and the Whale.* A counselor working with parents attempting to understand and cope with their adolescent child's suicidality might consider reviewing *Boy Interrupted,* and the parent of a trans child might find *Cowboys* meaningful and relevant. I have found that discussion of films offers a wonderful way to open clinically relevant areas that have not previously been explored.

One of the best experiences of my professional life was spending a year teaching graduate students in psychology at Yonsei University in Seoul, South Korea. I taught a course on psychopathology using *Movies and Mental lIllness* as a primary text. A modified syllabus for this course in presented in Appendix 2. In addition, Appendix 3 lists a number of websites that your students will find interesting, relevant and useful.

I occasionally discuss obscure films when a small section relates in a meaningful way to the points made in the chapter. There are also classic films such as *Psycho, A Clockwork Orange,* and *One Flew Over the Cuckoo's Nest* that have tremendous pedagogical value, and I take great pleasure in introducing a new generation of students to these movies. In addition, films such as *Pelle the Conqueror* or *Antonio's Line* are occasionally included, even when there is no direct connection to psychopathology, because the films are provocative and moving and are good illustrations of psychological phenomena. For detailed examples of these and other films depicting character strengths, resilience, and various positive psychological phenomena, I recommend a book I coauthored with Ryan Niemiec, *Positive Psychology at the Movies: Using Films to Build Character Strengths and Well-Being,* which discusses over 1,500 films. Ryan will be publishing a new edition of this book in the future as sole author; he is primarily interested in positive psychology, and I am primarily interested in psychopathology, and we have each agreed to serve as the single author for the book we feel most comfortable writing – that is, *Movies and Mental Illness* for me, and *Positive Psychology at the Movies* for Ryan.

Many readers will disagree with the ratings I have assigned films included in Appendix 6. However, it is important to remember that my ratings are based *primarily* on the pedagogical value of the film, and only secondarily on the film's artistic merit.

I am including my email address below, and I hope both professors and students will write to me after reading this book. I also hope those readers who share my enthusiasm about movies as a teaching tool will recommend additional films that I can include in the next edition of *Movies and Mental Illness*.

Danny Wedding, PhD, MPH
danny.wedding@gmail.com

Chapter 1

Films and Psychopathology

For better or worse, movies and television contribute significantly to shaping the public's perception of the mentally ill and those who treat them.

Steven E. Hyler

For contemporary audiences, attending movies is an experience that provides catharsis and unites the audience with their culture in much the same way that the tragedies of Sophocles and Aeschylus performed these functions for 5th-century BC Greek audiences.

Glen Gabbard and Krin Gabbard (1999)

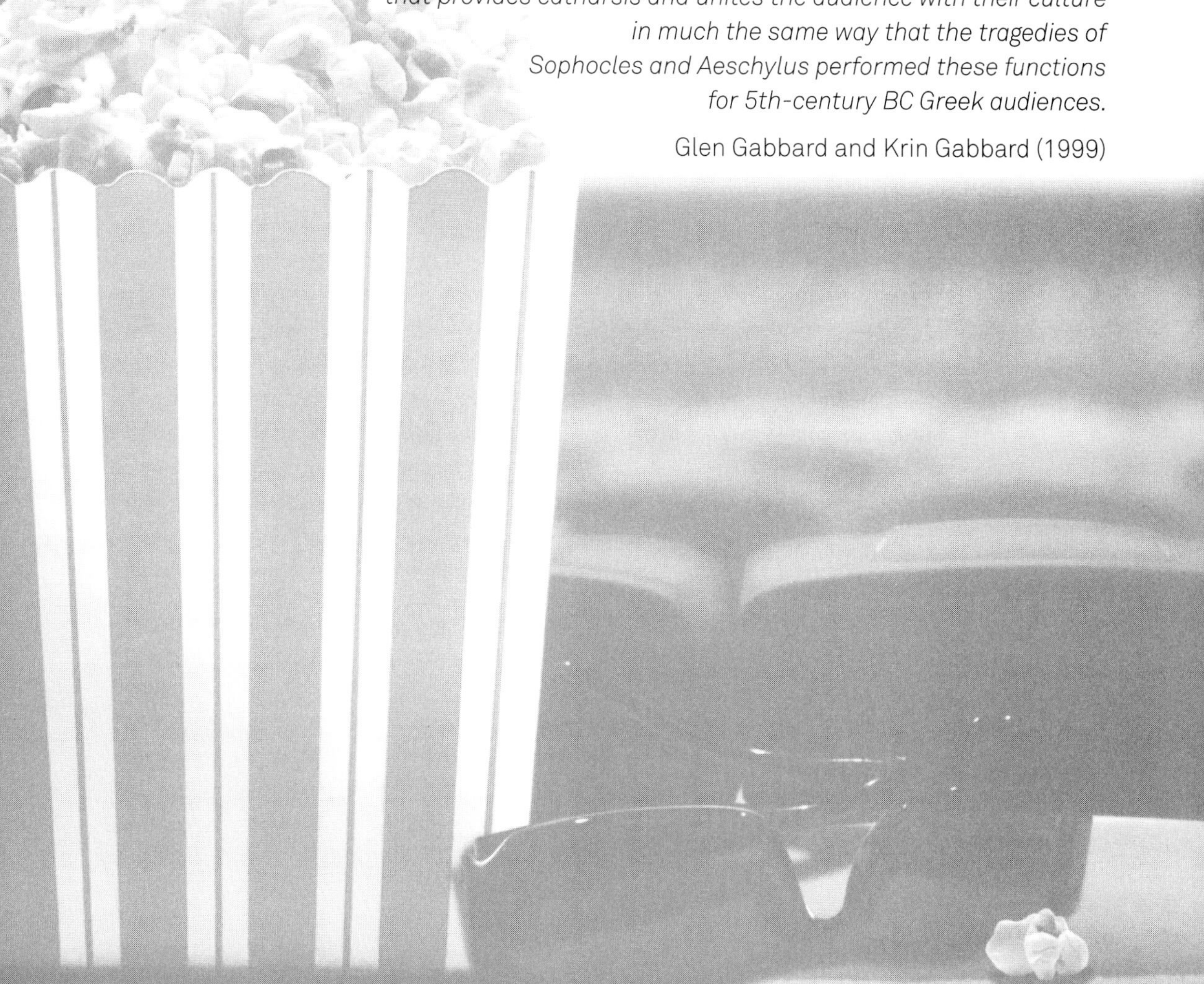

Introduction

In all human perceptual experience, nothing conveys information or evokes emotion quite as clearly as our visual sense. Filmmakers capture the richness of this visual sense, combine it with auditory stimuli, and create the ultimate waking dream experience: a movie. The viewer enters a trance, a state of absorption, concentration, and attention, engrossed by the story and the plight of the characters. When someone is watching a movie, an immediate bond is set up between the viewer and the film, and all the technical apparatus involved with the projection of the film becomes invisible as the images from the film pass into the viewer's consciousness. The viewer experiences a sort of dissociative state in which ordinary existence is suspended, serving as a psychological clutch (Butler & Palesh, 2004) in which the individual escapes from the stressors, conflicts, and worries of the day. This trance state is further enhanced in movie theaters where the viewer is fully enveloped in sight and sound, and in some instances, experiences the sense of touch through vibration effects. No other art form pervades the consciousness of the individual to the same extent and with such power as cinema. Many consider movies to be the most influential form of mass communication (Cape, 2003).

Hollywood took the original invention of the cinematic camera and invented a new art form in which the viewer becomes enveloped in the work of art. The camera carries the viewer into each scene, and the viewer perceives events from the inside as if surrounded by the characters in the film. The actors do not have to describe their feelings, as in a play, because the viewer directly experiences what they see and feel.

To produce an emotional response to a film, the director carefully develops both plot and character through precise camera work. Editing creates a visual and acoustic **gestalt**, to which the viewer responds. The more effective the technique, the more involved the viewer. In effect, the director constructs the film's (and the viewer's) reality. The selection of locations, sets, actors, costumes, and lighting contributes to the film's organization and shot-by-shot **mise-en-scène** (the physical arrangement of visual images). Arısoy and Gökmen (2021) have described the ways in which lighting can be used creatively to enhance both significance and fear in horror films, using *Dogtooth* (2009) as an exemplar film.

The Pervasive Influence of Films

Humans are creatures whose lives cry out for meaning and purpose, and we impose meaning even on random and unconnected events. In 1944, psychologists Fritz Heider and Marianne Simmel made a simple animated film using two triangles, a circle, and a box. Each shape moved, seemingly in a random manner. They asked people to watch the short film and describe what was happening. Inevitably, these research subjects "interpreted the picture in terms of [the] actions of animated beings, chiefly of persons" (p. 243). In short, viewers *created a story*, even when none existed. *We need stories in our lives*, and movies provide a compelling vehicle for sharing these stories. David Carroll has noted,

> By creating stories of our lives, we construct the salient features of our social identity, our sense of identity in relation to the important others in our lives. Our ability to construct stories that highlight the central features of our lives is an essential part of what it means to be a human being living in a social world. (Carroll, 2013 , p. 121)

Film has become such an integral part of our culture that it is the mirror in which we see ourselves reflected every day. Indeed, the social impact of film extends around the globe, and movies produced in Hollywood are watched in movie theaters in Europe, Asia, South America, and Africa, often in remote and surprising locations. Traveling is a personal passion, and I was surprised – and delighted – when I gave international lectures and discovered that many people in my audience had watched and loved many of the films I cherish.

The widespread popularity of online movies, streaming video (e.g., Netflix, Amazon Prime, Hulu), nominally priced Redbox rentals on street corners, the use of unlimited rentals for a monthly fee, and in-home, cable features like On-Demand make hundreds of thousands of movies available and accessible to anyone in the world (and certainly anyone with Internet access). We are no longer limited solely to the film selection and discretion of the corner video store. In addition, people now have wide access to films beyond Hollywood, including access to films from independent filmmakers, even those from developing countries. Moreover, with the affordability of digital video, neophyte and/or low-budget filmmakers can now tell their stories within the constraints of a much more reasonable budget without sacrificing quality (Taylor & Hsu, 2003); this increases the range of topics and themes that can be covered. Award-winning films such as *Gravity* (2013), *Rust and Bone* (2012), *The Revenant* (2015), and *Life of Pi* (2012) were all shot using digital video. However, some directors, such as Quentin Tarantino and Christopher Nolan, have been adamantly opposed to digital video, with Tarantino claiming, "If I can't shoot on film, I'll stop making movies" (Bramesco, 2016).

The current ubiquity of movie streaming is illustrated by the success of companies like Netflix, and Blockbuster's decision not to buy Netflix in 2000 has gone down as one of the biggest boardroom mistakes in corporate history. In 2010, Blockbuster filed for bankruptcy after losing $1.1 billion; at that time, Netflix was worth around $13 billion (Graser, 2013). Netflix's stock value has dramatically increased since then, although competition in the streaming market also has increased markedly, with companies like Disney, Amazon, and Apple all competing with Netflix.

Films have a greater influence than any other art form. This influence is felt across age, gender, nationality, and culture – and even across time. Films have become a pervasive and omnipresent part of our society, and yet people often have little conscious awareness of the profound influence the medium exerts.

Films are especially important in influencing the public perception of mental illness, because many people are uninformed about the problems of people with mental disorders, and the media tend to be especially effective in shaping opinion in those situations in which strong opinions are not already held (Heath, 2019). Although some films present sympathetic portrayals of people with mental illness and those professionals who work in the field of mental health (e.g., *The Three Faces of Eve*, *David and Lisa*, *Ordinary People*, and *A Beautiful Mind*), many more do not. Individuals with mental illness are often portrayed as aggressive, dangerous, and unpredictable; psychiatrists, psychologists, nurses, and other health professionals who work with these patients are often portrayed as "arrogant and ineffectual," "cold-hearted and authoritarian," "passive and apathetic," or "shrewd and manipulative" (Niemiec & Wedding, 2006; Wedding, 2017). Psychiatrists are often negatively portrayed in the cinema (Gabbard & Gabbard, 1999), and psychoanalysts have been ridiculed and misrepresented in numerous films (Sabbadini, 2015).

Films such as *Psycho* (1960) perpetuate the continuing confusion about the relationship between schizophrenia and dissociative identity disorder (formerly multiple personality disorder); *Friday the 13th* (1980), *Nightmare on Elm Street* (1984), and *The Adopted One* (2020) all perpetuate the pernicious misconception that people who leave psychiatric hospitals are violent and dangerous; movies such as *The Exorcist* (1973) suggest to the public that mental illness is the equivalent of possession by the devil; and films like *One Flew Over the Cuckoo's Nest* (1975) make the case that psychiatric hospitals are simply prisons in which there is little or no regard for patient rights or welfare. These films in part account for the continuing stigma of mental illness. Many of these themes are explored in Sharon Packer's book *Mental Illness in Popular Culture* (Packer, 2017).

Stigma is one of the reasons that so few people with mental problems receive help (Corrigan, 2018). The National Institute of Mental Health (NIMH) estimates that only half of those with mental disorders reach out for help with their problems, even though many current treatments for these disorders are inexpensive and effective (NIMH, 2023). In addition, there is still a strong tendency to see patients with mental disorders as the cause of their own disorders – for example, the National Alliance for the Mentally Ill (NAMI) has polling data that indicate that about one in three US citizens still conceptualizes mental illness in terms of evil and punishment for misbehavior.

Psychiatrist Peter Byrne (2009) has pointed out that films rarely portray mental illness or mental health practitioners accurately, but he also makes the compelling point that the job of a director is to create a film that will generate revenue for producers and investors, and it is not necessarily their job to educate the public. Byrne has described five rules of movie psychiatry:

1. Follow the money: Filmmaking is a commercial enterprise and producers may include inaccurate representations in their films to "give the public what they want".
2. Film begets film: Every new film draws on previous films within the genre.
3. Skewed distribution hides more films than censorship ever did.
4. There are no mental health films, just mental illness ones.
5. If it bleeds, it leads: Violence, injury and death often ensure prominence of a story in both news and film. (Byrne, 2009, pp. 287–288)

Byrne's points are well-taken, although I would challenge Number 4, because Ryan Niemiec and I wrote a book titled *Positive Psychology at the Movies* (Niemiec & Wedding, 2014) in which we document over 1,500 movies that display character strengths and other healthy aspects of human psychology, including positive mental health. This edition of *Movies and Mental Illness* also describes many films that offer positive depictions of mental health, and Dr. Niemiec has followed up our positive psychology book with a 2020 article in the *Journal of Clinical Psychology* titled "Character Strengths Cinematherapy: Using Movies to Inspire Change, Meaning, and Cinematic Elevation" (Niemiec, 2020).

Positive Psychology at the Movies is clearly an exception, however. Most books, like *Movies and Mental Illness*, focus on negative depictions of mental illness. Johnson and Walker (2021), as editors of a recent book titled *Normalizing Mental Illness and Neurodiversity in Entertainment Media: Quieting the Madness*, examine those films in which portrayals of mental, emotional, and developmental disabilities succeed.

Movies can portray powerful role models that can be especially meaningful for children and young people. *Black Panther* (2018) and *Black Panther: Wakanda Forever* (2022) are two examples. Both films are based on positive representations of Black culture. Zakia Gates (2022) noted that *Black Panther* promotes belief in Black power, excellence, and intelligence, and the film offers a role model of a Black female scientist, in the character of Suri. They note that there are few such models of Black male scientists, and ask: "If LeBron James conducted a critical analysis using physics and mathematics to make a 3-point shot, then what is the likelihood that young Black males' interest in the STEM programs would increase?" (p. 115).

Cinematic Elements

A film director must consider countless technical elements in the making of a film, often orchestrating hundreds of people, many of whom monitor and pass down orders to hundreds or thousands of other collaborators. However, there are three general phases involved in making a film.

The time spent prior to filming in the **preproduction phase** is often seen as the most important. Many directors *storyboard* (draw out) every shot, and choreograph every movement for each scene to be filmed. Countless meetings with each technical supervisor (e.g., cinematographer, costume designer, set designer, electrician) are held to facilitate preparation, coordination, and integration. The director will also scout out locations, work to cast appropriate actors for the various roles, and may rework the screenplay.

In the **production phase**, the director attempts to film their vision, working closely with the actors and actresses to encourage, stimulate, guide, or alter their work, while carefully monitoring camera angles, lighting, sound, and other technical areas.

In the **postproduction phase**, editing and laying out the musical score and background sounds are major areas of focus. The director integrates each of these elements while working to honor the original purpose, message, and underlying themes of the film.

Some of the most important cinematic elements are summarized with film examples in Table 1. Of course, these three phases exclude

Table 1. Film elements with movie examples

Film element	Explanation	Classic example	Recent example
Themes	Overall meaning, messages, motifs (e.g., love, good vs. evil)	*It's a Wonderful Life* (1946)	*Once Upon a Time in Hollywood* (2019); *The Tale* (2018)
Cinematography	Visual appeal, framing, camera work, lighting	*Lawrence of Arabia* (1962)	*Roma* (2018); *1917* (2019); *Nightmare Alley* (2021); *Oppenheimer* (2023)
Pacing	Movement, fluidity	*Jaws* (1975); *Fargo* (1996)	*1917* (2019); *Marriage Story* (2019)
Sound	Music, score, sound effects	*Ben-Hur* (1959); *Jaws* (1975)	*Bohemian Rhapsody* (2018); *Star Wars: Tales of the Jedi* (2022)
Mood	Tone, atmosphere	*M* (1931)	*The Snowtown Murders* (2012); *The Lighthouse* (2019)
Art	Set design, costumes	*Star Wars* (1977)	*Little Women* (2019); *West Side Story* (2021)
Dialogue	Conversation, modes of communication	*Annie Hall* (1977); *Pulp Fiction* (1994)	*Green Book* (2018); *Belfast* (2021)
Acting	Character portrayal, depth and quality, casting	*The Philadelphia Story* (1940)	*Joker* (2019); *Nomadland* (2020); *The Power of the Dog* (2021)
Editing	Continuity, transitions	*Citizen Kane* (1941)	*Ford v. Ferrari* (2019); *Tick, Tick ... BOOM!* (2021)
Screenplay	Storyline, plot; original or adapted to the screen	*One Flew Over the Cuckoo's Nest* (1975)	*The Power of the Dog* (2021); *Minari* (2020)
Direction	All elements together, quality of film overall	*A Clockwork Orange* (1971)	*Parasite* (2019); *The Power of the Dog* (2021)

countless other tasks involving financing, budgeting, marketing, and other business, administrative, consulting, and legal aspects. A mental health consultant may be used with certain films and may play a key role in any phase, particularly involving fine-tuning the screenplay and helping the director and actors understand psychological and related phenomena; I believe mental health consultants should be sought out for *every* film portraying a psychological condition or a therapeutic encounter. Unfortunately, such consultants are sorely underutilized in cinema. However, the directors of films such as *A Beautiful Mind*, *Antwone Fisher*, and *Analyze This* did use psychologists and/or psychiatrists as consultants. Stephen Sands, a pediatric neuropsychologist at Memorial Sloan Kettering Cancer Center in New York was a technical adviser for *Analyze That* (2002), starring Billy Crystal as a psychiatrist and Robert De Niro as a mobster. "De Niro was so eager to accurately portray mental illness that he visited a psychiatric hospital where Sands worked and participated in a group therapy meeting" (Stringer, 2016).

Directors attempt to artfully integrate the technical elements of sound, camera, and lighting fluidly with the plot, themes, pacing, and tone of the film, while eliciting quality acting performances. Danis Tanovic, director of a film that won the Academy Award for Best Foreign Language Film, *No Man's Land* (2001), about the Bosnian-Serbian war, speaks to many of these elements as he describes the shock and disharmony of the war that he attempted to depict in his film:

> This shock is something I have reproduced through my film. On one side, a long summer day – perfect nature, strong colors – and on the other, human beings and their black madness. And this long, hot summer day reflects the atmosphere of the film itself. Movements are heavy, thoughts are hard to grasp, time is slow and tension is hiding – hiding but present. When it finally explodes, it is like fireworks – sudden, loud, and quick. Panoramic shots of landscape become unexpectedly mixed with nervous details of action. It all lasts for a moment or two, and then tension hides again, waiting for the next opportunity to surprise. Time slows down again. (Danis Tanovic, quoted in the DVD insert for *No Man's Land*)

Changes in color and sound significantly impact the viewer's experience of a film. Butler and Palesh (2004) offer the example of Steven Spielberg's manipulation of these cinematic elements in *Saving Private Ryan* (1998). In addition to screams turned slowly into sobs or mumbles, colors are subdued to an almost black-and-white appearance so that when red is introduced in the battle scenes amid the muted background, the depiction of the reality of war becomes even more vivid for the viewer.

For the most skilled directors, virtually everything that the camera "sees" and records is meaningful. The sense of subjective experience produced by a sequence of **point-of-view** shots facilitates the viewer's identification with the film's characters, their perceptions, and their circumstances. Extreme **close-up shots** and a variety of **panning techniques** facilitate the importance of an emotional expression or inner conflict or develop pacing for the film. **High-angle and low-angle shots** give emphasis to character control, power, strength, weakness, and a variety of other dynamics. For example, in *American Beauty* (1999), high-angle shots are used at the beginning of the film focused on Lester Burnham (Kevin Spacey) to indicate a passiveness and submission to authority prior to his transformation to a strong-willed, commanding character. In *The Shawshank Redemption* (1994), a high-angle shot of Andy Dufresne in the rain with his arms raised symbolizes redemption and makes the character appear Christ-like (see Figure 1). High-angle shots were also often used in Alfred Hitchcock's films, and they – like his cameo appearances – became part of his cinematic signature.

Contrast this image with a different low-angle shot also reminiscent of the crucifixion of Christ in *Cool Hand Luke* (1967; see Figure 2).

Each viewer possesses unique perceptual preferences, prior knowledge about the film's content, and preconceptions about the images the film contains that mediate their perceptions

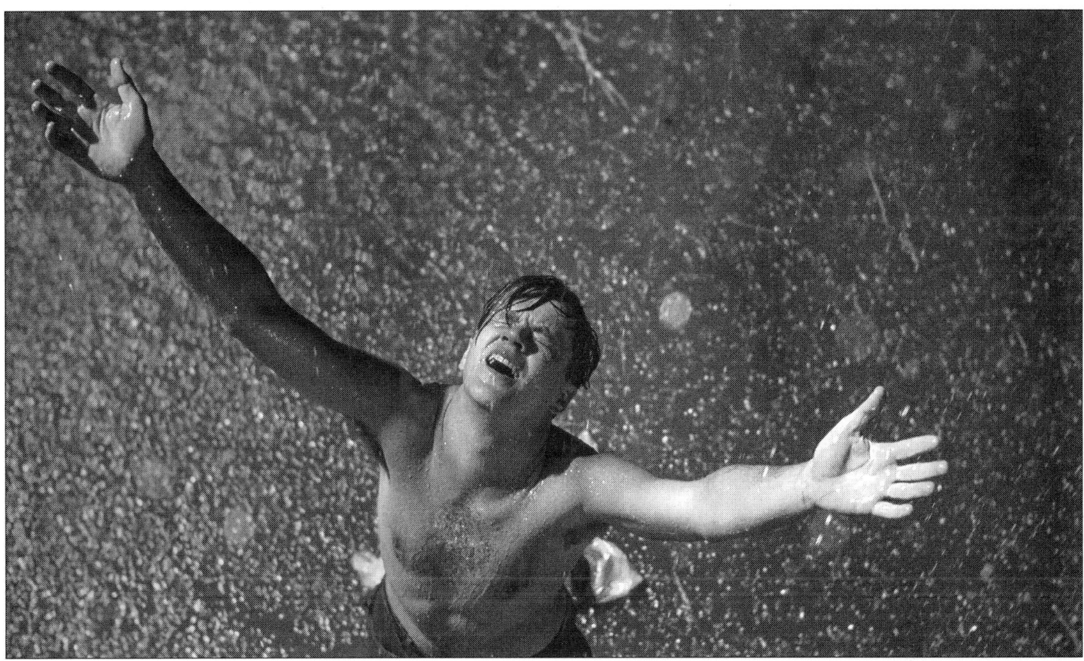

Figure 1. High-angle shot from *The Shawshank Redemption* (1994, Castle Rock Entertainment). Produced by Liz Glotzer, David V. Lester, and Niki Marvin. Directed by Frank Darabont.

and experience. Rarely, if ever, do any two viewers have an identical experience when viewing the same film. Each viewer subjectively selects, attends to, and translates the visual and acoustic images projected in a theater into their own version of the story. Often viewers are affected by, or identify with, the film's characters so strongly that it appears clear that the defense mechanism of **projection** is present. This process is facilitated when the viewer can anticipate the storyline, the plot, or the outcome. The avid moviegoer quickly realizes familiar themes, similar settings, and "formulas" for plots and endings across a variety of films.

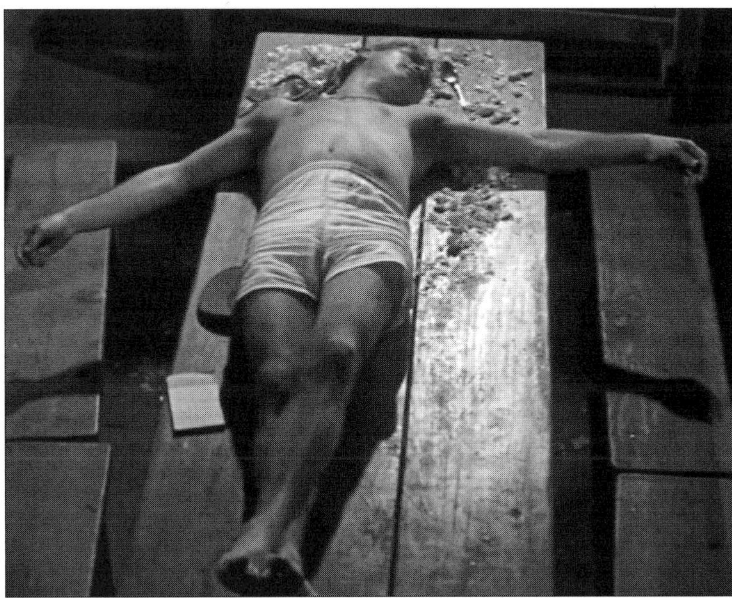

Figure 2.
Low-angle shot from *Cool Hand Luke* (1967, Jamel Productions). Produced by Gordon Carroll and Carter De Haven Jr. Directed by Stuart Rosenberg.

The Close-Up

When we see an isolated face on the screen, our consciousness of space is suspended, and we become vividly aware of all of the nuances of emotion that can be expressed by a grimace or a glance. We form beliefs about a character's emotions, moods, intentions, and thoughts as we look directly into their face. Indeed, many of the most profound emotional experiences (such as grief) are expressed much more powerfully through the human face than through words. Consider the dynamic film, *Amélie* (2001), in which director Jean-Pierre Jeunet purposefully chooses characters (as he does for all his films) who have very expressive faces. There are numerous close-ups of several of the characters' faces throughout the film. He explains that he wants to have characters who are interesting for the viewer to see. In turn, this enhances viewer interest and character development.

Director Woody Allen uses close-up shots smoothly and effectively, and they are a hallmark of many of his films. Some of the close-up images of Cate Blanchett playing the role of Jasmine in *Blue Jasmine* (2013) are unforgettable, and they linger long after the viewer has left the theater (see Figure 44).

This ability to share and comprehend subjective experiences through empathic interpretation of the language of the face is clear in early **silent films**, and these films still have the power to evoke strong emotions. In fact, many early directors of silent films, confronted with the development of "talkies," feared that the addition of sound would place a barrier between the spectator and the film and restore the external and internal distance and dualism present in other works of art. The principles of observing emotional nuances can be extended from the human face to the background and surroundings in which the character moves, and a character's subjective vision can be reproduced by a film as objective reality. For example, film can show a frightened, paranoid individual, enhancing the effect by portraying distorted, menacing houses and trees. This technique was used in the expressionist film *The Cabinet of Dr. Caligari* (1920).

What we see in a facial expression is immediately apparent to the spectator without the distraction of words, and a good actor can convey multiple emotions simultaneously. It has been shown repeatedly that real people playing themselves are less convincing than actors. This is true with instructional films, advertisements, and docudramas, as well as feature films. In *Ordinary People* (1980), director Robert Redford tried to cast a psychiatrist as the therapist, but the effect was unconvincing. Redford finally decided to cast actor Judd Hirsch in the role, and the film ended up winning an Academy Award for Best Picture, and Hirsch received a nomination for Best Actor. A notable exception was *One Flew Over the Cuckoo's Nest* (1975), a film in which a bona fide psychiatrist played the role of the hospital director, and filming occurred on the grounds of an actual psychiatric facility, Oregon State Hospital.

Quentin Tarantino is an expert in the extreme close-up shot, and there are numerous examples in Tarantino films, such as *Reservoir Dogs* (1992), *Pulp Fiction* (1994), the two *Kill Bill* films (2003, 2004), and *Django Unchained* (2012). It is almost impossible to forget the scene in *Kill Bill 2* in which the bride rips out Elle's one remaining eye and crushes it between her toes. The "Here's Johnny" close-up of Jack Nicholson peering through the door he just hacked open in *The Shining* (1980) has become iconic. Other films noted for close-up shots include *There Will Be Blood* (2009), *The Godfather* (1972), *Full Metal Jacket* (1987), *The Seventh Seal* (1957), *Psycho* (1960), *Persona* (1966), *The Good, the Bad and the Ugly* (1966), and *The Silence of the Lambs* (1991). Jordan Peele's *Get Out* (2017) effectively uses close-up shots to convey the protagonist's terror as he begins to realize the reality of the situation in which he finds himself (see Figure 3).

Identification

As a film is being projected onto a theater screen, we project ourselves into the action and identify with its protagonists. At one time it was thought

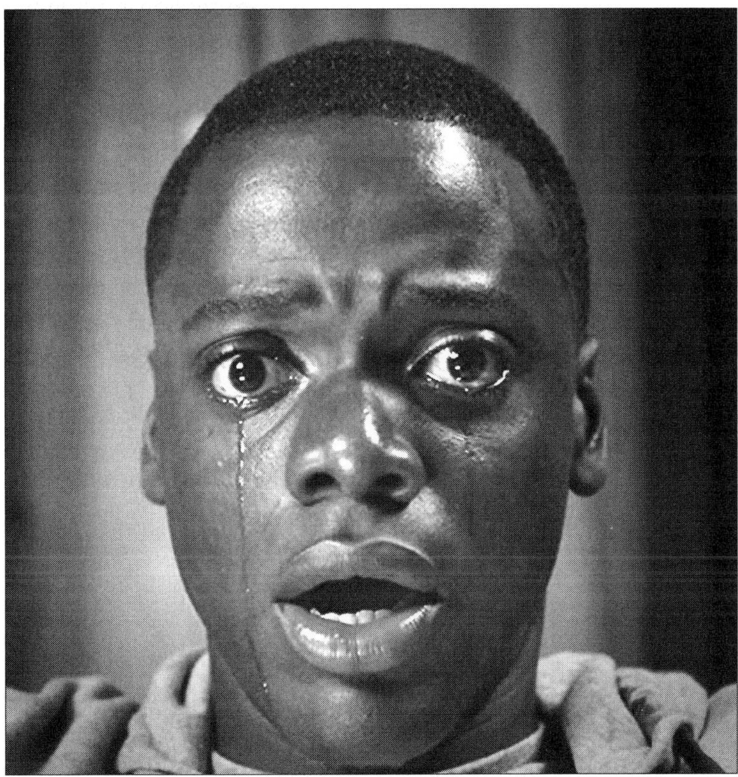

Figure 3.
Close up shot from *Get Out* of Daniel Kaluuya, playing the role of Chris Washington (2017, Universal Pictures, Blumhouse Productions, QC Entertainment, Monkeypaw Productions, Dentsu, Fuji Television Network). Produced by Jason Blum, Marcei A. Brown, Phillip Dawe, Gerard DiNardi, et al. Directed by Jordan Peele.

that to maintain the attention of viewers, a film had to have a central character and theme. At times, this central figure has been an antihero. However, directors such as Robert Altman and Quentin Tarantino have experimented with techniques in which they rapidly shift among short vignettes that may be only loosely linked with a storyline or central character. Altman's *Short Cuts* (1994) and Tarantino's *Pulp Fiction* (1994) are two examples of this approach. *Crash* (2004), directed by Paul Haggis, was so expert at interweaving stories to enhance meaning and viewer engagement that it won an Academy Award for Best Picture, among many other awards. *Love Actually* (2003), starring Hugh Grant, Martine McCutcheon, Liam Neeson, and Laura Linney, weaves together the romantic lives of eight couples whose lives are linked in complex ways that none of them fully understand or appreciate. Another example of this approach is *Cloud Atlas* (2012), a film in which multiple actors play multiple roles in vignettes that are loosely but meaningfully connected. The film addresses the obscure links between past, present, and future events. Critics were divided over whether it was entirely successful; however, I found the film engaging and provocative.

Suture

Viewers integrate separate, disjointed photographic images into coherent scenes and weave different scenes into the whole film experience without conscious effort or appreciation of the complicated psychological processes involved. **Suture**, to use a medical metaphor, occurs when cutting or editing is necessary, and the resulting cinematic gaps are "sewn" shut by viewers.

Film scholar Shohini Chaudhuri (2006) notes,

> The healing of narrative can only happen after the wound has been inflicted; and the more wounded we are, the more desperate we become for meaning and narrative. We can see this at work in *Psycho* (1960), where we follow and identify with Marion Crane until she is murdered halfway through the film in the famous shower scene, where every

> cinematic cut appears to be the stab of a knife. This inflicts a traumatic wound on the viewer who is left with no-one to identify within the empty motel except the cinematic enunciator. So desperate is our need for meaning and narrative that we then identify with Marion's murderer, Norman Bates, when he arrives to dispose of her body and her belongings. We even feel anxious for him when, momentarily, Marion's car refuses to sink into the swamp. Suture is the "hook" by which the film accomplishes this entrapment of the viewer. (Chaudhuri, 2006, p. 50)

According to suture theory, instead of asking, "Who is watching this?" and "How could this be happening?" viewers tacitly accept what is seen on the screen as natural and "real," even when the camera's gaze shifts abruptly from one scene, location, or character to another. Suture works because cinematic coding makes each shot appear to be the object of the gaze of whoever appears in the shot that follows. The most cited example of suturing is the **shot/reverse shot**, in which each of two characters is alternately viewed over the other's shoulder. The Coen brothers are noted for their use of the shot/reverse shot technique (e.g., *No Country for Old Men* [2007]).

Sound

Sound can create tension and evoke powerful emotions. It is a critical part of movies, and some sound scores have become iconic (e.g., *Jaws* with only two notes, repeated and becoming louder; the haunting theme music from *The Good, the Bad and the Ugly*). When sound comes from within a film and is appropriate to the events happening on the screen (e.g., screaming teenagers in a horror film), the sound is called **diegetic**; when sounds are added in postproduction, such as a musical score, the sounds are **nondiegetic** (e.g., the *Star Wars* theme, the sounds that accompany the shower scene in *Psycho*, or commentary by an omniscient narrator). Typically, both kinds of sounds are included in films. Baumgartner et al. (2006) studied the emotional power of music by using functional magnetic resonance imaging (FMRI) to assess how our brains respond to affective images (fearful or sad pictures), either alone or combined with emotional musical excerpts. Subjects' emotional experiences were markedly enhanced when sound was added to the images presented.

> The combination of sound and images showed increased activation in many structures known to be involved in emotion processing (including for example amygdala, hippocampus, parahippocampus, insula, striatum, medial ventral frontal cortex, cerebellum, fusiform gyrus). In contrast, the picture condition only showed an activation increase in the cognitive part of the prefrontal cortex, mainly in the right dorsolateral prefrontal cortex. Based on these findings, we suggest that emotional pictures evoke a more cognitive mode of emotion perception, whereas congruent presentations of emotional visual and musical stimuli rather automatically evoke strong emotional feelings and experiences. (Baumgartner et al., 2006, p. 151)

Representation of Psychological Phenomena in Film

Film is particularly well suited to depicting psychological states of mind and altered mental states. The combination of images, dialogue, sound effects, and music in a movie mimic and parallel the thoughts and feelings that occur in our stream of consciousness. Lights, colors, and sounds emanate from the screen in such a way that we readily find ourselves believing that we are experiencing what is happening on the screen.

In *Secrets of a Soul* (1926), German director Georg Wilhelm Pabst dramatized psychoanalytic theory with the help of two of Freud's assistants, Karl Abraham, and Hanns Sachs, and depicted dream sequences with multilayered superimposition (achieved through rewinding and multiple exposures). Freud himself did not want his name connected with the project and had misgivings about the film's ability to convey the nuances of psychoanalytic process. In a letter to Abraham, Freud wrote, "My chief objection is still that I do not believe satisfactory plastic representation of our abstractions is at all possible" (Freud, cited in Greenberg, 1993, p. 19). Freud remained skeptical about the cinema all his life. This perspective is in direct contrast to that of the late, renowned filmmaker Stanley Kubrick, who noted, "If it can be written, or thought, it can be filmed."

Film is frequently used to objectively portray subjective states such as dreams. The best example of this is Hitchcock's collaboration with Salvador Dali on the dream sequence in *Spellbound* (1945). Hitchcock wanted to "turn out the first picture on psychoanalysis." He was determined to break the traditional way of handling dream sequences through a blurred and hazy screen. Hitchcock wanted dreams with great visual sharpness and clarity, and images sharper than those in the film itself. He chose Salvador Dali as a collaborator because of the precision of the artist's work. Hitchcock originally wanted to shoot *Spellbound* in the open air and in natural light, but he wound up shooting the film in the studio to cut costs. *Spellbound* depicts the cathartic recovery of repressed memories, and an emotional experience intense enough to eliminate the hero's amnesia. This is a psychological process depicted in film since its early days and a motif found in many other Hitchcock films such as *Vertigo* (1958) and *Marnie* (1964). A detailed psychological analysis of Hitchcock's films can be found in O'Hara (2017).

Films can also be used to interweave fantasy and reality, and a director may intentionally set up situations in which the viewer cannot tell if the film portrays reality or the unconscious fantasies of a character. Examples of this technique include Ingmar Bergman's *Persona* (1966), Federico Fellini's *Juliet of the Spirits* (1965), Luis Buñuel's *Belle de Jour* (1966), Robert Altman's *Images* (1972), and Derek Cianfrance's *Beasts of the Southern Wild* (2012). Director David Lynch has made this approach his trademark with such films as *Mulholland Drive* (2001), *Lost Highway* (1997), *Blue Velvet* (1986), and *Eraserhead* (1977). One of the most striking recent examples is found in Robert Eggers' film *The Lighthouse* (2019; see Figure 4). This fascinating black-and-white movie was an artistic success; unfortunately, the pathology portrayed in the film is atypical and obscure, and it will not teach students much about the etiology or the presentation of mental illness.

"Hark Triton, hark! Bellow, bid our father the Sea King rise from the depths full foul in his fury! Black waves teeming with salt foam to smother this young mouth with pungent slime, to choke ye, engorging your organs til' ye turn blue and bloated with bilge and brine and can scream no more ..."

Willem Dafoe's character berating his assistant in *The Lighthouse* (2019)

Processes such as thinking, recalling, imagining, and feeling are not visible, but the language of the **montage** and camera techniques such as **slow fades** can suggest these invisible processes. Also, the film can be edited in such a way that the viewer is forced to think about psychological phenomena. The inclusion of images with symbolic meaning, such as a hearse passing by or the well-known chess game with death in *The Seventh Seal* (1957), can evoke certain moods or prepare the viewer for events that are about to occur. Symbolic sounds, such as a baby crying, can have a similar effect. Another example is the leitmotif that is played when Darth Vader and the Imperial Army enter a scene in any of the *Star Wars* films; it clearly conveys evil, danger, and power.

Another symbol often used in films is the mirror. When a character is filmed looking in the mirror, it can represent self-reflection, insight, a new identity emerging or changing, or even a narcissistic preoccupation with oneself. *Monster's Ball* (2001) uses mirrors and other reflective objects to symbolize self-distortion and negative self-perception in the two lead characters who are numb to their own lives. Mirrored images depict Marlon Brando's broken and distorted character in *Last Tango in Paris* (1972);

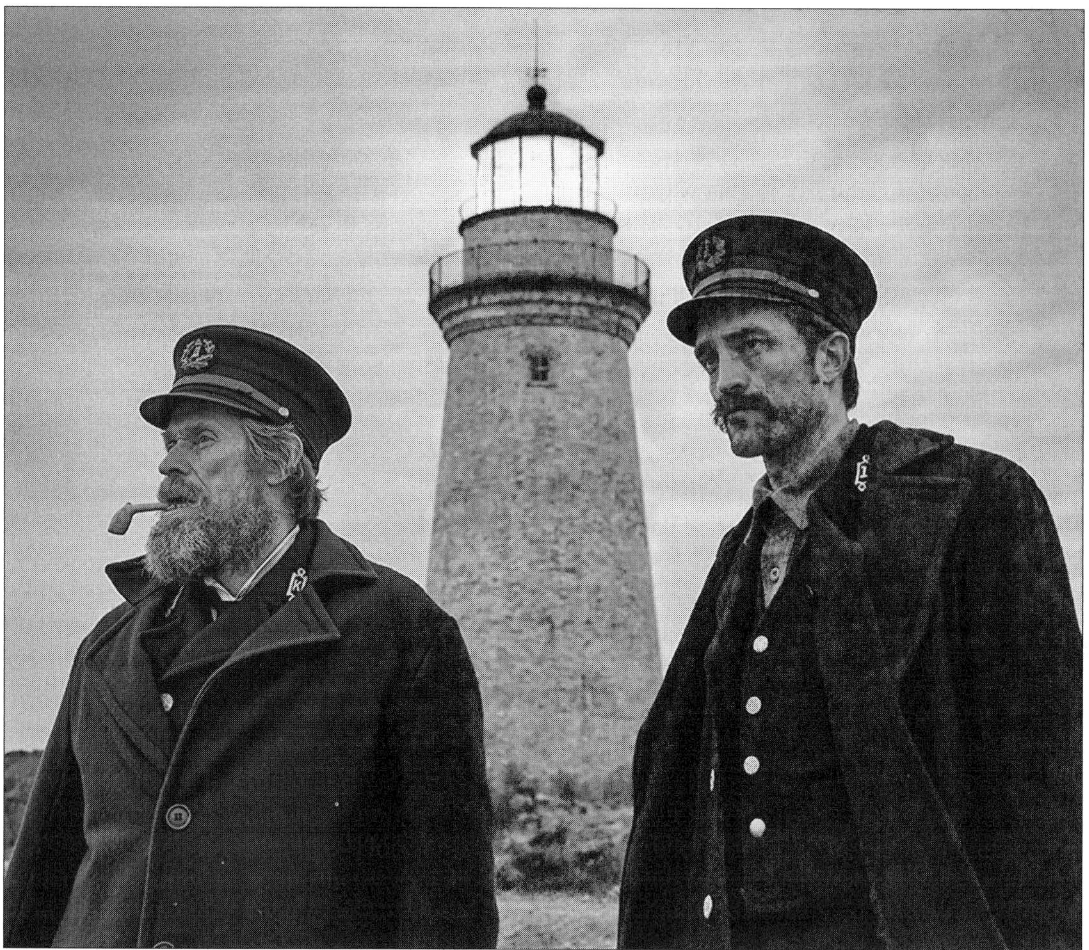

Figure 4. *The Lighthouse* (2019, A24, Maiden Voyage Pictures, New Regency Productions, Parts and Labor, RT Features). Produced by Chris Columbus, Eleanor Columbus, Robert Eggers, Issac Ericson, et al. Directed by Robert Eggers.

self-deprecation in *American Splendor* (2003); self-criticism in *Soldier's Girl* (2003); deterioration in *Ben X* (2007), *Black Swan* (2010), and *Focus* (2001); self-reflection and distortion in *Chloe* (2010); and externalization of blame in a dramatic, comical scene in *25th Hour* (2002). Director Andrei Tarkovsky made a classic film titled *The Mirror* (1975) in which mirrors trigger memories in a dying man.

Films offer numerous examples of unconscious motivation and **defense mechanisms**, involuntary patterns of thinking, feeling, or acting that arise in response to the subjective experience of anxiety. **Acting out** in reaction to stress or inner conflict is present in *The Hammer* (2010), *Intimacy* (2000), *You Can Count on Me* (2000), and *Lantana* (2001), and in Michael Douglas's response to the stress in his life in *Falling Down* (1993). **Altruism** can be seen in *Patch Adams* (1998), and in the character of the doctor who devotes himself to the indigent people of India in *Streets of Joy* (1994). **Denial** is dramatically illustrated in Katharine Hepburn's and Ellen Burstyn's gripping roles as drug addicts in *Long Day's Journey into Night* (1962) and *Requiem for a Dream* (2000), respectively, as well as the Oscar-winning film *The White Ribbon* (2009), and most of the townspeople in both *The Village* (2004) and *Dogville* (2003). **Intellectualization** is present in *Lorenzo's Oil* (1992), and **suppression** is apparent in *A Dangerous Method* (2011), *Rabbit Hole* (2010), *The United States of Leland* (2003), *Caramel*

(2007), and *Kill Bill: Vol. 2* (2004), and is commonplace in *Gone With the Wind* (1939).

"I'll think about it tomorrow. Tara! Home. I'll go home, and I'll think of some way to get him back! After all, tomorrow is another day!"

Suppression illustrated in *Gone With the Wind* (1939)

Psychological concepts are occasionally linked to specific films, and a salient example is found in the 1944 movie *Gaslight* starring Ingrid Bergman and Charles Boyer. Boyer, Bergman's husband in the film, manipulates the gas lights in their home, causing them to dim. When his wife remarks on the dimming lights, he attempts to convince her that she is imagining the phenomenon and the changes are all in her mind. Eventually, Bergman's character comes to question her sanity. Ingrid Bergman won the 1945 Academy Award for Best Actress for her performance (later she would go on to win the Best Actress award for *Anastasia* [1956] and Best Supporting Actress for *Murder on the Orient Express* [1974]).

The term "gaslighting" is now widely used by both therapists and laypeople to refer to systematic psychological manipulation achieved by lying to a victim. Writing in *Psychoanalytic Dialogues,* Glen Gabbard (2017) described helping a patient deal with her grief following the 2016 presidential election:

> Why would anyone vote for a guy who thinks it's fine to sexually assault women?" I had no answer for her question. I didn't get it, either. I still don't get it. In my role as a psychoanalyst, how could I possibly be helpful in this situation? The tools of my trade seemed useless. To try to explain the meanings of her reaction as derivatives of earlier experiences would be a form of gaslighting. It would invalidate an authentic reaction that millions of people were having in the aftermath of the election. All I could do was empathize and commiserate with her. (Gabbard, 2017, p. 385)

Psychoanalyst Orit Badouk Epstein (2019) describes how the concept of gaslighting was relevant to her treatment of a patient with dissociative identity disorder, and notes,

> The revival of the word and its modern interpretation is highly relevant to our work with clients who have been abused, in particular, clients with a poor sense of agency and those who have survived horrendous mind control, torture, and group abuse. (Epstein, 2019, p. 347)

Films illustrating gaslighting include *Solitary* (2009), *Rosemary's Baby* (1968), *Unsane* (2018), *The Woman in the Window* (2021), *The Invisible Man* (2020), and *The Girl on the Train* (2021).

The COVID-19 pandemic had a dramatic impact on the film industry. Movie theaters were closed, film festivals were cancelled, and film releases were postponed until the pandemic passed. Many of us who were virtually housebound spent 2020 and 2021 watching films to cope with the crisis. Writing about Alfred Hitchcock, physician Jules Lipoff (2020) notes,

> At the onset, our response was denial – this virus won't spread, and then that it won't be that big a problem, or that it isn't much worse than the seasonal flu. Thornhill in *North by Northwest* felt the same way. He thought that being mistaken as a spy was a problem that he could run away [from]. Likewise, we have made mistakes, not heeding advice fast enough, hesitant to change our lives in such a rapid fashion. But like Thornhill, we are resilient, and I can already anticipate the climax of this film – that we will be pushed harder than we could have imagined and that we will survive. And of course, survive we did. (Lipoff, 2020)

The Depiction of Psychological Disorders in Films

This book is organized according to the categories of mental disorders in the fifth edition of the *Diagnostic and Statistical Manual of Mental*

Disorders (DSM-5; American Psychiatric Association [APA], 2013) with appropriate film examples. Despite some misgivings about the medicalization of psychosocial problems and the lack of attention to individual differences, almost 90% of psychologists regularly consult the DSM-5 (Raskin et al., 2022).

Table 2 presents an overview of well-recognized and accepted disorders and some of the best representations of them in cinema. Watching any of these films will provide the viewer with insights into the presentation of the disorder portrayed.

Table 2. DSM-5 categories and examples of movies that portray them

Category	Classic film examples	More recent film examples
Neurodevelopmental disorders: Intellectual disability	*Sling Blade* (1996); *Of Mice and Men* (1939, 1992); *Dominick and Eugene* (1988); *Charly* (1968); *Forrest Gump* (1994); *To Kill a Mockingbird* (1962)	*Marvrellos* (2015); *The Peanut Butter Falcon* (2019); *Intelligent Lives* (2018); *Magic Life of V* (2019)
Neurodevelopmental disorders: Autism spectrum	*David and Lisa* (1962); *Rain Man* (1988)	*Temple Grandin* (2010); *Extremely Loud and Incredibly Close* (2011); *Life, Animated* (2016)
Neurocognitive disorders	*On Golden Pond* (1981); *Iris* (2001); *A Song for Martin* (2001)	*The Leisure Seeker* (2017); *Head Full of Honey* (2018); *The Father* (2020)
Substance-related and addictive disorders	*The Lost Weekend* (1945); *Clean and Sober* (1988); *Drunks* (1995); *Walk the Line* (2005); *Half Nelson* (2006)	*Krisha* (2015); *Honey Boy* (2019); *Judy* (2019); *The Way Back* (2020)
Schizophrenia spectrum and other psychotic disorders	*Taxi Driver* (1976); *The Fisher King* (1991); *Clean, Shaven* (1994); *A Beautiful Mind* (2001)	*Take Shelter* (2011); *Horse Girl* (2020); *The Adopted One* (2020)
Depressive disorders	*Red Desert* (1964); *Ordinary People* (1980); *The Hours* (2002)	*A Single Man* (2009); *Helen* (2009); *Melancholia* (2011); *Cake* (2014); *Manchester by the Sea* (2016); *February's Dog* (2022)
Bipolar disorders	*Mr. Jones* (1993); *Michael Clayton* (2007); *Crooked Beauty: Navigating the Space Between Beauty and Madness* (2010)	*Silver Linings Playbook* (2012); *Infinitely Polar Bear* (2015); *Touched with Fire* (2015); *No Letting Go* (2015)
Anxiety disorders	*Vertigo* (1958)	*The Perks of Being a Wallflower* (2012); *Dear Evan Hansen* (2021); *The Woman in the Window* (2021)
Obsessive-compulsive disorders	*As Good as It Gets* (1997)	*Matchstick Men* (2003); *The Aviator* (2004); *Phoebe in Wonderland* (2008)
Trauma- and stressor-related disorders	*The Deer Hunter* (1978); *Coming Home* (1978); *The Fisher King* (1991); *The Prince of Tides* (1991)	*Waltz With Bashir* (2008); *The Hurt Locker* (2008); *Antichrist* (2009); *The Dry Land* (2010); *The Magic Life of V* (2019)

Table 2. Continued

Category	Classic film examples	More recent film examples
Somatic symptom disorders	*Persona* (1966)	*Thérèse* (2004); *Hollywood Ending* (2002)
Dissociative disorders	*The Three Faces Of Eve* (1957); *Psycho* (1960); *Fight Club* (1999); *Primal Fear* (1996); *Me, Myself, and Irene* (2000)	*Unknown White Male* (2005); *Peacock* (2010); *Split* (2016)
Paraphilic disorders	*Lolita* (1962)	*The Woodsman* (2004); *Secretary* (2002); *Pervert Park* (2014)
Gender dysphoria	*Boys Don't Cry* (1999)	*Tomboy* (2011); *Cowboys* (2020); *Transhood* (2020)
Feeding and eating disorders	*The Best Little Girl in the World* (1982)	*Primo Amore* (2004); *Black Swan* (2010); *To the Bone* (2017); *Swallow* (2019); *The Wonder* (2022); *The Whale* (2022)
Sleep–wake disorders	*My Own Private Idaho* (1991)	*Insomnia* (2002); *The Machinist* (2004); *Inception* (2010)
Disruptive, impulse-control, and conduct disorders	*Marnie* (1964)	*Klepto* (2003); *2 Days in Paris* (2007)
Adjustment disorders	*The Wrong Man* (1957)	*Best in Show* (2000); *The Upside of Anger* (2005)
Sexual dysfunctions	*Bliss* (1997)	*Rust and Bone (2012); The Sessions (2012); Good Luck to You, Leo Grande (2022)*
Personality disorders	*Compulsion* (1959); *Fatal Attraction* (1987)	*We Need to Talk About Kevin* (2011); *Blue Jasmine* (2013); *The Iceman* (2012); *The Good Nurse* (2022)

Note. DSM-5 = *Diagnostic and Statistical Manual of Mental Disorders*, 5th edition.

Psychopathology in Different Film Genres

The depiction of mental illness in films most commonly appears in three popular genres: the drama, the horror film, and the suspense film. Often the most effective portrayals of mental illness are those that infuse surreal and expressionistic images into a montage that is realistic and plausible, powerfully conveying the "interior" of a character's psyche.

The popular genre of **drama** is the most fertile ground for psychopathology to be portrayed in movies in a very realistic, engaging way. Every chapter in this book has numerous examples of dramatic films depicting psychological disorders. The range is vast, and it extends from the slow-moving drama of *The Human Stain* (2003) and the disjointed, complex drama of *21 Grams* (2003), to the affectively engaging dramas of *12 Years a Slave* (2013) and *Captain Phillips* (2013).

An early film that served as a prototype for **horror** films, Wiene's *The Cabinet of Dr. Caligari* (1920), is highly expressionistic, and it established a precedent for setting macabre murders in mental institutions. Like dozens of films that followed, it linked insanity and the personal lives of psychiatrists, and implied that mental health professionals are all "a little odd." Evidence of the enduring effects of these themes is found in the successful and highly acclaimed film *The Silence of the Lambs* (1991) in which Anthony Hopkins plays a mentally deranged and cannibalistic psychiatrist. The various *Saw* (2004, 2005, 2006, 2007, 2008, 2009) movies and *House of 1000 Corpses* (2003) portray psychopathic villains who are clearly out of touch with reality, as does the dreadful trilogy of films that tell the story of *The Human Centipede* (2009, 2011, 2015).

Shand et al. (2014) have discussed the popularity of horror films and television programs, and the ways in which these media promulgate stigma. They note,

> Directors of horror movies certainly know how to push our psychological buttons. Horror films use several vehicles to create the unsettling feeling that we all know so well. Common filming techniques, sets, and editing help to create desired reactions, achieved in the horror genre through dark lighting, gruesome make-up, point of-view violence, and jump-cuts that cause an on-edge experience. (Shand et al., 2014, p. 423)

The seminal films of Alfred Hitchcock provide the best examples of the **suspense** genre. They are unique in the way they engage viewers and pander to their anxieties in subtle, unrelenting, and convincing ways. Many of Hitchcock's films, noted for their stylized realism, invariably evoke a sensation of vicariously pulling the viewer "in" to the plight of the characters as a not-so-innocent bystander, through a carefully edited montage of a variety of objective and subjective camera shots. Hitchcock's filmography reflects not only a fascination with pronounced and extreme psychopathology (e.g., *Psycho*, 1960), but more importantly, an appreciation of more subtle psychological phenomena such as acting out, reaction formation, idealization, repression, and undoing. These defense mechanisms are depicted in Hitchcock's films *Shadow of a Doubt* (1943), *Spellbound* (1945), and *Marnie* (1964). Hitchcock's style is immensely popular and has been imitated frequently by other directors such as David Lynch, M. Night Shyamalan, Brian De Palma, and Roman Polanski. Brian De Palma has acknowledged that Hitchcock's *Vertigo* (1958) was the inspiration for De Palma's film *Obsession* (1976) (Starkey, 2022).

Other examples of excellent suspense films include Robert Redford's *All Is Lost* (2013), Sean Durkin's *Martha Marcy May Marlene* (2011), Jordan Peele's *Get Out* (2017), and Ben Affleck's *Argo* (2012). *Argo* won an Academy Award for Best Picture.

Mental illness is also depicted, although less often, in the genre of **documentary** films. Frederick Wiseman's *Titicut Follies* (1967) and *Capturing the Friedmans* (2003) illustrate clear cases of psychopathology. It is interesting to contrast the former movie with the horror film *Bedlam* (1945) or "docudramatic" films such as *The Snake Pit* (1948), *Pressure Point* (1962), and *One Flew Over the Cuckoo's Nest* (1975), all dealing with mental institutions and the treatment of people with mental illness. At least two heralded films, *The Three Faces of Eve* (1957) and *Sybil* (1976), provide viewers with full-scale case histories and the struggles between patient and psychiatrist. *OC87: The Obsessive Compulsive, Major Depression, Bipolar, Asperger's Movie* (2010) documents filmmaker Bud Clayman's struggles with a variety of mental health concerns.

The **comedy** genre has its share of films portraying psychopathology. *Drop Dead Fred* (1991), *What About Bob?* (1991), *High Anxiety* (1977), *Scotland,* and *PA* (2001) all portray psychological aberrations, with quirky humor used to defuse the sense of anxiety produced by the behavior of the lead characters in each of the films. Director Woody Allen has made a career out of portraying anxiety, neuroticism, and somatization in various films such as *Hannah and Her Sisters* (1988) and *Hollywood Ending* (2002), but he later turned to subtle, dark, and complex psychopathology, as seen in the portrayal of personality disorders in *Match Point* (2005), *Vicky Cristina Barcelona* (2008), and *Blue Jasmine* (2013).

Misconceptions and Stereotypic Themes in Films

Otto Wahl, an authority on media psychology, summarizes the media's portrayal of mental illness in his book *Media Madness: Public Images of Mental Illness* (Wahl, 1995): "Overall, the mass media do a poor job of depicting mental illness, with misinformation frequently communicated, unfavorable stereotypes of people with mental illness predominating, and psychiatric terms used in inaccurate and offensive ways" (pp. 12–13). This is due to **media framing**, a concept that refers to the way media presents and organizes information that leads to interpretations by the public. In the case of mental illness in films, media framing is overwhelmingly negative and usually inaccurate (Goffman, 1986; Sieff, 2003). The media frames for mental illness are typically narrow and distorted, frequently presenting those with mental illness as violent, dangerous, simplistic, disillusioned, and/or innocent. This is troubling for at least two reasons: (1) Mental health literacy levels for the public are low (Orchowski et al., 2006); (2) Research has shown that people's primary source of information about mental illness is mass media (Wahl, 1995).

Steven Hyler (Hyler et al., 1991) has provided a compelling analysis of the portrayal of mental illness in films. Hyler and his colleagues describe six common stereotypes that perpetuate stigma. The first of these is that of the mental patient as **rebellious free spirit**. Examples of this portrayal can be found in films such as *Frances* (1982), *Nuts* (1987), *The Dream Team* (1989), *The Couch Trip* (1989), *An Angel at My Table* (1990), *Shine* (1996), *K-Pax* (2001), *Asylum* (2005), and most clearly in *One Flew Over the Cuckoo's Nest* (1975). The stereotype of the **homicidal maniac** is present in many of the slasher/horror films described earlier. However, the authors point out that this stereotype can also be traced back as far as D.W. Griffith's 1909 film *The Maniac Cook*, in which a psychotic employee attempts to kill an infant by cooking the child in an oven.

The patient as **seductress** is seen in films such as *The Caretakers* (1963) and *Dressed to Kill* (1980), and most clearly in the 1964 film *Lilith*, which stars Warren Beatty as a hospital therapist who is seduced by a psychiatric patient played by Jean Seberg. The further stereotype of the **enlightened member of society** is linked to the work of writers such as R. D. Laing and Thomas Szasz and is illustrated in films such as *King of Hearts* (1966) and *A Fine Madness* (1966). The **narcissistic parasite** stereotype presents people with mental disorders as self-centered, attention seeking, and demanding. It is reflected in films such as *What About Bob?* (1991), *Annie Hall* (1977), *High Anxiety* (1977), and *Lovesick* (1983).

Finally, the stereotype of **zoo specimen** is perpetuated by films that degrade people with mental illness by treating them as objects of derision or a source of amusement or entertainment for those who are "normal." Films that exemplify this stereotype include *Bedlam* (1948) and *Marat/Sade* (1966). A variation on this theme occurs in Brian De Palma's *Dressed to Kill* (1980), in which a psychotic and homicidal psychiatrist murders a nurse in a surrealistic amphitheater-like setting, with dozens of other patients sitting in the gallery and watching in silent approval.

Hyler (1988) describes three dominant themes in film that contribute to stereotypes about the etiology manifestation of mental disorders. The first is the **presumption of traumatic etiology**. This theme reinforces the belief that a single traumatic event is the cause of mental illness. Examples include the amnesia experienced by Gregory Peck that was eventually shown to be related to his role in the childhood death of his brother (revealed by Hitchcock in a dramatic and unforgettable flashback scene) in *Spellbound* (1945), and the dissociative identity disorder that resulted when a child was required to kiss the corpse of her dead grandmother in *The Three Faces of Eve* (1957). Other examples of this theme are found in films such as *Suddenly, Last*

Summer (1959), *Home of the Brave* (1949), *Nuts* (1987), and Robin Williams' character in *The Fisher King* (1991). *The Magic Life of V* (2019) is a recent documentary film that documents how the horrors of the past are carried into the future and can affect one's entire life.

Hyler's second theme is that of the **schizophrenogenic parent.** This is a widely held misconception that holds parents (most often, the mother) accountable for serious mental illness in their children. NAMI has worked hard to dispel this unfounded but pervasive belief, but it is deeply rooted in popular culture and commonplace in films. Examples include *Agnes of God* (1985), *Face to Face* (1976), *Sybil* (1980), *Carrie* (1976), *Frances* (1982), *Fear Strikes Out* (1957), and *Shine* (1995).

"Insanity runs in my family.
It practically gallops."

Mortimer Brewster (Cary Grant)
in *Arsenic and Old Lace* (1944)

The third misconception discussed by Hyler is that **harmless eccentricity is frequently labeled as mental illness and inappropriately treated.** We see this theme most vividly presented in the film *One Flew Over the Cuckoo's Nest* (1975). Jack Nicholson's character, Randle P. McMurphy, is charismatic, flamboyant, and colorful. The only diagnosis that seems at all appropriate is that of antisocial personality disorder, although it is not even clear that this is justified. However, once in the system he cannot get out, and he is eventually treated with electroconvulsive therapy (ECT) and lobotomy, presumably as a way of punishing his misbehavior in the name of treatment. The same theme is found in two films released in 1966, *King of Hearts* and *A Fine Madness*, and in the film *Chattahoochee* (1990).

A related theme, that treatment in mental health facilities is a form of social control, is reflected in the work of Thomas Szasz (e.g., in books such as *The Myth of Mental Illness* and *Psychiatric Slavery*; Szasz, 1974, 1977). It is also reflected in films depicting excesses in treatment, such as the aversion therapies portrayed in *A Clockwork Orange* (1971). For a list of 12 misconceptions perpetrated in movies, accompanied by film examples see Appendix 4. Appendix 5 looks specifically at the mental health profession and delineates a list of both balanced and unbalanced portrayals of psychotherapists.

Another myth, although one not specifically addressed by Hyler, is the belief that **love will always conquer mental illness**. This myth is promulgated by films like *Shine* (1996) and *Benny & Joon* (1993). Although the benefits and buffering effects of love are important for anyone coping with mental illness or addiction, the reality is that some people with these disorders do not improve no matter how much they are loved. The pernicious corollary to this myth is that if people who are mentally ill do not improve, it must be because they simply were not loved enough.

Jane Pirkis et al. (2006) reviewed the literature on the portrayals of mental illness in contemporary films and television programs, and an American Psychiatric Association (APA) summary of their article notes that

> On-screen portrayals are frequent and generally negative and have a cumulative effect on the public's perception of people with mental illness and on the likelihood of people with mental illness seeking appropriate help ... There is a need for the mental health sector and the film and television industries to collaborate to counter negative portrayals of mental illness, and to explore the potential for positive portrayals to educate and inform, as well as to entertain. (p. 523)

Psychopathology and its representation in films will be discussed in some detail in the chapters that follow. In general, I follow the nosology of the American Psychiatric Association's DSM-5, while also including diagnostic codes from the *International Classification of Diseases* (ICD), whenever appropriate. Appendix 6 includes a filmography broken down by diagnostic category. Readers who take time to review even a few of the films included in Appendix 6 will find that the experience will supplement and enhance their understanding of psychopathology.

Movies and Pedagogy

I have used films and film clips as teaching tools for the past 40 years, most often to teach psychopathology to medical students and graduate students in psychology. My students are always grateful for the opportunity to see vivid and visual examples of the concepts I describe in the classroom, and they find the conditions I talk about in lectures come alive with screen depictions.

William Altman et al. (2017), in an interesting article titled "Russell Crowe Is a Better Teacher Than You: Movies Outperform Paper Assignments or Teaching-as-Usual," describe multiple experiments that demonstrate the utility of films in the classroom. They conclude, "The key to learning was the feature film. Feature films provide a thorough context that offers concrete examples of abstract concepts. This helps students learn, especially in an area as rich as abnormal psychology" (Altman et al., 2017, p. 1).

Alexander Swan (2021) has also written about the utility of films as teaching tools in the psychology classroom, and in his chapter, he describes his podcast, *CinemaPsych*. My own thoughts about the use of films in the classroom are more fully developed in a chapter I wrote with two Thai colleagues from Chiang Mai University School of Medicine (Wedding et al., 2017). Anne Ferrari (2021) has described how the stigma of mental illness could be reduced by incorporating celebrity narratives in her abnormal psychology course.

Nick Wilson and colleagues (2014) reviewed 503 films to select a *top 10* list of movies they believed would facilitate learning by medical students taking a psychiatry clerkship. Their top-rated films were: For depressive and anxiety disorders: *Ordinary People* (1980) and *Silver Linings Playbook* (2012); for illicit drug use: *Trainspotting* (1996), *Winter's Bone* (2010), *Rachel Getting Married* (2008), and *Half Nelson* (2006); for alcohol use disorders: *Another Year* (2010) and *Passion Fish* (1992); and for schizophrenia: *The Devil and Daniel Johnston* (2006) and *An Angel at My Table* (1990). The complete list of the films they reviewed, along with commentary and hyperlinks, can be found at https://www.otago.ac.nz/wellington/otago072475.pdf.

Hall and Friedman (2015), writing in *Academic Psychiatry*, have argued that films in the *Star Wars* saga can be used to teach students about "borderline and narcissistic personality traits, psychopathy, PTSD, partner violence risk, developmental stages, and of course Oedipal conflicts" (Hall & Friedman, 2015, p. 726).

Kuhnigk et al. (2012) specifically addressed the utility of films in the psychiatry clerkship, and found that the combination of a film, a lecture, and a patient interview provided a powerful learning experience, and one that was highly rated by students. Matthew Alexander (2009) has discussed the ways films can be used to enhance the sensitivity of medical students and psychiatry residents to "couples struggling with communication, conflict resolution, affairs, addictions and many other aspects of the couple's odyssey" (p. 183).

Sampogna et al. (2022) noted that over the past 10–15 years, "the percentage of graduates choosing a career in psychiatry has been significantly reduced," and she calls for novel methods to teach psychiatry, writing,

> Another innovative solution is the use of movies as an educational tool. Watching movies and videos with students may allow them to discuss misconceptions about mental disorders in a relaxed setting (i.e., not in the patient's presence) and whether the clinical descriptions are accurate or not. Using videos to teach particular topics to medical students has been shown to result in improved recall of those situations. (p. 35)

Datta (2009) reported on the successful use of films in a third-year psychiatry clerkship at King's College in London, finding that medical students rated the use of film in the classroom beneficial and enjoyable. Akram et al. (2009) found that using movies to portray mental illness encouraged medical students to consider psychiatry as a potential career specialty. Kalra (2011) used the film *Stigmata* (1999) to teach residents about diagnostic dilemmas and diagnosis, and Cape

(2009) discussed the ways in which movies could be used to teach addiction medicine, noting, "There is a responsibility of the teacher to use this tool with care so as not to perpetuate the mythologies of addiction as often portrayed within commercial cinema" (p. 213).

Recupero et al. (2021) examined the use of film in a behavioral medicine course for physician assistants, and specifically examined the utility of movies in teaching students how to conduct a mental status examination. They conclude, "Movies depicting psychiatric illness and substance use disorders can be a fun and highly effective tool for helping students to learn and develop competency in the performance of mental status examinations." Wilson et al. (2013) have made a similar argument for incorporating films in nursing education, and Markie Blumer (2010) makes the same argument for the use of films in training marriage and family therapists.

Ozcakir and Bilgel (2014), writing in the *Journal of Palliative Medicine*, have documented the ways in which the movie *Wit* can be used to sensitize students to the issues of death, dying, and palliative care. I have used *Wit* in my own work with medical students in the context of a course in medical ethics.

Dartmouth professor Steven Schlozman has authored a remarkable little book titled *Film* (2021). I brought Steve to lecture to my medical students at the American University of Antigua. Describing his book, he writes,

> Our world is inundated by film. Our best stories are told on movie screens, on televisions, on smartphones and laptops. *Film* argues that on-screen storytelling is the most ubiquitous format for art to intersect with health and well-being, offering a way for us to appreciate, understand and even celebrate the most nuanced and complex notions of what it means to be healthy through the stories that we watch unfolding. Clinicians use film to better understand their patients, and individuals use film to better understand themselves and each other. ... Film can be used by clinicians and healthcare practitioners to better understand patients; by individuals to better understand themselves and others; and – perhaps most important of all – by societies as a tool in the fight against the stigma of illness. (Schlozman, 2023)

Children and Screen Time

Almost everyone in the United States now has easy access to a smartphone, laptop, or tablet, and the influence of screen time on children has become a hotly debated issues. The American Academy of Pediatrics (AAP) has taken a clear position on the potentially harmful effects of screen time for children, arguing there should be *no* screen time at all for children until 18 to 24 months, except for video chatting, and they maintain children ages 2 to 5 should get an hour or less of screen time per day (Pappas, 2020). However, there is strong evidence that US families with very young children routinely exceed these guidelines (Chen & Adler, 2019), and screens are often used as substitutes for babysitters. Video chatting is a salient exception, but toddlers benefit most from video chatting with grandparents and other extended family members when another adult is present to facilitate the interaction.

Though screen time recommendations for the youngest kids now make exceptions for video chatting, the evidence also suggests that toddlers find this medium confusing and that they struggle to make sense of video chat unless they have help from an adult who is physically present. In one study by Troseth and her colleagues, 2-year-olds were assigned to either watch a prerecorded video intended to teach them new words or to engage in a word-learning video chat session with an experimenter. In half of the cases, the child's parent simply sat with the child. In the other half, the parent followed the experimenter's directions, modeling interactions with the video screen. A live video chat kept the kids' attention better than a prerecorded video, but only kids whose parents participated alongside them were able to learn new words from the screen (Pappas, 2020).

In marked contrast to AAP guidelines, Konca (2022) studied the homes of children ages 3-6 living in Turkey, and found they lived in "digitally rich" environments, averaging more than 3 hours of screen time each day. Xie et al. (2021) examined Latino American families and found that the presence of grandparents in the home was positively correlated with increased screen time, which averaged more than 2 hours per day.

Roberston et al. (2022) noted that rates of depression, self-harm, suicide attempts, and suicide deaths rose sharply among US children and adolescents after 2012, and they attempted to identify screen time correlates for this increase. They found that,

> Youth spending 2 or more hours ... a day with screen media were more likely to fit criteria for depressive disorders, self-harm, and suicidal ideation or attempts, even after adjustment for demographic covariates. For anxiety disorders, associations with digital media use (social media, texting, gaming, and online videos) were stronger than with screen time generally. (Roberston et al., 2022, p. 530)

In a similar study, Preyde et al. (2022) examined screen time in hospitalized adolescents and found that a high percentage reported 5 or more hours of daily digital medial use. Pizzo et al. (2020) speculated that youths who spent more time using screens were more likely to have poor mental health, while time spent engaged in active behaviors (i.e., physical activity, socializing, and reading) would be associated with better mental health. Their study found that a history of mental illness and current depression in mothers was associated with less time spent engaged in active behaviors and more time spent using screens among the 357 youth they studied.

Nagata et al. (2022) conducted a methodologically sophisticated study that examined the relationship between social media and conduct disorder in children between the ages of 9 and 11. They found that exposure to more than 4 hours of total screen time per day was associated with a higher prevalence of conduct disorder (69%) and oppositional defiant disorder (ODD; 46%).

Otto Wahl (2009) argues that children as well as adults are affected by the ways in which media portray people with mental illness. He notes,

> Studies of television, films, cartoons, and other media suggest that images and references to mental illnesses are relatively common in children's media and that such images are more often negative than positive ones. The image of persons with psychiatric disorders as unattractive, violent, and criminal, for example, appears common in children's media, and references to mental illnesses are typically used to disparage and ridicule. (p. 249)

Gender and Movies

Movies promulgate gender stereotypes, and there are compelling data to document that films often portray women in demeaning, subservient, and secondary roles, while men are more often shown to be competent, self-confident, and assertive. This pernicious practice has its roots in early films such as *Gone With the Wind* (1939) in which Rhett Butler (Clark Gable) treats Scarlett O'Hara (Vivien Leigh) with obvious contempt after using his charm to win her over earlier in the film. His comment, "Frankly, my dear, I don't give a damn," has become iconic.

The Bechdel-Wallace test (BWT) originated in a drawing by feminist cartoonist Alison Bechdel in her cartoon strip *Dykes to Watch Out For*. It is often simply referred to as the Bechdel test, but the artist prefers to share credit with the friend who originally came up with the idea. The test is applied to determine if a movie is worth seeing, and it involves three simple criteria:

1. Does the film have at least two named women?
2. Do the women talk to each other?
3. Does their conversation deal with something other than a man?

Marcus Appel and Timo Gnambs (2022) designed a creative study that was reported in

Psychology of Popular Media. They analyzed female characters in the 30 worldwide highest grossing movies per year, for the past 40 years (i.e., 1,200 films). Their core data came from the Bechdel Test Movie List (https://bechdeltest.com), and they supplemented these findings with analyses of high grossing movies that were not included in the public citizen–scientist database. Appel and Gnambs (2022) found that "The BWT was passed by 49.58% of the 1,200 most popular movies of the past 40 years. As a point of comparison, 95.31% of coded movies passed the reverse BWT (based on a subset of 341 movies), speaking to a much stronger representation of men than women" (p. 3). They go on to note,

> Humans acquire gender-related knowledge, norms, social roles, and behavioral patterns from the symbolic environments that media provide .... Decades of media effects research on group representations and stereotypes show that media can have manifest consequences in real life . ... Stories are particularly influential, as they can absorb audience members and transport them into narrative worlds, reducing their willingness and ability to critically reflect on settings, characters, or storylines. ... Changing the popular symbolic environments of feature films could be one means to approach gender equality in real life. (Appel & Gnambs, 2022, p. 5)

It is interesting to note that the genesis of the Bechdel-Wallace test was likely Virginia Woolf's novel *A Room of One's Own* (1929). Woolf wrote,

> All these relationships between women, I thought, rapidly recalling the splendid gallery of fictitious women, are too simple. ... And I tried to remember any case in the course of my reading where two women are represented as friends. ... They are now and then mothers and daughters. But almost without exception they are shown in their relation to men. It was strange to think that all the great women of fiction were, until Jane Austen's day, not only seen by the other sex, but seen only in relation to the other sex. And how small a part of a woman's life is that. ...

A variation on the Bechdel-Wallace test was developed by Holly Tarquini. Called the F-Rating, it is a feminist classification system that asks if films are written or directed by one or more women, and whether female characters contribute significantly to the story. Films that meet all three criteria (writing, directing, significant female characters) are awarded a triple F rating. Examples of triple F films include *The Dressmaker* (2015), *Thirteen* (2003), *The Babadook* (2014), *Monster* (2003), *We Need to Talk About Kevin* (2011), *Winter's Bone* (2011), and *The Piano* (1993).

Kyle Killian (2022) has written that "The representation of superheroines in comic books and comic book movies tends to subscribe to the patriarchal logic of the male gaze, with male subjects looking at women as hypersexualized objects and corporeal spectacles" (p. 106). However, films like *Black Widow* (2021) and *Black Panther: Wakanda Forever* (2022) may be changing the way that female superheroes are perceived.

Making Movies Around the World

Films are made in countries around the world, and many cities promote film festivals. However, the United States towers over all other countries in terms of film productivity, and exporting films is a major contributor to the US gross domestic product. Figure 5 shows that dramas, comedies, romance, and action films were the most frequently produced genres, and the United States holds a dramatic lead over all other countries in terms of film productivity (Bioglio & Pensa, 2018).

Bioglio and Pensa (2018) applied a novel method for measuring the influence of films, directors, actors, and actresses, to the Internet Movie Database (IMDb). These researchers analyzed 47,000 international films to produce a list of milestone films in the history of cinema. They also analyzed 20,000 directors and almost 400,000 performers and ranked these individuals.

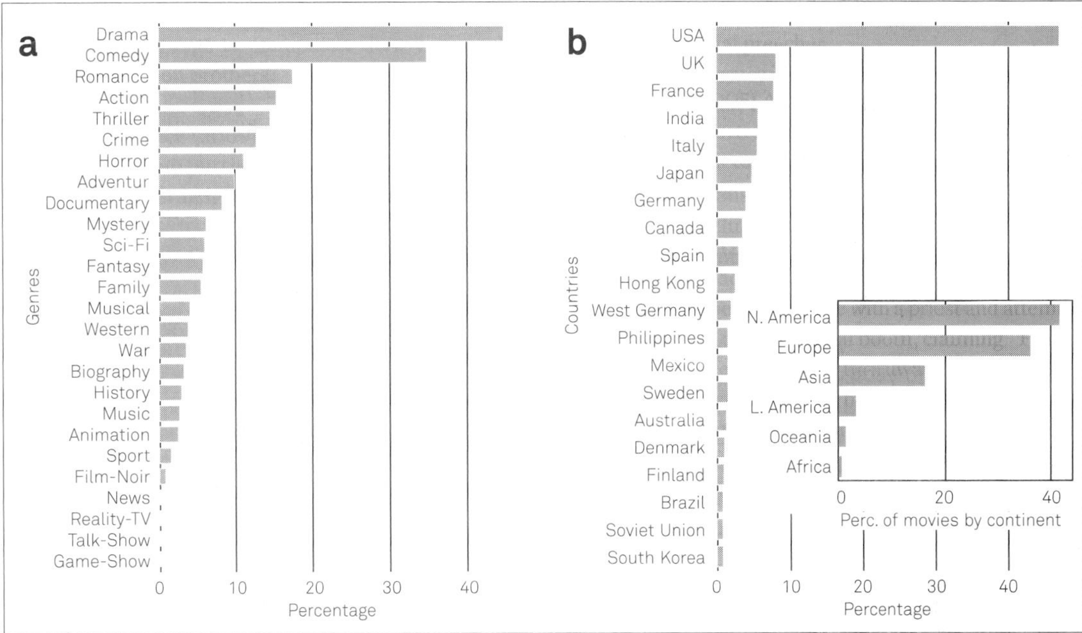

Figure 5. (a) Films ranked by genre; (b) Films ranked by productivity, country, and continent. From "Identification of Key Films and Personalities in the History of Cinema From a Western Perspective," by L. Bioglio & R. G. Pensa, 2018, *Applied Network Science, 3*(50), p. 6, https://doi.org/10.1007/s41109-018-0105-0. CC BY 4.0. Reprinted with permission.

They note,

> We have proposed a different metric for evaluating the career of directors, actors and actresses, inspired by the Medal Ranking System used in Olympic Games: a person gains a "gold" point for each movie directed/acted that reaches the top 5% influence in its year of release, a "silver" point for each movie in the best 5 to 10% ranking and a "bronze" point for each movie in the best 10 to 15% ranking, still in comparison with the other movies released during the same year. Personalities are then ranked according to the number of points gained, evaluating most precious metals more highly. (Bioglio & Pensa, 2018, p. 21)

This was a prodigious undertaking; however, the authors acknowledged that their analysis was biased toward European and North American movies, because their data were derived from IMDb, a database that focuses on Western culture.

The Bioglio and Pensa analysis of films suggested 20 films that were the most influential in their view (see Table 3).

Bioglio and Pensa also listed the top 20 directors using their methodology, along with the number of gold, silver, or bronze points that were collected by each, along with the year of their first and last movies, and the number of films directed in total (see Table 4).

A list of the top 20 actors, along with the number of gold, silver, and bronze points they earned, is found in Table 5.

A list of the top 20 actresses, along with the number of gold, silver, and bronze points they earned, is found in Table 6.

One should not make too much of these data because of the novelty of the approach taken by Bioglio and Pensa, but their lists should provide a stimulus and satisfying fodder for late-night discussions of the most important films, directors, actresses, and actors.

Table 3. The 20 most influential films according to the analysis of Bioglio & Pensa (2018)

Rank	Title
1	*The Wizard of Oz* (1939)
2	*Star Wars* (1977)
3	*Psycho* (1960)
4	*King Kong* (1933)
5	*2001: A Space Odyssey* (1968)
6	*Metropolis* (1927)
7	*Citizen Kane* (1941)
8	*The Birth of a Nation* (1915)
9	*Frankenstein* (1931)
10	*Snow White and the Seven Dwarfs* (1937)
11	*Casablanca* (1942)
12	*Dracula* (1931)
13	*The Godfather* (1972)
14	*Jaws* (1975)
15	*Nosferatu, eine Symphonie ...* (1922)
16	*The Searchers* (1956)
17	*Cabiria* (1914)
18	*Dr. Strangelove or: How I ...* (1964)
19	*Gone with the Wind* (1939)
20	*[Battleship] Potemkin* (1925)

Note. Most of these films were produced in the United States. From "Identification of Key Films and Personalities in the History of Cinema From a Western Perspective," by L. Bioglio & R. G. Pensa, 2018, *Applied Network Science, 3*(50), p. 12, https://doi.org/10.1007/s41109-018-0105-0. CC BY 4.0. Reprinted with permission.

Movie Theaters Versus Streaming Video in Your Home

Many of us have spent some of the best hours of our lives in movie theaters, and yet theaters increasingly must compete with streaming video for viewer time. High-definition television screens and surround sound audio units make the home viewing experience approximate the conditions associated with theater viewing, and films are increasingly being offered at the same time or soon after they are released in theaters. Netflix was the first company to refuse to participate in the longstanding tradition of providing theaters with an exclusive right for the initial release of new films, and instead releases films the same day they become available in theaters. Despite the convenience of home viewing, many cinephiles – like myself – find the theater experience vastly preferable. Fröber and Thomaschke (2021) have dubbed this the *cinema context effect*, and they note that movie theaters are dark cubes that protect the viewer from the outside world, and a large auditorium makes going to the movies a social experience. However, fewer than one in 10 films that are produced will be released in theaters, so there are many more choices for home viewing. These authors conclude by noting, "The present results provide clear-cut empirical evidence that a movie theater context is indeed boosting the cinematic experience in terms of an increase in a variety of aesthetic emotions" (p. 540), and they agree with Susan Sontag who wrote, "To see a great film only on television isn't to have really seen that film" (Sontag, 1996).

Celebrities and Mental Illness

It has been clearly documented that suicides by celebrities can produce a contagion effect. For example, after Robin Williams committed suicide, researchers compared

> the number of suicide deaths and the method of suicide in the 30 days before and after Aug. 11, 2014, and for the same time period in 2012 and 2013. In 2012–2014, there was an average of 113–117 suicide deaths per day; after Williams' suicide, the average rate increased to 142 suicide deaths per day, something not observed in 2012 or 2013. Approximately two-thirds of the people who died by suicide immediately after the actor's death used the same method of suicide as Williams. (National Institutes of Health, 2019)

Table 4. The top 20 directors according to Bioglio & Pensa (2018)

Rank	Name	Gold	Silver	Bronze	Career	No. of movies
1	Alfred Hitchcock	22	9	4	1925–1976	47
2	Steven Spielberg	18	3	2	1964–2020	33
3	Brian De Palma	14	5	0	1968–2012	29
4	Howard Hawks	12	4	3	1927–1970	39
5	John Ford	12	4	2	1917–1966	59
6	Martin Scorsese	11	6	2	1967–2014	33
7	Ingmar Bergman	11	2	1	1946–1986	33
8	Stanley Kubrick	11	1	1	1953–1999	13
9	Gerald Thomas	11	1	1	1958–1992	33
10	Ishiro Honda	10	8	2	1954–1990	30
11	Fritz Lang	10	1	2	1919–1960	33
12	Quentin Tarantino	10	1	0	1987–2015	13
13	David Cronenberg	10	1	0	1975–2014	19
14	Michael Curtiz	9	12	7	1922–1961	77
15	Raoul Walsh	9	5	4	1914–2010	57
16	John Carpenter	9	5	2	1974–2010	18
17	Clint Eastwood	9	4	4	1971–2016	34
18	Tim Burton	9	2	2	1985–2019	17
19	John Landis	9	2	1	1973–2010	19
20	Robert Rodriguez	9	2	0	1992–2014	18

Note. Gold, silver, and bronze points awarded for ranking of movie in top 5%, 5% to 10%, and 10% to 15%, respectively (see Bioglio & Pensa, 2018); Career = first film to last film in the Internet Movie Database (IMDb). From "Identification of Key Films and Personalities in the History of Cinema From a Western Perspective," by L. Bioglio & R. G. Pensa, 2018, *Applied Network Science, 3*(50), p. 15, https://doi.org/10.1007/s41109-018-0105-0. CC BY 4.0. Reprinted with permission.

Table 5. The top 20 actors according to Bioglio & Pensa (2018)

Rank	Name	Points: Gold, Silver, & Bronze	Career	No. of movies
1	Samuel L. Jackson	24, 5, 6	1981–2017	82
2	Clint Eastwood	18, 6, 4	1955–2013	54
3	Tom Cruise	18, 4, 3	1981–2017	41
4	Arnold Schwarzenegger	18, 3, 3	1976–2015	38
5	John Wayne	16, 10, 9	1930–1976	112
6	Willem Dafoe	16, 7, 5	1983–2014	57
7	Bruce Willis	16, 6, 3	1987–2016	62
8	Vincent Price	16, 5, 4	1938–1991	75
9	Demond Llewelyn	16, 2, 0	1963–1999	18
10	Ward Bond	16, 1, 4	1929–1959	73
11	Robert De Niro	15, 13, 7	1968–2016	75
12	Sean Connery	15, 8, 10	1957–2003	52
13	Jack Nicholson	15, 8, 4	1958–2011	54
14	Harrison Ford	15, 6, 3	1968–2015	45
15	Danny Trejo	15, 3, 3	1987–2015	74
16	Christopher Lee	14, 15, 7	1948–2014	105
17	Robbie Coltrane	14, 3, 0	1980–2012	37
18	Johnny Depp	14, 2, 4	1984–2017	52
19	Steve Buscemi	13, 7, 4	1986–2016	70
20	James Stewart	13, 6, 4	1935–1991	64

Note. Each item contains the number of gold, silver, and bronze points collected, the year of the first and last movies (at time of analysis), and the total number of films in which the actor had a role. From "Identification of Key Films and Personalities in the History of Cinema From a Western Perspective," by L. Bioglio & R. G. Pensa, 2018, *Applied Network Science, 3*(50), p. 18, https://doi.org/10.1007/s41109-018-0105-0. CC BY 4.0. Reprinted with permission.

Table 6. The top 20 actresses according to Bioglio & Pensa (2018)

Rank	Name	Points: Gold, Silver, & Bronze	Career	No. of movies
1	Lois Maxwell	16, 2, 0	1947–1988	27
2	Carrie Fisher	11, 3, 0	1975–2015	34
3	Maureen O'Sullivan	11, 2, 2	1930–1986	43
4	Halle Berry	10, 2, 4	1991–2017	29
5	Drew Barrymore	9, 6, 3	1980–2015	45
6	Lin Shaye	9, 5, 6	1978–2016	61
7	Cameron Diaz	9, 2, 2	1994–2014	29
8	Julianne Moore	8, 5, 4	1990–2017	49
9	Faye Dunaway	8, 5, 3	1967–2007	41
10	Beth Grant	8, 4, 3	1987–2015	41
11	Jamie Lee Curtis	8, 4, 3	1978–2014	33
12	Julie Christie	8, 4, 2	1963–2012	27
13	Sigourney Weaver	8, 3, 5	1977–2016	46
14	Joan Crawford	8, 3, 4	1925–1970	57
15	Maggie Smith	8, 3, 3	1962–2015	43
16	Frances Bay	8, 3, 1	1978–2014	35
17	Mary Ellen Trainor	8, 2, 6	1984–2003	23
18	Cloris Leachman	8, 2, 4	1955–2003	38
19	Judi Dench	8, 2,1	1965–2016	33
20	Natalie Portman	8, 1, 1	1994–2017	28

Note. Each item includes the number of gold, silver, and bronze points collected, the year of the first and last movies (at time of analysis), and the total number of films in which the actress had a role. From "Identification of Key Films and Personalities in the History of Cinema From a Western Perspective," by L. Bioglio & R. G. Pensa, 2018, *Applied Network Science, 3*(50), p. 18, https://doi.org/10.1007/s41109-018-0105-0. CC BY 4.0. Reprinted with permission.

However, celebrity self-disclosure can also have positive effects (Calhoun & Gold, 2020). For example, many famous individuals have shared their own challenges with mental health problems, or those of close family members. Lady Gaga was raped when she was 19, and she has spoken openly about her struggles with posttraumatic stress disorder (PTSD); Adele, Chrissy Teigen, Gwyneth Paltrow, and Brooke Shields have each shared stories about their experiences with postpartum depression; Dakota Johnson, Emma Stone, and Sarah Silverman all have had panic attacks; Carrie Fisher has struggled with both bipolar disorder and drug addiction; Dwayne Johnson has had to deal with a history of depression; Winona Ryder has been plagued by both anxiety and depression, and she has a history of arrest for shoplifting. Princess Diana spoke openly about her struggle with bulimia, and the number of women seeking treatment for bulimia increased dramatically. All of these stories serve to normalize the experience of mental illness and to encourage members of the public to seek treatment.

Actress and activist Glenn Close has been especially outspoken about the importance of mental health treatment, and she has set up a nonprofit organization called Bring Change to Mind (https://bringchange2mind.org/). The organization exists to encourage dialogue about mental health and to raise awareness, understanding, and empathy. Close began to speak out publicly about mental illness after her sister Jessie was diagnosed with bipolar disorder and her nephew with schizoaffective disorder. The nephew, Calen Pick, is featured in a public service announcement, *Schizo*, that has been seen by millions of people (Bring Change to Mind, 2022). The story of Glenn Close and her sister is told in their book, *Resilience: Two Sisters and a Story of Mental Illness*.

Some Films and Some Characters Defy Easy Classification

Although I have tried to pick excellent teaching films, some movies have characters that defy our attempts to label them. A recent example is *Oppenheimer* (2023), Christopher Nolan's magnificent exploration of the life and challenges faced by J. Robert Oppenheimer, father of the automatic bomb (Figure 6). The film is based on a biography by Kai Bird and Martin J. Sherwin, American Prometheus: *The Triumph and Tragedy of J. Robert Oppenheimer*. (Prometheus was a demigod who offended Zeus by giving fire to mortals; he was punished by being chained to a rock where an eagle fed each day upon his liver, only to have it grow back each night. Eventually, Prometheus was freed by Hercules.)

Nolan's film hints at some of the mental health problems Oppenheimer confronted during his very distinguished career. In graduate school he suffered a substantial depression characterized by dramatic and, at times, bizarre behavior (Werner, 2005). While training in the Cavendish Laboratory in Cambridge, he is alleged to have poisoned an apple that he left to be eaten by his mentor, Patrick Blackett. Fortunately, he has second thoughts and returned to the lab to retrieve the apple before it was eaten. At one point in the mid-20's, Oppenheimer was diagnosed with **dementia praecox**, a condition that today we call schizophrenia.

> **"I remembered the line from the Hindu scripture, the Bhagavad Gita; Vishnu is trying to persuade the prince that he should do his duty, and to impress him, takes on his multiarmed form and says, 'Now I am become Death, the destroyer of worlds.'"**
>
> **J. Robert Oppenheimer learned Sanskrit to more fully appreciate the *Bhagavad Gita***

Oppenheimer was clearly a genius – like John Nash – and we are reminded that mental health challenges can affect any of us. The fact that his life and his various diagnoses could fit any one

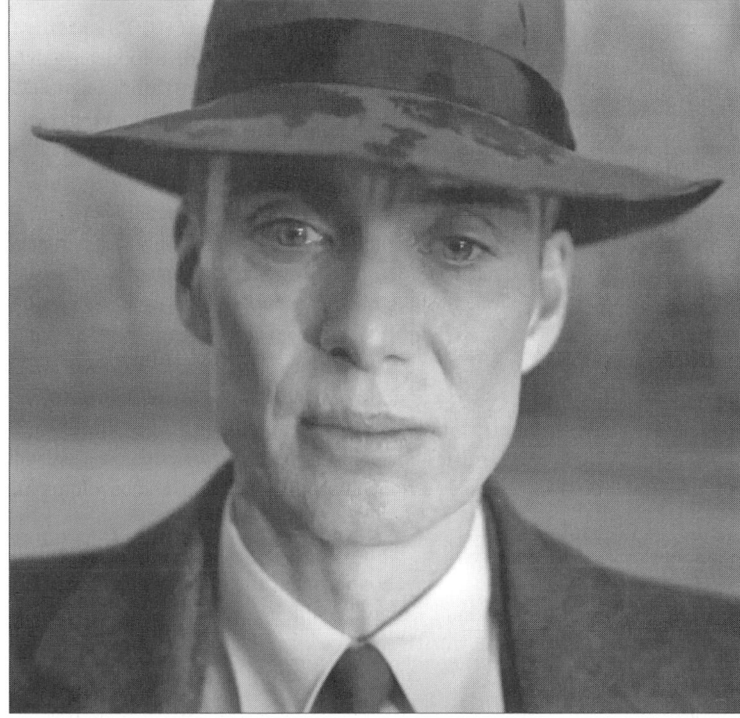

Figure 6.
Oppenheimer (2023, Universal Pictures). Produced by Emma Thomas, Charles Roven, Christopher Nolan. Directed by Christopher Nolan.

of three chapters in this book (schizophrenia spectrum disorders, mood disorders, or post-traumatic stress disorder following the bombings at Hiroshima and Nagasaki) underscores the complexity of the brain and behavior.

It is interesting to note that Oppenheimer gave an invited address at the 63rd annual meeting of the American Psychological Association in San Francisco in 1955. He remarked,

> Psychology, to everyone who works in the field, is felt to be a new subject in which real progress and real objectivity are recent. Physics is, perhaps, as old as the sciences come; physics is reputed to have a large, coherent, connected corpus of certitudes. This does not exist in psychology, and only the beginnings of it, the beginnings of things that are later going to be tied together, are now before us. (p. 128)

Mental Illness, Mental Health, and the Human Condition

Arango et al. (2021) developed a **comprehensive atlas of risk and protective factors** for mental disorders in which they identified numerous predictors for various mental disorders. The most robust predictors were as follows: for **dementia**, risk factors included type 2 diabetes mellitus, depression, and low frequency of social contacts; for **opioid use disorders**, tobacco smoking; for **nonorganic psychotic disorders**, cannabis use and childhood adversities; for **depressive disorders**, widowhood, sexual dysfunction, childhood physical and sexual abuse, job strain, obesity, and sleep disturbance; for **autism spectrum disorder (ASD)**, maternal overweight pre/during pregnancy; for **attention-deficit/hyperactivity disorder (ADHD)**, maternal pre-pregnancy obesity, maternal smoking during pregnancy, and maternal overweight pre/during pregnancy; while for **Alzheimer's disease**, the sole robust protective factor was high physical activity.

Mental illnesses, like those listed above, are among the most fascinating phenomena a filmmaker can depict on screen. There is, of course, much more to the human condition than psychopathology and what is going wrong with individuals. The positive aspects of human beings – happiness, achievement, talents, character strengths, interests, etc. – should not be viewed as mutually exclusive from mental struggles and disorders. Indeed, both can co-occur, and certainly one (i.e., positive psychology) can frequently benefit the other (i.e., mental disorders). In fact, while mental disorders are associated with lower levels of happiness, most people with mental disorders are happy. Elevated levels of distress do not preclude happy moods, and happiness does predict recovery from mental disorders (Bergsma et al., 2011).

In another book, *Positive Psychology at the Movies: Using Films to Build Character Strengths and Well-Being* (Niemiec & Wedding, 2014), Ryan Niemiec and I focus on what is right with people, and review nearly 1,500 cinematic portrayals of triumph, virtue, and positive influence. We use the VIA Classification system from the work *Character Strengths and Virtues* (Peterson & Seligman, 2004) of 24 universal character strengths, and discuss important cinematic examples of each (e.g., creativity, curiosity, kindness, fairness, etc.). Indeed, there is an overlap with the discussion here, as individuals with mental illness have character strengths and virtues (like all people) and often use their strengths to overcome mental adversity. Character strengths buffer people from vulnerabilities that can lead to depression and anxiety, such as the need for approval and perfectionism (Huta & Hawley, 2010). The specific character strengths of hope, kindness, social intelligence, self-regulation, and perspective buffer against the negative effects of stress and trauma (Park & Peterson, 2009). Such films are often truer to the human condition, as they are less likely to offer one-dimensional portrayals or shock-value sensationalism, and more likely to reveal the complexity and intrigue of what it means to be human. Films like *A Beautiful Mind* (2001) offer a compelling portrayal of schizophrenia, but this film also illustrates the character strengths of love, bravery, and perseverance. See Table 7 for examples of films that speak clearly to both dimensions of the human condition.

Table 7. Films portraying psychopathology as well as character strengths and virtues

Film	Psychopathology	Virtue	Character strength(s)
Elling (2001)	Anxiety disorder	Courage	Bravery and perseverance
Away From Her (2006)	Dementia	Humanity	Love
Mishima: A Life in Four Chapters (1985)	Suicide	Temperance	Self-regulation
Canvas (2006)	Schizophrenia	Wisdom and transcendence	Creativity and hope
The Soloist (2009)	Schizophrenia	Wisdom	Creativity
Insomnia (2002)	Sleep disorder	Courage	Bravery and perseverance
American Beauty (1999)	Mood disorder	Transcendence	Appreciation of beauty
It's a Wonderful Life (1946)	Adjustment disorder	Transcendence	Gratitude and hope
A Clockwork Orange (1971)	Personality disorder	Wisdom and transcendence	Curiosity and appreciation of excellence

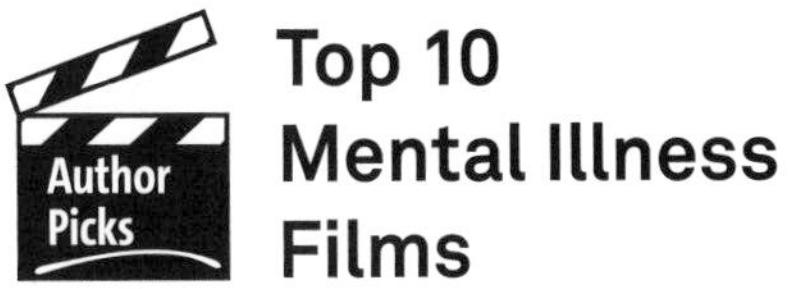

Top 10 Mental Illness Films

The Lost Weekend (1945)
Vertigo (1958)
Psycho (1960)
A Clockwork Orange (1971)
One Flew Over the Cuckoo's Nest (1975)
Apocalypse Now (1979)
A Beautiful Mind (2001)
Black Swan (2010)
Silver Linings Playbook (2012)
The Father (2020)

Chapter 2

Neurodevelopmental Disorders

My name is Temple Grandin.
I'm not like other people.
I think in pictures, and I connect them.

Temple Grandin

Movies and Persons With Disabilities

Like films portraying people with psychological disorders, films depicting individuals with disabilities can perpetrate misconceptions and stereotypes. These films are often shocking, inaccurate, implausible, and/or overly sentimental. From one vantage point, the person with a disability might be the subject of cheap jokes and bullying; from another angle, the portrayal can be patronizing or melodramatic. Such stereotyping can be made worse by casting actors without a disability who are expected to "fake it," or by having writers base their stories on stereotypes when they have no personal experience interacting with people with disabilities. Such contrived portrayals miss the uniqueness of the individual and lead to the misconception that all people with a particular disability are the same (e.g., the belief that all people with autism behave in a certain way).

Disabilities often are used as a plot device, and the character of the person with the disability is not developed fully in the story. For example, *The Other Sister* (1999) is a romantic comedy depicting the intellectual and developmental struggles of Carla Tate (Juliette Lewis) as she works hard to become an independent adult. However, many film critics found the film offensive and argued that intellectual disability was being used as a gimmick for the plot. The comedy *The Ringer* (2005) received similar criticism (Crawford, 2007). In this Farrelly brothers' film, Steve Barker (Johnny Knoxville) is desperate for money and decides to enter the Special Olympics to beat the reigning champ in the racing event. Special Olympics International supported the film, and consequently there are over 150 Special Olympics athletes in the film, with a handful having important supporting roles. Some stereotyping is present, including the use of the offensive word "retard" and the depiction of a person of average intelligence faking an intellectual disability with a false voice, unlikely behavior, mussed hair, and a contrived laugh. On the other hand, the film normalizes intellectual disability by showing that people with an intellectual disability experience normal emotions and activities – we see them struggling to compete, laughing, and supporting others; in addition, several of the characters with intellectual disability use sarcasm and wit to provide clever comic relief.

Films have also frequently perpetrated the misconception that individuals with a disability are more likely to be violent. Films like *Sling Blade* (1996) and *The Village* (2004) clearly convey this message. In fact, the opposite is true: Research has documented that those people with an intellectual disability, for example, are less likely to be aggressive than the "typical" individual. A similar misconception is that people with disabilities necessarily display outrageous behavior or exceptional talents. This can go in the negative behavior direction (e.g., smearing feces) or the positive behavior direction (e.g., savant/genius level talents). The film *The Black Balloon* (2008) is an example of the former while *Rain Man* (1988) is an example of the latter. Of course, both ends of the continuum are possible, but they are clearly not the norm, as some films suggest.

Stereotypes of women with disabilities have been categorized into four types by Norden (1994): the **sweet innocent** in *Stella Maris* (1918), the **obsessive avenger** in *Freaks* (1932), the **civilian superstar** in *Interrupted Melody* (1955), and the **bitter sibling** in *What Ever Happened to Baby Jane?* (1962). Norden also discusses realistic depictions of women with disabilities in *The Other Side of the Mountain* (1975), *Gaby: A True Story* (1987), and *Passion Fish* (1992).

Many films portray people with disabilities as asexual, and it is assumed that their disability precludes the ability to have a full and joyful sexual life. Esmail et al. (2010) found that viewing and discussing a documentary titled *Sexability* (2012) helped foster discussion and dispel stereotypes about the sexual lives of disabled people.

> Individuals with disabilities are commonly viewed as asexual due to a predominately heteronormative idea of sex and what is considered natural. A

> lack of information and education on sexuality and disability [is] a major contributing factor towards the stigma attached to disability and sexuality ... [and] stigma can lead individuals to internalize concepts of asexuality and may negatively impact confidence, desire and ability to find a partner while distorting one's overall sexual self-concept. (Esmail et al., 2010, p. 1148)

Films like *Crip Camp* (2020), and television programs like *Glee* can help educate the public. Three remarkable films released in 2012 were especially helpful in changing public attitudes about disability and sexuality: *The Sessions* portrays a disability rights activist in an iron lung who is determined to have a sex life and gets permission from his priest to do so; *Hyde Park on Hudson* shows a disabled FDR having an affair with his cousin; and *Rust and Bone* depicts a woman with a double amputation having a passionate sex life with her muscular lover. *The Sessions* is especially useful in portraying Helen Hunt's sex worker character sympathetically, showing her to be a highly trained professional, and someone offering an important service. In Europe, therapists offering sexual services to disabled people are increasingly labeled "sexual assistants" rather than sex workers, and they are forming powerful political alliances with members of the disability community (Geymonat, 2019).

People with disabilities – like almost everyone else – like being loved, held, hugged, kissed, and fondled, and many can and do enjoy orgasms.

De Moura et al. (2020) collected questionnaire data on *men* with spinal cord injuries (SCIs), and found,

> 90% made medium to large sexual adjustments, both physically and psychologically. The results of the present study demonstrated that men with SCI maintained an active sex life and unchanged sexual desire. [However] most men with SCI were not advised about physical and psychological sexual adjustments when adapting to sex, both physical and emotional. (p. 615)

Likewise, Rezaei-Fard et al. (2019) conducted a randomized clinical trial studying *women* with SCIs and discovered that the simple application of *permission, limited information, specific suggestions, and intensive therapy* (PLISSIT; a staged intervention model developed by Jack Annon) led to significant increases in sexual desire, arousal, lubrication, orgasm, and sexual satisfaction, along with a reduction in pain associated with sexual activity (Rezaei-Fard et al., 2019, p. 511).

Ian Freckelton (2013) has described some of the legal and ethical issues that confront therapists referring to sexual surrogates, noting that it is complicated and difficult for therapists to broker sexual contacts between patients and surrogates, even when these services would be beneficial and are needed.

> In some jurisdictions, arrangements involving sexual surrogate therapy (especially where the therapist benefits from it financially) may not be lawful. Further, in spite of many assertions one way and the other, there are no data enabling evaluation of the success rates of the interventions of sexual surrogates or sex workers. ... It is also unclear whether sexual surrogates' adherence to an ethical code effectively ameliorates the potential for countertherapeutic consequences from the commodification of intimacy, and it is far from straightforward to identify what steps should be taken by the referring health practitioner to select a suitable provider of sexual services to their patient or client, and then to monitor whether the arrangement is achieving its objectives. (Freckelton, 2013, p. 643)

Despite a few sex positive disability films, Botha and Harvey (2022) argue that films about acquired physical disability continue to produce negative stereotypes about disability, and they note "characters need to be complex, all-rounded individuals, with disability being only one facet of their personhood."

For information on the Reel Abilities Film Festival, the largest disabilities festival, which is held in several US cities, see their website (https://reelabilities.org/). For free short films starring (and in some cases, created by) individuals with different disabilities, go to https://sproutflix.org.

The Optimal Portrayal of Persons With Disabilities in Film

It is challenging for filmmakers to offer a portrayal of persons with disabilities that is accurate, substantive, and entertaining. Filmmakers are improving, however, and better films are being made. This may reflect enhanced societal awareness about the lives of people with disabilities.

There is no "perfect" portrayal of a person with an intellectual disability, an autism spectrum disorder, or a similar condition. However, there are several factors that are important for filmmakers to consider as they ponder potential film projects; viewers, too, can take such factors into consideration when making choices about the films they will watch.

I believe an optimal portrayal of persons with disabilities will contain all – or at least most – of the following elements:

Humanizing: The film offers unique insight into who the human being is – the person "beyond" the disability. This means that the film takes a person-first approach.

Dynamic: Viewers will witness – and be able to identify – many important aspects of the individual's life from the film, including positive traits, deficits, positive relationship and environmental factors, and negative relationship and environmental factors.

Balanced: The filmmaker strikes a balance between overemphasizing the disability, disorder, or deficits and oversentimentality or glorification of it.

Meaningful: The best films offer a compelling and substantive story about the characters they portray. In many cases, these are stories and characters that are inspiring and that depict the person with a disability transcending their disability or disorder.

Film is a type of entertainment, and this remains the main reason people view movies. However, even very entertaining films can still educate the viewer.

Neurodevelopmental Disorders

The DSM-5 categorizes neurodevelopmental disorders into seven broad categories: **intellectual disabilities**, **communication disorders**, **ASD**, **ADHD**, **specific learning disorder**, **motor disorders**, and **other developmental disorders**. Neurodevelopmental disorders are characterized by early onset in development (typically before a child enters grade school) and impairment in functioning in important life activities such as self-sufficiency, socializing with others, learning, and working. These disorders often co-occur and overlap. This chapter focuses on those conditions most frequently portrayed in films: intellectual disabilities, ASDs, ADHD, and to a lesser degree, communication disorders and motor disorders.

Intellectual Disability

The term "intellectual disability" has replaced the pejorative term "mental retardation." Rosa's Law, an unanimously supported, bipartisan bill signed into US federal law in 2010, removes the terms "mental retardation" and "mentally retarded" from federal health, education, and labor policy. It replaces those words with "individual with an intellectual disability" and "intellectual disability." The DSM-5 and ICD-11 have also made these changes. The American Association on Intellectual and Developmental Disabilities considers intellectual disability from a dimensional perspective and notes that disability is a state of functioning that exists within the fit between a person's capacities and the context in which they function, as opposed to the previous term "mental retardation," which viewed disability as a defect within the person (Wehmeyer et al., 2008). These scientists explain how this change in terms improves the accuracy in describing individuals as well as the social impact:

> The changing understanding of disability ... has marked impact on how society responds to people who manifest intellectual disability. The adoption of the term intellectual disability implies an understanding of disability consistent with an ecological and multidimensional perspective and requires that society respond with interventions that focus on individual strengths and that emphasize the role of supports to improve human functioning. (Wehmeyer et al., 2008, p. 317)

In short, use of the term "intellectual disability" emphasizes a *person-first* approach.

According to the DSM-5, intellectual disability is prevalent in about 1% of the population. The range of intellectual disability extends from mild to profound and has historically been defined in terms of scores on tests of intellectual ability. However, DSM-5 rejects the arbitrary use of IQ scores, in favor of clinical assessment of adaptive functioning, using historical categorical labels (mild, moderate, severe, and profound). Deficits in adaptive functioning include not meeting the expected standards for a child of their age or cultural group in communication, not using community resources, lacking self-direction, limited academic skills, or experiencing problems with leisure, health, or safety. There are numerous causes of intellectual disability – these include drug or alcohol abuse in the mother, chromosomal or genetic disorders, or lack of oxygen during a difficult delivery.

Today, a child diagnosed with an intellectual disability is usually kept at home and integrated into the school system when they reach school age. Schools, the design of buildings, and community support organizations are becoming increasingly **inclusive** for individuals with intellectual (and other) disabilities, integrating them into society-as-usual. Innovative approaches in early intervention when the child is in their first few years of life have a significant impact and can help the child improve intellectually and adaptively and reach the goal of functioning as independently as possible with minimal support. With appropriate training, most adults with intellectual disability live productive, independent lives.

Michael Gill (2012) has written about the politics of **masturbation training**, arguing that it is a suitable expression of sexuality for people with intellectual disability, helping them avoid pregnancy, disease, and sexually transmitted infections. Teaching seriously mentally challenged individuals to avoid public masturbation is a part of the training, which Gill maintains should be "programmed, restricted and professionalized" (p. 472).

Down syndrome was first described in 1862 by a British physician, J. Langdon Down. Down had to leave school at age 14, but he had an experience when he was 18 that shaped his eventual medical career.

> I was brought into contact with a feeble minded girl, who waited on our party and for whom the question haunted me – could nothing for her be done? I had then not entered on a medical student's career but ever and anon... the remembrance of that hapless girl presented itself to me and I longed to do something for her kind. (Ward, 1999, p. 19)

"Mongolian idiocy" was once used to describe individuals with intellectual disability, but it was clearly a pejorative term. In 1961, the journal *Lancet* looked for a less insulting term for the condition and settled on Down syndrome.

Down syndrome is the most common genetic cause of intellectual disability, and most but not all individuals with Down syndrome have a below-average IQ. This is a disorder caused by the individual having three chromosomes 21; the incidence is approximately 1 per 800–1,000 live births (Hodapp & Fidler, 2021). These children have distinctive physical characteristics that often include hypotonia, midface depression, and short ear length. People with Down syndrome have frequently been victims of stereotyping and prejudice. In the early 1960s, about 10% of all residents who were institutionalized had Down syndrome. They were institutionalized because it was thought that anyone with Down syndrome needed to live apart from the rest of society. This has been shown to be a very inaccurate stereotype. Families of children with

Down syndrome have become pioneers in the understanding of developmental disabilities, and institutionalization has become far less common.

Me, Too

I hesitated to include this film in this section because the primary character, while having Down syndrome, may not have an intellectual disability. (However, there are other characters in the film who clearly have an intellectual disability and are well portrayed in the film.) The protagonist of *Me, Too* (2009) is played by actor Pablo Pineda, an award-winning Spanish actor who has Down syndrome. Pineda portrays Daniel, a young man who has just earned a bachelor's degree (like Pineda himself, who earned a bachelor's degree in educational psychology, the first person in Europe with Down syndrome to accomplish this) and is working in his first job for regional social services. Daniel does his work well and has good adaptive functioning. There are some elements that suggest adaptive limitations, such as the fact that he continues to live with his mother, and at times he has difficulty tying his shoes, although he sometimes pretends to struggle with the latter in a strategic way to get a love interest to help him, allowing him to be in closer proximity to her. There are other instances in which Daniel uses his social intelligence, humor, and Down syndrome to his advantage, such as when he purposefully displays inappropriate behavior in an elevator with two strangers and his work colleague with the intention of embarrassing his colleague. When the colleague claims that Daniel is "faking it," the strangers are shocked that she would say such a thing about a person with a "handicap," and she and Daniel then roar with laughter at the humor and subtlety of the situation. Daniel is often reflective and observant and displays clear social intelligence in his interpretation of a woman's inner experience when he asks her: "Is that why you have such a sad expression on your lips?"

The drama in the film centers on Daniel falling in love with a work colleague (someone who does *not* have an intellectual disability). As he pursues her, they develop a friendship and engage in activities such as dancing, traveling, swimming, and having fun at the beach. She likes Daniel and acknowledges that she loves him; however, Down syndrome acts as a barrier to an intimate relationship, which is what he wants. She is forthright about her feelings, and says they cannot be a couple, but they can be close friends. Daniel is disappointed, but he understands the situation. He maintains resilient in response to social barriers and others' perceptions of him.

Daniel is aware of his Down syndrome and describes the physical characteristics associated with the syndrome to others. When asked about the severity level of his intellectual disability and whether he has a more minor form, Daniel replies with humor: "No, not at all. I'm Down syndrome from head to toe." When asked why he is doing so well, he explains the reason is his mother talked to him a lot when he was young about diverse topics such as history and politics, frequently asked him questions, and made sure he went to school. Daniel spends his time learning another language, working out, swimming, socializing with family, listening to hypnosis recordings to help him stop smoking, and continuing to learn.

The actor Pineda is an active advocate for the Down syndrome community. When interviewed about his role in the film and his experience of living with Down syndrome, he replied that he views the condition as just "another personal characteristic."

I highlight *Me, Too* as an exemplary film for filmmakers interested in depicting intellectual disability, and as a stellar example for educators and professionals teaching and exploring the topic and working with individuals with intellectual disabilities.

Monica and David

The marriage between the title characters, both of whom have Down syndrome, is the subject of the documentary *Monica and David* (2009). The film portrays the daily life of this couple, including their desires, hopes, and family interactions.

Monica and David initiated their wedding following years of a loving relationship they spent living apart. After a successful wedding and California honeymoon, they move in together along with Monica's mother and stepfather. Both characters have their own limitations – including cognitive impairment, obsessive-compulsive behavior, and adaptive limitations. Each tries to improve: Monica learns to cook, and David learns to regularly test his blood sugar and self-administer his insulin. There are scenes of tension – such as when the whole family moves into a bigger home – and scenes demonstrating deep caring, such as when David offers insight, support, and a "loving playfulness" for his wife after she explains she has written an honest and emotional letter sharing her anger with her biological father who abandoned her.

Monica's mother shares the rewards of being so close to her daughter and son-in-law and explains that she enjoys spending time with them. She also shares the difficult balance she must maintain between protecting David and Monica from exploitation, while at the same time not wanting to control and restrict them too much. She wonders and worries about how they will get by when she and her husband are no longer around – who will help support or care for them? How will they be treated by society? This film, directed by Alexandra Codina, won Best Documentary Feature at the Tribeca Film Festival, and was nominated for an Emmy for outstanding informational programming.

Forrest Gump

The now classic film *Forrest Gump* (1994) portrays 40 years in the life of a man who has a marginal IQ of 75, but whose innocence, innovation, and common sense make him wise. Forrest's condition would be classified as **borderline intellectual functioning**, and he would be tested for a learning disability.

This superb film begins with Forrest, played by Tom Hanks, telling his life story. When Forrest is a child, his mother (Sally Fields) believes in him and is determined that he should have a full, complete life. Forrest has a weak spine and needs to wear leg braces. He is forced to run from other children to protect himself, so that even with the leg braces he becomes an outstanding runner. Eventually, a local football coach spots Forrest and signs him to play college football. He begins a brilliant career that eventually leads him to the army and service in Vietnam. He wins a medal and becomes a table tennis star. After being discharged from the army, Forrest goes into the shrimp business and becomes a millionaire. Forrest has a life-long friend, Jenny Curran (Robin Wright Penn), who often came to his aid as a child. As an adult, he can help her as she and her son cope with disability and death resulting from AIDS.

Drill Sergeant: "Gump! What's your sole purpose in this army?"
Forrest Gump: "To do whatever you tell me, drill sergeant!"
Drill Sergeant: "God damn it, Gump! You're a goddamn genius! This is the most outstanding answer I have ever heard. You must have a goddamn I.Q. of 160. You are goddamn gifted, Private Gump."

***Forrest Gump* (1994)**

Even with a limited intelligence and modest academic ability, Forrest can feel good about himself and who he is – a simple man who leaves his mark on the world. The development of his self-esteem has its roots in his childhood and his mother's confidence in him. The friendship with Jenny encourages him. Because of the support of these two women, it never occurs to Forrest that he might not succeed.

Shorty and *Radio*

Two films that portray adult males with intellectual disabilities who are accepted and integrated into the community of a football team are the documentary *Shorty* and the feature film *Radio*.

Shorty (2003) tells the story of Walter Simms (nicknamed "Shorty"), a man with Down syndrome, who for 28 years has been an important member of the Hampden-Sydney College community – the football team, the college campus, and the larger community. The film follows Shorty in his daily work and his interactions with coaches, players, students, and others at the college. He is often called part of the family. Shorty's passion for the football program is so strong that his one birthday wish is that Hampden-Sydney College defeats their archrival, Randolph-Macon, in the 107-year rivalry known as "The Game." Despite his cognitive limitations, Shorty exhibits tremendous zest and energy and is loving and humorous with everyone in his life. Whenever Shorty is around, people seem happier. The film also depicts Shorty's induction into the Hampden-Sydney College Athletic Hall-of-Fame and his acceptance speech.

When the real-life Shorty was initially approached about the potential for making of this film, he was hesitant and humble, saying he did not think he had enough personality for a film to be made about him. The community and filmmakers disagreed, finding him to be charming, friendly, passionate, humorous, caring, honest, brave, and hopeful. The film was made by actor Danny Aiello's production company, Revolution Earth; when interviewed about the film, Aiello explained that he wanted to make a film about the regular life of a person with Down syndrome and to educate the public about this disorder.

Inspired by a true story, *Radio* (2003) is the story of Coach Harold Jones (Ed Harris) who takes in a young man, Radio (Cuba Gooding Jr.), and makes him an assistant coach for the football team. Though he is never given a diagnosis in the film (other than the label "slow"), Radio clearly has an intellectual disability. At the beginning of the film, Radio barely speaks a word, mostly uttering sounds, is hunched over in posture, and walks around with a shopping cart for several miles to get groceries. He lives alone with his mother and is completely isolated. He is never given a chance in life. Early in the film, Radio is cruelly ridiculed and mistreated by several football players. One player continues his cruel taunting of Radio, but he accepts the criticism without complaining. Given an opportunity to help the football team, Radio agrees and begins to talk much more, interacts with others, and helps the team in significant ways; in fact, he becomes a symbol of inspiration for the players, and his life changes. Coach Jones goes out of his way to help give Radio opportunities; he defends Radio in front of the community and integrates him into the school system. When the coach is asked why he is helping Radio, he responds: "It's the right thing to do." The story speaks to the courage and sacrifices of two men who influence one another and in turn grow in courage and dedication. Coach Jones admits part of his dedication and care for Radio arises from childhood shame for not taking action to protect a boy with a disability who was being tortured.

Dominick and Eugene

Dominick and Eugene (1988), directed by Robert M. Young, is a movie about twin brothers Dominick (Tom Hulce) and Eugene Luciao (Ray Liotta), who live together in a low-income Pittsburgh neighborhood. Dominick ("Nicky") experienced brain trauma as a child and is developmentally disabled. He also has a learning disability and memory problems. The story begins as the twins approach their 26th birthday. Nicky is interested in the Hulk; Eugene ("Gino") is completing medical school and has been accepted into a California residency program. Gino, who feels responsible for his brother and who is afraid to tell him about his plans to move, is frequently angry with Nicky. The movie depicts the change in the brotherly relationship as each matures and responds to his respective need to live separately. It also highlights the strength of people with intellectual disabilities.

Dominick: "Gene, tell me about when we were born."
Eugene: "You were born first. And 12 minutes later I was born. You are the big brother. Our mother died when we were born. Our father worked in the steel mill."
Dominick: "And you and me was always together. Our father had to go away. I fell down and hurt my head and that is why I can't remember."

***Dominick and Eugene* (1988)**

Other Films Portraying Intellectual Disability

The film *I Am Sam* (2001) depicts an adult, Sam (Sean Penn), with intellectual disability and some autistic behaviors who lives independently. He thinks very concretely and has difficulty with any task requiring abstract thought. His reading and math ability are limited. Sam lives in an apartment with his 7-year-old daughter, Lucy, whom he has cared for since birth. Sam has assumed responsibility for raising Lucy with the help of a neighbor. He has not had contact with any family members. He has several friends who also have developmental disabilities who provide support to Sam and his daughter. The father and daughter have the same intellectual abilities, and they enjoy playing in the park, singing songs, and reading together. When Lucy surpasses her father's intellectual capacity, she is embarrassed by his limited cognitive abilities. She struggles to cope with classmates and friends making fun of Sam and frequently tells her friends she is adopted. At a birthday party planned by her father, Lucy becomes distraught over her father's child-like behavior. Child Protective Services eventually takes Lucy away from her father.

> **"You don't know what it is when you try, and you try, and you try, and you never get there!"**
>
> **Sam expressing the challenges of his life in *I Am Sam* (2001)**

Ira Wohl's film *Best Boy* (1979) is a documentary that examines the life of Wohl's cousin, Philly, a man with an intellectual disability who has spent his entire life living with, and being protected by, his parents. The film beautifully documents the concerns of Philly's parents about who will take care of him after their death, a common theme in films depicting parents of children with intellectual disabilities. Philly's father dies while the film is being made, and his mother reluctantly allows Philly to become involved in an adult day services program. In addition, the film does a beautiful job portraying the emotional richness of Philly's life and the strong bonds that have been formed between this man and his family. Ira Wohl produced a moving sequel to *Best Boy* titled *Best Man: 'Best Boy' and All of Us Twenty Years Later* (1997). This film brings the viewer up to date on the life of Philly, who now lives in a group home in Queens. He has a full and meaningful life, and he is shown preparing for a significant, albeit delayed, rite of passage – his bar mitzvah.

The challenges and concerns of parents who have young children (or adult children) with Down syndrome is a common theme in films about intellectual disabilities. Examples can be found in *Praying With Lior* (2008, UK), *The Memory Keeper's Daughter* (2008), *Girlfriend* (2010), *Me, Too* (2009), and particularly in *Monica and David* (2009). *Any Day Now* (2012) is a sensitive film describing the attempt of a gay couple to provide a loving home for a boy with Down syndrome and the challenges they confront as they deal with bigotry and stereotypes. This powerful film is based on a true story.

Some films depict a character with a disability who significantly influences other characters, as in the comedy *There's Something About Mary* (1998). The protagonist's brother Warren (W. Earl Brown) has intellectual disability and autistic tendencies. He exhibits **echolalia**, perseverates in his play, displays finger-flicking behavior, and wears earmuffs to block out disturbing sounds. He clearly likes the lead character, Ted (Ben Stiller), but when Ted touches him near his ears, Warren's sensitivity leads to a violent reaction – he picks Ted up and spins him around before throwing him down on the coffee table. It is an upsetting incident, but the whole family realizes that it happened due to a triggering event and was not due to malevolence on Warren's part. Mary (Cameron Diaz) lives near Warren and remains an active part of his life. She volunteers and spends time with Warren and other people with disabilities. Mary is not simply a "do good" person; she is also a good sister. The antagonists in the film attempt to fake being "good," but eventually their manipulations fall short. In addition, although Warren has a significant disability, he does do comical and outrageous things. Since this film is a comedy, and all of the other nondisabled characters do things that are comical, it does not appear that the director has singled out Warren. His behavior clearly influences the lives of the other characters.

Characters with intellectual disabilities can also be found in Philip Seymour Hoffman's socially awkward character, Jack, in *Jack Goes Boating* (2010), and in the films *Caramel* (2007, Lebanon) and *The Secret Life of Bees* (2008).

Films sometimes show people with disabilities, particularly intellectual disability, being exploited by others. In *Amélie* (2001), one character is ridiculed and mistreated by his boss in front of others. Though he is depicted with an intellectual disability, his character is more developed as he takes charge of a fruit stand, demonstrates competence in this new role, enjoys painting with a friend, and experiences a deep appreciation of life. In one of the many disturbing scenes in *Gummo* (1997), a girl with an intellectual disability is sold to young boys for sex.

The Importance of Tying Your Own Shoes (2009) is an animated documentary that portrays the lives of four adult artists with Down syndrome. The film aims to dispel stereotypes and highlight the achievements of the protagonists (Avni et al., 2011).

A few older films have poignantly illustrated the difficulties – and sometimes the beauty – in the lives of people who have an intellectual disability, such as *Charly* (1968), *A Day in the Death of Joe Egg* (1972), and *Of Mice and Men* (1939, 1992). There are also reprehensible films, such as *Tropic Thunder* (2008), that deliberately use offensive language to get laughs at the expense of people with intellectual disabilities. Timothy Shriver (2008) in the *Washington Post* described the film this way: "By all accounts, it is an unchecked assault on the humanity of people with intellectual disabilities – an affront to dignity, hope and respect."

Flowers for Algernon is a made-for-TV film released in 2000 based on a 1966 novel by Daniel Keyes. The film portrays an intellectually challenged man who undergoes a surgical procedure to raise his IQ. The operation is a success, but there are negative and positive changes in the protagonist's life. Ghoshal and Wilkinson (2017) have described the dubious ethical decisions that were made in the novel and film, as well as the difficulty in obtaining informed consent from people who are intellectually disabled.

Intelligent Lives (2018) portrays the lives of three young adults with intellectual disabilities and argues for inclusive public policies that help people with intellectual limitations participate in regular school programs, find meaningful work, and enjoy intimate relationships. Actor Chris Cooper narrates the documentary and shares the story of his own son, Jesse, who was able to succeed in public schools until his premature death at age 17. Psychology students seeing the film will be challenged by the film's critique of the utility of intelligence tests.

"The IQ test told us nothing about Jesse's potential. About who he was as a person. Can any attempt to measure intelligence predict a person's value or potential to contribute meaningfully to the world?"

Chris Cooper discusses the limits of traditional intellectual assessment, in *Intelligent Lives* (2018)

Short Films

Several **short films** have been made about people with an intellectual disability, some of which can be accessed online, such as the whimsical *3:15 to Brunswick* (2012, Australia), the charming *Be My Brother* (2009, Australia), the honest *Between Sasquatch and Superman* (2010), and a film with several intersecting stories, *Beyond Borders* (2009, Belgium). The film *Waiting for Ronald* (2003) is discussed in Chapter 5; *Jacob's Turn* (2010) depicts a 4-year-old boy's early experiences on a T-ball team with "typical" kids; and *Hannah* (2010) is a striking film with no dialogue and no characters other than the dancer-athlete Hannah Dempsey, a young woman with Down syndrome displaying significant strength, endurance, and suave finesse as she conquers snowy mountain landscapes, ocean waves, and chilling temperatures while downhill skiing, spinning, swimming, and sprinting.

The Ups of Downs (2002) is a short documentary depicting the unique interests, talents, and personality of Danny, a young man with Down syndrome, who leads a very active and productive life. Danny performs and dances in a theatrical group, and he is the lead singer of a hardcore band with which he performs live shows sporting his red, spiked hair. He has a girlfriend with whom he regularly has sex; dabbles in photography; is a prolific painter; and he drinks beer when socializing with friends. "It's very, very important to let me speak," says Danny, referring to his desire for people to be patient with his slow and sometimes unclear speech. In the film, the filmmaker asks Danny, "Do you know that not everyone allows Down syndrome people to be born?"

> **"I am a free person and I need my own life ... because having my own life is very, very important."**
>
> **Danny in *The Ups of Downs* (2002)**

Danny is not the only person with Down syndrome featured in short films and music videos. In addition, there is Cam Lasley, a talented rapper with music videos such as *Against These Walls*. There is also the popular Australian rock band, Rudely Interrupted, in which five of the six members have a major disability, including intellectual disabilities (e.g., two members have Down syndrome), other developmental disabilities, ASDs, blindness, and deafness. The documentary *Rudely Interrupted* (2009) follows this inspiring band on a world tour that includes the first performance by any band in front of the United Nations. The one person without a disability is Rohan Brooks, the band manager and one of the guitarists. The film portrays the strengths of everyone in the band as well as the challenges brought forth by each of their disabilities. The band comes together as a unit to offer strong musical performances as well as support to one another when one of the band members is struggling.

Autism Spectrum Disorder

Autism spectrum disorder (ASD) is a complex neurodevelopmental disorder characterized by early onset difficulties in social communication and interaction, unusually restricted, repetitive behavior and interests. The condition is usually diagnosed before the age of 3 years and typically lasts through the lifespan (Pellecchia et al., 2021). ASD occurs four times more frequently in males than in females and occurs in 1 in 54 children in the United States (Maenner et al., 2020). Approximately 75% of persons with ASD also have an intellectual disability, and about half do not communicate verbally. The worldwide incidence of ASD is approximately 1%, and the number of children diagnosed with the disorder has been growing dramatically since the 1980s. At least part of this increase can be attributed to enhanced awareness of the disorder. ASD is largely inherited, and there is little evidence linking the condition to specific environmental exposures. However, advanced maternal age and diabetes in the mother during pregnancy are established risk factors. It is also clear that ASD is a complex problem that requires special treatment and family support.

Problems in social interaction and communication and restricted, repetitive patterns of behavior are the primary symptoms of ASD. Many children with ASD are not able to maintain eye-to-eye gaze, respond with facial expressions, or use normal body posture and gestures. As children with autism grow older, they do not typically develop peer relationships appropriate to their developmental level. They often do not express pleasure in other people's happiness or participate in interpersonal give and take. These children's behaviors can be frustrating to parents because of a clear and visible lack of emotional warmth. There is often a delay and sometimes a complete lack of development of spoken language. If there is speech, there is impairment in the ability to initiate or sustain a conversation with others. Their use of language is often repetitive or idiosyncratic. As children, they may not be able to engage in make-believe play or social imitative play appropriate to their developmental level.

Other symptoms of ASD are repetitive and stereotyped patterns of behavior, interests, and activities. For example, children may rock for hours, twist their fingers, rub their hands on their legs, spin, or repeat complex body movements. People with ASD compulsively adhere to specific, often nonfunctional, routines or rituals. The children are frequently preoccupied with objects rather than people. A child with autism may be fascinated with a motor, a piece of equipment, a model automobile, or train schedules. The child may spend hours taking an object apart and putting it together again.

Most adults with ASD continue to be inattentive to social convention, lack social skills, have few or no friends, and typically do not marry. They may also be troubled by chronic anxiety. The repetitive behavior and movements found in children with ASD usually persist into adulthood.

In addition to treatment with medication, behavior modification, and individualized educational approaches, the family plays a critical role. Most families need support in helping their child with autism, and implementing treatment programs within the home to help the child generalize from the home to an academic setting is often useful. Parents learn how to teach their children appropriate social and communication skills and behavior modification techniques. Family therapy is sometimes also recommended to help the family cope with the stress and problems associated with raising a child with ASD.

The prognosis for children with ASD is mixed. If a child begins to acquire language, is socially responsive, and shows improvement in cognitive skills by the age of 5–7, the child will have a better prognosis than those children who do not. The diagnosis of ASD is rarely made before the age of 3 years; however, Saint-Georges et al. (2011) examined family movies of children younger than 18 months. Three groups were studied: children with autism (AD), intellectual disability (ID), and typical development (TD). These researchers wanted to study "interaction synchrony," and they found that deviant autistic behaviors appear before 18 months. Parents feel the lack of interactive initiative and responsiveness of their babies and try to increasingly supply soliciting behaviors. Thus, we stress that credence should be given to parents' intuition as they recognize, long before diagnosis, the pathological process through the interactive pattern with their child.

Because the manifestations of autism vary tremendously across patients, depending on the severity of the condition, the child's age, and their developmental level, the DSM-5 now classifies autism as a **spectrum disorder**. The diagnosis of ASD includes children and adults who would have previously been diagnosed as people with high-functioning autism or **Asperger's disorder**. Temple Grandin is clearly an example of someone with an ASD who is functioning at an extremely high level (e.g., she has a PhD, she lectures around the world, and she has published numerous books; see the section Autism and *Temple Grandin*, in this chapter). People with this condition are frequently labeled as odd and eccentric. However, language skills are intact, and cognitive development is not delayed.

Ron Suskind (2014a, 2014b) has described the poignant developmental regression of his son Owen at age 3: Owen was subsequently diagnosed with regressive autism, which affects about a third of children with the ASD diagnosis.

> My wife, Cornelia, a former journalist, was home with him – a new story every day, a new horror. He could barely use a sippy cup, though he'd long ago graduated to a big-boy cup. He wove about like someone walking with his eyes shut. "It doesn't make sense," I'd say at night. "You don't grow backward." Had he been injured somehow when he was out of our sight, banged his head, swallowed something poisonous? It was like searching for clues to a kidnapping. (Suskind, 2014b)

Ron and his wife Cornelia learned that they could connect with Owen by watching old Disney movies.

> Owen's only activity with his brother, Walt, is something they did before the autism struck: watching Disney movies. "The Little Mermaid," "Beauty and the Beast," "Aladdin" – it was a boom time for

> Disney – and also the old classics: "Dumbo," "Fantasia," "Pinocchio," "Bambi." ... It is hard to know all the things going through the mind of our 6-year-old, Walt, about how his little brother, now nearly 4, is changing. They pile up pillows on our bed and sit close, Walt often with his arm around Owen's shoulders, trying to hold him – and the shifting world – in place. (Suskind, 2014b)

Despite his difficulties with communication, even as a child, Owen was a remarkable artist who could draw Disney characters with remarkable accuracy and detail. His story is documented in the highly recommended film *Life, Animated* (2016).

In a fascinating recent study, Elena Tenenbaum and her colleagues used tablet computers to present movies specifically designed to elicit behaviors associated with risk for ASD. Children responded to the movies, and the researchers calculated the ratio of syllabic vocalizations to all vocalizations. Those children producing more *nonsyllabic* vocalizations were 24 times more likely to be diagnosed with ASD, compared with children who exhibited typical development. "Children with ASD were less likely to produce words, less likely to produce speech like sounds, and more likely to produce atypical sounds while watching these movies" (Tenenbaum et al., 2020).

Rasmussen and Jiang (2019) played the animated movie of Heider and Simmel (1944) to subjects on the ASD and normal controls (see the section on The Pervasive Influence of Films). Participants with higher autism traits reported lower levels of social interaction on this simple task – that is, *they were far less likely to create stories* or attribute meaning to the random movements of geometric shapes.

There is considerable overlap between the diagnosis of ASD and obsessive-compulsive disorder, and a symptom like compulsive hand-washing can be found in either disorder. Bedford et al. (2022) have addressed the challenges of differentiation, assessment, and treatment for these two disorders. Likewise, Ghaziuddin and Ghaziuddin (2021) have noted that comorbidity is common in people with autism, and both bipolar disorder and schizophrenia can occur in people who have been diagnosed and labeled on the autism disorder spectrum.

Some clinicians have become wealthy by setting up diagnostic imaging centers and claiming that neuroimaging technology can be used to diagnose ASD with 80–90% accuracy. Almost all professional societies and research experts have rejected these claims (Thibault et al., 2019).

Malynnda Johnson (2021) has written a chapter examining the way Sherlock Holmes is portrayed in the media, noting that he is often labeled a psychopath, sociopath, and, more commonly, autistic. Although Holmes is an odd character, I find arguments that he might be on the autism spectrum less than compelling.

"Kids get a lot of labels – dyslexic, ADHD, autism – and people get hung up on the label. Well, these labels are not precise diagnoses ... [People] get so hung up on the deficit, they forget about developing the strengths."

Temple Grandin in an interview with *Great Falls Tribune* reporter Briana Wipf, January 7, 2014

Adam (2009) is a film about a high-functioning 29-year-old man with ASD who falls in love with his neighbor Beth. Adam has a fixated interest in astronomy, and this reaches the savant level, because he knows more about this subject than almost anyone else. When he first invites Beth to come to his room, it is literally an invitation to watch the planets move as they are projected on his bedroom wall. Because of Adam's limited social skills, he is intimidated by an upcoming job interview, and Beth coaches him, teaching him how to maintain eye contact with the interviewer and demonstrate enthusiasm about the potential new job. Adam is aware of many of his social limitations, his excessive focus on logic and facts, and his tendency to take everything literally. He has difficulty with the analogies people use, and he does not understand social nuances or jokes, or how to respond to the emotions of others. When he gets stressed or nervous, he talks rapidly and provides many more details than the situation or interaction calls for. The film demonstrates some of the challenges inherent in loving someone with this condition. It is a rare and accurate depiction of what *Diagnostic and Statistical Manual of Mental Disorders,* 4th edition (DSM-IV; APA, 1994) termed Asperger's disorder.

The movie *Mozart and the Whale* (2005) is based on the real-life story of Jerry and Mary Newport, two high-functioning people with ASD. Jerry Newport is a savant who can calculate numbers and dates and who was unaware that he had a form of autism until he saw *Rain Man.* He subsequently organized support groups around the country. Mary has prodigious artistic talents. The title for the movie is based on a Halloween party where Jerry was dressed as a whale expressing his adoration of *Free Willy.* Mary arrived in the guise of Nannerl Mozart, the brilliant musician whose life was overshadowed by her famous brother. The difficulties in their relationship and their struggles to live a quality life are documented in their publications, presentations, and various television programs. The movie deals with the development of a meaningful relationship between the characters Donald and Isabelle despite their opposing personalities and the symptoms associated with their disorders. For example, when Donald nervously brings Isabelle to the cluttered apartment he shares with an array of uncaged birds, she announces in her typically forthright manner, "This is about sex" – an approach too direct for Donald. Isabelle is extremely labile and emotionally insecure, creating legitimate doubt as to whether she, more than Donald, can ever handle a permanent relationship. The film received mixed reviews but has the advantage of having been written by individuals who have the disorder.

In *Breaking and Entering* (2006), Will (Jude Law) and his live-in girlfriend, Liv (Robin Wright Penn), raise a young adolescent girl, Beatrice (Poppy Jones), who has an ASD. Beatrice displays behaviors typical of ASD, including limited social skills, repetitive behaviors (endlessly watching herself on video), and being upset by changes in her environment or routine. She also demonstrates sensory issues related to music. When stressed, she closes her eyes and repeats words. She thinks concretely and has an unusual collection of batteries. Her behavior places strain on Will and Liv's relationship. Liv becomes closer to Beatrice, while Will avoids the situation by working and distancing himself from the two of them.

American Splendor (2003) is about Harvey Pekar (Paul Giamatti), a comic book writer whose friend and coworker is a man (Toby Radloff) with what was formerly called Asperger's. Toby is socially awkward, has a monotone voice, and restricted patterns of interest and behavior. Toby is a self-proclaimed "world-class nerd" who wears a button reading "Genuine Nerd" and proudly recounts once driving over 200 miles to see the movie *Revenge of the Nerds.* Overall, the portrayal is realistic and challenges the viewer's stereotypes about Asperger's.

The Horse Boy (2009) is a documentary of two parents (a journalist–author and a professor–scientist), Rupert Isaacson and Kristin Neff, who travel to remote areas throughout Mongolia searching for shamans and reindeer herders to bring healing to their young son, Rowan, who has an ASD. Rowan is incontinent and has horrible tantrums, after which he is inconsolable. He spends hours lining up objects. The film educates the viewer about autism and emphasizes its genetic links; however, it also notes the interaction of genetics with environmental factors. The film clearly depicts the resolute love the parents have for Rowan and their bravery and open-mindedness in pursuing novel treatments and alternative healing. While on this long journey and through various interactions with shamans, Rowan experiences some changes – for example, he becomes more social – and after the trip his incontinence disappears, he develops new social skills, and he begins to regularly ride horses. Rupert is clear to say that he is not arguing that he found a "cure" for ASD; however, his son did experience healing. Rupert documents his son's changes – and notes that he does not know specifically what accounted for the changes (it could have been the vastly different environment and culture or the shamanistic rituals or some other change in Rowan's life) – as well as the positive impact the trip had for their family. The film includes interviews with Simon Baron-Cohen, Steve Edelson, and Temple Grandin, all of whom comment on the nature and treatment of autism.

"Why does autism have to be a limitation? Why can't it be a gateway to healing?"

Rupert Isaacson sees his son benefit from a unique connection with a horse, in *The Horse Boy* (2009)

Equine therapy is discussed quite positively in this film. However, this form of therapy for ASD remains controversial. Two recent meta-analyses have produced positive results with small effect sizes (Dimolareva & Dunn, 2021; Drobonikuv & Mychailyszyn, 2021). The first paper notes,

> The meta-analyses indicated small effect sizes related to improvements in social interaction and communication and reduction in autism spectrum disorder symptoms. Additionally, there was little evidence for a relationship between dosage and effect size. In conclusion, AAIs [animal-assisted interventions] appear to offer small improvements in social interaction and communication for children with Autism, which may be comparable to activities used in active control conditions. (Dimolareva & Dunn, 2021, p. 2436)

Recently, Caitlin Peters and colleagues (2022) compared equine-assisted occupational therapy for ASD children, with a therapy-as-usual control group who simply worked in a garden. They summarize their study by noting, "This study provides preliminary evidence that horses can be integrated into occupational therapy for youth with ASD to improve social and behavioral goals" (p. 4114).

Temple Grandin herself, in a chapter coauthored with four other colleagues (Grandin et al., 2015), has weighed in on the value of animals in the lives of individuals living with an ASD diagnosis, writing,

> Animals play many roles in the lives of persons with autism spectrum disorder (ASD). For some persons with ASD, animals can provide strong social supports both as companions and as service animals. For others, animals may provide a unique catalyst for therapeutic success. (p. 225)

This Is Nicholas – Living With Autism (2019) is one of the most recent and most powerful films to document the challenges associated with life on the autism spectrum – as well as the way these challenges can be successfully overcome. The film opens with Nicholas and his mother describing his Asperger's symptoms. The family lives in Emily, Ireland, and they narrate the film with beautiful Irish accents. At age 13, Nicholas developed echolalia, repeating phrases like "thank you" over and over. His father described his son's behavior as being like "a record player that got stuck." The film beautifully illustrates the critical importance of family, school, and community support. Nicholas is not the best exemplar of someone with autism because his presentation is complicated by marked depression and occasional hallucinations of "a black figure." He also hears voices telling him, "Don't listen to your mother or I will kill you." However, with the support of his family and the Railway Preservation Society of Ireland (RPSI), Nicholas develops a fascination with and an encyclopedic knowledge of steam trains. Nicholas also learns Buteyko breath training and appears to benefit. He becomes fascinated with video cameras, and eventually earns a college degree in media studies, going on to win international prizes in China and the United States; the latter prize is presented to him in Hollywood, and he is accompanied to receive the award by his sister. The film concludes with Nicholas's words: "I'm full of confidence in the future." Any parent with a child diagnosed with ASD is likely to find comfort in this uplifting film.

It is fascinating to learn that the actor Anthony Hopkins was diagnosed with Asperger's (a now outdated term for individuals with ASD who are high functioning) in 2014, when he was 77 years old. He noted, "I could never settle anywhere. I was troubled and caused trouble, especially in my early years … I don't go to parties; I don't have many friends." The *Autism Key* website notes that "individuals with Asperger's often exhibit remarkable rote memory skills and tend to be focused on a few very narrow interests (Autism Key, 2020). In Hopkins' case, these traits have proven advantageous as an actor" (Distractify, 2020). The same article goes on to note,

> Hopkin's ability to memorize lines has astounded some of Hollywood's most powerful and influential directors. Cast and crew members of the 1997 film *Amistad* couldn't believe that the actor was able to memorize a seven-page courtroom monologue and deliver the entire speech in a single take. After that, director Steven Spielberg reportedly only referred to Hopkins as Sir Anthony, and not Tony. (Distractify, 2020)

Rain Man

While many people in the autism community have grown tired of the synonymous connection between the word "autism" and the film *Rain Man* (1988), the film continues to be the quintessential media example of raising awareness about the condition. Part of the weariness is perpetration of the misconception that all people with an ASD have **savant** abilities.

Rain Man won Academy Awards for Best Actor, Best Director, Best Picture, and Best Original Screenplay. The film stars Dustin Hoffman as Raymond Babbitt and Tom Cruise as Raymond's younger brother, Charlie. The drama opens with Charlie, a cynical hustler in his mid-20s, unemotionally learning of his father's death. Charlie and his father had been estranged for many years. Charlie's father only left a 1949 Buick to his youngest son, but he left $3 million in a trust fund for a secret beneficiary.

Charlie traces the beneficiary and discovers that he has an older brother, Raymond, who has an autism spectrum disorder and lives in the sanatorium Walbrook. Raymond's world is bound by the rituals of watching television programs and eating certain foods on certain days. The books and baseball memorabilia in his room must be in order, or Raymond becomes agitated and begins reciting the Abbot and Costello routine, "Who's on First?" When the sanatorium administrator refuses to give Charlie half of the inheritance, Charlie removes his brother from Walbrook.

Charlie wants to return to the coast, but Raymond refuses to fly. The story unfolds as Charlie and Raymond cross the country in their father's Buick. Their adventures include seeing an accident, after which Raymond refuses to travel on interstate highways, and a day spent in a motel because Raymond refuses to go out in the rain. Raymond has many idiosyncrasies, such as having maple syrup on the table before the pancakes are served, insisting upon snacks of apple juice and cheese balls, imitating any noise he hears, and being preoccupied with television. One of Raymond's most significant symptoms is his tendency to constantly repeat the same word or phrase.

Raymond has savant abilities, which occur in only about 10% of people with ASDs (and in less than 1% of those without autism). When this occurs, the individual usually scores low on standardized IQ tests but has one or two outstanding talents, such as calculating dates, drawing, or musical performance (see the section Autistic Savants). Raymond can memorize several pages of a telephone book after just one reading, and he quickly memorizes baseball statistics. When a box of toothpicks falls open, Raymond almost intuitively knows how many toothpicks are on the floor. Upon discovery of Raymond's unusual memory and mathematical skills, Charlie decides to capitalize on these to recoup his business losses through gambling in Las Vegas. When Raymond inadvertently makes a date with a prostitute, Charlie teaches his brother how to dance. When the woman fails to show up, Raymond dances with Charlie's girlfriend, Susanna (Valeria Golino), who gives Raymond his first kiss.

Charlie develops an appreciation for the complexity of the illness when Raymond becomes upset after being frightened by the noise of a smoke detector. The movie ends when Charlie, who has developed a sensitivity and love for his brother, turns down a $250,000 settlement and lets his brother voluntarily admit himself back into Walbrook.

Overall, this is a technically correct portrayal of a character with an ASD – Raymond has all the correct mannerisms, tics, and tendencies of any number of real-life people with autism. The story surrounding the characters is also realistic – many families were separated by institutionalization as people with disabilities were simply erased from family memory. (For example, Charlie never knew he had an older brother.)

Rain Man does reinforce the misconception that "it's an institution or nothing" for people with significant disabilities. However, the assumption that someone like Raymond would be happiest in a large institution is foolish. Although the familiarity and smooth routines often occurring in an institutional setting enhance Raymond's comfort and adaptation, people like Raymond can also live fully, successfully, and happily in their own homes, with individualized supports as needed and with housemates of their own choosing.

In *Silent Fall* (1994), a retired child psychiatrist (Richard Dreyfuss) works with Tim Warden (Ben Faulkner), a young boy with ASD who was a witness to his parents' murder. Tim rocks, enjoys spinning and movement, twirls and fidgets with his fingers while watching them in front of his face, and has limited communication through grunting and moaning noises. He displays a distant look in his eyes with flat affect and adheres to rigid rules such as never eating anything that is round. He communicates through cards, nonverbal signals, drawings, and figures. He displays **echolalia**, repeating others' speech at certain times while impersonating them. He bangs his head against the wall when he gets upset or stressed.

August Rush (2007) is a film about an orphan, August Rush, played by Freddie Highmore, in search of his musician parents. It turns out that August, who is mute and has behaviors characteristic of a person with ASD (though he may not meet the full diagnostic criteria for the disorder), has inherited his parents' musical ability; in fact, he is a savant who teaches himself to play a guitar almost immediately after picking one up. He eventually winds up training at the Juilliard School where he astonishes the faculty with his precocious musical ability. Predictably, he becomes reunited with his parents by the end of the film.

Leonardo DiCaprio plays Johnny Depp's autistic younger brother in *What's Eating Gilbert Grape?* (1993). This character is not a savant, and he certainly is no saint; however, he is realistically portrayed as a needy, younger sibling growing up in a family that loves him.

In the classic *To Kill a Mockingbird* (1962), a young Robert Duvall makes his film debut as Boo Radley, a neighbor with ASD who kills a man to protect two young children. His diagnosis is never mentioned, and it would not have been recognized as autism at the time the film was made.

Molly (1999) is a disappointing film about a woman with ASD. Molly (played by Elisabeth Shue) undergoes experimental surgery that temporarily brings her back to normal functioning; her brain eventually rejects the cells used in the operation, and she returns to her earlier level of functioning. Molly's brother, Buck, initially avoids and fears his sister and agrees to try anything to make her better, but this enthusiasm is followed by disappointment in the surgery's failure. The film ends with a stereotypic "change-of-heart" ending when Buck arranges for Molly to live with him.

The Boy Who Could Fly (1986) tells the story of a young girl, Millie Michaelson (Lucy Deakins), who moves to a new house and neighborhood after the death of her father who had committed suicide following a diagnosis of cancer. She copes with her grief by becoming involved with the boy who lives next door, a boy with ASD who spends much of each day on his roof, preparing to fly. His parents were killed in a plane crash, and the boy developed his fixation of the idea of flying immediately after their death.

Autistic Savants

Although not a characteristic feature of ASD, approximately 10% of individuals with this diagnosis display special talents such as reproducing any tune by memory after only hearing it once or memorizing long strings of numbers. Savant skills typically occur in one of five specific domains: Mathematics, art, music, mechanical ability, and calendar calculating. Exceptional music ability is the most common savant skill, and savant skills occur approximately 4 times more frequently in males than females (Treffert, 2000).

Alexander Luria, a Russian neuropsychologist, followed the case of Solomon Shereshevsky for over 30 years, and described him in *The Mind of a Mnemonist* (1968). Shereshevsky had **fivefold synesthesia**, a condition in which stimulation of any one of his senses triggered a response in the other five.

Stephen Wiltshire is a British autistic savant who can reproduce detailed drawings of cityscapes from memory, often after flying over cities like New York, Tokyo, and Rome in helicopters. His pen-and-ink drawings sell for thousands of pounds, but he needs help to simply find his way around the towns he can recreate on canvas with such amazing detail.

Bouvet et al. (2017) report a case of a patient with synesthesia and savant abilities. She perceived sounds as colors and had extraordinary talent in astrophysics. However, like many people on the autism spectrum, she found social interaction difficult, she performed poorly in school, and she became easily confused. Because of these symptoms, she had been previously (mis)diagnosed with schizophrenia. There are numerous other case reports of savant talents. Ogun et al. (2022) describe the case of a 27-year-old undergraduate with hypercalculia. Neuroimaging revealed a lesion in their right parietal lobe white matter.

The Rainman Twins (2008) is a made-for-TV documentary that introduces viewers to Flo and Kay Lyman, the world's only known identical twin autistic savants. The documentary sympathetically portrays their adulation for TV personality Dick Clark, and it provides numerous examples of their prodigious memory abilities.

Numerous other films have portrayed characters on the ASD who have savant talents including *Adam* (2009; astronomy), *Mozart and the Whale* (2009; math), and *August Rush* (2007; music).

A Korean television series, *Extraordinary Attorney Woo*, portrays a gifted attorney who is profoundly autistic, but successful nonetheless. Another popular television program, *The Good Doctor,* depicts a surgery resident with autism spectrum disorder and a savant syndrome; the character's autism often helps him solve seemingly intractable surgical dilemmas. The show introduced millions of people to the challenges presented by autism spectrum disorder, but some experts maintain the character of Gregory House on the hospital drama *House* represents a more accurate version of how someone who has ASD but is very high functioning might behave (Iati, 2023). Stern and Barnes (2019) asked a simple research question: Does watching *The Good Doctor* affect knowledge of and attitudes toward autism? Their findings were somewhat surprising.

> Individuals' knowledge and attitudes about autism spectrum disorder (ASD) work together to shape the stigma held about ASD. One way that this information is communicated to the public is through popular media; however, little is known about the effectiveness of fictional depictions of ASD in educating and shaping attitudes about ASD. The purpose of this research was to investigate the impact media has on knowledge about and attitudes towards ASD, compared to that of a college lecture on the subject. Exposure to one episode of a fictional drama depicting ASD, compared to watching a lecture, resulted in more accurate knowledge, more positive characteristics associated with ASD, fewer negative characteristics associated with ASD, and a greater desire to learn more about ASD. (Stern & Barnes, 2019, p. 2581)

Autism and *Temple Grandin*

Temple Grandin (2010) is a movie about a remarkable woman, portrayed in the film by Claire Danes. When Temple first goes to her aunt's home in Arizona, she initially must put a sign on her door so she will know which room is hers. She experiences tremendous stress when the sign is removed, and she copes by running outdoors and putting herself in a "squeeze

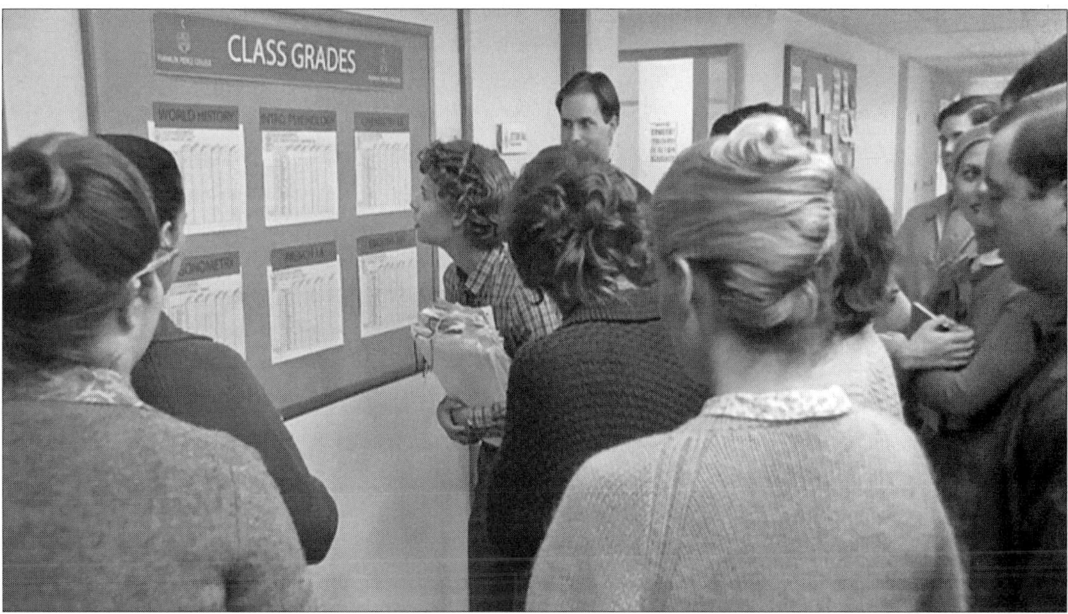

Figure 7. *Temple Grandin* (2010, HBO Films, Ruby Films, Gerson Saines). Produced by Gil Bellows, Dante Di Loreto, Anthony Edwards, and Scott Ferguson. Directed by Mick Jackson.

machine," a device her uncle uses when inoculating cattle. She develops a similar device in her college dormitory room, and later at an autism conference attempts to explain how the device was soothing: "Being held by another person is scary but rolling or being held by surfaces reproduces the calming effect that ordinary children get from a hug." However, she continues to experience the challenges associated with being a person with ASD (e.g., she is threatened by an automatic sliding glass door in a supermarket). Later in the film, "going through doors" becomes a metaphor for overcoming the challenges Temple faces in her day-to-day life; Betty Goscowitz (the friendly wife of the owner of a slaughterhouse with "a grandson who's artistic") symbolizes how others in the life of a person with an ASD can be helpful. Temple Grandin (the person on whom the film is based) provides a useful commentary on the DVD. She reports that antidepressants she began taking in 1980 have been helpful in eliminating most of her panic attacks and helping her deal with her anxiety in those situations that she finds overly stimulating. Imaging studies of Grandin's brain and neuropsychological tests reveal exceptional nonverbal intelligence and spatial ability, enhanced brain volume, a left lateral ventricle much larger than the one on the right, and an abnormally large amygdala. She obtained a perfect score on Ravens Progressive Matrices, a widely used measure of nonverbal intelligence. Figure 7 shows Grandin upset by the discovery that she had received an "F" grade for one of her papers. Grandin has written a chapter describing her own challenges in finding suitable employment, with recommendations for both parents and employers (Grandin, 2020).

Attention-Deficit/Hyperactivity Disorder

Children and adolescents are frequently diagnosed with ADHD. Diagnosis of ADHD using the DSM-5 requires evidence of "a persistent pattern of inattention and/or hyperactivity-impulsivity which interferes with functioning or development" (APA, 2013, p. 59). Six or more symptoms of inattention must be present and/or six or more symptoms of hyperactivity and impulsivity. Common symptoms of inattention are failure to attend to details, difficulty sustaining attention, failure to listen, difficulty following through with tasks such as homework, difficulty organizing tasks, avoidance of any task that requires sustained mental effort, losing things, easy distraction, and forgetfulness. Symptoms of hyperactivity and impulsivity include fidgeting, leaving one's seat at inappropriate times, running or climbing in inappropriate situations, the lack of ability to engage in quiet leisure activities, always being "on the go," talking excessively, blurting out answers to questions, difficulty in waiting for one's turn, or frequent interruption. At least some of these symptoms must have been present before the age of 12 years for someone to qualify for the diagnosis. Clinicians must specify if the disorder involves inattention or hyperactivity/impulsivity or both conditions, and they must specify severity level (mild, moderate, or severe).

Dory, the blue fish in *Finding Nemo* (2003), is a character who displays many of the symptoms of ADHD. While Dory describes herself as having a neurological condition of short-term memory loss, the behavior she exhibits parallels the inattentive qualities of ADHD. Dory is forgetful and often loses track of her current task or activity, and she is easily distracted, such as when she becomes preoccupied with a baby jellyfish, a distraction that leads her and Nemo into danger. She impulsively approaches various fish in the sea and often displays hyperactive behavior as she swims, as if "driven by a motor," another classic quality of ADHD.

In another children's film, *Winnie the Pooh* (2011), many of the characters may have a psychological disorder - Tigger has ADHD symptoms (also evident in *The Tigger Movie* [2000]), Piglet is anxious, Eeyore is depressed, Owl has obsessive-compulsive disorder (OCD), and Pooh has a binge eating behavior. While we may not agree with each of these being a full-blown disorder (remember that a formal diagnosis requires that the symptoms must cause serious distress or impairment or affect the individual's everyday functioning), some symptoms are present in each character.

Many adult characters display symptoms of ADHD. John Cusak portrays an air traffic controller who was once diagnosed with ADHD, in the film *Pushing Tin* (1999). He attempts to use his ADHD to focus his attention on his work; however, at times it leads to recklessness. Clark Griswold (Chevy Chase), in the National Lampoon films *Vacation* (1983) and *Christmas Vacation* (1989), portrays many of the symptoms of ADHD, such as distractibility, impulsivity, and especially inattention. The Mr. Bean character (played by Rowan Atkinson) from the TV series of the same name and the film *Mr. Bean's Holiday* (2007) is another comedic figure who exhibits the inattentive and impulsive characteristics of ADHD. *Charlie Bartlett* (2007) is a film about a teenage boy who gets diagnosed with ADHD and is prescribed Ritalin. He becomes quite high and runs naked through the streets. Realizing the power of the drug, he arranges to sell it to his classmates in the boys' bathroom.

Love and Other Drugs (2010) stars Jake Gyllenhaal as a pharmaceutical salesman with ADHD who becomes romantically involved with Anne Hathaway, a woman with Parkinson's. Writing about this film in *PsycCRITIQUES*, Linda Young notes,

> Can a no-strings-attached sexual relationship morph into a healthy, lasting love relationship between two self-focused twenty-somethings? *Love and Other Drugs* provides a platform for exploring this question, complicated by the issue of living with a degenerative disease. Both the main characters, Jamie and Maggie, have self-focused, dismissive parents; compounding their mutually low self-regard are Jamie's negative schema around attention deficit disorder (ADD) and Maggie's hopelessness around Parkinson's. They both feel like damaged goods and use their good looks and charm to grab fleeting affirmations in their no-strings sexual relationships. Although some of the dialogue is sanguine, iconic real-life couples like Christopher and Dana Reeve and Roger and Chaz Ebert are a testament to this film's optimistic view of love against the odds of physical degeneration. They, and this film, just might help all of us learn how to love better. (Young, 2011)

Thumbsucker and ADHD

In the award-winning coming-of-age film *Thumbsucker* (2005), 17-year-old Justin Cobb (Lou Pucci) comforts himself by sucking his thumb but is also highly distressed by his infantile habit and his inability to stop his obsessive behavior. As an awkward, self-conscious teenager, his psychological stress leads to failure on a debate team, deficient performance in school, and a break-up with his girlfriend. Justin's dentist, Perry Lyman, confronts Justin about his thumb sucking and uses hypnosis to make the thumb distasteful. Justin's frustration increases when he is unable to find an adequate substitute for his thumb sucking. A well-meaning, but ill-informed school counselor diagnoses Justin as having ADHD and strongly recommends a stimulant (Ritalin) as treatment. After starting the stimulant, Justin's behavior improves, and he begins to excel on the debate team. The transition from a shy and socially inept teenager to debate team star is dramatic. Watch for a young Keanu Reeves in the role of the well-intentioned orthodontist.

Errors in diagnosing ADHD are common, and careful evaluation is critical before the diagnosis is made. If ADHD is present, treatment should include counseling in addition to medication. This film demonstrates the negative outcomes associated with a misdiagnosis and inappropriate medication. It is unlikely that Justin had ADHD, and it is certainly unlikely that he would have had legal access to the amount of Ritalin he eventually wound up taking.

Communication Disorders

Communication disorders involve deficits in language, speech, and communication. A Best Picture Academy Award winning film, *The King's Speech* (2010) illustrates **stuttering** (also called childhood-onset fluency disorder; see Figure 8). In the film, Colin Firth portrays King George VI of the United Kingdom (Bertie) who suffers from stuttering and is helped by Lionel Logue (Geoffrey Rush), a speech therapist (see Figure 8). Prior to consulting with Logue, Bertie attempts many unsuccessful treatments (e.g., trying to speak with marbles in his mouth). Logue's approach, however, is warm, insightful, and challenging, and certainly an approach that promotes self-acceptance, which is one of the

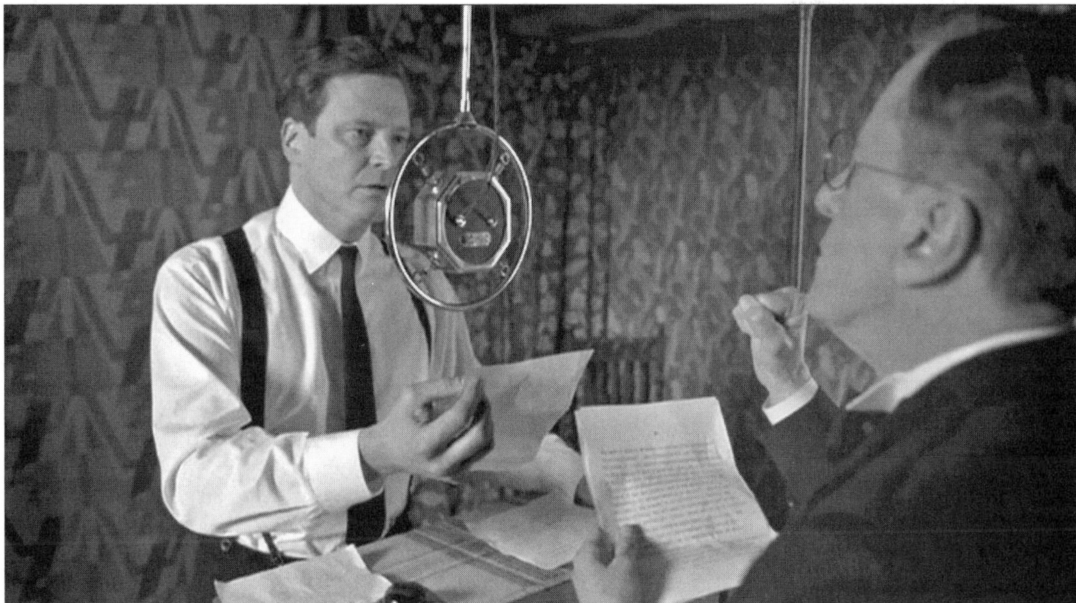

Figure 8. *The King's Speech* (2010, Weinstein Company, UK Film Council, et al.). Produced by Paul Brett, Iain Canning, Charles Dorfman, Simon Egan, et al. Directed by Tom Hooper.

more current approaches to stuttering, in addition to a nonavoidance approach in which the person who stutters is encouraged to embrace communication (Ghiselli & Davis, 2011; Jackson, 2006). King George can forge a meaningful "therapeutic" relationship with Logue, who engages Bertie in a variety of innovative techniques (e.g., reading aloud while listening to music with headphones, so he cannot hear himself speak). Figure 8 depicts Logue coaching Bertie using one of his idiosyncratic methods. In their *PsycCRITIQUES* review of the film, Ghiselli and Davis (2011) observe that these techniques have been used by actors and actresses who stutter, such as Marilyn Monroe, which led to her whispery, sexy voice; they go on to say,

> These techniques do not cure stuttering, but instead mask stuttering. Additionally, people who utilize these techniques may become dependent on them to avoid or conceal their stuttering. This experience is oftentimes referred to as "covert stuttering." Although the outside world may view covert stuttering as the stutterer transcending his or her speech impediment, it can also come at an emotional and psychological cost because the person who stutters (PWS) may not be expressing themselves in the way and with the words that they desire. (Ghiselli & Davis, 2011)

The film was written by a person who struggles with stuttering, David Seidler, and was directed by Tom Hooper. Due to the popularity, acclaim, and critical success of the film, *The King's Speech* is likely to promote public awareness about stuttering, just as *Rain Man* promoted public awareness about ASD. While both films have flaws, *The King's Speech* helps to educate the public about the realities and struggles of stuttering. Ghiselli and Davis (2011) also observe,

> Although stuttering is often regarded as a speech disorder that must be overcome and avoided, one must also remember that it is still a component of a person's identity that, like any other facet of the self, should not only be acknowledged, but also appreciated. Despite the incongruences between *The King's Speech* and what we now know about the origins of stuttering and its treatment, it is clear from a sociological point of view that the film has provided a positive role model for the stuttering community, as well as a solid base from which to educate others about stuttering. (Ghiselli & Davis, 2011)

With Logue's help, King George was able to overcome his stuttering and deliver a "call to action" radio address in 1939, which marked England's declaration of war upon Germany.

Stuttering affects about 5% of children, and anxiety is a frequent concomitant of stuttering. A provocative study suggests that transcranial direct current stimulation (tDCS) may reduce both stuttering and anxiety (Aval, 2021), but the research needs replication.

Billy Bibbit is hospitalized on a psychiatric ward in *One Flew Over the Cuckoo's Nest* (1975), although his primary problem is stuttering, not mental illness. He had to drop out of college after failing ROTC: "I c-c-couldn't take it. Wh-wh-wh-whenever the officer in charge of class would call roll, call 'Bibbit,' I couldn't answer" He adds, "You were supposed to say, 'Here sir,' and I never c-c-could get it out." Billy once had a girlfriend, "And even when I pr-proposed, I flubbed it," he says. "I said, 'Huh-honey, will you muh- muh- muh- muh- muh ..' till the girl broke out l-laughing." One of the saddest moments in this Milos Foreman film occurs when Billy commits suicide.

Two other films that depict characters with speech impediments are *The Straight Story* (1999) and *Liam* (2000). *The Straight Story* is a David Lynch film about Alvin Straight, a 73-year-old man with chronic health problems who decides to ride a power lawnmower from Iowa to Wisconsin to reunite with his estranged brother. This movie, based on a true story, is significantly different from Lynch's other films. I mention it here because Sissy Spacek, who plays Straight's daughter Rose, has a significant speech impediment. Spacek used a mechanical device in her mouth to alter her pronunciation, and she met the real Rose Straight on the set and tried to model her speech to match that of Ms. Straight.

Liam tells the story of a 7-year-old boy growing up in Liverpool. He has a marked speech impairment, but is charming and loveable, nonetheless.

Kenneth St. Louis (2020) compared the stigma associated with three conditions: mental illness, stuttering, and obesity. He found that the greatest stigma was associated with mental illness, and the least with obesity. Stuttering fell between these two. He notes, "Impressions and knowledge of – as well as experience with – stigmatized conditions can inform public awareness campaigns and individual clinical programs dealing with stigma" (St. Louis, 2020, p. 2023).

President Biden's lifelong struggles with stuttering have been well documented, and he stands as a remarkable example of someone who overcame childhood communication struggles to achieve remarkable success as a political leader. His courageous acknowledgement of his lifelong struggle with stuttering has helped lessen the stigma associated with this disorder.

Another major diagnosis that falls under the communications disorder category is language disorder, which is characterized by persistent difficulties in the acquisition and use of language, due to deficits in comprehension or production. *The Wild Child* (1970, France) depicts a young boy who was found living on his own in a French forest in 1798. This feral child was unable to speak, read, write, or walk. He would easily have met the criteria for a language disorder, but he also exhibited signs of an intellectual disability and ASD. Based on a true story, the film was directed by the famous filmmaker François Truffaut, who stars in the film as Dr. Jean Itard, the child's teacher.

Where the Crawdads Sing (2022) is a recent, engaging film about an abandoned girl named Kya who raised herself in the marshlands of North Carolina. She is known as "Marsh Girl" to the local community. Kya develops normal language because she is raised with parents and four siblings; one by one, family members leave, and eventually her alcoholic father abandons her at age 10, and she is left to deal with life – and puberty – on her own. She becomes romantically involved with a local boy who abandons her when he goes off to college. She then begins to have sex with another man who winds up marrying a different woman. Kya becomes the main suspect when the second lover is found dead. The storyline is implausible; Kya only goes to school 1 day, and she never returns after the other children make fun of her because she cannot spell "dog." Her first boyfriend teaches her to read, and she becomes an autodidact and amateur biologist, eventually publishing four books about the marshlands of North Carolina. The film is based on the novel of the same name by Delia Owens. Several critics panned the movie, but both the film and the book have received widespread praise from the public.

Motor Disorders

Motor disorders include **tic disorder**, **developmental coordination disorder**, and **stereotypic movement disorder**; however, tic disorders are the most recognizable motor disorder in films. A tic is a sudden, rapid, recurrent, nonrhythmic event that can occur in movement or in vocalization. Tourette's disorder is the dominant type of tic disorder and occurs when both motor and vocal tics are present for more than a year, even though the frequency may increase and decrease over time. Tic disorders appear at around 5 or 6 years of age and most often decrease in severity and frequency as a child ages. Individuals with tic disorders often have comorbid psychiatric disorders including ADHD, OCD, anxiety, depression, learning disabilities, and ODD (McGoldrick, 2017).

The documentary *I Have Tourette's but Tourette's Doesn't Have Me* (2005) depicts several children speaking about their experiences with the condition. The children express themselves directly with humor, charm, and insight, and describe their experiences in the home, school, and social environments. *The Tic Code* is a movie that displays a mentoring relationship between two individuals with Tourette's disorder – a child prodigy and an adult musician. Tourette's disorder is also evident in characters in the films *Maze* (2000); *Niagara, Niagara* (1997); *Front of the Class*

(2008); and *Phoebe in Wonderland* (2008). In the last film, a young girl diagnosed with both Tourette's and OCD displays vocal tics as she barks out inappropriate phrases to her neighbor. Unfortunately, the depiction of Tourette's disorder, especially vocal tics (e.g., cursing), is routinely used for cheap comic relief as in *Deuce Bigalow: Male Gigolo* (1999).

Cerebral palsy is not a DSM-5 diagnosis, but it is a significant central motor disorder that affects muscle tone, movement, and posture. The prevalence is approximately 1.5 per 1,000 live births in high-income countries, and more than double that in low- and middle-income countries (McIntyre et al., 2022). The risk for cerebral palsy is greatest for children born prematurely.

Characters with cerebral palsy are found in several films, such as *Dance Me to My Song* (1998, Australia), *Music Within* (2007), *Oasis* (2002, South Korea), *Storytelling* (2001), and *My Left Foot* (1989, Ireland). This last film is the story of Christy Brown, a successful artist and author with cerebral palsy who grows up in a poor working-class family in Ireland. Brown was never idle and, using only his left foot to paint and write, could cope with painful feelings, confront social struggles, transcend isolation, and express himself through his art.

Rory O'Shea Was Here (2005) depicts the friendship, dependence, struggles, and joys of two young men, Rory and Michael. Rory has muscular dystrophy, and Michael has cerebral palsy. This drama displays genuine interaction and care between friends, as well as their arguments and disagreements. A resounding core theme of the film is the ability of these two men to use the physical strengths of each other to cooperate in solving problems and be more successful as a team than they could ever be as separate individuals. *Magnifico* (2003, Philippines) displays a family under significant stress. With limited finances, the grandmother becomes ill and needs costly medical care, the eldest son loses a precious academic scholarship in Manila, and the daughter has cerebral palsy. She displays significant muscle rigidity and shaking and is unable to speak other than with occasional grunting sounds. The family takes care of her basic needs but does not go out of their way to discover her interests, passions, and strengths. The other son, Magnifico, is a young, kind, and devoted child who is eager to improve his family's situation. He applies his creativity and love to help each member of the family – for example, he discovers what his sister is interested in (e.g., attending a carnival) and puts her on his back and takes her to experience the various carnival rides. Magnifico's impact on his sister, family, and ultimately the larger community, is significant.

"Okay, listen. I got something wrong with me. That's the first thing to know. I twitch and shout a lot. It makes me look like a damn freak show. But inside my head is an even bigger mess. I can't stop twisting things around, words and sounds especially. I have to keep playing with them until they come out right."

Lionel Essrog (Ed Norton) describes his Tourette's in *Motherless Brooklyn* (2019)

Motherless Brooklyn (2019), directed by and starring Ed Norton, features a lonely private detective afflicted with Tourette's syndrome who sets out to solve the mystery associated with his best friend's murder. The film is set in the 1950s, and Ed Norton is magnificent in the role. He has significant tics that accompany his verbal outbursts, and he has learned that "gum makes it better." His Tourette's is exacerbated by stress and becomes markedly more pronounced after his boss is shot. He is unable to avoid touching women whenever he is anxious, and he can't avoid repeatedly blowing out the match when he attempts to light a cigarette for a woman in a bar. Norton's character smokes marijuana to cope with his Tourette's.

Crip Camp (2020) is a remarkable movie supported and sponsored by Barack and Michelle Obama. The film documents the development and history of a summer camp (Camp Jened) for students with disabilities (see Figure 9).

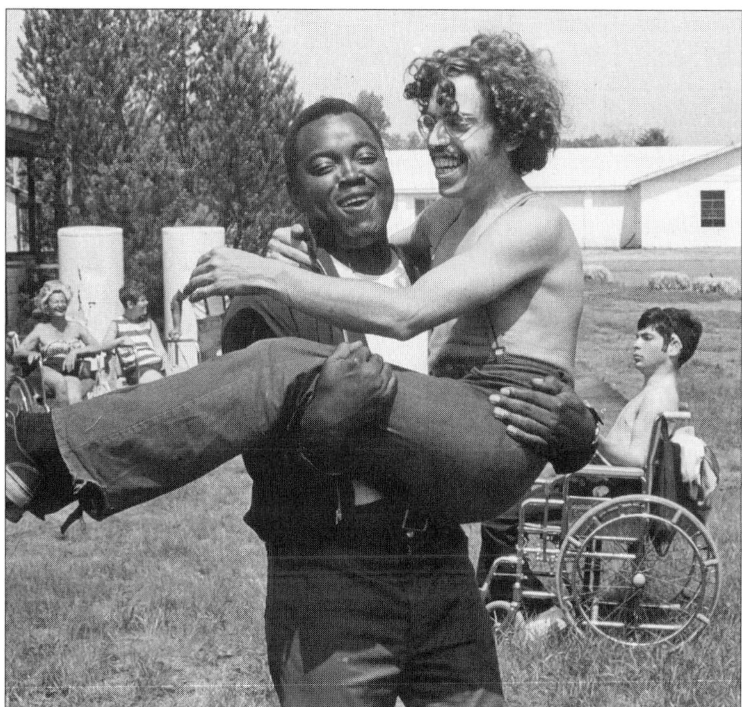

Figure 9.
Crip Camp (2020, Good Gravy Films and Higher Ground Productions). Produced by Rachel Antell, Sara Bolder, Ben Braun, Josh Braun, et al. Directed by James Lebrecht and Nicole Newnham. Executive Producers Barack and Michelle Obama.

Crip Camp includes a dozen or so activists telling their stories, and every story is engaging. The movie documents parallels to the civil rights movement and the women's movement, and shows how the movement was energized by a decision to move its headquarters to Berkeley. The diversity in the camp is highlighted, and campers are open and candid about their interest in and desire to have full sexual lives. Every mental health professional should watch this film, as well as President Obama's interview with the directors and key actors in the film.

Ernesto Morales and colleagues (2016) have noted that masturbation by people with handicaps is a "little discussed topic, but a ubiquitous reality." They interviewed adults with upper limb disabilities and documented the substantial difficulties individuals experienced when attempting to masturbate. They advocate promoting sexual autonomy via masturbation, and they offer specific solutions including "hospital programs, guides, training, adaptation of sex toys, and legalization of appropriate sexual assistance" (p. 417).

International Films: Neurodevelopmental Disorders

Many films do not present a character who happens to have a disability where the disability is treated as just another aspect of the character's life. An exception are films by French director Jean Pierre-Jeunet, whose *Amélie* (2001, France) and *The City of Lost Children* (1995, France) depict such characters and suggest that their meaningful contributions far outweigh the significance of their intellectual disability.

Pauline and Paulette (2001, Belgium) is an award-winning Belgian comedy–drama. Pauline (Dora van der Groen) is a 66-year-old woman with an intellectual disability who has been cared for by her sister Martha. When Martha dies, her younger sisters, Paulette (Ann Petersen) and Cecile (Rosemarie Bergmans), become responsible for Pauline. Both sisters are busy in their own lives. According to Martha's will, her wealthy estate will only be divided into three equal parts if one of the sisters looks after Pauline. If they decide to place her in an institution, Pauline will be the only heir. This film depicts a family's dilemma and difficulties when faced with making decisions about loved ones. It also highlights the reality of intellectual disability and underscores the degree of love and commitment required by family members to take care of another family member who has an intellectual disability. In contrast to the film *I Am Sam* (2001), this movie focuses more on character development (e.g., kindness, curiosity, creativity, playfulness, and love).

Adam Elliot, director of the popular Australian clay animation films, *Harvie Krumpet* (2003, Australia) and *Mary and Max* (2009, Australia), references and depicts neurodevelopmental disorders in his films, usually in a comical and inoffensive manner. In the former Academy Award–winning film, Harvie is diagnosed with Tourette's disorder and incorrectly assumed to have an intellectual disability. Despite suicidal intentions, a brain tumor, testicular cancer, being struck by lightning, and suffering growing senility, Harvey remains optimistic. The film is narrated by Geoffrey Rush. *Mary and Max* uses the voices of Toni Collette and Philip Seymour Hoffman, in the roles of Mary and Max, respectively, to portray a long-distance, pen pal friendship. Max is labeled with Asperger's syndrome, which is correctly described as "a neurobiological, pervasive developmental disability"; however, Max prefers to simply refer to himself as an "aspie." He explains that he finds people confusing and has never had a friend, and he describes his mind as literal and logical. He has trouble understanding the emotions of others, cannot interpret people's faces, is hypersensitive to sound, likes solving problems, and has trouble expressing his own emotions. Mary goes to college to study "disorders of the mind" and later writes a book about Asperger's, which offends Max and temporarily stifles their friendship. Both films are charming and highly recommended.

The negative impact of institutionalization is clearly outlined in the documentary, *Her Name Is Sabine* (*Elle s'appelle Sabine;* 2007, France). This is an honest and vivid portrait of Sabine Bonnaire, a woman with ASD who is the sister of a famous French actress Sandrine Bonnaire, who wrote and directed the film. The film depicts the present-day life of Sabine, interspersed with family history and home movies. Prior to hospitalization, Sabine lived at home with her mother and sisters, and she flourished. She engaged in various creative arts, music and crafts and studied topics like geography. After her sisters moved out of the home, she traveled to visit them independently; however, she increasingly began to exhibit disruptive behaviors. Her aggressive and destructive outbursts became so significant that her family decided to place her in a psychiatric hospital when she was 28 years old, and she stayed there for 5 years. Sabine languished and suffered in the hospital. During family visits, it was clear she was heavily medicated; she is barely able to speak, and she is profoundly lethargic. Physically, she shifted from slim and attractive to obese and unkempt, and she hunches over with her mouth gaping open. She communicates in screams and cursing, and she drools, picks her nose, and looks dazed. In addition, while institutionalized, she became untrusting and self-injurious; she banged her head, became aggressive, was often mute and was troubled by intrusive thoughts. She began to claim that she would marry a firefighter and raise children. After leaving the hospital, some of these behaviors improved; however, much of the physical and psychological damage persisted, and her social functioning remained limited at the time of the filming.

"Is the decline in her abilities inherent in her condition? Will she ever be without medication?
Will we take that trip again? Can the damage of institutionalization ever be repaired?"

Filmmaker Sandrine Bonnaire wondering about her sister, in *Her Name Is Sabine* (2007)

The Dead Mother (*La Madre Muerta;* 1993, Spain) portrays Leire, a mute, young girl with characteristics of intellectual disability and ASD, who is the only witness to a burglar who breaks into her house and kills her mother. Twenty years later, Leire is in an institution and by chance the criminal sees her and, fearing she might turn him in, kidnaps her and holds her for ransom. Leire displays flat affect and muscle rigidity. She is easily distracted by details (e.g., a crack on a wall, bubbles in a bathtub, and her own hands), has poor eye contact, and reacts to loud noises. While living in the institution, Leire displays a traumatic response to blood and shakes and cries when a boy falls and cuts himself. She is not toilet trained, and she is obsessed with chocolate, which makes her vulnerable to manipulation and exploitation. She rarely, if ever, laughs. She displays some adaptive difficulties, such as difficulty in dressing, and she is unable to bathe herself. Leire is an innocent character whose behavior stands in marked contrast to the pathological criminals around her.

The Black Balloon (2008, Australia) depicts the challenges, joys, stressors, and coping patterns of a family raising a child, Charlie, who was diagnosed with an intellectual disability, autism, and ADHD. Charlie giggles constantly, makes strange noises, taps repeatedly, rocks, and engages in various repetitive behaviors. The film displays several dramatic incidents such as Charlie running out of the house and down several blocks of his neighborhood in his underwear; wiping his feces all over the floor, his clothes, and body; placing his brother's girlfriend's tampon in his mouth; making a scene in a busy grocery store by rolling around on the floor; smashing a window when punished; and masturbating at the table during a birthday celebration. The impact on the entire family is significant, and each family member copes in their own way, communicating with Charlie and connecting with the family unit. The film will help viewers understand and appreciate the challenges associated with raising a child with a severe ASD. The film accurately depicts the conflicting emotions of love and anger and the explicit and implicit tensions that exist in family interactions. The film's director, Elissa Down, grew up with two brothers who were coping with ASD, and it is likely that this experience contributed to the film's integrity, honesty, and veracity.

In another Australian film, *Somersault* (2004), a young female protagonist encounters a boy with ASD. He is passive and taciturn with blunted affect and is shown studying emotions on cards with his mother.

"All's I know is he's my own, and you're weak as piss if you don't look after your own."

Charlie's father's response when asked whether he ever wished Charlie was "normal," in *The Black Balloon*

Ben X (2007, Belgium) is a subtitled Flemish film about a young man, Ben, who is taciturn, quirky, and awkward in his interactions. He is quick to take things personally. He displays a wide range of symptoms, presenting an interesting differential diagnosis challenge for health profession students seeing this film. Ben sees a range of doctors, each of whom give him different diagnoses and descriptors for his symptoms, ranging from "emotionally dysfunctional," "a bit stressed," "a light form of psychosis," and "sensitive," to "Asperger's syndrome." The film does portray **equine therapy**, an emerging treatment that is sometimes used successfully with ASDs. Ben's struggles with emotions and social interaction, and his sensitivity to sound and touch, support a diagnosis of ASD. In addition, he is quick to identify small details but has trouble seeing the bigger picture. In many situations, he has no idea how to interact or make a connection; for example, after a girl has traveled across town to meet him, he sits next to her but is unable to muster the courage necessary to speak to her, and he just runs away. He is often judged, teased, and called names by other students. The film depicts two brutal bullying scenes that are humiliating, abusive, and torturous. He is so affected by this social abuse and disconnection that he becomes preoccupied with suicide; he begins to plan his own death, and he eventually attempts suicide by jumping off a boat.

Despite the emotional turmoil some of these scenes will cause in some viewers, the film has a surprising and uniquely redemptive ending that makes the painful earlier scenes more rewarding. The film leaves the viewer with the message that one sometimes must go to great lengths to effect substantive social change.

Lighthouse of the Whales (*El Faro de Las Orcas;* 2016, Spain) is a film about a mother from Madrid who travels to Argentina after seeing a documentary about the therapeutic value of animals, and specifically orca whales. Her son improves, and the mother and the Argentine ranger predictably fall in love. The film is based on a true story.

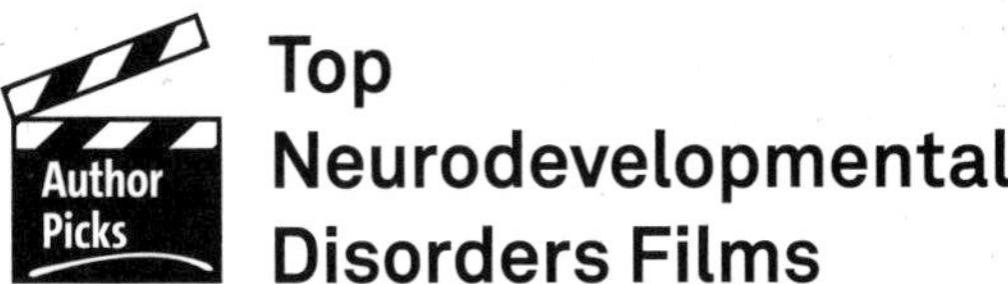

Top Neurodevelopmental Disorders Films

Intellectual Disabilities

Forrest Gump (1994)
Pauline and Paulette (2001)
Monica and David (2009)
Intelligent Lives (2018)

Communication Disorders

The King's Speech (2010)

Autism Spectrum Disorder

Temple Grandin (2010)
Life, Animated (2016)
This Is Nicholas – Living With Autism (2019)

Motor Disorders

Motherless Brooklyn (2019)
Crip Camp (2020)

Chapter 3

Schizophrenia Spectrum and Other Psychotic Disorders

My name is John Nash!
I'm being held against my will!
Someone call the Department of Defense!

John Nash (Russell Crowe) in *A Beautiful Mind* (2001)

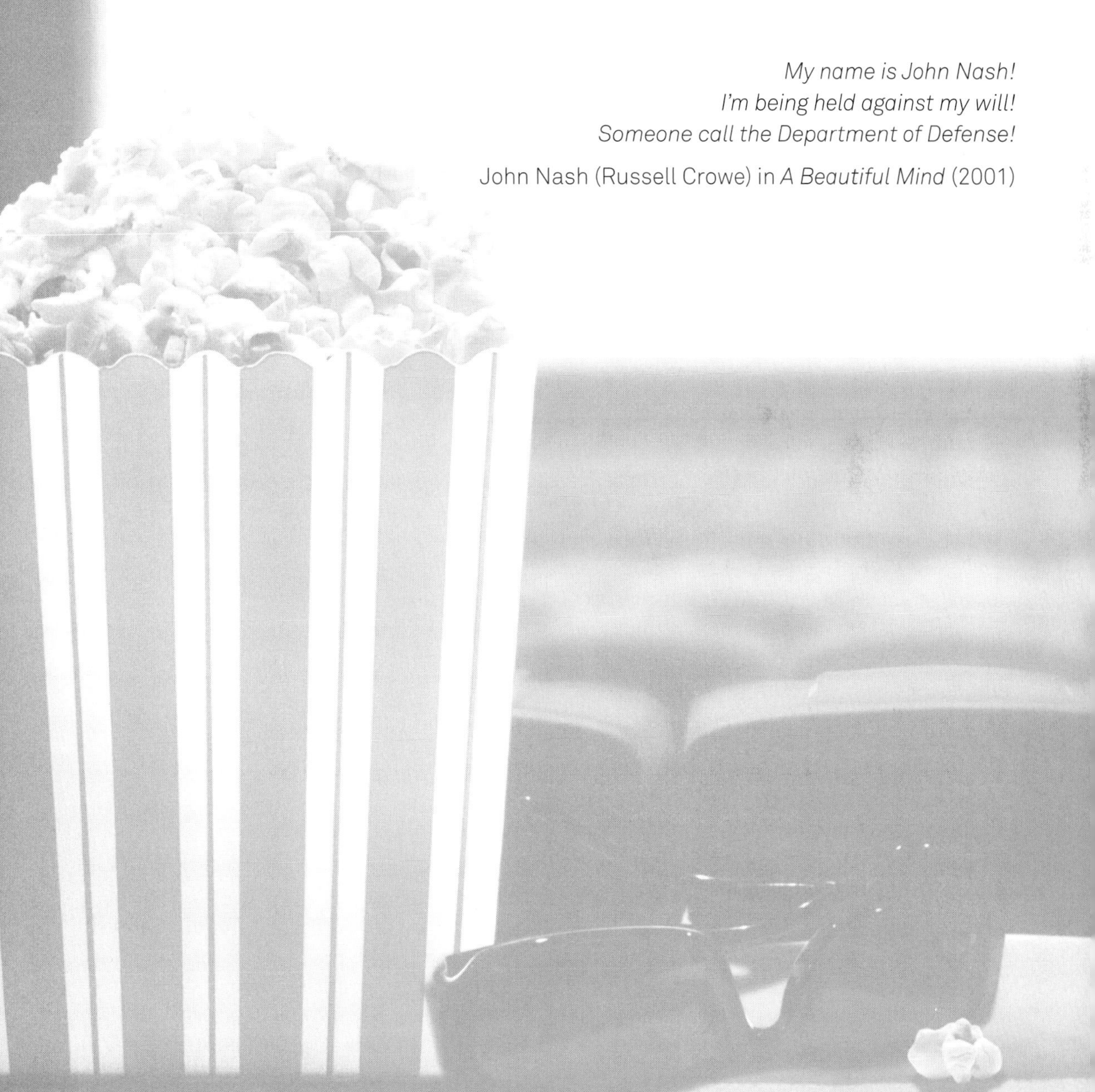

Psychotic Disorders

The DSM-5 now classifies schizophrenia as a spectrum disorder, in much the same way that autism was redefined as a spectrum disorder. This practice recognizes that psychotic symptoms vary in severity along a continuum. *The key features of psychotic disorders are delusions, hallucinations, disorganized thinking, abnormal behavior, and negative symptoms.* **Delusions** are fixed beliefs that resist change, despite evidence contrary to the delusion. Delusions are often paranoid, grandiose, erotomanic (e.g., romantic fixation on a celebrity or public figure), or somatic. People with delusions may or may not meet the diagnostic criteria for schizophrenic spectrum disorder. Delusions often take the form of a belief that someone else has control of one's thoughts and/or behavior.

Hallucinations are perceptual experiences that distort reality or exist without a realistic stimulus. They are most often auditory in nature; *the presence of olfactory or gustatory hallucinations should always trigger a referral for evaluation by a neurologist.* People with psychotic disorders also frequently present with **disorganized thinking** that most often takes the form of distortions in speech such as loose associations, tangential thinking, or "word salad."

Movement may also be distorted in psychotic disorders. This sometimes takes the form of **catatonia**; catatonia may result in either marked diminution of activity, or exaggerated motor activity. It is sometimes difficult to distinguish catatonic excitement from the mania that accompanies bipolar disorder. **Waxy flexibility**, the tendency of a patient to maintain a position or posture once the position has been established, is one of the defining features of catatonic stupor.

Delusions, hallucinations, and movement disorders are all considered **positive symptoms**. In contrast, the **negative symptoms** associated with psychotic disorders are less salient and dramatic; however, they can be just as limiting for the individual with the disease. The most common negative symptoms associated with psychotic disorders are diminished emotional expression and a lack of motivated, purposeful activity. Patients with negative symptoms appear vacant and hollow; they may avoid eye contact and often sit for long hours without engaging in meaningful activity. They may wander aimlessly, say little, and appear to have no interest in other people or other activities.

Recent research involved showing movies portraying emotional bonding and loss to stimulate oxytocin in patients with schizophrenia versus healthy controls. Lower baseline oxytocin levels were observed in females, and oxytocin reactivity in response to the films was significantly higher in the schizophrenia group. These findings suggest that oxytocin may be a modulator of socioemotional function in people who develop schizophrenia (Speck et al., 2019).

Note that the diagnosis of schizotypal personality disorder is considered part of the schizophrenia spectrum, but the DSM-5 discusses this disorder most fully in the chapter on personality disorders. We take the same approach – readers will find film examples of schizotypal personality in Chapter 13.

Anyone interested in a first-hand account of life with schizophrenia will benefit from reading the book *Mental Traveler: A Father, a Son, and a Journey Through Schizophrenia* (Mitchell, 2020). This book is a memoir of the life and death of author's son, Gabriel Mitchell, who struggled with schizophrenia for 20 years until his suicide at age 38. The book will be especially meaningful for parents and caregivers who love someone coping with this disease.

The Diagnosis of Schizophrenia

Schizophrenia usually first occurs during late adolescence or early adulthood, although it sometimes – but rarely – begins in childhood or middle to late adulthood. Even though the frequency of the illness is approximately equal in men and women, symptoms in males occur earlier than in females. Peak onset occurs in the early- to mid-20s for males and mid- to late-20s for females. In general, the outcome of the illness is worse with earlier onset.

For a person to be diagnosed with schizophrenia, certain symptoms must be present. According to the DSM-5, there must be continuous signs of the disturbance for at least 6 months and, for 1 month (the active phase), two or more of the following must be present: delusions, hallucinations, disorganized speech, grossly disorganized or catatonic behavior, or negative symptoms. In addition, at least one of the symptoms must be the presence of delusions, hallucinations, or disorganized speech (i.e., the presence of catatonic behavior and negative symptoms alone would not be sufficient to justify the diagnosis). The individual's ability to function in work, social relations, and self-care decreases during the active phase and rarely returns to the individual's premorbid level of functioning.

"The nightmare of schizophrenia is not knowing what's true. Imagine if you had suddenly learned that the people, the places, the moments most important to you were not gone, not dead, but worse ... they've never been. What kind of hell would that be?"

Dr. Rosen educating Alicia Nash about her husband's schizophrenia, in *A Beautiful Mind* (2001)

Patients with schizophrenia spectrum disorder frequently have systematized delusions or frequent hallucinations related to a single theme (e.g., hearing denigrating voices). These individuals are often extremely anxious, angry, or argumentative, and may become violent. However, there is *not* the strong relationship between violence and schizophrenia that many people expect (and which movies suggest is common). When violence does occur, it most often occurs in young males with a history of violent behavior who are nonadherent to their medication regimens, or with those individuals whose illness is complicated by substance abuse.

Elaine Walker and her colleagues examined early childhood home movies from families in which one child developed schizophrenia. Trained observers rated facial affect in the children who became schizophrenic and their nonschizophrenic siblings. For females, there were consistently fewer expressions of joy in the preschizophrenic children than in their same-sex siblings who did not develop the disorder. This difference was present at every age, but only for females. However, both preschizophrenic males and preschizophrenic females displayed greater negative affect than their nonschizophrenic same-sex siblings (Walker et al., 1993). A subsequent study demonstrated a higher rate of neuromotor abnormalities and poorer motor skills in the preschizophrenic subjects in the first 2 years of life, with deficits noted predominately on the left side of the body (Walker et al., 1994).

Schizophrenia and *A Beautiful Mind:* Realities, Misconceptions, and Recovery

A Beautiful Mind (2001) is based on the biography of the same title by Sylvia Nasar, written about the life of John Forbes Nash Jr., a Princeton professor who won the Nobel Prize for Economics in 1994. John and Alicia Nash have noted in interviews that they are satisfied with the final film product. Dr. Nash was often on the set of *A Beautiful Mind* and consulted with Russell Crowe and Ron Howard in the production process. Although the film is true to the spirit and major events of John Nash's life, it does leave out some of the less flattering details, such as his divorce and remarriage to Alicia and an arrest history.

The film gives the viewer a vivid glimpse of what it feels like to experience schizophrenia. Ron Howard accomplishes this by depicting life from the perspective of John Nash's character and the unfolding of his genius, while temporarily omitting the fact that Nash is hallucinating characters including secret military agents and an imaginary roommate. When the film is halfway over, the viewer learns that much of what has been witnessed from Nash's perspective is unreal. This underscores the fact that oftentimes individuals are completely unaware that they are experiencing hallucinations or delusions, and that others are not experiencing the present moment in the same way. *Shutter Island* (2010) takes a similar perspective with the protagonist, played by Leonardo DiCaprio; however, the overall effect is not as successful.

> **"Often what I feel is obligation ... or guilt over wanting to leave, rage against John, against God. But then I look at him and I force myself to see the man that I married, and he becomes that man. He's transformed into someone that I love, and I'm transformed into someone that loves him. It's not all the time but it's enough."**
>
> **Alicia Nash in response to a question about how she is coping with her husband's illness, in *A Beautiful Mind* (2001)**

A Beautiful Mind depicts the horrors, traumas, and suffering of schizophrenia, and but it also illustrates that people with schizophrenia can sometimes live a normal life, certainly outside of mental institutions, sometimes functioning as well as anyone in society. The film has educated millions of viewers about the realities and challenges of schizophrenia. However, it has flaws and may mislead viewers in significant ways. For example, auditory hallucinations are more common and occur far more frequently than visual hallucinations, yet visual hallucinations are portrayed as one of John Nash's most salient symptoms, and the public is left to believe that this is a standard presentation for those with schizophrenia. Director Ron Howard was working in a visual medium, and therefore he chose to emphasize visual phenomena. The film may also mislead viewers because it shows John Nash overcoming his illness by putting himself on a "diet of the mind" (i.e., he learned to simply ignore his hallucinations and delusions); this may have worked for John Nash, but it is highly unlikely to work for the average person coping with this illness. Finally, the film depicts Nash receiving insulin shock therapy (Figure 10), although many viewers mistakenly assume he is receiving electroconvulsive therapy (ECT).

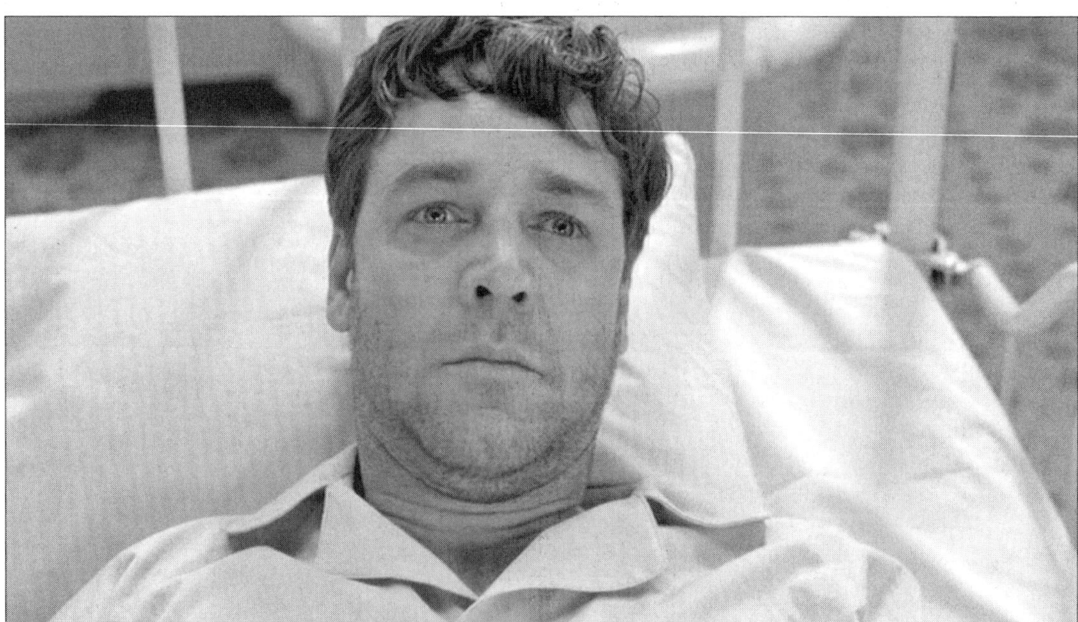

Figure 10. *A Beautiful Mind* (2001, Universal Pictures, Dreamworks, Imagine Entertainment). Produced by Brian Grazer, Todd Hallowell, Ron Howard, Karen Kehela, et al. Directed by Ron Howard.

The film digs deep into the challenges associated with treatment and rehabilitation of a person coping with a severe mental illness. Few films have done as good a job depicting the impact of a schizophrenia spectrum disorder upon healthy family members. The latter part of the film depicts John Nash's wife, Alicia, playing a key role in helping him "live with the realities of schizophrenia." She helps him remember to take his medications. She works longer hours, takes a significant role in child rearing, and manages household chores, all in support of her husband's recovery.

> **"He's been injected with a serum. I can see him because of the chemicals enlisted in my bloodstream when my implant dissolved. I couldn't tell you; it was for your own protection."**
>
> **John Nash during a relapse after not taking his medication in *A Beautiful Mind* (2001)**

Relapse is common in people with schizophrenia, due to numerous challenges, such as depression associated with recovery, the reality of remembering to take medications several times per day, and the multiple unpleasant side effects of the medication. This film is an accurate depiction of the difficulty of compliance with medication regimens, and it shows the impact of psychotropic medications on John Nash's ability to work, his difficulties in taking care of his son, and his sexual performance.

It is a challenge for the person with schizophrenia to adapt and become integrated into the community. The depiction of John Nash's struggle to adapt is another strength of the film. Stress triggers his delusions, and he longs to give up and escape the stress of social interactions, but he also has moments of grace and meaningful connection with others.

The film shows the public's fears about schizophrenia and examines the illness's impact on Nash's friends. His best friend goes to Nash's house, but he is visibly nervous, hesitant in his speech, and laughs uncomfortably. Another friend watches Nash closely when Nash enters the office. Other reactions are more negative: Some students at the university make fun of Nash and mimic his awkward gait and posture, while others stare in disbelief at his odd behavior.

Finally, this movie illustrates the quandary posed when patients with several psychiatric illnesses such as schizophrenia are not able to give informed consent (Jacobson, 2011). Patients with schizophrenia are frequently paranoid and suspicious of the treatments offered to them. In these cases, a family member like Alicia Nash can provide the consent necessary for physicians to hospitalize and treat a seriously disturbed patient. While less dramatic, simply getting a patient to give consent for something as simple as a COVID vaccination can be challenging (Raffard et al., 2022).

A Beautiful Mind can be compared with the film *Proof* (2005), starring Anthony Hopkins as a world-class mathematician with schizophrenia working at an elite university. *Proof* also depicts the impact of schizophrenia on family members (in *Proof*, the father–daughter relationship is emphasized). Frederick Frese, a psychologist and professor of psychology who had a schizophrenia spectrum disorder, reviewed this film for *PsycCRITIQUES* and reported that *Proof* "does an excellent job of capturing what is happening in the mind as it experiences the expanded horizon of meaningfulness that occurs in schizophrenia" (Frese, 2006).

Other Movies About Schizophrenia Spectrum Disorders

Among people diagnosed with schizophrenia spectrum disorder, paranoid patients are the most likely to commit acts of violence. This is a common subtype portrayed in films; it is popularized in films such as *A Beautiful Mind* (2001), *Donnie Darko* (2001), *Gothika* (2003), and *The Adopted One* (2020). In contrast, the documentary *People Say I'm Crazy* (2004) is a remarkably honest and real portrayal of the daily life of a courageous man coping with paranoia and schizophrenia spectrum disorder.

Incoherent speech and disorganized behavior are common with schizophrenia spectrum disorders. These patients rapidly shift from one idea to another; often these ideas are unrelated. They may also express inappropriate emotion, such as laughing on a sad occasion (e.g., during a funeral). They usually have very strange mannerisms and are extremely socially impaired. Robin Williams' character in *The Fisher King* (1991) and Geoffrey Rush's portrayal of David Helfgott in *Shine* (1996) both illustrate these symptoms. Ralph Fiennes' title character in *Spider* (2002) is another excellent example of this type of schizophrenia spectrum disorder.

Some patients with schizophrenia spectrum disorders display **catatonia**. For example, catatonic persons may appear to be in a stupor, completely unaware of their environment. They may maintain one posture for a long time, crawl into a fetal position, hold an arm in a bizarre position, or sit stiffly in a chair; it may be difficult to move the individual because of the muscle rigidity. At times, these individuals become excited or agitated but slip into previous mannerisms. At times they are mute. The film *Awakenings* (1990) is a dramatic portrayal of catatonia (although this film depicted a neurological rather than psychiatric condition). Many films depicting psychiatric institutions have one or two characters (often in the background) who display catatonia, as in *K-Pax* (2001) and *House of Fools* (2004).

Other patients with a diagnosis of schizophrenia will not hallucinate or have delusions, but they will display social withdrawal or eccentric behavior. Eugene Levy's character, Mitch, in *A Mighty Wind* (2003) illustrates this phenomenon. Mitch sits alone and stares for hours in a drab motel room; displays psychomotor retardation; exhibits blank, distant, and quizzical facial expressions; and has inappropriate social skills, yet he does not appear to be in the active phase of a schizophrenia spectrum disorder. These are residual effects. The viewer learns Mitch had previously been hospitalized for severe depression, anger outbursts, and eccentric behavior, though an actual diagnosis is never given.

Stranger Than Fiction (2006) stars Will Ferrell as Harold Crick, an IRS agent who leads an insipid life until he begins to hear someone narrating his life and telling him he is going to die soon. Harold recognizes the voice; it was the voice of an esteemed author he had heard on television. He begins to look for the author to convince her that she cannot end the story by having the protagonist die.

Dr. Mittag-Leffler: "I'm afraid what you're describing is schizophrenia."
Harold Crick: "No, no. It's not schizophrenia. It's just a voice in my head. I mean, the voice isn't telling me to do anything. It's telling me what I've already done ... accurately, and with a better vocabulary."
Dr. Mittag-Leffler: "Mr. Crick, you have a voice speaking to you."
Harold Crick: "No, not TO me. ABOUT me. I'm somehow involved in some sort of story. Like I'm a character in my own life. But the problem is that the voice comes and goes ..."
Dr. Mittag-Leffler: "Mr. Crick, I hate to sound like a broken record, but that's schizophrenia."

A physician argues with Will Ferrell's character about his diagnosis, in *Stranger Than Fiction* (2006)

Three Christs (2020) is a movie adaptation of Milton Rokeach's 1964 book *Three Christs of Ypsilanti*. The book and the film revolve around interactions between three psychiatric inpatients, all of whom believe they are Jesus Christ. Each of the patients is diagnosed with paranoid schizophrenia. The film takes place in the 1950s and is useful for illustrating some of the primitive treatments applied in psychiatric hospitals. One of the three patients (Cassel, played by Peter Dinklage) winds up committing suicide. The psychologist in the film, Dr. Alan Stone (played by Richard Gere), is sympathetically portrayed. I read the book many years ago as a graduate student and remember enjoying it. The movie was less satisfying. Anyone seriously interested in the original case will want to read Rokeach's book and an article by Donald Capps

(2010), describing the youngest patient, Leon Gabor, who,

> met the challenges that the procedure posed by creative elaborations of his delusional system, especially through the adoption of a new name that gave the initial appearance of the abandonment of his Christ identity but in fact drew on aspects of the real Jesus Christ's identity that were missing from his earlier self-representation. (p. 560)

The Professor and the Madman (2019) is also based on a book with the same name by Simon Winchester. The film has a stellar cast, including Mel Gibson and Sean Penn. The film and the book both revolve around the life of James Murray, a scholar who collaborated with a physician, Dr. William Minor, who had murdered a man but who was found not guilty by reason of insanity and committed to the Broadmoor Criminal Lunatic Asylum. The two men collaborated to produce the *Oxford English Dictionary*, and Dr. Minor submitted more than 10,000 dictionary entries. However, Minor's mental health continued to deteriorate, and one of his delusions was that he was being abducted to sexually assault young children. Minor ensured this could not happen by cutting off his penis. Here too, the book was better than the movie. (Years ago, I attended the International Congress of Psychology in Beijing. The program for the Congress was replete with typographical errors. I attended a session on "Self-Genital Mutilation," a serious psychiatric problem. However, the typesetter had dropped the "S" in self, so the program read "Elf Genital Mutilation." A colleague leaned over and remarked, "I didn't even know the little bastards had genitals!")

Patricia Owen (2012) identified 41 English language movies released between 1990 and 2010 in which a major character was coping with the challenges associated with schizophrenia. Most of these characters were White and male, and most had positive symptoms. Delusions were the most common symptom, followed by auditory and visual hallucinations. Violence was commonplace: Nearly a third of these characters were homicidal, and approximately one in four committed suicide. In addition, one in four of the films suggested an early traumatic event was responsible for the schizophrenia spectrum disorder being portrayed. Owen concluded,

> The finding that misinformation and negative portrayals of schizophrenia in contemporary movies are common underscores the importance of determining how viewers interpret media messages and how these interpretations inform attitudes and beliefs both of the general public and of people with schizophrenia. (Owen, 2012, p. 655)

Family Dynamics and Schizophrenia Spectrum Disorder

In the 1960s and 1970s, a popular theory implicated dysfunctional family communication patterns in the etiology of schizophrenia. Communication within the family of a person with schizophrenia was believed to be indirect, unclear, incongruent, and growth impeding. Communication within these families was thought to be distorted and based on "double messages" that occurred when a child received two opposing messages from the parent and was placed in a **double bind**. For example, a parent might say, "Come here and give me a hug," and when the child responded, the parent would tense up and push the child away. The child then would feel that pleasing the parent was an impossible no-win situation and would develop schizophrenia in response to this psychological bind. The **schizophrenogenic family** was characterized as being severely fused. Members of these families never adequately separated or developed into individuals, and thus the family had no boundaries. This view of distorted family communication has been discounted as a cause of schizophrenia.

Even though no one seriously believes that parents "cause" their children's schizophrenia spectrum disorder, this misconception persists in both popular culture and contemporary cinema.

Peter Winter's mother in *Clean, Shaven* (1993) is portrayed as cold, aloof, and withdrawn; there is a clear implication that she is at least in part responsible for her son's illness. Likewise, the movie *Shine* (1996), Scott Hick's fascinating film about the life of child prodigy and pianist David Helfgott, clearly implicates David's father as the root of his son's subsequent mental illness. The father is alternately loving and hateful, telling his son, "No one can love you like me!" while at the same time actively working to limit his son's future and potential. A similar theme can be found in the 1962 film *David and Lisa*, in which David's mother – a woman focused on appearances – makes some efforts to support David but ends up appearing insensitive to her son's abilities and problems. The father is depicted as passive, distant, and unavailable to David in his younger years. Both parents are ineffective in dealing with David's problems, and the film suggests there is a link between the dysfunctional parental communication and David's mental illness.

Sweetie (1989) is Jane Campion's debut film. It beautifully illustrates how very difficult it can be for a family to cope with a member who has a serious mental illness. The film presents a realistic portrayal of schizophrenia.

Strange Voices (1987) is a made-for-TV movie starring Valerie Harper as the mother of a first-year college student named Nicole who has her initial breakdown shortly before starting her first semester. Once on campus, she hears voices, becomes paranoid, and behaves in inappropriate ways. Nicole is diagnosed with schizophrenia, but she throws away her medication because it makes her feel "like a stone." In her dorm, she plays her stereo loudly to drown out the voices she hears. She is admitted to a psychiatric facility, but after a 72-hour-hold she is discharged against medical advice (AMA). After returning home, she accidentally starts a fire in the kitchen. She is admitted to a psychiatric hospital for a second time, but after a few days escapes and winds up being homeless. Nicole is arrested after not being able to pay for a meal she eats at a diner. A friendly social worker eventually tracks down her family, and they come to take her home. Nicole's father blames himself because an aunt in his family was odd and eccentric, and she eventually committed suicide; the father realizes it is likely that his "Aunt Lily" was schizophrenic, and he thinks he is genetically responsible for his daughter's illness. At a family support group meeting, Nicole's mother learns that one third of men and two thirds of women living on the street meet the criteria for a diagnosis of schizophrenia. A psychiatrist acknowledges the limits of his ability to help, remarking, "I feel guilty too because I'm part of a psychiatric community that has largely shunned schizophrenia and its victims because we feel powerless in the face of it." The film ends positively after Valerie Harper's character visits a group home and sees young people making genuine contributions despite their diagnosis. Although Nicole's presentation is atypical (e.g., Nicole's onset is immediate and dramatic rather than insidious), the film might be interesting for someone with a child recently diagnosed with schizophrenia. In addition, the movie dramatically illustrates the stress that a family must endure when they have a child who has a serious mental illness.

The Primary Misconception: People With Mental Illness Are Frequently Violent

One of the most profound yet common stereotypes in contemporary cinema is the connection filmmakers draw between mental illness and violence. This misconception is strongest in films that portray schizophrenia spectrum disorder. It is often not explicitly stated in the film; however, the plotline and ensuing messages are usually clear to the viewer: They see a character being treated for a psychological problem, or they see a character begin to deteriorate with mental illness, and the next thing the viewer sees is that person perpetrating a violent act. This is unfortunate because the public is not educated on the relationship between violence and mental illness, and many individuals, influenced by media reports, are likely to exaggerate their own personal risk when interacting with someone who has a mental illness. The reality is that *people with mental illness are far more likely to be the victim of a violent act than to be the perpetrator of violence*; moreover, research also shows that mental illness is neither a necessary nor a sufficient cause for violence (Stuart, 2003). The data are mixed as to whether people with mental illness are more or less likely to react with violence than the public. Yet filmmakers use this stereotype, as it provides a clear understanding of what is often unspeakable and perplexing; it is a way to clear up ambiguity and to make sense of the human psyche.

"I was Mr. Nobody till I killed the biggest somebody on earth ... I was nothing and [then] I was a big shot."
"There was no emotion in my blood, there was no anger, there was nothing. It was dead silence in my brain, dead cold quiet. He looked at me, he looked past me. Then I heard my head, [it] said do it, do it, do it, over again."

Mark Chapman explaining his murder of John Lennon, in *The Killing of John Lennon* (2006)

Films portraying the assassination of public figures are a clear example of filmmakers leveraging this idea. Two in particular – *The Killing of John Lennon* (2006) and *The Assassination of Richard Nixon* (2004) – portray men who obsess over a public figure and subsequently murder or attempt to murder because of a strong delusional process. Both men are scruffy, irritable, quirky, socially awkward, and withdrawn. Each has a deep insecurity and inferiority and anger toward some aspect of the social system (e.g., consumerism, politics), and each uses violence to deal with these frustrations. Each is a fascinating, accurate portrayal of the internal dialogue and reasoning that fosters a grandiose delusional state.

In *The Killing of John Lennon*, Mark Chapman is very grandiose and paranoid, displaying mood changes and delusional explanations for his behavior. He shows no remorse or regret and believes he later received a message from God to plead guilty. In the end, both films leave the viewer with a powerful sense that there is a connection between schizophrenia/delusions and violence/murder.

"That little guy can't do it anymore. He just can't do it anymore ... because there's a cancer in the system. The whole system has a cancer and I'm being punished because I resist. But somebody has to resist, just somebody has to resist."
"I know what it's like to not be respected, to be lied to, and to be treated like a great big nothing."

Samuel J. Bicke's (Sean Penn) delusions that led to his assassination attempt on Richard Nixon, in *The Assassination of Richard Nixon* (2004)

Another film that makes people fear those with mental illness is *Keane* (2004), a movie in which a man frantically searches for his daughter whom he has lost at a Port Authority bus terminal in New York City. Damian Lewis as the protagonist, a man with a schizophrenia spectrum disorder, does a marvelous job portraying how he struggles to hold reality together even while he continues to deteriorate. Nevertheless, the aspects of the film that most viewers will remember are the scenes of intense and bizarre behavior. In one scene, William Keane chases and attacks a stranger in a parking garage.

William H. Macy's portrayal of a man losing touch with reality in *Edmond* (2005), written for the screen and the stage by David Mamet, is equally chilling. Edmond breaks up with his wife and slowly deteriorates as he starts to wander the streets of New York City looking for sex. As he begins to self-destruct, his loneliness, isolation, instability, and lack of responsibility and empathy become clear. The viewer will easily remember standout scenes of Edmond impulsively screaming at a woman who does not listen to him on the subway and his murder of a waitress after having sex with her. He later rationalizes his killing as the result of too much coffee, and he claims that there are just too many people in the world.

There are hundreds of suspense and horror movies about "psychotic killers" who are on a rampage, usually attacking women. While entertaining for some, these films typically have nothing to do with any mental disorder, and they perpetuate the stigma associated with mental illness. The term "psychotic" is used to induce fear and suggest unpredictability. Pictures such as *The Caretakers* (1963), *The Silent Partner* (1979), *Alone in the Dark* (1982), *Angel in Red* (1991), *Cape Fear* (1991), and *The Adopted One* (2020) have contributed to shaping the stigma experienced by people with mental illness.

Two horror/thriller films that portray characters deteriorating with mental illness who consequently become violent are *May* (2002) and *Love Object* (2003). *May* is a macabre, well-acted character study of a veterinary technician whose best friend is her doll. As she continues to fail at intimate and social relationships, she becomes psychotic and begins to kill to get ideal body parts that she combines to form a whole. In *Love Object*, a young man believes his lifelike sex doll is real and comes to believe he is being controlled and attacked by the doll; these delusions deepen and extend to violence in the outside world.

Even the portrayal of schizophrenia in the widely popular *A Beautiful Mind* (2001), albeit helpful in educating the public in many ways, also highlights scenes in which John Nash becomes violent or dangerous to his wife and to their newborn baby - particularly when he is in a paranoid state. Other classic examples of this stereotype include Annie Wilkes, the delusional character played by Academy Award winner Kathy Bates, who tortures a writer she is obsessed with in *Misery* (1990), the isolated female protagonist in Roman Polanski's *Repulsion* (1965, UK), and Robert De Niro's classic role as a delusional killer, Travis Bickle, in *Taxi Driver* (1976).

The most recent film to promote the pernicious myth that schizophrenia causes people to become homicidal is *The Adopted One* (2020), a movie in which a troubled child kills his adoptive parents and subsequently spends 30 years in a mental institution. After he murders a guard and escapes from the institution, he kills numerous additional people, most often with a hammer, often smiling while killing his victims. The film opens with a doctor telling the protagonist, Jonathan, "based on your psychiatric evaluation, our belief is that you have schizophrenia," and then there are multiple flashbacks showing Jonathan as a child, pushing another child down the stairs, drawing pictures with themes of violence and murder, and eventually killing his abusive adoptive parents when he is 8 years old. There is an incoherent and inexplicable connection between Jonathan and his psychiatrist, Dr. Woods, who gives him keys to escape the institution and later provides him with a home and protection. Words alone are insufficient to fully explain just how insulting this film is to people with mental illness, and how shamelessly it exploits the public's belief that people with schizophrenia are murderous maniacs who go on extended homicidal rampages whenever they are released from psychiatric hospitals.

Schizophrenia Spectrum Disorders in Contemporary Films

Schizophrenia

Can films educate students and the public about the realities of schizophrenia spectrum disorders? In one study, a video was constructed with segments from popular movies depicting inaccurate and accurate portrayals of schizophrenia (Owen, 2007). The researchers randomly assigned college students to either a video presentation or a traditional lecture on schizophrenia, and later tested the students' knowledge of schizophrenia. The results showed knowledge improvement following both the movie clips and the lecture; however, the movie clips had a greater corrective effect for female students.

Canvas

This 2006 film from first-time director-writer Joseph Greco is an outstanding portrayal of the paranoid symptoms that are often associated with schizophrenia spectrum disorders. It is based on some of Greco's experiences growing up with a parent coping with the symptoms of schizophrenia. Indeed, some individuals in the mental health community believe actress Marcia Gay Harden's portrayal of a character with schizophrenia is the most accurate in film history. Harden plays Mary Marino who desires to be close to her husband and son, but who finds that her illness is a significant obstacle to achieving this goal. She regularly has auditory hallucinations and tries to drown out the sound, first with running water, and later by pouring water on her forehead. She displays inappropriate affect (e.g., laughing at the dinner table during conversation about a serious matter), embarrasses her son by running after the bus saying that she was concerned about his safety, and she is socially unaware of the discomfort her symptoms cause others with whom she interacts. In a memorable scene, Mary runs around in the rain, fear-struck and paranoid as she wakes up the neighbors searching for a wiretap. The film references the Baker Act (also called the Florida Mental Health Act), a law that can be invoked by judges, police, physicians, or mental health professionals, and which allows for involuntary examination of individuals who have mental illness and who are believed to be likely to harm themselves or others or who neglect their own basic needs. Mary is routinely picked up by the police when her paranoid behavior puts her safety at risk.

Important themes in the film include the loss of a family member (to institutionalization), the struggles associated with coping with mental illness, and the challenge of finding hope at the most trying of times. The realities of severe mental illness are not minimized – Mary is often in and out of the hospital, she frequently stops taking her medication, and her illness has a profound impact on her family. Her husband obsesses about building a boat, and her son begins to avoid school. Nevertheless, each of the three taps into an outlet of creativity to cope with the situation – each has a different "canvas," whether it be painting, knitting, or construction and building.

"When you paint, they go away."
"Who?"
"The voices."

Mary Marino interacting with another patient in *Canvas* (2006)

The film is a wonderful portrayal of the impact of mental illness on the family; it is also tender, hopeful, and positive, with an ending that is neither contrived nor forced.

The Soloist

The Soloist (2009) is an outstanding film starring Jamie Foxx as Nathaniel Ayers, a homeless man and brilliant musician who has schizophrenia. Robert Downey Jr. plays the Los Angeles Times columnist Steve Lopez, the reporter who stumbles upon Ayers playing a broken violin on the street next to a statue of Beethoven. Intrigued by Ayers, Lopez writes a series of stories about him, and their relationship develops into a lasting friendship. *The Soloist* does an excellent job at portraying the symptoms of schizophrenia and the resulting impact on daily functioning and social interaction. Director Joe Wright emphasizes auditory hallucinations through a haunting series of various voices that increase in intensity, tone, and frequency; unlike in the film *A Beautiful Mind* – and truer to the reality of schizophrenia – visual hallucinations are de-emphasized. Ayers exhibits a significant level of paranoia but shows a modest degree of symptom awareness when he observes that he might "make a spectacle" of himself. Lopez encourages Ayers to take medication; however, Ayers refuses. A counselor advises

Lopez that Ayers cannot be forced to take medication unless he is a danger to himself or others. The film flashes back to scenes in Ayers' childhood when he isolated himself in a dark basement repeatedly practicing his music, and to his early symptomatic days at the Juilliard School before his illness forced him to drop out of that prestigious academy.

Unfortunately, the film falls into the prevalent trap of perpetrating the misconception that all people with schizophrenia eventually become violent and dangerous. Of course, a person with a mental illness can be violent, like anyone else. The problem is that filmmakers notoriously make disorders such as schizophrenia spectrum disorders synonymous with violent, dangerous, and often lethal behavior. The everyday moviegoers and consumers of mental health films looking for education about a disorder that they or a family member have been diagnosed with are then misled, simply because filmmakers want to enhance the drama of the film. Unfortunately, it is the dramatic and violent scenes that viewers will remember.

Bug

The William Friedkin film *Bug* (2006), based on a play, is an excellent, moody, mysterious, and raw depiction of mental illness. Most of the film takes place in one room, which heightens emotions, gives the viewer a claustrophobic feel and forces them to focus on the characters. An emotionally wounded and exhausted woman, Agnes (Ashley Judd), lives in a small motel room and uses cocaine with her occasional lesbian lover. Her only child vanished several years ago at age 9 and she has been struggling with an abusive husband, Jerry (Harry Connick Jr.), who was recently released from prison. Agnes befriends a strange man, Peter, who claims he is able "to sense things." Peter is a highly intuitive person with keen social intelligence; he quickly and correctly realizes that Agnes is someone who has suffered a lot in her life. He also senses that she has a "bad" husband, and he quickly notices times when she has lied to him. But he also believes her motel room is infested with microscopic bugs. Soon the room is filled with bug traps, sprays, fumigation devices, and even a microscope. He takes his own blood samples and points out the bugs that are multiplying. He later painfully explains that he had been kicked out of the military because of his paranoid beliefs. Peter's next step in eliminating the "bugs" is to cover the entire rooms in tin foil, from top to bottom including all the furniture and household items. He claims that the tin foil scrambles the "signals" of the bugs, making it impossible for them to communicate. He shares extensive details about his persecutory delusions, describing special experiments, prototypes, biochips, and military testing conducted on a global scale.

Peter's psychiatrist arrives at the motel explaining that Peter has been hospitalized for 4 years at an Army hospital where he was diagnosed as a "delusional paranoid with schizophrenic tendencies." After resisting the psychiatrist's advice, Peter brutally and repeatedly stabs him. In a scene reminiscent of another film portraying schizophrenia (*Clean, Shaven*), Peter graphically yanks out his teeth believing there is a transmitter in his gums. Agnes, a vulnerable, traumatized, and lonely woman desperate for a connection, begins to share Peter's psychotic beliefs (i.e., shared psychotic disorder or *folie à deux*). The tension accelerates, and the mental status of both characters continues to deteriorate, culminating in a decision to set themselves on fire to destroy the bugs. This film is an excellent portrayal of schizophrenia, and it provides salient examples of tactile and visual hallucinations and paranoia; however, it also perpetuates the myth that people with mental illness are always violent.

Take Shelter and *Revolution #9*

These are two excellent films that illustrate late-onset psychosis. Each film demonstrates the symptoms of schizophrenia that are left untreated, causing significant decline in the protagonists' functioning and social well-being.

Take Shelter (2011) is a Gus Van Sant film that features Curtis, a small-town construction worker. Curtis begins to experience symptoms of night terrors that specifically target him and his daughter. He experiences hallucinations and delusions; he subsequently conducts research on mental illness and concludes that he has symptoms of schizophrenia. He believes terrible storms are coming and observes signs of storms that no one else can see; he sees figures in the storm, sees flocks of birds that are not there, and hears storms that are not present. His coworkers notice and remark on his strange behavior. His symptoms result in a decision to take time off from work to build a tornado shelter. He sees a counselor who tells him she can listen to him but cannot prescribe medication. Curtis receives mild antianxiety medication from his family doctor, yet avoids communicating about his symptoms with his wife. The film reviews some of the family history of Curtis and points out that his mother left him in a parking lot at age 10, and he was found a few days later eating trash out of a dumpster. His mother was diagnosed with paranoid schizophrenia and taken to a state hospital, and Curtis was raised by his father (who had recently died, exacerbating the stress Curtis was experiencing). Interestingly, the age of onset of symptoms for both mother and son was in their mid-30s. As the film concludes, the whole family can see a massive storm looming, as if to symbolically challenge the viewer's assumptions about Curtis and his presumed illness. While the film is excellent and one of the better portrayals of schizophrenia, there is one episode of violence, which contributes to the misconception that all people with mental illness are violent.

Revolution #9 (2001) is a dramatic and unsentimental illustration of paranoid schizophrenia and the complexities and failings of the US health care system. James Jackson is a freelance writer-reviewer who was recently engaged. As he goes about his work and social life, he begins to realize something is wrong, but he believes his problems are external (i.e., other people are causing his problems). His exhibits diminished eye contact, angry facial expressions, and agitation. He thinks that his fiancée's brother's son is sending him messages, that his fiancée is involved, and that his coworkers are rearranging his desk behind his back. James's writing becomes muddled and confused. His confusion and paranoia escalate as he believes that others are manipulating him. After a month of gradual deterioration, he becomes convinced that a perfume commercial for Revolution 9 contains hidden messages and was made especially for him. He says to his fiancée: "look at that ... they're good aren't they ... it's a code, it hits you underneath." He watches the commercial repeatedly – completely consumed and paranoid. He later stalks the director of the commercial, calling him, creating anonymous, threatening pictures, and he then tricks the director into participating in an interview that ends in violence. A common thread of his social interactions is his belief that he is the subject of a grand conspiracy that involves his fiancée, coworkers, hospital staff, a judge, and others he meets. He is admitted to a hospital and placed on medication for 2 weeks. He is later released and becomes suicidal.

Revolution #9 is particularly effective in depicting the impact of mental illness on the protagonist's fiancée. She expresses concern, agitation, and helplessness, and while she perseveres in trying to get him help, he gives her almost no reason to sustain hope. She persuades him to visit a psychiatrist, but he walks out, defensive, and angry. She repeatedly compromises and ends up giving up her job because of her efforts to help her fiancé.

Director Tim McCann confuses the viewer with humor, and close-up shots are used to enhance the feeling of claustrophobia. McCann also skillfully manages sounds – for example, he stifles sounds, cuts out words, and uses rapid nondiegetic sound. This effect contributes to the cinematic depiction of the progression of schizophrenia. The film offers a sympathetic portrayal of mental health professionals and shows them as competent and knowledgeable about the condition they are treating. The film also provides a rare glimpse of how the mental health community (along with insurance companies) tries to take care of mentally ill people within the cost-benefit constraints of modern health care. The film also depicts manipulation and exploitation by insurance companies determined to avoid paying for necessary care.

Black Swan

Darren Aronofsky's *Black Swan* (2010) is a provocative and unforgettable film starring Natalie Portman, who won an Academy Award for Best Actress for her portrayal of Nina Sayers, the Swan Queen. Sayers is a ballerina who gradually decompensates as she competes for, wins, and then prepares for the lead role in the ballet *Swan Lake*, which ends in a dramatic finale. She is under tremendous pressure to succeed in the highly competitive world of ballet, and the stress of competition is complicated by a dysfunctional relationship with her mother (played by Barbara Hershey, in a role depicting a woman who gave up her career in ballet after her daughter was born) and sexual harassment by her director. She also experiences the drug ecstasy for the first time and has a lesbian encounter with Lily, her doppelgänger and the dancer who plays the role of the Black Swan. While Nina's character presents a diagnostic quandary because she exhibits symptoms associated with several disorders, she clearly exhibits anorexic and bulimic behavior, and she has a history of scratching herself to the point where she bleeds (i.e., excoriation). It is also clear that she is delusional and psychotic; however, the film is unrealistic insofar as someone experiencing a psychosis as profound and as complicated as that experienced by Portman's character would never be able to perform at the prominent level required by the lead role in *Swan Lake*. Nadine Kaslow, 2014 president of the American Psychological Association and the staff psychologist for the Atlanta Ballet, called the film "intense and disturbing and fascinating and mysterious" (abc News, 2010). Reviewing the film for *PsycCRITIQUES*, Keith Oatley and Ryan Niemiec (2011) note, "She presents a diagnostic conundrum, meeting some of the diagnostic criteria for a number of psychological conditions, including schizophrenia, obsessive-compulsive disorder, anorexia, bulimia, dissociative disorder, and major depression." The dramatic climax of this psychologically complex film is seen in Figure 11.

Nina: "I came to ask for the part."
Thomas Leroy: "The truth is when I look at you all I see is the white swan. Yes, you're beautiful, fearful, and fragile. Ideal casting. But the black swan? It's a hard fucking job to dance both."
Nina: "I can dance the black swan, too."
Thomas Leroy: "Really? In four years, every time you dance, I see you obsessed getting each and every move perfectly right, but I never see you lose yourself. Ever! All that discipline for what?"

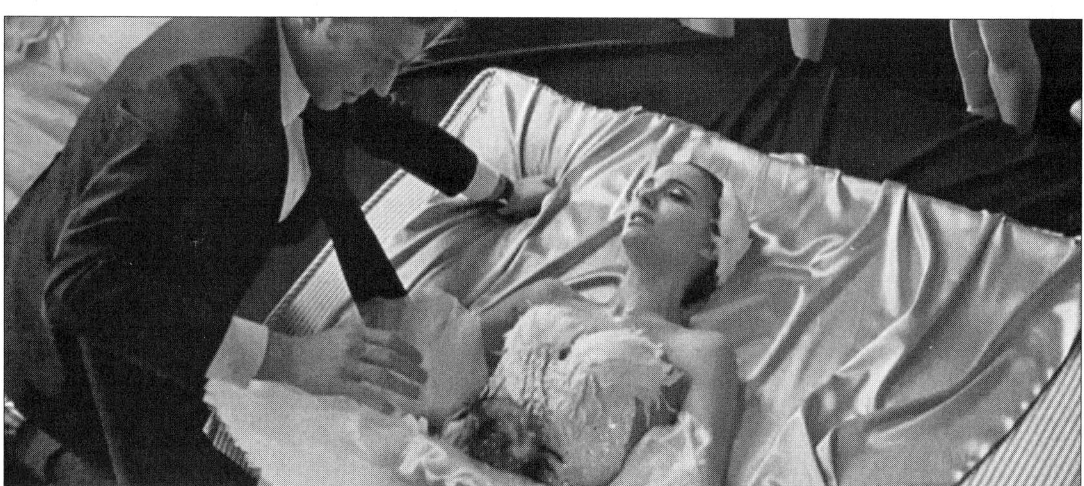

Figure 11. *Black Swan (2010*, Searchlight Pictures, Cross Creek Pictures, Protozoa, Phoenix Pictures, Dune Entertainment). Produced by Jon Avnet, Bradley J. Fischer, Scott Franklin, Jerry Fruchtman, et al. Directed by Darren Aronofsky.

Nina: [whispers] "I just want to be perfect."
Thomas Leroy: "What?"
Nina: "I want to be perfect."
Thomas Leroy: [scoffs] "Perfection is not just about control. It's also about letting go. Surprise yourself so you can surprise the audience. Transcendence! Very few have it in them."
Nina: "I think I do have it in me."

Dialogue between Thomas Leroy and Nina in *Black Swan* (2010)

Spider

The viewer realizes this is a deeply psychological movie as they see the opening credits. Inkblots, like those used with the classic psychological assessment tool, the Rorschach Test, are integrated into the opening. The viewer is thus invited to "interpret" and challenge what they are seeing from the very start to the ambiguous ending.

Director David Cronenberg sets the tone of this 2002 film in the first scene, which depicts "the flow of humanity" - an arriving train, the hustle of activity, and a multitude of people heading toward their own destinations - contrasted with the lead character, Spider (Ralph Fiennes), slowly stepping off the train, disoriented and isolated from everyone else. This dark and dreary film maps out the psychological terrain of a man with schizophrenia. Spider has minimal dialogue, so the viewer learns about his inner world through his facial expressions, body language, and utter isolation.

The adult character Spider, played by Ralph Fiennes, has been discharged from an institution and attempts to integrate into a group home. He has many symptoms of schizophrenia, including delusions, mumbling and disorganized speech, incoherent and grossly disorganized behavior, an unclean and disheveled appearance, and negative symptoms including severely flattened affect and shuffling gait.

Ingeniously, Cronenberg places the present-day Spider character in all of the memory scenes as Spider tries to reassemble his past. The adult Spider is shown observing his parents and himself as a boy interacting with the world. Some of these memories are false, and some are accurate, but neither the viewer nor Spider himself knows the truth. To make matters more complicated, Spider fuses the identities of his memories as well as his past and present, which results in further confusion and distortion.

This is also a good depiction of childhood schizophrenia as we see the young boy distort reality, express the paranoid belief that his father and his father's lover killed his mother, and the boy's complete isolation from social contact.

"You're by yourself too much. You need some mates. When I was your age, I had mates. Every young lad needs ... some mates."

Bill Cleg (Gabriel Byrne) speaking to his delusional son, in *Spider* (2002)

Throughout the film, several metaphors are used to portray Spider's struggle to recognize reality and the disintegration of that reality into psychosis. In one scene, Spider is carefully putting together an extraordinarily complex puzzle of hundreds of pieces, and in a later scene after putting together some painful memory fragments, he angrily destroys the puzzle, throwing the pieces to the floor in the day room. Broken mirrors, pieces of glass, and twine, used to create a spider's web, symbolize his mental state.

K-Pax

In this 2001 film, Kevin Spacey plays Prot, a man claiming to be from the planet K-Pax who has traveled to Earth by light beams. At the outset, we see Prot appear in a busy train station among sparkles of light. Soon he is falsely accused of a crime and admitted to a psychiatric institution. The psychiatrist, Dr. Powell (Jeff Bridges), takes an interest in working with Prot when he learns Prot is unresponsive to conventional psychiatric medications. As their relationship progresses, Dr. Powell learns much about the identity of Prot and the differences between K-Pax and Earth. Prot offers extensive (and savant-like) explanations of his planet's rotational patterns, discusses the ways in which men and women procreate on his planet, and gives descriptions of the differences between the planets. Many of Prot's delusions are bizarre, which keeps him from being given a diagnosis of delusional disorder. The viewer essentially has two options at this point: Prot is either a man with schizophrenia or a spiritual guide from another planet. We can view the film accepting the former as true to help us understand the predicament in which a delusional patient finds himself. He is completely trapped by his delusions and does not have a way out; the painful challenge of this is that the patient is not aware he is delusional. Viewers who choose the latter option are choosing a fascinating, inspirational take on the film, while at the same time buying into the misconception that the person with mental illness is an "enlightened member of society" (Hyler et al., 1991). It is worth noting, however, that some cultures do indeed believe that a person with schizophrenia is an enlightened member of society; therapists and educators should appreciate and acknowledge such cultural beliefs and spend time exploring these beliefs with their patients.

The situation in *K-Pax* gets more complex. As Dr. Powell questions Prot about where he comes from and where he has visited this planet, another diagnostic explanation emerges. We learn through flashbacks and hypnotic regression that Prot is Robert Porter, a man who found the bodies of his murdered and raped wife and child, and then experienced the trauma of encountering the killer in his home and breaking the murderer's neck. Prot then washes his bloody hands with a water hose (hence his water phobia) and attempts suicide in a nearby river. The viewer is left to assume Prot was found and taken to the psychiatric hospital. Consequently, additional diagnostic considerations emerge, such as PTSD and dissociative fugue. His sudden travel, assumption of a new identity, and inability to recall his past (other than under hypnosis) make a compelling case for the diagnosis of dissociative fugue.

In the end, Prot becomes catatonic – unresponsive and rigid as he is pushed around in a wheelchair – providing further evidence to support a diagnosis of schizophrenia.

Horse Girl

Alison Brie stars in *Horse Girl* (2020), a convincing portrayal of the insidious onset of schizophrenia (Figure 12). Brie's character, Sarah, is a

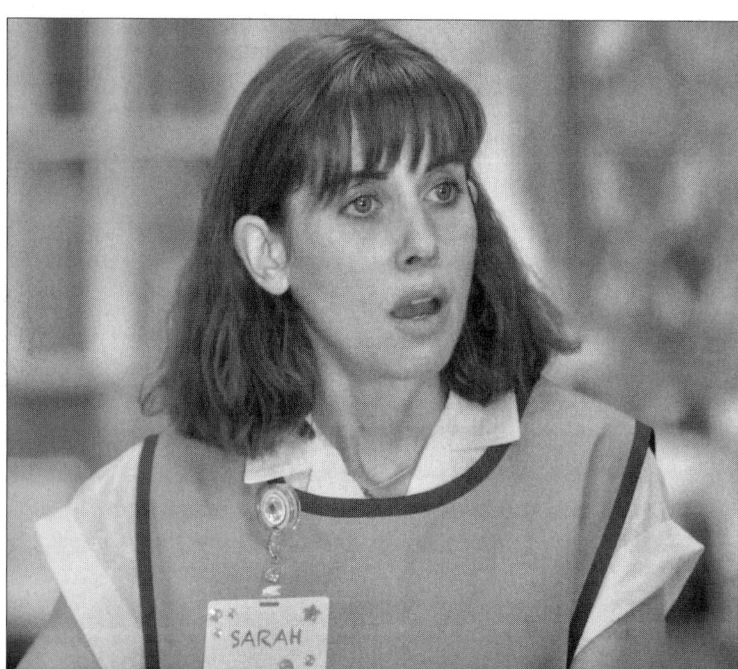

Figure 12.
Horse Girl (2020, Netflix). Produced by Jeff Baena, Alison Brie, Alana Carithers, Jay Duplass, et al. Directed by Jeff Baena.

polite young woman who works with her only friend, played by Molly Shannon, in a fabric store. Sarah loves horses and a crime show called *Purgatory*, and she attends Zumba classes, but otherwise does not have much of a life. She does have a kind roommate who tries to be helpful, but who cannot fathom why Sarah behaves so oddly. The roommate fixes Sarah up with her boyfriend's buddy, and Sarah and the boy develop a romantic connection. However, he also finds Sarah's fixation with *Purgatory* a bit strange, and he is frightened by her odd behavior and her absolute conviction that aliens exist and abduct people. Sarah is also quick to buy into Internet conspiracy theories. As the movie unfolds, we see Sarah unravel and become increasingly ill, and her father shares a family history of schizophrenia which has been hinted at but never explained.

Horse Girl was cowritten by Alison Brie and inspired by her own family history of mental illness. Her grandmother had been diagnosed with paranoid schizophrenia, and Brie herself has struggled with depression.

Delusional Disorders

Contrary to widespread belief, a delusional disorder is not synonymous with schizophrenia, it is not a subtype of schizophrenia, and hallucinations are not a predominant feature. Delusional disorder is, however, one of the less severe conditions on the schizophrenia spectrum. The delusions experienced by someone with a delusional disorder are not bizarre; instead, they involve situations of everyday life, such as being poisoned, followed, or loved, when in fact this is not happening. The delusions can be erotomanic, grandiose, jealous, persecutory, somatic, or a combination of these types. A person with delusional disorder can usually function well in their daily life.

Lars and the Real Girl (2007) is an exceptional portrayal of delusional disorder. Ryan Gosling portrays Lars, a taciturn, aloof young man who lives in a detached residence near his brother's family. Lars does everything he can to avoid social contact, intimacy, and conversation. One day he purchases a lifelike doll on the Internet, names her Bianca, and comes to believe Bianca is his actual girlfriend. He takes Bianca to parties, to church, and to family dinners, and he treats her with respect, telling her his innermost secrets and feelings. Interestingly, the small community decides to join Lars' delusion, talking to, spending time with, and even fighting over who will be able to interact with her. It is this community support that fosters Lars' connections with real people until he feels safe enough to let the delusion go.

In contrast to my belief that Lars meets the criteria for delusional disorder, psychologist Larry Leitner (2008), reviewing this movie for *PsycCRITIQUES*, argues that Lars is "a tender and decent man who probably would earn a DSM diagnosis of schizoid, avoidant, or perhaps even schizotypal personality disorder." (Part of the joy of watching films with mental health themes is debating differential diagnoses with your colleagues.) Leitner goes on to write,

> Through this relationship, he actually becomes at ease with people. The movie emphasizes two things that are critical in life-changing psychotherapy. First, others need to trust the client's innate self-healing potential. It also takes others who are willing to enter into and honor Lars's experiential world to allow for Lars to self-heal. If these others had lacked the ability to connect with Lars's experience, he would have been labeled psychotic, would have been given drugs, and easily could have never recovered. (Leitner, 2008)

A less powerful example of one or more characters who might meet criteria for delusional disorder (although more information is needed) is found in the film *Confessions of a Superhero* (2007). This independent film offers a glimpse into the lives of the characters who walk along the Hollywood Walk of Fame posing for pictures for tips, as characters such as Superman, Batman, Wonder Woman, and Hulk, Some of these individuals are aggressive and get arrested, such as Batman, portrayed by a man who has a secret past and may have worked for the mafia; the film shows Batman describing his problems with anger control, and some of his sessions with a psychiatrist are depicted. The man portraying Superman is shown to be obsessed with his character; he persistently believes he has a mother who was an actress who sent him to various psychiatric facilities; other characters are shown challenging this belief system.

In *The Truman Show* (1998), no psychotic disorders are portrayed. However, this Peter Weir movie is a useful teaching tool in understanding delusional disorders. It flips the essence of a delusion. The film is about the unreal life of Truman Burbank. Everything around him has been created for him (or, better stated, created for the public viewing his reality show) – all the people in the city, all the buildings, the streetlamps, the water, even the sun! It is all an extensive production set for a television show, yet Truman accepts his town of Seahaven as his reality; it is all he has known from birth to young adulthood. His name is appropriate as he is the only "true man" because everyone else, including his wife, best friend, mother, and father, are set actors. Eventually, Truman senses that he is trapped in a "world within a world" and tries to escape this contrived reality.

"We accept the reality with which the world is presented to us."

Christof (Ed Harris)
in *The Truman Show* (1998)

Imagine that there was no television show, and that Seahaven was like any other town; in this scenario, would Truman's behavior be seen as delusional? All of his behavior would be seen as paranoid: His questioning and threatening of his wife with a knife, his suspicious looking around the store, his pausing in the middle of the street and stopping traffic. Most of the world around him would be incorporated into his delusional framework. He would include various environmental elements in his delusions: The camera equipment that suddenly falls from the sky, the rainwater that just rains down on him and then follows him when he steps out of it, the observation of inconsistency in his wife's behavior. Further paranoid behaviors are exhibited when he follows his wife, and he questions whom he can trust. Truman explains that he believes his whole life is "building to something" and that he needs to escape to Fiji for a while. We would interpret this as delusional thinking. Instead, Truman does what a person with delusional disorder does not typically do. He challenges his own perception of reality, and this is what sets him free.

They Might Be Giants (1971) stars George C. Scott and Joanne Woodward. Scott's character is a man who just lost his wife; he copes by developing the delusion that he is Sherlock Holmes. Woodward plays a psychiatrist (named Watson!) who treats him by becoming his assistant.

Lucy in the Sky (2019) stars Natalie Portman as Lucy Cola, an astronaut who has seen Earth from space, and who can't adjust to normal life after returning to her NASA job and her family. The film is loosely based on the story of Lisa Nowak, a woman who attempted to kidnap another female astronaut after an affair with a NASA colleague fell apart. A psychiatrist who assessed Nowak offered diagnoses of bipolar disorder, obsessive-compulsive disorder, and Asperger's syndrome, but none of these seem as compelling as **delusional disorder, erotomanic type**. Students will learn more from reading about Lisa Nowak's life than from watching this film.

The Wonder (2022, Ireland) is a difficult film to classify because it involves multiple examples of pathology: anorexia, misuse of position and power, brother–sister incest, and parental neglect and abuse. However, there is also unambiguous evidence of a shared delusional disorder involving a religious theme, as so often occurs with such disorders (Hanevik et al., 2017).

The film revolves around a young girl in a remote Irish village who is alleged to have stopped eating four months earlier, subsisting solely on "manna from heaven" (see Exodus 16). An English nurse and a nun, also a nurse, are brought to the village by the town elders to witness the girl and document her condition (see Figure 13). An elderly physician has given her a potion that he believes to be a secret formula that eliminates the need for nutrition; a priest believes the girl's prolonged fast is evidence of a miracle. Eventually the girl's life is saved by the nurse (played by Florence Pugh). I won't spoil this complex and fascinating film with a plot summary, but it is highly recommended.

> **Nurse Wright: "She has anemia, dropsy, scurvy, pellagra ..."**
> **Dr. McBrearty: "You are a nurse. Please don't make a diagnosis. You're paid to watch, not to intervene ... you're overstepping, Madam."**
>
> **An arrogant physician berates a nurse desperately trying to save her patient's life, in *The Wonder***

Other Films Portraying Psychotic Disorders

People with schizophrenia spectrum disorders often get stereotyped as being the crazy person on the street, which generalizes to the misconception that all eccentric behavior is crazy. Films depict such instances with minor characters that may or may not have much impact on the plot, but nevertheless this misconception helps shape the stigma associated with mental illness. In *Cinema Paradiso* (1988), one man who appears to have schizophrenia makes a serious claim to a public square at a certain time each evening. Each day, he runs around a small area of the street he believes he owns, exclaiming, "The square is mine. It's twelve o'clock, the square is mine!" refusing to allow anyone to step into this area. Later in the film (many years later), he continues the behavior, claiming "It's my square. It's

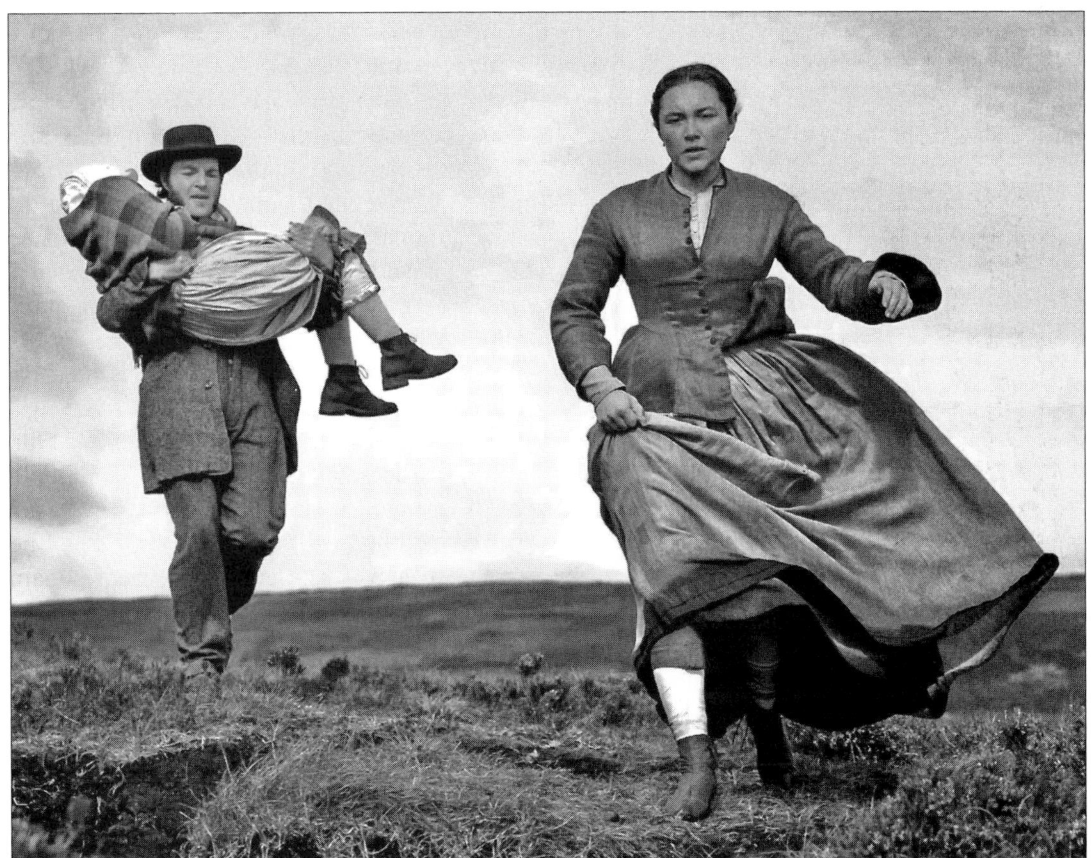

Figure 13. *The Wonder* (2022, Element Pictures, Element, Screen Ireland, House Productions). Produced by Len Blavatnik, Danny Cohen, Emma Donoghue, Ed Guiney, et al. Directed by Sebastián Lelio.

mine. The square is mine." Though these are not critical scenes in the film, the eccentricity and subsequent label do not go unnoticed by the viewer.

At times, the psychosis depicted in films is a brief break with reality (i.e., a **brief psychotic disorder**), often with an obvious trigger. Consider the Bernardo Bertolucci film *The Dreamers* (2003), in which a young man triangulates with a pair of enmeshed fraternal twins (male and female). At one point, when the young man and the female twin are about to have sex, she begins to hear her twin brother in the next room with another woman. She breaks with reality screaming to the young man, "Who are you? What are you doing in my room? Get out!" while pounding on her brother's wall. The next morning, after a restful sleep, she is coherent and once again oriented to reality. If her symptoms lasted longer than 1 day, she would be likely to receive a diagnosis of brief psychotic disorder. The experience of the female twin in *The Dreamers* is like the experience of a character in *Jesus of Montreal* (1989, Canada/France) who has a psychotic break in the subway, in which he suddenly begins to blurt random, abstract sentences to strangers and then passes out; in such cases, one would immediately wonder if there were an underlying medical cause for the syncopal episode.

Shared psychotic disorder (also called *folie à deux* [French for "a madness shared by two"]), a condition emphasized in DSM-IV but not included in DSM-5, occurs when an individual develops a delusion in the context of a close relationship with someone who already has a delusion. Shared psychotic disorder is seldom depicted in films; however, the film *Birth* (2004) is a notable exception. This independent film features Nicole Kidman as Anna, who encounters Sean, a young boy with the delusion that he is the incarnation of Anna's deceased husband. Anna is skeptical at first, but as she begins to spend time with Sean, she begins to believe him, sharing his delusion. Of course, no other characters believe this could be anything but a delusion, and the boy is later confronted by Anna's late husband's lover, who claims the husband would have sought out others first. This breaks the delusional framework – and the boy, who "only feels love" for Anna – disappointedly tells Anna he is not the husband. Her *folie à deux* no longer possible, Anna moves on with her life.

Another example of a film portraying *a folie à deux* is the independent film *Apart* (2011), in which a teenager coming out of a coma gets sucked into the delusional belief system of his girlfriend. *Who's Afraid of Virginia Woolf?* (1966) also portrays spouses who appear to have characteristics of a shared psychotic disorder involving a son who never existed.

Rahman et al. (2013) describe the case of infanticide of a 4-month-old infant by starvation and dehydration: "The mother suffered from schizoaffective disorder, and the father was diagnosed with shared psychotic disorder (*folie à deux*) by forensic assessment" (p. 1110).

John Cassavetes' film *A Woman Under the Influence* (1974) presents some challenging differential diagnosis questions. With Mabel Longhetti (Gena Rowlands), there is some evidence for **schizoaffective disorder,** as she is clearly not in touch with reality and has various mood problems; however, it is unclear whether she experiences her psychosis for more than 2 weeks without any mood symptoms. In addition, she meets a hallmark borderline personality criterion – an intense fear of abandonment – and she self-mutilates. She is called chronically nervous by others, including her own child, and an anxiety disorder diagnosis would have to be considered too. More information would be needed to be able to ensure a proper differential diagnosis.

Psychotic disorder due to a general medical condition can be seen in *Synecdoche, New York* (2008). Philip Seymour Hoffman portrays Caden Cotard (the name "Cotard" is a direct reference to Cotard's syndrome, a nihilistic or negation delusion). This is a rare neuropsychiatric disorder in which the individual holds a delusional belief that they are dead or do not exist. The character Cotard struggles with several existential, relationship, and life problems, bordering on the somatic and delusional, with accompanying mood disturbances. The actual diagnosis is not certain, due to the surrealistic filmmaking and complexly layered plot of filmmaker Charlie Kaufman.

There are a few **classic genre films** that portray schizophrenia spectrum disorders, and Martin Scorsese and Francis Ford Coppola have each directed numerous films over the decades that depict these disorders. Coppola's film *Apocalypse Now* (1979), which is a commentary on the conflicts in the human heart – rational versus irrational and good versus evil – stars Marlon Brando as the infamous Colonel Kurtz, an officer who drops out of the Vietnam War, takes the law into his own hands, and makes his home in the jungle. Kurtz is described throughout the film as "mad"; this label does not provide much information, but the viewer witnesses moments of insight and brilliance as well as psychosis in this character. Kurtz had witnessed terrible atrocities during the war, and he believed that such horrors could not be explained in words, noting: "Horror and moral terror are your friends. If they are not, they are enemies to be feared. They are truly enemies." His dying words are some of the most famous in movie history: "The horror, the horror."

Martin Scorsese directed *The King of Comedy* (1982), a dark comedy about a famous talk show host, Jerry Langford (Jerry Lewis), who is hounded by his fans.

> **"It's better to be king for a night than a schmuck for a lifetime."**
>
> **Robert DeNiro as Rupert Pupkin, in *The King of Comedy* (1982)**

The film focuses on two fans: the unknown stand-up comic Rupert Pupkin (Robert De Niro) and his friend (Sandra Bernhard). Pupkin is an obsessive, out-of-touch man who lives in a fantasy world filled with imaginary successes. His delusions become even more pronounced when he has a one-time, "forced" conversation in a cab with Jerry and convinces himself that this is evidence of a substantive and meaningful friendship. His delusions deepen, and he becomes motivated to do anything necessary to support and maintain his delusional beliefs (e.g., kidnapping Jerry).

Terry Gilliam's 1991 film *The Fisher King*, stars Robin Williams as Parry, an obsessed yet benign street person. Parry believes himself to be a knight whose mission is to save the Holy Grail. Throughout the film, Parry has several hallucinations, including seeing friendly "little people" who communicate with him regularly and give him guidance. The Red Knight is a frightening hallucination that appears at times of extreme stress or when he is reminded of his personal tragedy.

In *Sophie's Choice* (1982), Sophie (Meryl Streep), Nathan (Kevin Kline), and Stingo (Peter MacNicol) become inseparable friends, with Sophie and Nathan maintaining a turbulent romantic/sexual relationship, and Stingo eventually falling deeply in love with Sophie. Sophie and Stingo struggle to understand Nathan's eccentric, erratic behavior, which at various times involves intense love, suspiciousness, anger, hostility, and paranoia. Initially, Nathan merely is an unstable, "moody" person who claims to be a Harvard graduate and an overworked research biologist. As the story unfolds, the viewer learns that Nathan has been diagnosed with schizophrenia, and he is only marginally coping with life. His symptoms are exacerbated by amphetamines and cocaine, and his psychotic thinking leads to vicious accusations and unpredictable behavior. His bizarre behavior becomes more pronounced as his interpersonal stress increases and his denial is challenged. It is unclear how much Nathan's drug use influences his symptoms; if it were determined that his symptoms developed during or within a month of his substance intoxication or withdrawal, he would qualify for a **substance/medication-induced psychotic disorder** diagnosis.

One of the most vivid cinematic portrayals of psychiatric decompensation occurs in *The Caine Mutiny* (1954). Humphrey Bogart plays Lieutenant Commander Philip Francis Queeg, the obsessive-compulsive captain of a World War II destroyer. The ship's crew silently watches the deterioration that occurs as Queeg is put under increasing pressure, and eventually a junior officer, Lieutenant Barney Greenwald (José Ferrer), takes command. Greenwald is later court-martialed, and the film's most dramatic moment comes when Queeg cracks under the stress of the courtroom examination while playing with steel ball bearings, as he does when he is anxious.

> **"Ah, but the strawberries! That's, that's where I had them. They laughed at me and made jokes, but I proved beyond the shadow of a doubt, and with, with geometric logic, that, that a duplicate key to the wardroom icebox did exist."**
>
> **Captain Queeg in *The Caine Mutiny* (1954)**

Other films that illustrate psychotic disorders - some with more success than others - include *404* (2011), *Angels of the Universe* (2000), Lars von Trier's unforgettable film *Antichrist* (2009), *Deranged* (2012), *Lilith* (2011), *Pi* (1998), *Secret Window* (2004), *Some Voices* (2000), *The Experiment* (2010), *The Jacket* (2005), *The Number 23* (2007), *Gigantic* (2008), and *The Adopted One* (2020).

International Films: Schizophrenia and Other Psychotic Disorders

Oil on Water (2009, South Africa) explicitly deals with the ways in which schizophrenia spectrum disorder affects a loving relationship; the protagonist - an artist - begins to decompensate about halfway through film. We first become aware of his illness when we see Japanese masks on the wall begin to speak. The voices escalate and become increasingly **ego dystonic**. The protagonist has a loss of libido, experiences both hallucinations and delusions, and becomes suicidal. The film ends with some somber statistics: "Over 51 million people in the world suffer from schizophrenia. More than 50% will attempt suicide at least once. Between 10 and 15% will succeed."

Two films from South Korea are particularly noteworthy for their portrayal of mental illness: *Save the Green Planet* (2003) and *I'm a Cyborg, But That's OK* (2006). In the former, a young man pursues individuals he perceives are aliens that come from Andromeda, and he must stop them from destroying the planet. He and his girlfriend capture these individuals and torture them; by doing so, he believes he is taking away their powers by going after their "sensitive zones" (eyes, feet, and genitals) and by limiting their telepathy (which aliens do through their hair). He is genuinely convinced that he is heroic and saving humans. He experiences several **ideas of influence** as seen in his correspondence with the aliens. In *I'm a Cyborg, But That's OK*, a young woman, Young-goon, is admitted to a psychiatric institution. She embodies a delusion that she is a cyborg and frequently communicates with clocks and vending machines. She refuses to eat, believing she will break down if she eats. She wears her dead grandmother's dentures to communicate and feels she must kill the staff, so she imagines shooting the doctors, nurses, and hospital staff with guns that are her fingers. In the memorable opening scene, while working on an assembly line, Young-goon matter-of-factly follows what her auditory hallucinations ("a broadcast") say to her - she cuts her arm, put wires in it, and then plugs the wires into the wall. The film also touches on the origins of Young-goon's psychosis: Her grandmother, also treated for schizophrenia, thought she was a mother-mouse caring for several baby mice and ate a diet of only radishes.

The depiction in *I'm a Cyborg, But That's OK* is a good illustration of the power of psychotic beliefs and the futility of a helping professional in challenging such beliefs when the professional is contending with the client's psychosis, culture-bound issues (the secrecy and shame of such beliefs thus leading to a lack of disclosure, as evidenced in this film), mutism, and the client's own lack of awareness of her own beliefs and their impact. Surprisingly, most of the psychological jargon and diagnoses are accurate in the film. As is the case for most films portraying psychiatric hospital wards, the portrayal of the psychiatric patients suggests that people with mental illness are wild and crazy, with some rolling around on the floor. It raises the question, should the emphasis of such films be to educate the viewer or help the viewer to better empathize? This film emphasizes the dramatic, the interesting, and the eccentric, revealing the character's innermost, highly distorted delusional beliefs; this helps the viewer empathize with the character, but the film sacrifices an opportunity to educate the viewer about the realities of mental illness and its treatment.

He Loves Me, He Loves Me Not (2002, France) might be the most effective and clear-cut use of the cinema to depict a **delusional disorder**. It is the directorial debut of French director Laetitia Colombani. First, viewers are completely taken in as they see reality from Angelique's (*Amélie's* Audrey Tautou) perception of her blossoming love relationship with a man named Loic. Midway through, the film rewinds, flashes back to the beginning, and then gives us the vantage point of Loic, who is a married doctor who barely knows Angelique exists. It is only as the second half of the film unfolds that the viewer can then backtrack in their mind to remember how Angelique perceived the relationship and compare that with what Loic sees and experiences. It is the latter that becomes reality. Thus, the viewer eventually realizes everything in the first half of the film is Angelique's delusion. The viewer learns she obsessively calls Loic, leaving multiple messages. Her obsessions with drawings, following him around, and writing notes, all reinforce and maintain her delusional framework.

The delusional person can readily function in society, as shown with Angelique taking care of her house, working a regular job, wearing appropriate attire, and communicating with others around her. Without knowing her thinking, we would not know she is delusional, particularly with her very sweet, often smiling, and innocent presentation. The film also depicts the risk in breaking the framework of a person's delusional mindset. It is here we see the stereotype of the violent psychiatric patient, as Angelique takes on the frame of mind "if I can't have him, no one will" and attempts to murder two innocent people.

"We all dream of a great love affair. I just dreamed a little harder."

Angélique describes her infatuation with her married physician lover, in *He Loves Me, He Loves Me Not*

Many films are ambiguous in their portrayal of delusional disorder, and they leave the viewer confused about whether the disorder is real or whether the character is simply idiosyncratic or eccentric. However, *He Loves Me, He Loves Me Not* is not at all ambiguous. The film maintains an honest and clear narrative about the disorder and stays with its purpose in showing drastically different truths, where one side is much "more real" than the other. Angelique's diagnosis of **delusional disorder, erotomanic type** is discussed in the end when she is taken to a psychiatric hospital. The filmmakers knew what they specifically wanted to achieve with this deeply psychological film, and they accomplished it.

The film *11'09"01 - September 11* (2002, UK/France/Egypt/Japan/Mexico/US/Iran) is what followed when producer Alain Brigand proposed to 11 renowned directors to each "create a film lasting eleven minutes, nine seconds and one frame - September 11 - around the events of September 11 and their consequences" (Spirituality & Practice, n.d.). He asked them to look toward their own cultures, memories, stories, and language in constructing their short film segments. The filmmakers include directors from Bosnia-Herzegovina, India, the United States, Japan, Egypt, Mexico, Iran, the United Kingdom, France, West Africa, and Israel. In one segment, Japanese director Shohei Imamura depicts a man who heads off to war as a soldier and returns home as a snake (in human form). He maintains and embodies this severe, bizarre delusion, slithering around, hissing like a snake, biting the woman who feeds him, and eating a live rat. He is eventually kept in a cage and then forced out of the home. Before slithering into a body of water, he is asked, "Does being a man disgust you that much?" In a terrifying and poignant way, this simple question (and the psychosis) speaks to the horror of war.

House of Fools (2002) is a Russian-Chechnyan film based on a true story. Set in 1996, during the first Chechen war, the film depicts a psychiatric hospital on the border of a war-torn area. The hospital staff flees due to conflict in Chechnya, leaving the patients to fend for themselves. Soldiers find refuge in the hospital and interact with the patients. As with most films depicting psychiatric institutions, there is a hodgepodge of psychopathology depicted. One patient, Jana, has hallucinations (or are they daydreams?) of herself in a video that portrays the famous singer Bryan Adams, who appears in the film as himself, often singing the lyrics "have you ever really loved a woman?" Jana has a **delusional disorder, erotomanic type**, as she believes Bryan Adams is her fiancé and that he is in love with her. Her room is covered in Bryan Adams posters. In a later scene, she naïvely believes the mock marriage proposal made to her by a soldier seeking refuge. Soon she finds herself in a bind, struggling to choose between the deceptive soldier and the delusion of Bryan Adams. In one scene, Jana is gripping broken glass so hard that her hand becomes cut and bloodied. She uses a fantasy of Bryan Adams to cope with the pain. Jana denies her illness, telling people she was once sick but is not anymore. Furthermore, she believes she is a teacher for her fellow patients, teaching them yoga and how to play the accordion. Jana tries to help other patients when they make mistakes or need guidance. Cinematically, the viewer sees her reality of bright colors and light where the staff and patients are dancing to her music. This cinematic technique – weaving from patient perception to reality – is used frequently in the film. Other patients include a person with delusions, a psychotic fire starter, a psychotic transvestite, a psychotic midget, and a person who is catatonic.

Something Like Happiness (2005, Czech Republic) portrays the complex dynamics among three adults who are friends from childhood: Tonik, Monika, and Dasha. A single mother of two, Dasha deteriorates into psychosis, neglects her children, and is only concerned about having a male companion. She is admitted to a psychiatric ward and becomes determined to become pregnant. In an upsetting scene, Dasha, upon being released from the ward, goes to her friend's home where her children have been properly cared for and interrupts the children's special party, grabbing them, forcing them into her car, and refusing to let them get their belongings.

Werner Herzog's *Aguirre, the Wrath of God* (1972, West Germany/Peru/Mexico) shows the Spanish conquistadors' search for the mythic treasure of El Dorado deep in the Amazon reaches of Peru. Aguirre is a defiant, competitive, powermonger who leads a mutiny. During long, fruitless journeys in the jungle, he loses touch with reality and develops a **delusional disorder, grandiose type**. His appearance becomes boggy eyed, shaky, hypervigilant, and preoccupied. Aguirre's grandiosity continues to increase as he speaks of getting larger ships for bigger conquests. He shows a blatant disregard for his men's needs and leads them to suffering and destruction. At one point he exclaims, "I, the wrath of God, will marry my own daughter," and speaks of ruling with her.

> **"If I, Aguirre, want the birds to drop dead from the trees then the birds will drop dead from the trees. I am the wrath of God. The earth I walk upon sees me and quakes. But whoever follows me and the river will win untold riches."**
>
> **Aguirre's delusions of grandeur in *Aguirre, the Wrath of God* (1972)**

As previously noted, filmmakers often link violence and psychosis. *Rampo Noir* (2005, Japan) is a collection of four short, surreal horror films – *Mars's Canal*, *Mirror Hell*, *Caterpillar*, and *Crawling Bugs* – which are adaptations and tributes to the Japanese poet Rampo. Each gives a distinct perspective on violence and a disturbing environment or situation relating to hell. Since each has a strong surreal component, they also provide unique perspectives on mental illness, violence, and psychosis. *Mars's Canal* uses no sound, except for static, and creates intentional defects in the visual image. The viewer sees surrealist images of a naked man along a landscape, violence with a naked woman, and darkness slowly creeping over a character's face (e.g., to show the slow deterioration that is often associated with mental illness). This segment ends with a quote from Rampo: "Reality is seen in dreams. What you dream at night is real." Another character portraying a link between psychosis and violence is the thief in *The Cook, the Thief, His Wife & Her Lover* (1989; see the section Violence in International Films: Violence and Physical and Sexual Abuse, in Chapter 15).

An Angel at My Table (1990), Jane Campion's film biography of New Zealand writer Janet Frame, is a compelling story of misdiagnosis and malpractice. Frame, an awkward, anxious, and socially inept adolescent, is misdiagnosed as having schizophrenia after an apparent panic attack, and winds up receiving shock treatment and being hospitalized for 8 years. She narrowly avoided receiving a frontal lobotomy, a popular treatment at the time.

Crimson Gold (2003, Iran) illustrates themes of classism, highlighting the distance and tension between the wealthy and the poor in modern-day Iran. Hussein is a taciturn pizza delivery man who delivers pizza to both rich and poor; however, when he is treated poorly and rejected – both when wearing a suit and tie and when dressed more casually – by a jewelry store manager, he explodes. It is interesting to note that in real life the lead actor had been diagnosed with schizophrenia; this is never mentioned or explicitly portrayed in the film, but it potentially helps account for the uncanny accuracy of the character's flat affect and distant behavior.

The disturbing film *Dogtooth* (2009, Greece) portrays a psychotic family. The spouses share their psychosis (i.e., they have a **shared psychotic disorder**), and their odd beliefs have a dramatic impact on their three children. The various characters all exhibit absurd, shocking, psychopathic, incestuous, and odd behavior. The film begins with the children listening to an audiotape of someone teaching a foreign language, but the words are being taught incorrectly. The parents teach the incorrect meaning of words throughout the film (e.g., "pussy" is a "bright light," and "zombie" is "a small yellow flower"). The children then begin a "game" of endurance in which each puts their finger under hot water, and the last to pull away is the winner. The father then blindfolds a security guard and drives her to the family home to engage in paid sex with his son (later in the film when this woman is killed, the father has his son fondle the son's two sisters to decide which one the son wants as a sexual partner). The father returns home from work in clothes he has deliberately tattered and colored with red food coloring and tells the family that a dangerous (domestic) cat in the neighborhood is attacking and killing people; the family then get on their knees and bark like dogs. One of the children, caught between reality and delusion, believes that to escape from the house she must extract a tooth (referred to as "the dogtooth"), and she smashes herself repeatedly in the face with a heavy barbell to extract the tooth. The film clearly depicts psychopathology and its impact on children and their development. Viewers who can handle consistently disturbing behavior may learn something from this film; however, it is not recommended for classroom teaching.

Although I believe students can learn much about psychopathology from watching international films, I am also sympathetic to the ideas Ethan Watters eloquently expressed in his book *Crazy Like Us: The Globalization of the American Psyche* (Watters, 2010). Watters argues that in addition to exporting movies and junk food, we have exported a model of mental illness that is inappropriate for much of the world.

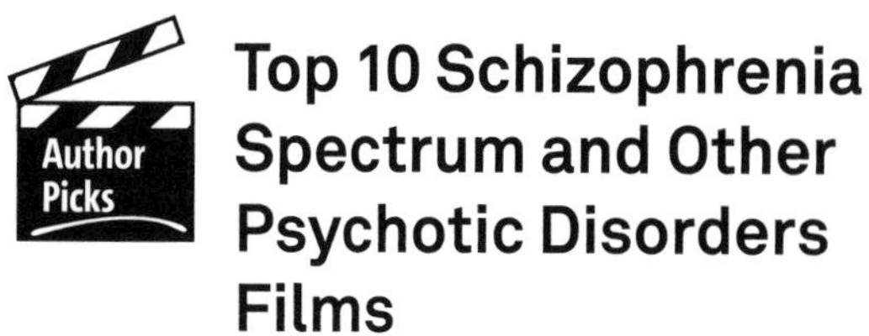

Top 10 Schizophrenia Spectrum and Other Psychotic Disorders Films

A Beautiful Mind (2001)
Clean, Shaven (1993)
Shine (1996)
Revolution #9 (2001)
Spider (2002)
He Loves Me, He Loves Me Not (2002, France)
Canvas (2006)
Lars and the Real Girl (2007)
The Soloist (2009)
Take Shelter (2011)

Chapter 4

Bipolar and Depressive Disorders

They call me Luna. Because my mind moves in tune with the lunar shifts. They call me a lunatic ... because my biological clock's a time bomb that ticks down to the minute the full moon's lit. And I just got out of the loony bin, and I haven't been taking my medication, so I'm about as unstable as if nitro raped glycerin. More insane than Batman's Riddler if Jim Carrey had played him without taking his Ritalin. I'll leave you riddles sicker than a crossword puzzle written by Jack the Ripper.

Marco rapping in group therapy, in *Touched With Fire*

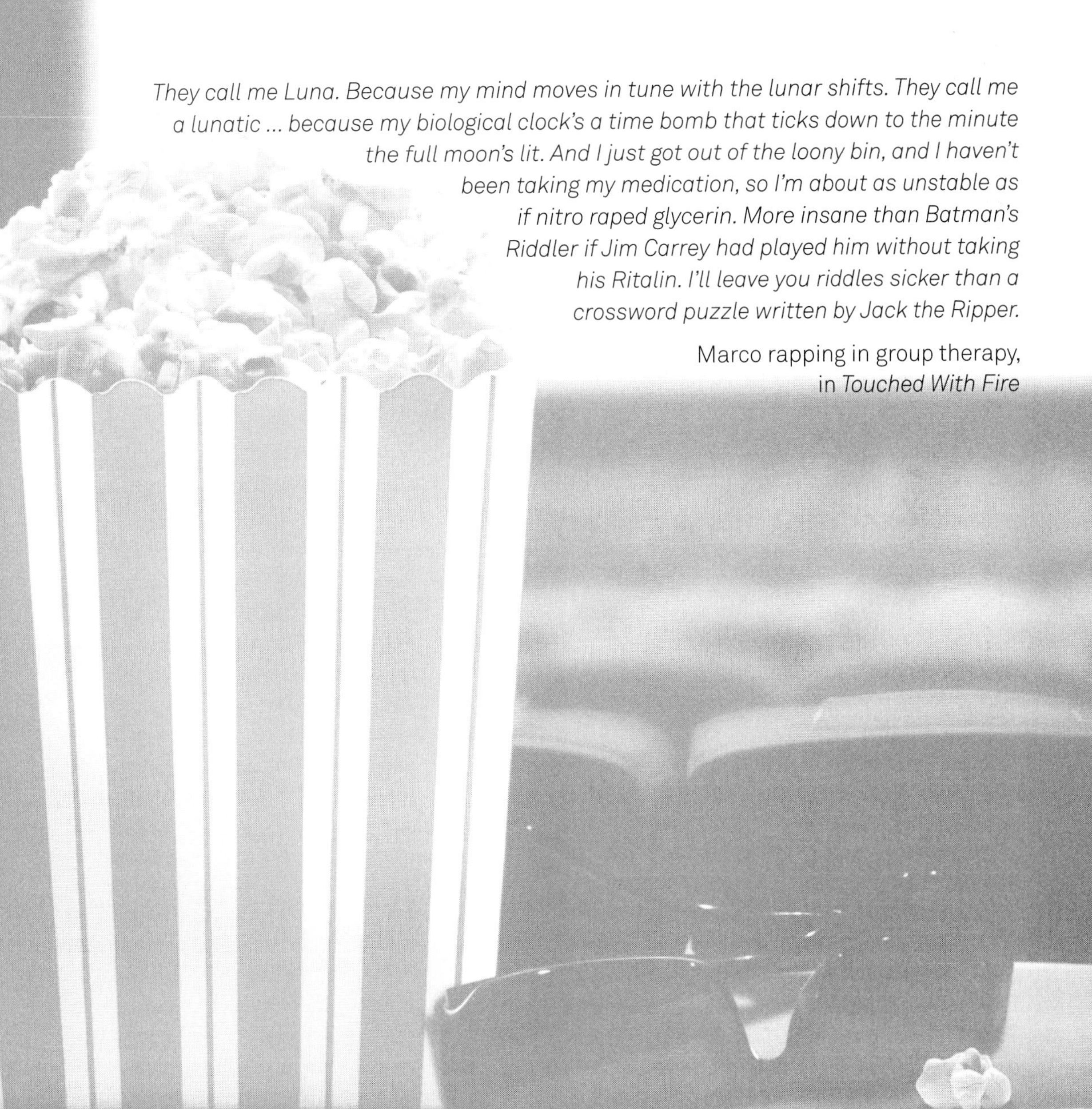

Depressive and Bipolar Disorders

Periods of depression are normal in most persons' lives. For example, failing an examination or the ending of a relationship often precipitates a predictable period of sadness. In addition, the feelings of high energy that accompany major events such as graduation or marriage are also common in everyday life. However, some illnesses involve affective states that resemble these normal periods of depression or elation, but they are different. The individual experiencing a mood disorder is consumed by negative emotions and is unable to alleviate them through normal coping mechanisms. These illnesses are characterized by emotions that are so intense they begin to dominate a person's life. Mood disorders include many different cognitive, emotional, and behavioral manifestations, but the overriding symptoms of all mood disorders are *emotional* in nature. The DSM-5 categorizes types of mood disorders in separate chapters, specifically as **bipolar and related disorders** (bipolar I, bipolar II, or cyclothymic) or as **depressive disorders** (disruptive mood dysregulation disorder, major depressive disorder, persistent depressive disorder [dysthymia], and premenstrual dysphoric disorder). As with all DSM-5 diagnoses, there are also diagnoses provided in both categories for substance/medication-induced, due to another medical condition, and other specified and unspecified disorders. Sadness, irritability, and somatic/cognitive changes that impact functioning are common features of both bipolar and depressive disorders; however, these categories of disorders differ from one another in their duration, timing, and etiology.

Depressive Disorders

Depressive disorders, one of the most common types of mental disorders, occur in approximately one in 10 adults in the United States each year. Most surveys show that depression is 2 to 3 times more prevalent in women, and the disorder is most common among young adults and adolescents (Goodwin et al., 2022). There is a relationship between depressive disorders and social class, and depressive symptoms are more common in individuals with fewer economic advantages.

A **major depressive disorder** is associated with depressed mood and a loss of interest or pleasure in daily activities. Sleep, eating habits, appetite, concentration, motivation, self-esteem, and energy level are the behaviors most often affected. An episode can range from mild (few symptoms) to severe, and in some instances major depressive episodes can be accompanied by delusions and hallucinations. Some people experience a **masked depression** in which they unconsciously mask their depression and experience physical aches and pains rather than traditional depressive symptoms. These physical manifestations of depression are often misdiagnosed as physical illnesses. Others experience an **agitated depression** where frustration and anger seem to dominate and cover up depressive symptoms. If chronically depressed moods, low self-esteem, and feelings of pessimism, despair, or hopelessness are present for 2 years without suicidal thoughts or limitations in functioning, the diagnosis of **persistent depressive disorder** is made. (This condition is still widely diagnosed as **dysthymia.**) While the diagnosis of major depressive disorder requires symptoms that last for at least a 2-week period, the diagnosis of persistent depressive disorder requires a history of depressed mood that has lasted for at least 2 years.

Touched With Fire (2015)

Touched With Fire (2015) stars Katie Holmes as Carla, and Luke Kirby as Marco, two deeply troubled poets who meet as inpatients in a psychiatric hospital. Carla has admitted herself accidentally, and she is dismayed to discover that she cannot simply discharge herself after a day of observation. Marco has been involuntarily admitted by his father. Both Carla and Marco have

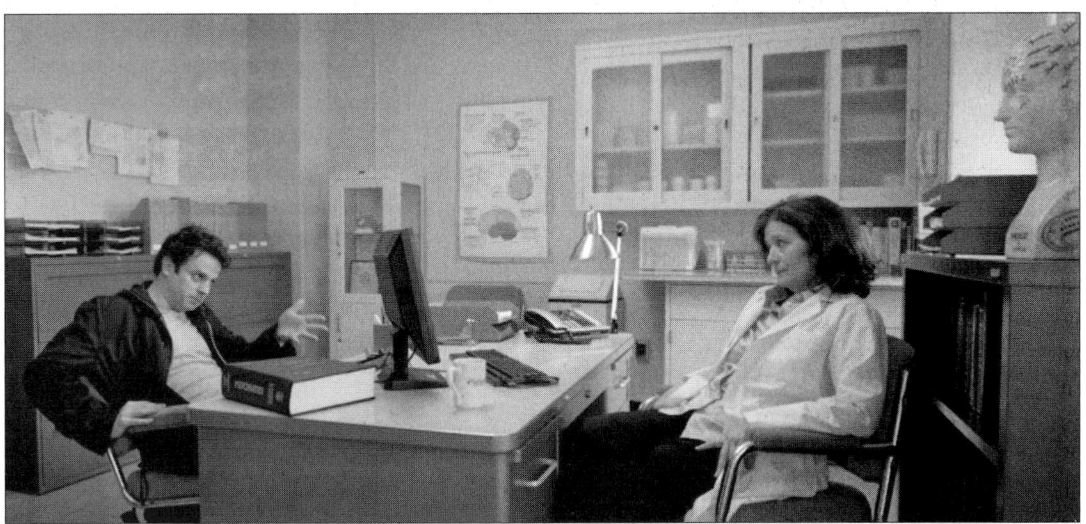

Figure 14. *Touched With Fire* (2015, 40 Acres & a Mule Filmworks). Produced by Jeremy Alter, Katie Holmes, Avy Kaufman, Spike Lee, et al. Directed by Paul Dalio.

a diagnosis of bipolar disorder, and they are on a ward with others with a similar diagnosis. Figure 14 show's Marco's intake interview (note the copy of Kaplan and Sadock's *Comprehensive Textbook of Psychiatry* sitting on the psychiatrist's desk).

Initially, the two poets do not get along; however, they soon begin having clandestine meetings late at night – neither can sleep – and their initial tension blossoms into romance. They eventually marry, and Carla becomes pregnant; however, she decides to have an abortion and leaves Marco after an argument in which he physically abuses her, and it becomes clear that he is not going to continue to take his medication. They have an amicable reunion at the end of the film when they meet in a bookstore for a joint poetry reading. The film is highly recommended for anyone interested in the relationship between bipolar disorder and creativity.

The Beaver (2011)

Jodie Foster directed *The Beaver,* and she costars with Mel Gibson, playing a supportive wife who has reached her wits end with her profoundly depressed husband (Gibson, playing the role of Walter Black). She kicks him out of the house, and he goes to a hotel where he becomes quite drunk and makes two suicide attempts; one attempt involves hanging himself from a shower curtain rod, and the other involves an attempt to jump from the balcony of his hotel. Both attempts failed, in part because of his profound intoxication. Walter has maintained a positive relationship with his youngest son, but his older adolescent son is estranged and hostile toward his father. Walter stops going to therapy and adopts a radical treatment plan for his depression: He stops speaking for himself and only communicates with others through a hand puppet (the Beaver; see Figure 15). The puppet has a different accent, a keen sense of humor, and it is decidedly upbeat and optimistic. The puppet berates Walter for his depression and his low energy; with encouragement from this **alter ego,** representing that part of Walter that wanted to get well, the protagonist proceeds to put his life back together. However, in a dramatic and surprising ending to the film, Walter severs his relationship with the Beaver by cutting off his arm with a buzz saw, finally realizing that he has always had the internal resources necessary for him to overcome his illness. This film was used as the exemplar for bipolar and depressive disorders in an earlier edition of *Movies and Mental Illness.*

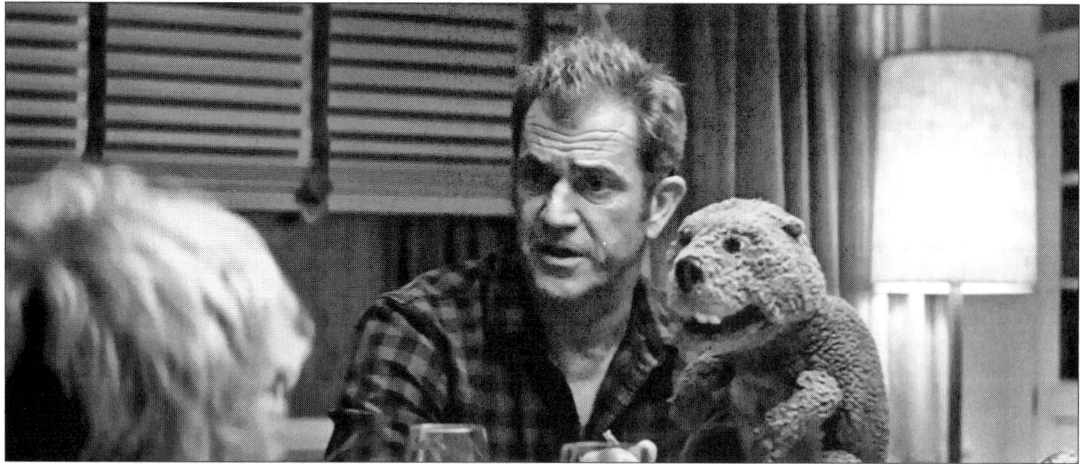

Figure 15. *The Beaver* (2011, Summit Entertainment, Participant Media). Produced by Steve Golin, Keith Redmon, and Ann Ruark. Directed by Jodie Foster.

> **"We reach a point where, in order to go on, we have to wipe the slate clean. We start to see ourselves as a box that we're trapped inside and no matter how we try and escape, self-help, therapy, drugs, we just sink further and further down. The only way to truly break out of the box is to get rid of it all together ... Starting over isn't crazy. Crazy is being miserable and walking around half asleep, numb, day after day after day. Crazy is pretending to be happy. Pretending that the way things are is the way they have to be for the rest of your bleeding life. All the potential, hope, all that joy, feeling, all that passion that life has sucked out of you. Reach out, grab a hold of it and snatch it back from that bloodsucking rabble."**
>
> **Walter Black in *The Beaver* (2011)**

Other Films Portraying Depression

Excellent portrayals of depression can be found in *Mind the Gap* (2004) and *Shopgirl* (2005). The first film interweaves several vignettes of characters honestly and earnestly struggling to change their lives. In one vignette, an African American man is clearly depressed, with considerable evidence of suppressed anger. He sits around watching television all day in his lonely apartment. He is riddled with guilt for having cheated on his wife and abandoned his son. He purchases a shotgun at a store and writes a suicide note telling his son that the son is not to blame. However, before pulling the trigger, he consults a priest who gives him some wise advice on the distinction between saying "I'm sorry" and asking, "Will you forgive me?"; the man then travels to speak face-to-face with both his ex-wife and his son to ask for their forgiveness in two powerful scenes. *Shopgirl*, based on actor–screenwriter Steve Martin's novella, is another film that offers a realistic, nonstereotyped portrayal of depression. In this film, a young, isolated, depressed woman, Mirabelle, falls in love with an older man; the film uses muted colors and positions Mirabelle's workstation in a way that highlights her isolation from the other workers.

In *American Splendor* (2003), comic strip writer Harvey Pekar (Paul Giamatti) displays the symptoms and behaviors associated with persistent depressive disorder. His dysthymia is expressed through agitation and negativity, and he kicks and breaks objects and sees life through a very pessimistic filter, frequently describing himself as "a nobody." He has a chronically furrowed brow that emphasizes his agitated affect and frustrated view of the world.

Harvey has few social skills; he is socially distant, unfriendly, and awkward, and acts inappropriately and has poor eye contact. Despite success with his comic books, he remains cynical and pessimistic; this theme is emphasized when he repeatedly appears on the David Letterman Show and comes across as a defensive misanthrope. Harvey denies having any sense of spirituality. He is lonely and makes a quick decision to marry after one meeting with a woman who travels from out of state to visit him; to the viewer, it seems obvious that these are two lonely people covering up their pain. Nevertheless, Harvey seems to have found a good match in his wife (Hope Davis) who also has a dysthymic quality; she is easily agitated, highly somatic, pessimistic, and suffers from hypersomnia.

Various coping strategies are exhibited in the film. When diagnosed with cancer, Harvey explores creative expression of the disease through comics. Responding in a less healthy way, Harvey exhibits characteristics of **hoarding disorder**: His home is dirty and cluttered; there are stacks of comic books everywhere; and he regularly goes to thrift stores and garage sales to acquire more "stuff."

In the emotionally intense *Monster's Ball* (2001), Hank (Billy Bob Thornton) and Leticia (Halle Berry) are two lost, self-hating people who become even more lonely and raw after each loses an only child – Hank's son commits suicide in front of him, and Leticia's son is hit by a car. Both parents had been physically and verbally abusive to their sons as they attempted to work through their inner turmoil and struggles. The film emphasizes how both characters are trying to escape from their internal hell; in some ways, the prison in which Hank works is a metaphor for their inner pain, loneliness, isolation, and futility. Hank quits his job at the prison, where he works with death row inmates, realizing the emotional toll his job has taken on his personal life. A relationship between the racist Hank and the beautiful Black woman Leticia begins, following an act of kindness by Hank when he aids a screaming Leticia he finds on the side of the road; he explains that he just felt like "doing the right thing" and that he is trying to get "outside of his insides." After becoming drunk, Hank and Leticia engage in raw, uninhibited sex "just to feel." Both are emotionally numb and overwhelmed by their personal pain; scenes of the two lovers interacting are juxtaposed with flashes of human hands reaching into a cage to release a bird desperately flapping its wings. Through their connection, which becomes more intimate and genuine over time, both characters find meaningful, expressive outlets for their depression, for the first time. Halle Berry won an academy award for best actress in a leading role for her portrayal of Leticia.

The Cooler (2003) is about Bernie (William H. Macy), an "unlucky" man, who works for a traditional, antisocial casino boss (Alec Baldwin). Bernie's job is walking around successful casino patrons to bring them bad luck. Bernie is "the cooler" because he turns winners into losers; his appearance at a table is enough to make a winning gambler quickly go bankrupt. He claims he can do this easily; "I just be myself." He is stuck in the past and trapped by it, unable to move on, since he is forced to use his "bad luck" to pay off his extensive gambling debt or be killed by the casino boss. When we look deeper beyond the plot, the viewers see that Bernie's personality is very self-critical, self-defeating, and negativistic. His "unlucky" quality is a self-fulfilling prophecy. He is isolated, lives alone, and is too passive to change his life.

The Cooler presents a classic **depressive triad**: The protagonist is *hapless* (unlucky), *hopeless*, and *helpless*. A cognitive therapy approach emphasizing the impact of one's thoughts, beliefs, and attitudes as affecting mood states is highlighted. Upon falling in love, Bernie's luck changes, he becomes assertive, and his presence at casino tables enhances the success of others. The power of attitude is an overriding theme in the film, and we see Bernie's negative attitude keeping him from love and luck, while positive attitudes bring him good luck and success.

In many ways, the story is clichéd – the fight for love to the death, escape from a tyrannical boss, and tremendous luck in the end save the heroes from their inevitable demise.

In *Scent of a Woman* (1992), Lieutenant Colonel Frank Slade exhibits many of the classic symptoms of a major depressive disorder and clearly would qualify for the diagnosis. He has both a depressed mood and a loss of interest and pleasure in everyday activities (**anhedonia**). Slade's angry comment "I have no life, I'm in the dark" clearly suggests his depression is related to his blindness, and the sentence captures the lack of meaning and purpose in his life. His daily activities, sitting alone and drinking himself into oblivion when he is not tormenting his 4-year-old niece, are clear indications of his loss of interest in life. It is a useful pedagogical exercise to list the numerous risk factors for suicide present in the character of Frank Slade.

Some people who are depressed are not pleasant and can be quite difficult to be around. They are often agitated and easily angered. This serves to hide their underlying need for help. Colonel Slade is irritable, intimidating, and verbally abusive to anyone who approaches him. Expression of this type of anger and abuse has a distancing effect on others, who naturally withdraw from unpleasant situations. Charles Simms, a college student hired to accompany the Colonel on a trip, does not want to stay with Slade after meeting him, and Simms dreads the weekend he is forced to spend with the Colonel.

Another interesting film depicting depression is the 1971 Academy Award–winning film *The Hospital* starring George C. Scott as Herbert Bock, a middle-aged, depressed, suicidal physician who is trying to cope with the mayhem of a crowded and disorganized institution, where negligence and confusion result in a series of deaths. Bock's personal life is as chaotic as the hospital he runs. He is recently divorced, alienated from his children, and suffering from both personal and sexual impotence. He had been believed to be a medical genius in his early career; however, at the point we are introduced to him in the film, he is washed up and discouraged. At one point in the film, Bock is seen sitting in his office, preparing to inject a fatal dose of potassium. He exclaims: "I've lost my reason for being ... my purpose!" and later when he is upset and drinking: "People are sicker than ever. We cure nothing. We heal nothing."

Bock demonstrates the classical symptoms of a major depressive disorder. His depressed mood is expressed through his explosive angry episodes and chronic irritability. He is **anhedonic** and expresses little interest in his patients, his profession, or any of the activities of daily living through which most of us find meaning and purpose. Bock cannot sleep, he feels worthless, and he is plagued by recurrent thoughts of suicide. Dr. Bock's behavior is remarkably like that of Lt. Colonel Slade – it is similar because both men are clinically depressed.

Marlon Brando plays a depressed man trying to come to grips with the meaning of his wife's suicide in Bernado Bertolucci's powerful film *Last Tango in Paris* (1972). The character of the coach's wife in Peter Bogdanovich's *The Last Picture Show* (1971) is clearly depressed, and her affect and behavior offer good teaching examples of depressed affect for students learning how to give a mental status examination. The despair that overcomes a man when he is abandoned by his wife is presented in the Australian film *My First Wife* (1984). Finally, Joanne Woodward gives a memorable performance as a depressed housewife in *Summer Wishes, Winter Dreams* (1973).

I highly recommend *Prozac Nation* (2001) as a film that illustrates the devastation caused by depression in a gifted but deeply troubled Harvard freshman (Lizzie) played by Christina Ricci. The film presents a compelling portrayal of Lizzie's slow descent into depression, and Lizzie provides an insightful description of her illness.

> Hemingway has this classic moment in *The Sun Also Rises* when someone asks Mike Campbell how he went bankrupt. All he can say is, "gradually, then suddenly." That's how depression hits. You wake up one morning afraid that you're going to live. (Lizzie, in the film *Prozac Nation*, 2001)

Lizzie knows she needs medication, but she also knows that it is not sufficient to solve her myriad personal problems. At one point she states, "I call this the crack-house where I come to score. Dr.

Sterling is my dealer. Seems like everyone's doctor is dealing this stuff now. Sometimes it feels like we're all living in a Prozac nation."

> **"If only my life could be more like the movies. I want an angel to swoop down to me like he does to Jimmy Stewart in *It's a Wonderful Life* and talk me out of suicide. I've always waited for that one moment of truth to set me free and change my life forever. But he won't come. It doesn't happen that way."**
>
> **Lizzie in *Prozac Nation* (2001)**

The Visitor (2007), directed by Tom McCarthy, is a sensitive portrayal of the human suffering associated with social isolation and with the restrictive immigration policies in the United States. The film stars Richard Jenkins as a depressed and ineffectual college professor who has never recovered from the death of his wife. Jenkins' character, Prof. Walter Vale, makes a half-hearted attempt to learn to play the piano, but lacks the energy, passion, and talent necessary to succeed at this task. Watching Vale interact with his colleagues and students reminds the viewer of Hamlet's lament, "O God, O God, how weary, stale, flat, and unprofitable seem to me all the uses of this world!" Vale's life has become weary, stale, flat, and unprofitable, and he finds meaning, purpose and some degree of contentment only when he stops contemplating his own unhappiness and becomes invested in helping a pair of undocumented workers, he finds living in his infrequently used New York City apartment. Walter's transition from a staid, discouraged, and unhappy college professor to someone genuinely interested in life and in others is symbolized by the transition from his desultory attempt to learn to play classical music on the piano, to his enthusiasm for the *djembe* (an African drum that he passionately plays in the subway in the film's last moments). The film illustrates both persistent depressive disorder and burnout, and it is a convincing demonstration of the therapeutic truism that one helps oneself most by learning to reach out and help others.

In *Manchester by the Sea* (2016), Casey Affleck stars as a depressed man working as a janitor in Boston after losing his children in a house fire he could have prevented. When his older brother dies, Affleck's character must take over raising his teenage nephew. This involves returning to Manchester, the home of his former wife and the site where his children died. The film is heartbreaking, and it perfectly captures the despair felt by people who lose their children.

Three Identical Strangers (2018) is a remarkable documentary-biography that chronicles the lives of triplets separated at birth and sent to live with different adoptive parents. By chance, two of the twins wind up at the same college, and quickly realize they are related. After learning

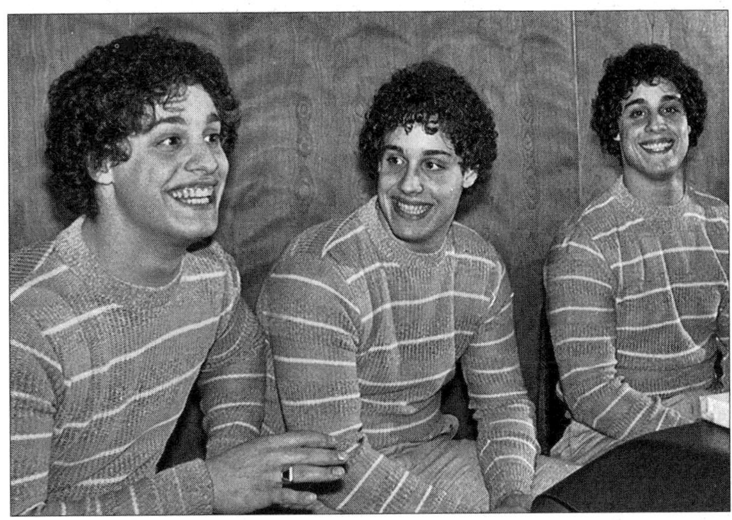

Figure 16.
Three Identical Strangers (2018, RAW). Produced by Tom Barry, Louise Dew, Poppy Dixon, Dimitri Doganis, et al. Directed by Tim Wardle.

about the reunion of the two college students, the third brother realizes he is also related and contacts the first two. Although the three are often seen in the film laughing and joking, there is a dark side to the story (see Figure 16). Their separation was planned and engineered by an unethical Yale psychologist working with a Jewish adoption agency; the psychologist, Dr. Peter Neubauer, wanted to do the definitive study of nature versus nurture. All three triplets struggled with depression, and one of them committed suicide. The research was profoundly unethical, rivaling the Tuskegee syphilis experiment, a study in which Black men with syphilis were left untreated, often dying horrible deaths.

Hyler (1988) has pointed out that many of the characters who appear depressed in films would meet the DSM-IV criteria for **adjustment disorder with depressed mood** rather than major depression. The examples Hyler cites include Jimmy Stewart's character in Frank Capra's *It's a Wonderful Life* (1946) and Henry Fonda's character in *The Wrong Man* (1956). In the latter film, Fonda becomes depressed after he is unjustly accused of murder.

Bereavement-related depression is a controversial condition due to the difficulty inherent in defining what a normal bereavement period should be. The DSM-5 lists it both as a disorder needing further study and as a condition that can be diagnosed in the trauma- and stressor-related disorders category (the actual label is **persistent complex bereavement disorder** and is coded as another specified trauma- and stressor-related disorder). I will discuss this further in Chapter 6.

Martin Manning (2017) has written about how traditional holiday movies depict depression and suicide. The reader seriously interested in learning more about the presentation of suicide in films will want to read *Suicide Movies: Social Patterns 1900–2009* (Stack & Bowman, 2012). This book reports a study analyzing more than 1,500 films released over a 110-year period that depict at least one suicide. In addition, it would be worthwhile to see *Walking Man* (2015), a short documentary film about a father and son, both coping with bipolar disorder, who walk across the state of Missouri to highlight the needs of people with mental illness and to underscore the state's genuine problem with adolescent suicide.

Bipolar and Related Disorders

Bipolar disorder occurs less frequently than depressive disorders but affects approximately 0.6% of the US population. Prevalence rates for bipolar disorder tend to be lower in other countries, but it is unclear if this reflects true differences in incidence or simply differences in diagnostic patterns and training for psychiatrists and other mental health professionals.

Unlike depression, bipolar disorders occur equally often among men and women. Like most mental disorders, the prevalence is greater in lower socioeconomic groups, in part because these illnesses interfere with a person's ability to work, and in part because the cost of the illnesses quickly depletes the economic resources of all but the very wealthy. Even wealthy clients can quickly become impoverished, however, because of the poor judgment and spending sprees often associated with manic episodes.

A **manic episode** is a distinct period of an abnormally and persistently elevated, expansive, or irritable mood, lasting at least 1 week, during which the mood disturbance causes marked impairment of work or functioning. The manic episode may range from mild to severe and may be accompanied by psychotic features. During manic episodes, people develop exaggerated sense of self-esteem, decreased need for sleep, and increased energy levels. These individuals often display a flight of ideas (jumping rapidly from one thought to another) and speak very rapidly.

A **hypomanic episode** results in a period of sustained elevated mood, lasting at least 4 days. This change is obvious to others and alters a person's level of functioning. However, a hypomanic episode is not severe enough to impair work or social functioning.

People with bipolar illnesses are often very likable. Their basic personality is usually outgoing, and they often work in people-intensive occupations such as sales. During a manic episode, they feel good about themselves, and their moods are contagious. They are often very generous and may buy strangers expensive gifts. Judgment is typically poor during a manic episode, and these individuals may gamble away their life savings or spend money they cannot afford to lose on an expensive vacation. They often have multiple sexual partners during their manic episodes. They also have endless physical energy, appear to function perfectly well without sleep, usually eat little, and may lose 30–40 lb (13.6–18 kg) within a few weeks. The potential for physical exhaustion during a manic episode is very real, and the long-term consequences of a manic episode can be devastating for families. For example, it may take years to pay back a debt or forgive infidelities.

Bipolar I illnesses are diagnosed when a person has *both* manic and depressive episodes and cycles from one to another. The depressive episode may last 3–6 months before the person swings to a manic phase. The diagnosis of **bipolar II** disorder is reserved for those who have primarily depressive episodes, with occasional hypomania. These patients do not have full-blown manic episodes. **Cyclothymic disorders** are found in individuals who never experience a major depressive or manic episode but who have had hypomanic and depressive symptoms that persist for at least a two-year period.

To address the overdiagnosis of bipolar disorder in children, **disruptive mood dysregulation disorder** was added as a new depressive disorder category for DSM-5. This label is applied to individuals who display severe temper outbursts behaviorally and/or verbally that are inconsistent with their developmental level and accompanied by persistent irritable or angry mood. It is recommended that this diagnosis be restricted to ages 7–18, those ages in which validity for the condition has been established. This condition is a tricky one to diagnose in films; to make the diagnosis one must have enough information to differentiate the condition from conduct disorder, ODD, bipolar disorders, and impulse control disorders.

Silver Linings Playbook

Silver Linings Playbook (2012) provides an excellent cinematic depiction of bipolar I disorder. It was nominated for numerous Academy Awards, and Jennifer Lawrence won the Academy Award and a Golden Globe Award for Best Performance by an Actress in a Leading Role for her portrayal of Tiffany, a distraught widow who deals with her grief by indiscriminate sex with strangers and with all her male coworkers.

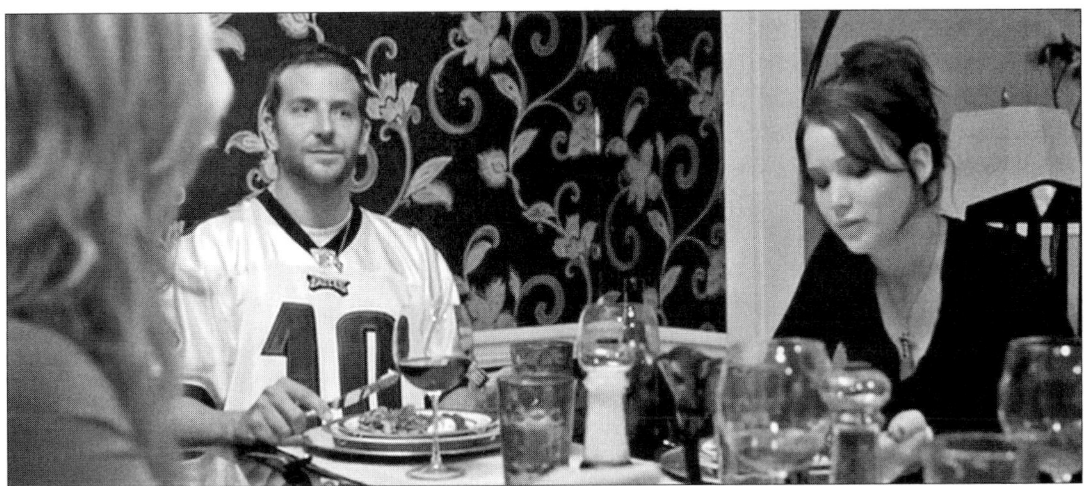

Figure 17. *Silver Linings Playbook* (2012, The Weinstein Company). Produced by Bruce Cohen, Bradley Cooper, Donna Gigliotti, and Jonathan Gordon. Directed by David O. Russell.

Bradley Cooper plays Pat, an unemployed high school teacher who has just been released from a psychiatric hospital where he spent 8 months after discovering his wife in the shower with another man, subsequently beating the man almost to death. Pat hopes to become reunited with his wife, but she has a restraining order in place and clearly no longer wants him in her life. There is clear sexual chemistry between Pat and Tiffany, and this leaves other family members feeling uncomfortable and tense in their presence (Figure 17).

Tiffany: "What meds are you on?"
Pat: "None. I used to be on Lithium and Seroquel and Abilify, but they make me foggy, and they also make me bloated."
Tiffany: "Yeah. I was on Xanax and Effexor. I wasn't as sharp."
Pat: "You ever take Klonopin?"
Tiffany: "Klonopin, yeah ..."
Pat: "What day is it? How about Trazodone?"
Tiffany: "Trazodone?"
Pat: "It flattens you out. I mean you are done. It takes the life right out of your eyes."

Pat and Tiffany compare notes for their reactions to several psychiatric medications, in *Silver Linings Playbook* (2012)

Pat is still manic after his release from the hospital. In one scene, he becomes visibly disturbed by what he perceives as an unsatisfactory ending of Ernest Hemingway's novel *A Farewell to Arms*. He throws the book through the window, shattering the pane, and then bursts into his parents' bedroom at 4:00 a.m. to share his disappointment with the way the book ends. This is a realistic portrayal of the way someone with bipolar I disorder might act. Unfortunately, the film only shows Pat behaving normally or in a manic phase, and the profound depression that accompanies bipolar I is never shown in the film. However, the film does illustrate the importance of peer and family support for someone coping with this disorder, and the film ends with an optimistic message about the possibility of recovery.

Mr. Jones

Alan Greisman and Debra Greenfield's 1993 film *Mr. Jones* is about a musician, Mr. Jones, played by Richard Gere, and his psychiatrist, Dr. Libbie Bowen, played by Lena Olin. *Mr. Jones* is a clear-cut illustration of bipolar I disorder. The film portrays Jones as elated, seductive, and euphoric. He is a charismatic man with tremendous personal charm. He persuades a contractor to hire him, proceeds to the roof, and prepares to fly after rhythmically pounding a few nails into the roof. Before climbing to the front of the roof, he insists that Howard, his newfound friend, accept a $100 bill. After realizing that Jones really believes that he can fly, Howard persuades him to move away from the beam where he is teetering. An ambulance arrives and takes Jones to a local psychiatric emergency unit, where he is released after a few hours. At the hospital, he is misdiagnosed and given inappropriate medications.

Mr. Jones: "I'd like to close my account, please."
Susan: "You just opened this account last week."
Mr. Jones: "Yeah, I'm a fickle kind of guy."
Susan: "Oh, my goodness."
Susan: "Okay, you have $12,752 in your account. Do you want that in hundreds?"
Mr. Jones: "I'll leave that up to your impeccable judgment ... but keep a hundred for yourself."

Richard Gere's character displaying the poor judgment characteristic of bipolar I disorder, in *Mr. Jones* (1993)

Next, Jones goes to a bank and withdraws over $12,000; he seduces the teller in the process, and then goes on a spending spree. He purchases a baby grand piano, checks into an expensive hotel, and then attends a concert. He is arrested and returned to the hospital after he disrupts the symphony by attempting to take over for the conductor as the orchestra is playing Beethoven's "Ode to Joy" – Jones is convinced that Beethoven would have wanted the piece played at a much faster tempo. Jones is once again hospitalized in a state of manic exhaustion, but this time he is accurately diagnosed and treated by psychiatrist Elizabeth (Libbie) Bowen.

Jones knows he has bipolar disorder. He was first diagnosed in late adolescence and had several hospitalizations. However, he refuses to take his medication because it makes his hands shake. It is during the "highs" or the manic phases that he feels best about himself. The rest of the time Jones is lonely and depressed. His lows are life threatening and result in several suicide attempts. The viewer can gain some insight into the impact of a mental illness on the promising career of a classical musician. In addition, the film illustrates the ways in which interpersonal relationships are affected by a condition such as bipolar disorder. Jones's one important prior relationship ended when a woman he loved could no longer deal with his mood swings.

Unfortunately, the rest of the movie involves the romantic relationship that develops between Dr. Bowen and Jones. Even though Dr. Bowen resigns from the hospital, underscoring the unethical nature of this doctor–patient relationship, the true impact of the psychiatrist's behavior is never addressed in the movie.

Other Films Depicting Bipolar Disorder

Some films describe characters with bipolar disorder but do not show them as symptomatic. In *The Last Days of Disco* (1998), for example, one character is stereotyped as "looney" and "crazy"; however, he is also depicted as compliant with lithium, and shown to be stable, kind, and balanced. *Garden State* (2004) also depicts a patient diagnosed with bipolar disorder. However, this patient becomes noncompliant with his medication and finds that his life improves dramatically when he is not taking lithium, and there is no apparent exacerbation of his bipolar symptoms. While **drug holidays** might be recommended by physicians on occasion, films of this sort mislead the public and suggest that these important decisions can be made without medical consultation. Matt Damon's character in *The Informant* (2009), a Steven Soderbergh film, is diagnosed with bipolar disorder, and he receives hospitalization and medication; his symptoms at least partially explain his illegal behavior and the web of lies that spiral out of control.

One of the best films depicting bipolar illness is *Call Me Anna*, a 1990 made-for-TV movie starring Patty Duke, who plays herself in this adaptation of her best-selling autobiography. The film traces her career and her battle with bipolar disorder and vividly portrays her mood swings and the accompanying personality changes she experienced. In real life, Patty Duke has become a vocal advocate for persons with mental illness.

Gena Rowlands plays a woman who appears to have a bipolar I disorder in the John Cassavetes film *A Woman Under the Influence* (1974). She is quite convincing during a manic episode, and there is a memorable scene in which a neighbor stops by to drop off his children and then decides that it is not safe to leave them with Rowlands. He does not know exactly what is wrong, but it is clear to him that *something* is not right. Unlike *Mr. Jones*, the actual diagnosis is never specified in *A Woman Under the Influence*, even though Rowlands character spends 6 months in a psychiatric hospital (see also the section Other Films Portraying Psychotic Disorders).

Another example of an apparent bipolar disorder is found in the Harrison Ford character in *Mosquito Coast* (1986), although that character's eccentric habits and obsessional style are adequate to support multiple diagnoses. In addition, the biographical film *Mommie Dearest* (1981) suggests that Joan Crawford had bipolar disorder.

Examples of the type of rapid speech, quick thinking, and impulsive behavior associated with a hypomanic episode can be seen in the college president character played by Groucho Marx in *Horse Feathers* (1932) and in *Good Morning, Vietnam* (1987), a film in which Robin Williams plays an Air Force disc jockey with a rapid and clever repartee that endears him to his military audience.

Blue Sky (1994) stars Jessica Lange and Tommy Lee Jones. Lange, who won an Academy Award for her role in this film, plays Carly

Marshall, a woman whose bipolar disorder (diagnosed with the then-appropriate term "manic-depressive disorder") gets her family in considerable trouble. She sunbathes topless and acts out sexually, and the film illustrates the profound effects of a disease like bipolar disorder on families.

> **"You take water, for example. Sometimes it's water, sometimes it's ice. Sometimes it's steam, sometimes vapor. It's always the same old H2O. It only changes its properties. Your mother's like that. She's like water."**
>
> **Henry Marshall (Tommy Lee Jones) tries to explain their mother's erratic behavior to his children, in *Blue Sky* (1994)**

Infinitely Polar Bear (2015) is a compelling and highly recommended film that shows how families are affected by bipolar disorder (see Figure 18). The movie is directed by Maya Forbes and pays homage to her father, Cam Stuart, who was diagnosed with "manic depression" in 1967. In the film, two young girls are left in the care of their father, a man recently released from a psychiatric hospital, while their mother attends graduate school. The film might be useful to show children learning how to cope with a parent diagnosed with bipolar disorder (Rosenfarb, 2016).

No Letting Go (2015) is a dramatic film based on the real-life story of screenwriter–producer Randi Silverman. The film is discussed at some length in Chapter 16; suffice it to say here that the movie will be deeply moving for anyone dealing with a child suffering from a mental illness. Timothy, the protagonist, initially presents with anxiety symptoms, but he is eventually diagnosed as someone coping with the challenges of bipolar disorder. His depressive symptoms are accurately depicted; however, the one scene in which he is portrayed as manic seems contrived. Therapists might want to prescribe the film for parents learning how to cope with the challenges presented by a child with a serious mental illness.

Two other films that present fairly accurate portrayals of bipolar I disorder are *Running with Scissors* (2006) and *Michael Clayton* (2007). In the first film, Annette Bening plays a bipolar

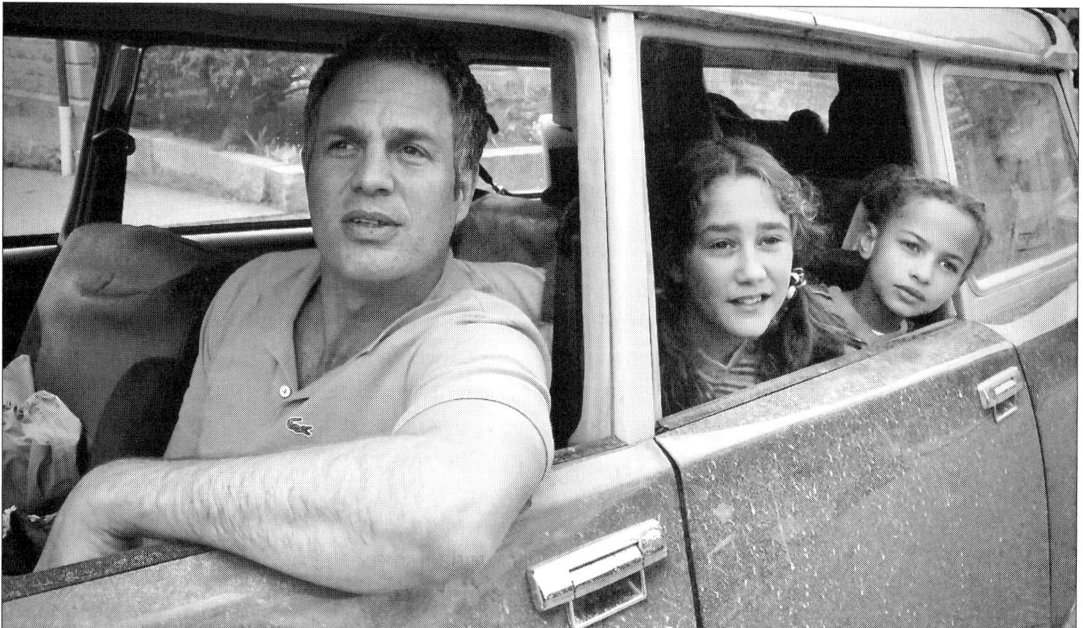

Figure 18. *Infinitely Polar Bear* (2015, Paper Street Films, Bad Robot, KGB Media, Park Pictures). Produced by J. J. Abrams, Sam Bisbee, Bryan Burk, Stewart Anderson, et al. Directed by Maya Forbes.

mother who turns over her son's life to her psychiatrist; in the second film, Tom Wilkinson portrays a senior attorney in a large law firm who becomes manic. Wilkinson's character displays inappropriate behavior (e.g., stripping in court), pressured speech, and grandiose thinking. His illness is controlled by medication, but he becomes quite ill when he stops taking his lithium, and the film illustrates the critical importance of adherence to medication regimens for anyone with this disorder.

In marked contrast to the films described above, the movie *Bipolar* (2014) is egregiously bad. The movie is a variant of the Dr. Jekyll and Mr. Hyde theme in which Harry Poole, a pleasant patient diagnosed with bipolar disorder, is treated with an experimental medication which makes him turn into "Edward Grey," an extraverted and dislikable man who becomes angry and homicidal. He turns on his physician when the doctor refuses to continue his medication, but he gets his hands on a surreptitious supply with the help of a voluptuous nurse who subsequently becomes his lover. There is evidence of a genetic basis for Harry's illness (his mother had committed suicide), and hypersexuality is present during manic episodes, but this film gets everything else wrong. In particular, the film erroneously suggests people with a bipolar diagnosis are violent and dangerous (e.g., Harry – when he becomes Edward – kills an innocent man who is using an ATM machine, murders a prostitute, shoots and kills his girlfriend, and he gleefully hands a gun to his father who subsequently kills himself). Edward gets revenge on the psychiatrist who initially treated him by knocking him out, tying him up, and forcing him to ingest a sugar cube laced with a massive amount of LSD. While high, the doctor plunges to his death after attempting to fly from the top of a building.

In the poetic, experimental film *Crooked Beauty: Navigating the Space Between Beauty and Madness* (2010), director Ken Paul Rosenthal weaves photographic images and the mercurial weather patterns of the San Francisco Bay area with voice-over storytelling and artwork by activist-artist Jacks Ashley McNamara, a woman who suffers from a severe mental illness. This short film is stunning as a positive psychology film, one that depicts psychological struggle and turmoil while simultaneously depicting resilience, creativity, humanity, and triumph (Niemiec & Wedding, 2014). In their *PsycCRITIQUES* review, Larry Leitner and Hideaki Imai (2011) cite studies that document that people with schizophrenia often can achieve better outcomes in treatment programs without medication. The pervasiveness of psychiatry and the medical model can sometimes lead to the alternative: "The client can be condemned to a lifetime of medication, many of which will shorten the client's lifespan by as much as 20 years" (Leitner & Imai, 2011). The film elicits important questions for psychologists and other providers about mental illness and its treatment.

"Take the best day you ever had and multiply it by a million."

A woman describing how good it feels to be manic, in *Of Two Minds* (2012)

Of Two Minds: Riding the Bipolar Roller Coaster (2012) is a documentary filmed over a 3-year period. It is built around interviews with three people who have first-hand experience with the highs and lows of bipolar disorder. The film was directed by Lisa Klein and her husband; Klein's sister suffered from bipolar disorder, so Klein had personal experience with the disorder. All three people interviewed are articulate and intelligent, although they disagree about the utility of medication in the treatment of their disorder. One man, an architect with a degree from Yale, became a crack addict, and once planned to attack a police officer using an ice pick to achieve "death by cop." All three individuals would be classified as having bipolar I, and each vacillates between extreme highs and desperate lows.

David Coleman, a screenwriter, and a man coping with bipolar disorder, has devoted an entire book to the analysis of the ways in which bipolar disorder is depicted in films. The cover of the book shows Bradley Cooper jogging in the film *Silver Linings Playbook.* Coleman's book is titled *The Bipolar Express: Manic Depression and the Movies,* and is highly recommended for anyone who wants to examine the specific portrayal of bipolar disorder in more detail (see review by Potts, 2015).

Theories of Mood Disorders

There are three main theoretical explanations associated with mood disorders: **Genetic theories**, which are useful in understanding familial tendencies; **Biological theories**, which explain the physiological changes and the rationale for pharmacotherapy and ECT; and **psychological theories**, which support the use of psychotherapy and other psychological approaches to treatment. The environment and external events are extremely crucial factors in the manifestation of mood disorders – for example, with the loss of a job or a recent divorce.

Genetic Theories

Twin and adoption studies have documented that there is a genetic vulnerability to mood disorders. Bipolar disorder has been shown to have an extremely high heritability estimate of 93% in identical twins (Kieseppa et al., 2004), and it is associated with a loss of approximately 10–20 potential years of life (McIntyre et al., 2020).

When researchers compared the incidence of mood disorders in identical twins (who share the same genetic code) with that of fraternal twins (who have different genetic material), the concordance rate was 67% for the identical twins and 15% for fraternal twins. The high concordance for identical twins has also been found in twins who were raised in different environments. There is a significant genetic component in mood disorders.

Biological Theories

The biological approach to mood disorders focuses on the activity of neurotransmitters in the limbic system. The neurotransmitters involved include **dopamine**, **serotonin**, **acetylcholine**, and **norepinephrine**. In depression, it is believed that there are fewer available neurotransmitters in the synaptic junction; in contrast, in mania there is an excess.

The limbic system also regulates the pituitary hormone, a key element in the complex endocrine system. Changes in the endocrine system also influence mood. There have been many studies documenting the changes in the functioning of the pituitary gland and thyroid that occur with mood disorders. Some depressed people have been found to secrete an excessive amount of **cortisol**, a hormone produced by the pituitary gland. Additionally, persistently low thyroid hormone levels have been noted in some cases of depression, and an elevated thyroid hormone level is present in some rapid cycling bipolar disorders.

Although psychiatry has embraced biological theories since the publication of DSM-III in 1980, surprisingly little progress has been made in identifying the biological bases for most major mental illness, and prevailing theories clearly have been shaped by government policies, rivalries between different academic programs and scientists, industry profit mongering, and television advertising (Harrington, 2019).

Psychological Theories

Psychological theories have always played a key role in the understanding and treatment of mood disorders. While depressive and bipolar disorders clearly have a biological basis, the psychodynamic conceptualization of these disorders provides a separate way of understanding the behavioral and emotional problems associated with these conditions. Many of the psychological features of depression are readily apparent in films.

The early psychoanalysts (e.g., Sigmund Freud, Karl Abraham) noticed that people with depression experienced **ambivalence** toward significant persons in their lives. That is, they often acted as if they loved and hated the same person. In *Scent of a Woman* (1992), Lieutenant Colonel Frank Slade is both affectionate and antagonistic toward his niece, brother, and other family members. He also becomes antagonistic and aggressive when Charlie Simms tries to help him.

Introjection, the unconscious "taking in" of qualities and values of another person or a group with whom emotional ties exist, was also identified as a characteristic feature of depression. In *Scent of a Woman*, Slade introjected the values of the military and continued to treat everyone as if they were subordinates who reported to him. Interestingly, Slade had been discharged from the military because of his overbearing behavior. Colonel Slade's difficulties in the Army were related to a long-standing history of untreated depression.

Regression, another characteristic of depression, refers to a return to an earlier pattern of behavior. During a depressive episode, childhood behavioral patterns may appear, and a person may act less mature. In *Scent of a Woman*, Slade's ongoing battle with a 4-year-old is not acceptable adult behavior for a retired colonel.

Denial, ignoring the existence of reality, is characteristic of persons experiencing a manic episode. These patients often stop taking their medication because they believe that there is nothing wrong with them. They reject any advice from family members and may become belligerent at any suggestion that they are ill. Jones had been hospitalized multiple times after he discontinued his medication in *Mr. Jones*, and he is smart enough to know it will happen again. However, each time, he convinces himself that this time will be different. This is a classic example of denial.

Cognitive behavior theorists have contributed significantly to understanding the depression experience. Aaron Beck (who died recently at age 100) has described a **cognitive triad** that is common in these patients. The triad consists of (1) perceiving oneself as defective and inadequate, (2) perceiving the world as demanding and punishing, and (3) expecting failure, defeat, and hardship (Beck, 1976). These "automatic thoughts" are readily apparent in *American Splendor* (2003), *The Cooler* (2003), *Scent of a Woman* (1992), *The Hospital* (1971), and in Julianne Moore's character in *The Hours* (2002).

Mood Disorders and Creativity

There is compelling evidence that mood disorders may be related to the creative process, and numerous artists, poets, and composers have been diagnosed as depressed or bipolar, or have biographies that suggest that these disorders were present. Dean Simonton, who has studied creativity and creative genius for over 40 years, notes that artists and those in professions involving skills that are subjective, intuitive, and emotive are more likely to have mental illness than those who are scientists or in professions using skills that are rational, logical, and formal (Ludwig, 1998; Simonton, 2009). Simonton adds that some creators can control their bizarre thoughts and use them productively. Similarly, Kay Redfield Jamison, a psychologist with bipolar disorder, notes that the periods of creativity in many individuals with this disorder typically happen during healthy periods in which the person draws upon the experiences that occurred in their manic, hypomanic, or depressed phase (Jamison, 1993). Jamison has a brief cameo appearance in Paul Dalio's film *Touched With Fire* (2015) in which she advises the two protagonists on the importance of medication.

Marco: "Van Gogh. Top member of the Bipolar Club. You see this?"
Nurse Amy: "Yes, it's beautiful!"
Marco: "You know why?"
Nurse Amy: "Why?"

Marco: "Because it's the painting of the sky he saw from his sanitarium window when he was manic."
Nurse Amy: "Really?"
Marco: "Yeah. You don't believe me, go look it up."
Nurse Amy: "I believe you."
Marco: "Well, when you go out tonight, and you look at the sky and you see how dull it is, think about if you would've medicated Van Gogh!"

***Touched With Fire* (2015)**

The Devil and Daniel Johnston (2006) is another compelling film illustrating a potential link between bipolar disorder and creativity. Johnston was a gifted musician and artist who spent much of his life in mental institutions. One of his hospitalizations resulted from a manic episode that occurred while his pilot father was flying a private two-seater plane following a music concert in Austin, Texas. Johnston became convinced that he was Casper the Friendly Ghost, removed the key from the plane's ignition, and threw it outside! His father was required to crash land the plane, but only minor injuries resulted.

Several actors and actresses have struggled with bipolar disorder, including Richard Dreyfuss, Patty Duke, Carrie Fisher, Linda Hamilton, Jean-Claude Van Damme, and Vivien Leigh. Examples of poets believed to have experienced mood disorders include William Blake, Ralph Waldo Emerson, Edgar Allan Poe, Lord Byron, Alfred Lord Tennyson, John Berryman, Sylvia Plath, Theodore Roethke, and Anne Sexton; examples of painters and composers with mood disorders include Vincent van Gogh, Georgia O'Keefe, and Robert Shuman (Jamison, 1993). Sylvia Plath's difficulties with depression are detailed in *Sylvia* (2003), the film adaptation of her semiautobiographical novel *The Bell Jar* (1979), in which Gwyneth Paltrow plays the title role. Novelist Virginia Woolf's mood disorder is portrayed in the highly recommended movie *The Hours* (2002). The troubled life of Beethoven is portrayed in the 1995 film *Immortal Beloved*. Vincent van Gogh's life, work, and mental illness (which may have been bipolar disorder) have been documented in the films *Vincent* (1987), *Vincent & Theo* (1990), and *Van Gogh* (1991). However, none of these matches the artistic achievement established by the 1956 film *Lust for Life*, in which Kirk Douglas plays van Gogh and Anthony Quinn plays the supporting role of Paul Gauguin. The final days of influential Nirvana lead singer–guitarist, Kurt Cobain, are portrayed in Gus van Sant's *Last Days* (2005) and *Kurt Cobain: About a Son* (2006); Cobain had been diagnosed with bipolar disorder and committed suicide in 1994. Wedding (2000) provides examples of the cognitive distortions found in the poems of Anne Sexton; these distortions are common in depressed and suicidal people.

There are several movies about Ernest Hemingway, as well as an excellent television miniseries by Ken Burns, but these films typically address earlier periods in his life, and rarely deal with his suicide. Hemingway won a Nobel Prize and a Pulitzer Prize, was married, and had homes worldwide. However, he did deal well with the indignities of old age, and he believed the ECT treatments he had received while hospitalized had robbed him of his creativity. He made several suicide attempts before finally shooting himself in the head in Idaho. He was 61 years old. There was a strong genetic history of depression, and his father had committed suicide with a gun when Hemingway was 29.

Shakespeare was fascinated by people who took their own lives, and his plays and their film adaptations provide a useful and fascinating way to approach the study of suicide. Major Shakespearean plays in which suicide is a prominent theme include *Romeo and Juliet*, *Julius Caesar*, *Hamlet*, *Anthony and Cleopatra*, *Macbeth*, *Othello*, and *King Lear*. There have been multiple film adaptations of each of these plays.

Feist et al. (2021) examined the relationship between psychopathology and creativity by having raters score biographies of eminent artists, scientists, and athletes on a three-point scale of psychopathology (*not present*, *probable*, and *present*). Raters were blind to the identity of the biographies they were rating, and the athletes served as a comparison group (famous but not creative). They found that,

> Apart from anxiety disorder, athletes did not differ from the U.S. population in lifetime rates of psychopathology, whereas artists differed from the population in terms of alcoholism, anxiety disorder, drug abuse, and depression. These data generally corroborate and replicate previous biographical research on the link between artistic creativity and life-time rates of psychopathology. (Feist et al., 2021, p. 1)

Creativity does not always have to come in the form of great art and writing – it can also present simply as creative thinking. This is known as **divergent thinking** – producing many ways to solve problems. In *Sherlock Holmes* (2009) and *Sherlock Holmes: A Game of Shadows* (2011), the character of Holmes may have a bipolar disorder as evidenced by episodes of depression and his intense, elevated mood periods. However, Holmes' character also happens to be an exemplary model of divergent thinking.

Suicide

Suicide and Depression

Suicide is the eighth most frequent cause of death throughout the world, but suicide rates vary widely between different countries. The suicide rate is low in the less prosperous countries and highest in the more affluent ones, such as Germany, Switzerland, and Sweden. However, the suicide rate is also high in all Eastern European nations. The suicide rates in the United States and Canada are in the middle range; however, suicide rates in the United States increased by 33% between 1999 and 2017 (Temko et al., 2020).

Among adolescents, suicide is the third most frequent cause of death. While men are more likely to commit suicide, women attempt suicide more frequently than men. Men are more successful in their attempts because they are more likely to choose a more lethal means (e.g., guns).

Mortality rates for suicide are generally higher in urban areas, and prevalence rates for suicide have been shown to be positively correlated with the size of cities. Although suicide has a low incidence in closely knit rural communities, the problem is more common among older persons, in areas where agriculture is in decline, and among workers who are immigrating into cities. The incidence of suicide increases with age, with older persons at greatest risk for killing themselves (National Institute of Mental Health [NIMH], 2003).

People with bipolar disorder are at least 15 times more likely to commit suicide than those in the general population and may account for one quarter of all completed suicides, according to DSM-5. (American Psychiatric Association, 2013, p. 131).

One of the best predictors of who will attempt suicide is a history of a psychiatric disorder. Those who are at the highest risk for suicide are those who have no hope. People who express hopelessness are more likely to commit suicide than those who have some hope for the future. The association between suicidality and hopelessness is stronger and more stable than the association of suicidality with the presence of depression and substance use disorders (Kuo et al., 2004). The lead characters in two films discussed earlier (see the section Depressive Disorders, in this chapter), *Scent of a Woman* (1992) and *The Hospital* (1971), each have a strong sense of hopelessness.

Representative Jamie Raskin (D-Maryland) lost his son, Tommy, to suicide on December 31, 2020. Tommy was a successful writer, vegan, animal rights activist, and Harvard Law School student with a photographic memory, but he also experienced hopelessness, and he was profoundly depressed. Remembering their son, Jamie and Sarah Raskin wrote,

> He began to be tortured later in his 20s by a blindingly painful and merciless "disease called depression," ... a kind of relentless torture in the brain for him, and despite very fine doctors and a loving family and friendship network of hundreds who adored him beyond words and whom he adored too, the

> pain became overwhelming and unyielding and unbearable at last for our dear boy, this young man of surpassing promise to our broken world.
>
> On the last hellish brutal day of that godawful miserable year of 2020, when hundreds of thousands of Americans and millions of people all over the world died alone in bed in the darkness from an invisible killer disease ravaging their bodies and minds, we also lost our dear, dear, beloved son, Hannah and Tabitha's beloved irreplaceable brother, a radiant light in this broken world.
>
> He left us this farewell note on New Year's Eve day: "Please forgive me. My illness won today. Please look after each other, the animals, and the global poor for me. All my love, Tommy." (Raskin, 2023)

Congressman Raskin's book *Unthinkable* was released in January 2023. In it, Raskin describes his regret that he didn't notice more signs of his son's withdrawal from life, and he regrets not asking Tommy directly if he was considering suicide. He notes, "We connected no dots. We were blindsided" (Raskin, 2023).

It is likely that Tommy Raskin's depression was exacerbated by COVID-19. Ettman et al. (2020) have documented a dramatic increase in depression symptoms during and following the pandemic, noting that,

> [the] prevalence of depression symptoms in the US was more than 3-fold higher during COVID-19 compared with before the COVID-19 pandemic. Individuals with lower social resources, lower economic resources, and greater exposure to stressors (e.g., job loss) reported a greater burden of depression symptoms. (Ettman et al., 2020)

Risk Factors and Antecedents

There are many risk factors associated with suicide. The demographic risk factors include being adolescent or elderly; male; White; separated, divorced, or widowed; isolated; and unemployed. Other risk factors include depression, alcoholism, bipolar disorders, and neurological disorders.

Unfortunately, even though risk factors and the antecedents of suicide have been well established, accurately predicting who will commit suicide is extraordinarily difficult. Most clinicians include a suicide assessment in their initial interaction with any client who has an emotional problem or a mental illness. An assessment for suicide focuses on three issues: intent, plan, and lethality.

Intent, or thinking about suicide, is a specific indicator of an impending suicide and probably the single most important predictor. Those people most intent on suicide have worse insomnia, are more pessimistic, and are less able to concentrate than those with less intent. In the film *Night, Mother* (1986), the entire story focuses on Jesse's plan to kill herself. Those individuals most intent on killing themselves are more often males, older, single or separated, and living alone. However, experts also know that intent is episodic, and that even if there is no intent today, there may be tomorrow. In *Dead Poets Society* (1989), there is no mention of Neil's intent, and the viewer is led to believe that he does not intend to kill himself; however, he eventually returns home, feels helpless, and convinces himself there is no way out of an untenable situation. If someone had recognized his intent or if he had reached out for help (e.g., by calling a suicide hotline), Neil might have been able to identify creative alternatives to suicide.

Most experts believe that even though a person is intent on suicide, there is almost always an underlying wish to be rescued. Thus, a person who is very intent on killing themselves may consciously or unconsciously send out signals of distress, evidence of helplessness, or pleas for help. Some of the verbal cues may be "I am going away" or "You won't be seeing much of me from now on." There may also be unusual behaviors such as putting one's affairs in order, giving away prized possessions, engaging in atypical acts, or becoming socially isolated. These behaviors are all present in *Scent of a Woman* (1992). Lt. Colonel Slade puts his financial affairs in order, visits his family, says goodbye, and has his "last fling" before he attempts to kill himself.

People who have a **plan** for committing suicide are more likely to kill themselves than those who have vague thoughts about not wanting to live. Clinicians are trained to determine whether their patients have a plan to kill themselves and how specific these plans are. An individual who does not have a plan is at lower risk than someone who knows how they can commit suicide, and who has access to the planned method. In *The Hospital* (1971), Dr. Herbert Bock plans to kill himself by injecting a lethal dose of potassium. He demonstrates both plan and intent, and, because of his easy access to potassium, he is clearly at considerable risk.

The **lethality** of the method is also an indicator of the risk of suicide. The more lethal the chosen means, the more likely it is that the person will commit suicide, especially if there is easy access to the method selected (e.g., guns in the home). The most lethal suicide methods are using guns, jumping off buildings and bridges, and hanging. Slashing one's wrists and ingesting 15 or fewer aspirins are common methods of attempting suicide, but they are seldom lethal. Other methods that carry a moderate to high risk of lethality are drowning, carbon monoxide suffocation, and deep cuts to the throat. In both *Scent of a Woman* (1992) and *Dead Poets Society* (1989), the lethality was high because guns were the means selected for the suicidal act.

Colin Firth portrays a gay man living alone in *A Single Man* (2009). Firth's character has recently lost his lover in an automobile accident. He is suffering, dysphoric, isolated, and suicidal. He displays several signs suggesting he is preparing to kill himself: He announces that "this day" will be different. He packs a gun and then gives unique, out-of-character compliments to his housekeeper and assistant, picking out details which he appreciates, both of which surprise the women and brighten their day. He shares his fears and notes the challenge of being fully honest.

Boy Interrupted

Boy Interrupted (2009) is an important and powerful documentary about a young man who committed suicide in his early teens in 2005. It was produced by his parents who are filmmakers. Evan Scott Perry was diagnosed with bipolar disorder after inpatient hospitalization due to a suicide attempt during which he stood on top of a tall building until a teacher talked him down. After inpatient treatment, Evan went to a center that focused on milieu therapy, which helped Evan tap into his "boy-ness," offering a shift from his current behavior in which he acted like an immature adult. Evan was highly moody and as a young child, and he seemed to act like two different people. He was preoccupied with death and suicide. He displayed aggression, periods of depression, intense emotions, and explosiveness, and he had difficulty managing his feelings. His poor impulse control and personal belief in his negative thoughts seemed to worsen. During his tantrums, he would destroy most items in his room. There was a family history of suicide by an uncle. Evan left a poignant suicide note marked with teenage angst, like the notes left by thousands of other teens. As one psychiatrist notes in the film, bipolar disorder is "psychiatry's cancer" – it kills people. In addition to being an emotional film, *Boy Interrupted* is thought-provoking and educational and represents a creative way to cope with an incomprehensible tragedy (i.e., make a film about the tragedy). The film is also important in depicting the impact of suicide on parents, siblings, friends, and the family unit. It shows that suicide is not without significant consequences and significant lasting impact on others (e.g., a grandmother of another suicide victim shares in the film that as a family member, "one never recovers"). The film emphasizes how the fantasy of family and friends simply saying wonderful things at the funeral of a suicide victim is both naïve and transient, while the pain and suffering of the living is ongoing and salient.

Seven Pounds

Will Smith initially worked with Italian director Gabriele Muccino to produce the movie *The Pursuit of Happyness* (2006), a moving portrayal of a man and his son who triumph over economic difficulties and homelessness. The actor and the director teamed up again to produce *Seven Pounds* (2008), a provocative and controversial movie in which the protagonist, Ben Thomas, attempts to atone for a single tragic mistake in an otherwise charmed life by committing suicide and giving away his home, his wealth, and various body parts (including his eyes and his heart) to seven decent and deserving individuals. In some obscure way, this allows Thomas to "undo" his responsibility for the death of his fiancée and the six other individuals killed in an accident that he clearly caused when attempting to read a Blackberry message at the same time he was driving a vintage Corvette far too fast. Thomas becomes romantically (but not sexually) involved with Emily Posa (Rosario Dawson), a woman who will die unless a suitable donor can be found, and she receives a heart transplant. Thomas works with a childhood friend to ensure that his heart goes to Emily, his eyes go to Ezra Turner (a blind, vegan telemarketer played by Woody Harrelson), and other needy individuals receive other body parts. The movie is overly sentimental, and there is ambiguous evidence of psychopathology in Will Smith's character; however, we do believe the film raises interesting questions about the movie industry's tendency to glamorize suicide, and it suggests that suicide can sometimes be an altruistic act. The movie illustrates that mental health professionals are hard pressed to identify suicidal thinking in any patient who denies it, and we believe the film can provide a springboard for lively class discussions about depression, suicide, and the societal responsibilities of directors and producers.

House of Sand and Fog

House of Sand and Fog (2003) offers a compelling illustration of the ways in which depression can present. The movie stars Jennifer Connelly as Kathy, a depressed, recovering alcoholic; Ben Kingsley as Behrani, a former high-ranking Iranian colonel working hard at two menial jobs to support his family; and Ron Eldard as Lester, a married police officer who protects Kathy and wants to start a new life with her. Director Vadim Perelman succinctly describes the dynamics of each character's psyche as follows: "Behrani wants up, Kathy wants in, and Lester wants out. Those are their motivations." Kathy's house is seized due to tax payment delinquency, and Behrani wins the house in an auction, thus beginning a complex web of morality, conflict, individual needs, and pursuit of one's dreams.

> **"The woman has come here and tried to take her own life. We must help her. She is a bird, a broken one. Your grandfather used to say the bird which flies into your house is an angel. You must look upon its presence like a blessing."**
>
> **Behrani giving advice regarding Kathy's first suicide attempt, in *House of Sand and Fog* (2003)**

Kathy lives alone in a house she and her brother inherited from their father. In one of the opening scenes, Kathy is sleeping when she is awakened by her advice-giving mother on the phone; after discussing the need for her to attend support group meetings, Kathy ends the conversation with a single tear streaming down her cheek and hangs up the phone. She then rises from her shaking waterbed (an early symbol of her instability) and begins to walk around her dirty house that includes a dripping faucet and a large stack of unopened mail blocking her front door. The opening scenes set up a depiction of an unsteady woman with a history of alcoholism who lives a sedentary, isolated, and unmotivated life. These scenes set the stage for Kathy's battles with alcoholism and depression.

Kathy's symptoms include agitation, numb and blunted affect, and social isolation. Early on, she alludes to her struggle with depression and remarks, "I'm trying not to harp on the negative." Kathy also has financial problems, and because she is unable to afford a motel for 2 days, she begins to live and sleep in her car, turning the engine on for heat. She finds some comfort and escape from her loneliness through an affair with a married man. As stress increases, she begins to smoke cigarettes again. There is a clear link between alcohol and depression, yet this begins with denial. Kathy says, "See, when I think of my sobriety I don't think about wine, alcohol was never a problem." She then begins to drink wine with a subtle smile. This is a break in her 2 years of sobriety, and it rapidly results in physical and emotional deterioration. This is a serious and severe relapse for Kathy, clearly triggered by the stress and chaos in her life.

Kathy's overt "cry for help" comes when she calls her brother, pleading with him to visit and support her: "I just feel lost, Frankie, I just feel lost." Her brother, a typical busy American, claims there are new things needing attention at his job and quickly gets off the phone. Kathy's despair continues to escalate. With tearfulness and bloodshot eyes from crying, Kathy purchases several miniature bottles of whiskey and some gasoline. She drinks the whiskey while driving and crying. Her depression and helplessness then lead to two suicide attempts. While despairing over the house she has lost, she tries to kill herself with a gun, pulling the trigger several times; however, the gun is not loaded. She is found, taken in and cared for by her rival Behrani and his family, and she attempts suicide a second time, swallowing several bottles of unnamed prescription medicine. She is saved again, this time because she is found early and forced to throw up most of the medicine.

Metaphors for depression abound in this film. The emergence of the moon and the setting or rising of the sun represent character transitions and shifts into different moods and mental states. As the title suggests, sand and fog are crucial elements in the film; one interpretation is that both represent the symptoms of depression. Sand is a naturally unsteady element representing the sinking nature of suicide. As Kathy sinks deeper into depression, fog is seen in many scenes, becomes thicker and more concealing until in one scene it surrounds the house. There are several camera shots of moving fog in which the fog quickly covers trees, mountains, water, and homes. This is like the rapid clouding associated with the negative thoughts, helplessness, and self-destructive behaviors one finds in depression. The film opens with life being cut down (trees) and concludes with a shot of a tree surrounded and protected by a fence.

The viewer is particularly challenged with this film, as they can empathize with both characters and can see the needs of both sides. As tension rises and conflict continues, this challenge becomes more complex, even to the point where a state of helplessness is induced in the viewer which mirrors the helplessness portrayed on screen.

The Hours

The Hours (2002) is a film of enormous psychological, emotional, and cinematic proportions. The film was nominated for Academy Awards for Best Picture, Best Director, and Best Adapted Screenplay. The all-star cast includes Nicole Kidman, Meryl Streep, Julianne Moore, Ed Harris, Claire Danes, Jeff Daniels, Toni Collette, John C. Reilly, and Miranda Richardson. The music was brilliantly composed by the renowned Philip Glass, and the script was adapted by David Hare. Ironically, one of the least known figures in this film is the most important – the director. This was director Stephen Daldry's second feature film, although his extensive work and awards in the London theater showed he was more than equal to the challenge of directing a movie.

"If I were thinking clearly, Leonard, I would tell you that I wrestle alone in the dark, in the deep dark and that only I can know, only I can understand my own condition."

Virginia Woolf (Nicole Kidman) talking to her husband, in *The Hours* (2002)

The film depicts three stories about three women who are closely connected although they live in different periods. Each woman struggles with both serious depressive symptoms and suicide issues.

Kidman plays the now celebrated novelist Virginia Woolf, struggling to write her soon-to-be-famous novel *Mrs. Dalloway* in the early 1900s while suffering with what would be identified today as bipolar disorder. The film dramatically begins and ends with the suicide of Virginia Woolf, who drowns herself in a quickly flowing river with heavy rocks in her pockets to weigh her down. Woolf's depression is emphasized in the film, though some mania symptoms are depicted, including her agitation, decreased need for sleep, poor judgment, and indecisiveness, such as when she decides to leave her house against doctor's orders with the intention to move to and live in London. She has a history of "fits," problems with mood, she hears voices, and she has made two suicide attempts. Although her life has been set up to protect her, the inner turmoil she experiences is simply too painful for her to continue to live. She smokes marijuana to calm herself, focus her thoughts, and numb the pain. Her suicide by drowning is depicted in Figure 19.

The character Laura (Julianne Moore) is living in a quaint neighborhood home in the 1950s. She reads *Mrs. Dalloway* with interest and passion, finding comfort and inspiration in the lead character. Laura's character is an enigma, but she is clearly depressed and overwhelmed by life and its demands. She is socially awkward and skittish, at times unsure of how to respond socially, and at other times standing near the door (after the doorbell rings) but not answering it. She is overwhelmed by easy tasks (e.g., baking a cake), and she is extremely critical of herself when she makes mistakes. Laura, like Woolf, feels alone and craves connections though she does not seem to know how to make them. She kisses her visiting neighbor, Kitty (Toni Collette), on the lips, clearly trying to connect with another person in a meaningful way. She spends a lot of time alone and experiences frequent crying spells. At one point, she decides to commit suicide, leaves her son with a babysitter and checks into a hotel – a suicidal dream is the catalyst that changes her mind. Life is too much for her to cope with and rather than committing suicide, she travels to Canada to restart her life, abandoning her husband and children.

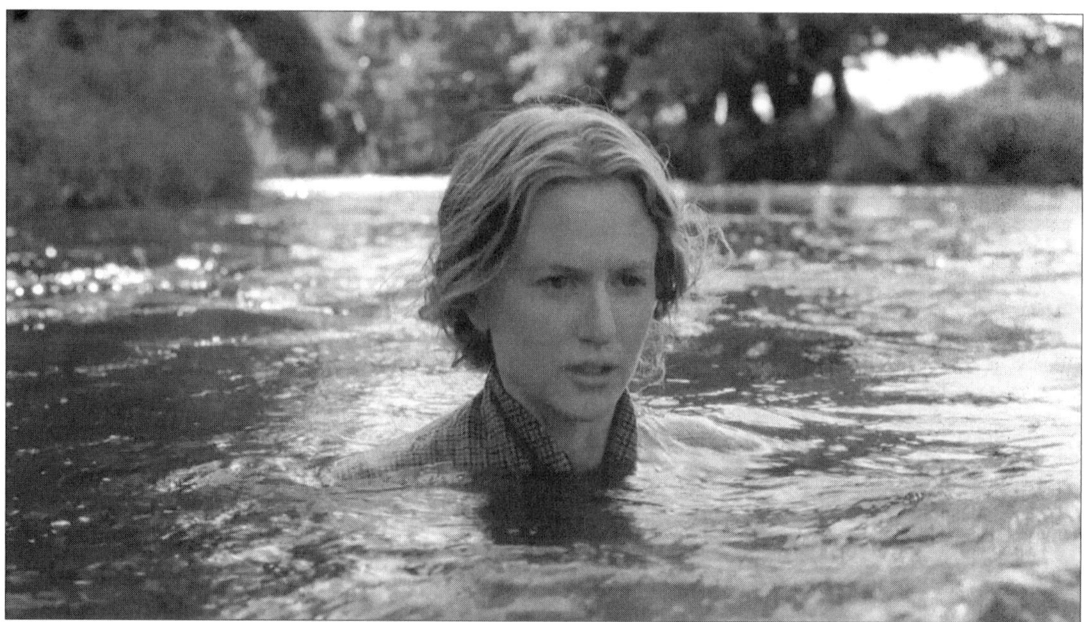

Figure 19. *The Hours* (2002, Paramount Pictures, Miramax, Scott Rudin Productions). Produced by Michael Alden, Robert Fox, Mark Huffam, Ian MacNeil, Scott Rudin, and Marieke Spencer. Directed by Stephen Daldry.

> **"There are times when you don't belong, and you think you're going to kill yourself. Once I went to a hotel. Later that night I made a plan. The plan was I would leave my family when my second child was born. That's what I did. I got up one morning, made breakfast, went to the bus stop, got on a bus, left a note ... What does it mean to regret when you have no choice? It's what you can bear. There it is. No one's going to forgive me. It was death. I chose life."**
>
> **Laura (Julianne Moore) explaining herself in *The Hours* (2002)**

The third interwoven story is set in New York City in 2001 and involves Clarissa (Meryl Streep), a woman trying to impress others and cover up her pain by throwing a party (just as in *Mrs. Dalloway*) for Richard (Ed Harris), her former lover, who is a prize-winning poet dying of AIDS. Clarissa is a strong woman who is socially confident and appears sure of herself. Her vulnerability is slowly disclosed through her struggles to help Richard, through her distant relationship with her partner of several years, and in her emotions that rush to the surface when she confronts a former lover (Jeff Daniels).

Clarissa covers her inner pain through self-sacrifice, trying to help Richard cope with his hallucinations, noncompliance with medication, depression, and cynicism. Ultimately, Richard commits suicide by allowing himself to fall from a high apartment window in front of Clarissa.

> **"I still have to face the hours, don't I? ... I mean the hours after the party and the hours after that."**
>
> **Richard (Ed Harris) alluding to his suicidal thoughts when speaking to Clarissa, in *The Hours* (2002)**

Dead Poets Society

Dead Poets Society (1989) stars the late Robin Williams as John Keating, an unconventional English teacher at a strict boys' preparatory school. This film was nominated for several Academy Awards. Set in 1959, this drama contrasts institutional values and individual creativity. By fostering "critical thinking" in his classroom, Keating broadens students' educational experience and their ability to think independently. The students also discover that when Keating was a student at the school, he started a secret society, the Dead Poets Society, dedicated to intellectual creativity. These students reactivate the society.

> **"We don't read and write poetry because it's cute. We read and write poetry because we are members of the human race. And the human race is filled with passion. And medicine, law, business, engineering, these are noble pursuits and necessary to sustain life. But poetry, beauty, romance, love, these are what we stay alive for."**
>
> **John Keating explains his love for poetry, in *Dead Poets Society***

One important conflict in the film is between Neil, a student who wants to be an actor, and his father, a domineering businessman who wants his son to be a doctor. Neil's father will not allow him to try out for a campus production of *A Midsummer Night's Dream*. Neil disregards his father's demands, goes to the audition, and is selected for the lead role. Keating encourages Neil to explore the relationship with his father and to enlist his father's support. Neil's father is enraged when he views his son's successful performance. Neil is immediately brought home, and in an act of desperation, believing that his father will never "allow" him to become an actor, Neil shoots himself with his father's gun. Keating becomes the scapegoat for Neil's suicide, and the school's administration uses the suicide as an excuse to fire the unconventional teacher. The film ends with the other students protesting Keating's dismissal.

Wristcutters: A Love Story (2006) opens with Zia, the lead character, slashing his wrists. He then finds himself in a purgatory, populated by other people who committed suicide. He considers killing himself again but suspects he will only wind up in a still worse setting. The film will teach you little about depression and suicide, and it insults the viewer's intelligence by making use of a cheap "it was all just a dream" plot device that explains everything away.

Harold and Maude (1971) is a cult classic that opens with Harold, a troubled teenager, pretending to hang himself. He routinely fakes suicide attempts, primarily to annoy his intrusive mother, and he amuses himself by attending funerals of people he has never met. At one of these funerals, he meets Maude, a 79-year-old woman who also enjoys attending funerals. These two unlikely companions become fast friends, and Harold professes his love for Maude shortly before she dies.

There is a memorable suicide by hanging in *The Shawshank Redemption* (1994), and few viewers can forget the Russian roulette games that prisoners of war are forced to play in *The Deer Hunter* (1978). A four-part HBO made-for-TV miniseries, *Olive Kitteridge*, also presents a compelling illustration of a misanthropic homemaker (played by Frances McDormand) grappling with suicidal ideation after the stroke and subsequent death of her pharmacist husband.

Other Films Dealing With Depression and Suicide

Many recent films portray protagonists who end their life, suggesting there is no trend to decrease the frequency of the portrayal of suicide in films; consider *Revolutionary Road* (2008), *The Reader* (2008), *Boy A* (2007), and the sacrificial suicide in *Gran Torino* (2008). An interesting educational exercise is to assign students to select two films portraying suicidality and write a paper comparing and contrasting method, etiology, risk factors, level of suffering, diagnoses, familial and social impact, and so forth.

Hopelessness and suicidal intent are well depicted in the film *Night, Mother* (1986), starring Sissy Spacek as Jesse and Anne Bancroft as the mother, Thelma. This film is a thought-provoking and gripping film adaptation of a Pulitzer Prize–winning stage play about suicide. The entire film takes place in the mother's home, where Jesse has lived since her divorce. As the play begins it is 6:05 p.m., and Jesse has just informed her mother that she plans to kill herself that night. The two women examine their lives as Thelma tries to protect her daughter from her decision. Jesse explains that she has no hope and ends her life at 7:45 p.m.

Whose Life Is It Anyway (1981) stars Richard Dreyfuss as Ken Harrison, a famous sculptor who becomes quadriplegic after a car accident. He becomes profoundly depressed and argues that he should be allowed to die. The hospital chief of staff (played by John Cassavetes) disagrees. Ken is given an injection of valium despite his clear refusal, and he can't do anything because of his paralysis. Similar themes involving the right to die are explored in *Me Before You* (2016), *Million Dollar Baby* (2004), *The Sea Inside* (2004), *You Don't Know Jack* (2010), *Johnny Got His Gun* (1971), *One True Thing* (1998), *Adam* (2020), and the extraordinary documentary *How to Die in Oregon* (2011).

Suicidal intent, hopelessness, cynicism, and serious depression are also depicted in the fascinating film, *Sunset Limited* (2011), which has a cast of two. This dialogue film between White (Tommy Lee Jones) and Black (Samuel L. Jackson) initially centers on Black trying to understand why White has just attempted suicide in a train station. White is a professor who displays sadness, anhedonia, fatigue, poor self-care, low appetite, insomnia, social isolation, severe work and relationship dissatisfaction, anomie, and a lack of meaning and purpose in life. He says he does not believe in anything any longer, that everything he previously believed in was "flimsy," and that he yearns for blackness, for silence, for nothingness, for death, for the end. He reports that both medication and group therapy for depression were unsuccessful. Black, at times, is encouraging, insightful, and challenging, occasionally using religious arguments to impact the atheist White. The film offers a compelling depiction of depression and shows the resistant power of the mind, the power of negative thoughts and beliefs on behavior, and the suffering that results.

Suicide makes for high drama, and it is a common theme in films. Some examples include the unforgettable Russian roulette death of the soldier who remained in Vietnam in *The Deer Hunter* (1978); the suicide by drowning of a young man who feels he cannot please his critical father in *The Field* (1990); the murder–suicide by a Marine recruit in *Full Metal Jacket* (1987); the lead character in the Roman Polanski film *The Tenant* (1976), who becomes suicidal after renting the apartment of a woman who in fact had recently committed suicide; the female protagonist (played by Greta Garbo) committing suicide by stepping in front of an oncoming train in *Anna Karenina* (1935); and the suicide staged to look like a hunting accident in *Mountains of the Moon* (1990). Japanese novelist Yukio Mishima, one of the most fascinating characters in contemporary literature, committed *seppuku* (ritualistic suicide), and his life and death are portrayed in the film *Mishima: A Life in Four Chapters* (1985). Peter Finch, playing Howard Beale, the mad prophet of the evening news, announces to the world that he will commit suicide on the air in 2 weeks and sees his ratings soar in the film *Network* (1976). In the independent film, *Eye of God* (1997), a young boy views his mother's suicide. He is left in acute stress, confusion, and terror, unable to speak and catatonic. Shortly after, he kills himself at the age of 14.

Million Dollar Baby (2004) stars Clint Eastwood, Hilary Swank, and Morgan Freeman. Swank plays the character of Maggie, a young woman boxer who is being trained by Eastwood's character. During a fight, Maggie's opponent hits her over the head with a chair while her back is turned, and Maggie subsequently becomes paralyzed. She begs her trainer to help her die "before the memory of the applause dies."

This is one of Clint Eastwood's finest films: Clint Eastwood won an Academy Award for Best Director, and Hilary Swank won the award for Best Actress at the 2005 Academy Awards. The movie presents the dilemma faced by health care professionals when working with a patient who wants to die, but it has been criticized by members of the disability rights community. Lutfiyya et al. (2009) wrote,

> The last section of the film portrays someone broken and defeated, struggling to end her life. With this surprising twist of storytelling, the movie wades into the murky philosophical waters of bioethics and the controversy surrounding the right to die. It also finds itself, whether by accident or by design, in the middle of a heated debate about what it means to live (or die) with a disability. (Lutfiyya et al., 2009, p. 225)

"I'm 32, Mr. Dunn, and I'm here celebrating the fact that I spent another year scraping dishes and waitressing which is what I've been doing since 13, and according to you, I'll be 37 before I can even throw a decent punch, which I have to admit, after working on this speed bag for a month getting nowhere may be the God's simple truth. Other truth is, my brother's in prison, my sister cheats on welfare by pretending one of her babies is still alive, my daddy's dead, and my momma weighs 312 lbs. If I was thinking straight, I'd go back home, find a used trailer, buy a deep fryer and some Oreos. Problem is, [boxing] is the only thing I ever felt good doing. If I'm too old for this, then I got nothing."

Maggie pleads with her trainer, in *Million Dollar Baby*

Often a failed suicide attempt is a means by which a director can heighten tension or set the stage for future character development. After Olivia (Patricia Clarkson) attempts suicide in *The Station Agent* (2003), her relationship with two other lonely characters deepens, and the three become close and mutually supportive friends. When Pu Yi, the last emperor of China, attempts to commit suicide by slashing his wrists in a railroad station restroom in Bernardo Bertolucci's *The Last Emperor* (1987), we get some insight into his character and a better sense of the despair he is experiencing. Alex Forrest (Glenn Close) attempts suicide by slashing her wrists in *Fatal Attraction* (1987), and the attempt is necessary to establish the extent to which she is willing to go to manipulate and control her lover. After Emmett Foley (Gary Oldman) shoots himself in the chest in the opening scenes of *Chattahoochee* (1989), we learn that he is afraid to die and not genuinely psychotic.

Suicide is sometimes romanticized in film, such as in the hauntingly beautiful *Elvira Madigan* (1967), in which two lovers decide on a double suicide. In *The Hairdresser's Husband* (1992), the female protagonist jumps to her death by drowning in order not to lose the happiness she has found with her new husband. *The Virgin Suicides* (1999) was Sofia Coppola's directorial debut. The story involves a repressed family with five daughters who commit suicide in response to their mother's overbearing control and repression. Unfortunately, this film supports the public misconception that suicide is caused by overcontrolling parents, when in fact it is the opposite that is more likely.

Finally, suicide is often treated as a humorous topic. Examples include Burt Reynolds' character in *The End* (1978), the multiple suicide attempts of Harold in the black comedy *Harold and Maude* (1972), the Italian judge who tries to get his sister to commit suicide in *Leap into the Void* (1979), the elaborate last supper for the impotent and suicidal camp dentist in *M*A*S*H* (1970), and the inadvertent death by hanging in *The Ruling Class* (1972).

There are also moments of humor in *The Skeleton Twins* (2014). Reviewing the film for *PsycCRITIQUES,* Joanne Steuer noted,

> This film is about twins, Milo (Bill Hader) and Maggie (Kristen Wiig), whose parents endowed them with the twin gifts of parental suicide and emotional abandonment during childhood and adolescence. Although they live on opposite coasts, Milo and Maggie attempt suicide on the same day. They survive and the film follows them as they attempt to recuperate from the experience. Tied to each other emotionally, they can easily hurt each other. This film is about depression, anger, love, and hurt. And although it is a difficult story, it is entertainment that is also psychologically correct. It gives life to the studies about the long-term effects of parental suicide and neglect. Funny and sad, *The Skeleton Twins* is an emotional roller-coaster and well worth the price of admission. (Steuer, 2015)

Eyes Upon Waking (2022) is based upon the director's life story. The film depicts a woman who is hospitalized following two suicide attempts.

Many films deal with the depression and suicidal desires that follow disabling medical conditions or accidents that result in paraplegia or quadriplegia. Botha and Harvey (2022), in a brilliant paper, argue that cinematic discourses contribute to the maintenance of ableist power and "continue to perpetuate hegemonic discourses, emotionally provocative, and caricatured portrayals of disability." They analyze three films to illustrate these points: *You're Not You* (2014), *Me Before You* (2016), and *Stronger* (2017). *You're Not You* is a movie about a concert pianist, Kate (played by Hilary Swank) who becomes suicidal and refuses treatment as her amyotrophic lateral sclerosis (ALS) progresses. *Me Before You* deals with a wealthy, handsome banker left paralyzed after an accident who falls in love with his perky young caregiver; he opts for euthanasia and leaves a fortune to her. *Stronger* (2017) tells the story of Jeff Bauman (Jake Gyllenhaal) who is a victim of the Boston Marathon bombing. Botha and Harvey note, "hegemonic discourses of loss, and the subsequent adjustment narratives are recurrent plot devices in filmic representations of acquired disability," and they document how these films perpetuate a "better dead than disabled" narrative (Botha & Harvey, 2022). They also show how the "disabled have been precluded from sexual citizenry because they have continuously been conceptualized as either undesiring or undesirable in lay consciousness, cultural imagery, and public policy." The film *Stronger* is an exception to this theme, and Gyllenhaal's character has a satisfying sexual relationship with his girlfriend that signifies a "progressive leap in the representation of disabled sex in film."

Prevention of Suicide

Since there are no clear predictors of suicide, there are no foolproof prevention strategies. Treatment of an acutely suicidal individual involves protecting them and connecting with that part in each person that wants to be rescued. Usually, a person who is suicidal is hospitalized and not allowed to be alone. Even in those instances, if a person wants to commit suicide, a hospital environment cannot prevent it, and many suicides have been completed in a protected environment. In the film *Crossover* (1983), a psychiatric nurse is plagued by self-doubt after one of the patients he works with commits suicide.

An important part in any suicidal person's care plan should include support from others and open communication. This is exhibited in the dark comedy, *It's Kind of a Funny Story* (2010), in which a 16-year-old admits himself to a psychiatric hospital for suicidality related to stress from his academic and social life. He reports depression and cessation of the medication Zoloft on his own accord. He shares a few vulnerabilities (fear of rejection, perfectionism, and people-pleasing behavior) with Bobby, an older patient played by Zach Galifianakis; these concerns are contrasted with more dramatic vulnerabilities such as a history of abuse, trauma, and drug abuse – conditions that characterize other patients in the hospital. Catastrophizing, magnification, and helplessness are further cognitive and emotional vulnerabilities of the protagonist. The film depicts the importance of open communication, the ability to both give and receive support, learning positive reframing, acts of kindness, role playing, self-expression through art, optimistic thinking, directly confronting one's difficulties, and establishing new connections, as distinct, healthy coping approaches to manage depression and stress.

Till et al. (2014) surveyed 943 individuals online and had them rate 50 preselected films, 25 of which included a suicide. They found,

> Individual film genre preferences seem to reflect risk factors of suicide, with film genres focusing on sad contents being preferred by individuals with higher scores on suicide risk factors. However, suicide movies are more enjoyed by viewers with higher life satisfaction, which may reflect a better ability to cope with such content. (Till et al., 2014)

Niederkrotenthaler and Till (2020) showed films to 158 young adults with depressive symptoms and suicidal thoughts. The sample was split into two groups: One group viewed a short film depicting a young person experiencing depression and suicidality, and the other group saw a thematically unrelated control film. Depressed mood was significantly lower in the intervention group, with a small to medium effect size. The authors found viewing films depicting suicidal thinking did not trigger or enhance similar thoughts in their 18- to 24-year-old subjects, and they suggest that viewing such films may have beneficial effects.

Ordinary People

Ordinary People (1980), an Academy Award winning film based on Judith Guest's novel by the same name, depicts the aftermath of a suicide attempt. Conrad Jarret, played by Timothy Hutton, is a sensitive teenager who has attempted suicide following a boating accident that killed his brother, Buck. Conrad could not overcome his guilt, attempted suicide, and was hospitalized for 4 months. The film begins following Conrad's return home and traces his struggle for personal redemption and his futile attempts to communicate with his parents. His father, Calvin, played by Donald Sutherland, is a successful tax attorney who tries to respond to Conrad's needs. His mother, Beth, played by Mary Tyler Moore, is well-intentioned but unable to meet her son's needs. Beth is the nucleus of a family in a crisis.

Upon his return from the hospital, Conrad is inattentive in class and distant with classmates. He is also ill at ease with his parents. His father encourages Conrad to contact a psychiatrist, and eventually he begins therapy with Dr. Tyrone Berger, played by Judd Hirsch. In therapy, Conrad explores his relationship with his parents. When Dr. Berger suggests that the entire family meet, Beth refuses. Throughout the movie, Beth's feelings toward her living son become obvious. Calvin begins to question his relationship with Beth and unsuccessfully tries to reengage his wife. Beth eventually leaves her husband and son, who come to terms with Beth's limitations and begin to rebuild their lives around their love for each other.

Other characters play an important role in the movie. Conrad's swimming coach quizzes him about his hospitalization, asks him whether he received shock treatment, and is demanding during training sessions. Conrad finally decides to quit the swimming team.

Another important character is Karen, a girl Conrad met at the hospital. While hospitalized, Conrad and Karen had a completely "open and honest" relationship. When Conrad contacts her at home, she is distant but appears to be in control. She is involved in school activities and maintains she no longer thinks about the problems that resulted in her suicide attempt. She also decides not to see a therapist. Karen's newfound confidence is startling to Conrad, who begins to question his own fragile condition. When he tries to contact her later, however, Conrad learns that she has committed suicide.

Karen's death forces Conrad to relive the boating accident that took Buck's life. At last, he can explain his guilt – he lived, and Buck did not. Conrad realizes that he was angry with Buck because he did not hang onto the boat. With the help of Dr. Berger, he experiences the intense pain of his loss and resolves his guilt.

If a suicide attempt is survived, the meaning of the attempt should be examined. Even though the viewer is not told whether Conrad has symptoms of depression, it is safe to assume that they were present prior to the suicide attempt. Conrad's suicide attempt was both an attempt to kill himself and a cry for help. His family fails to appreciate or respond to his distress over his brother's death. His mother is unable to relate to anyone, and his father is withdrawn from family interaction. Through a suicide attempt, Conrad got his family and friends to acknowledge his desperate situation.

Every suicide threat should be taken seriously. While attempting suicide is often an impulsive act, it is also an act of communication. If Conrad had possessed the necessary communication skills, he could have discussed his feelings and explored their meaning.

International Films: Depressive Disorders, Bipolar Disorders, and Suicide

The Son

The Son (2022) stars Hugh Jackman and Laura Dern, and there is a short section with Anthony Hopkins playing a distant and unpleasant father/grandfather. Jackman's character experiences great love for his son, but he finds himself behaving in ways that disgust him – i.e., he replicates many of the same behaviors exhibited by his own father. Jackman's character is coping with a teenage son (who has been living with his mother after his parents divorced) and a newborn, and the unhappy teenager asks to live with his father. His depression is palpable, and he has dropped out of school without telling his parents, spending every afternoon taking long, isolated walks. The son is hospitalized, and he begs his parents to take him out of the hospital – against medical advice. The parents capitulate to their son's demands and have him discharged, with somewhat predictable and disastrous results. The film received somewhat negative reviews (e.g., a 29% tomatometer review by top critics on Rotten Tomatoes), but I found it to be an accurate and pedagogically useful depiction of the ways in which depression presents in a teenager, and the film illustrates the perturbations that can ripple through a family with a mentally ill child, no matter how much love parents have for their children.

Melancholia (2011, Denmark), an intriguing, at times surreal and beautiful, and at times tragic and disturbing film, depicts Kirsten Dunst as a woman with severe depression. On occasion, this reaches levels where she struggles to function and take care of herself, and in one instance, she cannot lift her leg to get into the bath and doubles over on the floor. She also displays crying spells, inappropriate affect, and exhaustion. Her erratic and impulsive behavior is evidence of the need for differential diagnoses including bipolar and an impulse control disorder. Freud's comments on melancholia are applicable to the film:

> A profoundly painful dejection, cessation of interest in the outside world, loss of the capacity to love, inhibition of all activity, and a lowering of the self-regarding feelings to a degree that finds utterance in self-reproaches ... and culminates in a delusional expectation of punishment. (Scott, 2011)

Melancholia was written and directed by the controversial Lars von Trier, known to suffer from serious depression, which has, at times, significantly disrupted his filmmaking.

Respiro (2002, Italy) is a highly recommended Italian film about a woman whose behavior would meet criteria for the diagnosis of bipolar disorder. Her behavior is erratic, unpredictable, and frequently inappropriate (e.g., she invites her sons to go swimming with her in the nude). The people in her small Mediterranean fishing village insist that she be sent to Milan for psychiatric hospitalization after she releases a pack of mad, caged dogs that must be shot from the rooftops. She avoids psychiatric hospitalization when her oldest son helps her find refuge in a cave, and her husband and the villagers eventually come to miss her eccentric but life-affirming behavior.

The slow-moving but powerful Iranian film *Taste of Cherry* (1997, Iran) won the Palme d'Or at the Cannes Film Festival. The movie illustrates the grim determination of a man who has decided to take his own life, but who cannot find anyone to help him. He has dug a hole in the ground and plans to lie in the hole and die after taking a handful of pills; however, it is important to him that he find someone to fill up the hole after he has died. One person he attempts to persuade to take on this task asks a poignant question that leads to the suicidal man questioning his decision: "Do you want to give up the taste of cherries?"

In the graphic, disturbing film, *Suicide Room* (2011, Poland), Dominik is a wealthy normal adolescent with many friends. After kissing a classmate while drunk at a party, a stream of bullying is set off, mostly through electronic media. Life spirals out of control for Dominik. Eventually, he connects with a girl in the "suicide room," an online chat room. The room graphically depicts suicides and self-injurious behavior (cutting); one girl in the room explains she has not left her house for 3 years and that she only wishes for pain, abuse, and suffering, and that she has a fervent desire to die, all of which give her a sense of freedom. This influences Dominik to stay away from school. He stays locked in his room for 10 days where he engages in self-mutilation. His parents are disengaged, workaholic parents who attempt to help him but are limited in their parenting skills. While the film depicts atrocious events in the chat room, there are positives shown as well such as connection and shared pain. The film includes scenes of animation to depict Dominik's interactions as an avatar attempting to cope. Symptoms of depression, anxiety, insomnia, and negative thinking are illustrated. A psychiatrist makes a house call and speaks with Dominik behind the locked door to his room. Finally, his parents get into the room and take away his Internet connection; Dominik is devastated and experiences emotional withdrawal when he can no longer connect with his new chat room friends.

Turtles Can Fly (2004, Iran/France/Iraq), filmed on the Iraq–Turkey border, depicts an adolescent with severe PTSD, who is depressed, homicidal, and suicidal, clearly in reaction to the horrors and atrocities of war; the film does not hold back in depicting what happens to children in war-torn countries.

The Japanese film *Maborosi* (1995) shows how a young woman is affected after the senseless and random suicide of her husband, who chooses, without any apparent reason, to deliberately walk into the path of an oncoming train.

A Spanish film, *The Sea Inside* (*Mar Adentro*; 2004) stars Javier Bardem as a 26-year-old man who had become quadriplegic after a diving accident; he spends over 28 years only able to move his mouth. His lawyer supports his right to die; his friends try to talk him out of it. His father remarks, "There is only one thing worse than having your son die on you ... him wanting to die." The film raises interesting ethical issues for students in the health professions (Agrest, 2011).

Suicide Club (2002) is a Japanese film that explores the phenomenon of suicide and raises more questions than it answers. It assesses links between suicide and crime, music, violence, group contagion, internal compulsions, consumerism, evil, and various external factors. After 54 young girls mysteriously and collectively commit suicide by jumping in front of an oncoming subway train, mass hysteria and confusion develop, and several individuals and groups around the country take their lives. One scene depicts a group of students joking about creating a suicide club, and they gather at the edge of a building's roof, chanting to encourage each other to jump. One by one, they watch each other plummet to their death. The film illustrates the phenomenon of suicide **contagion** (de Leo & Heller, 2008; Hacker et al., 2008), a severe problem that is compounded by media such as the Internet (Mehlum, 2000). Contagion is also sometimes referred to as the **Werther Effect** (based on a spike in suicides in Germany after Goethe published *The Sorrows of Young Werther* in 1774).

Rain (2001) is a New Zealand film about a young girl coming of age as she interacts with family and neighbors on a beach. The film is included in this chapter because of the girl's depressed mother, an alcoholic who acts out sexually and only seems to be happy when she is drinking. Drinking clearly helps her escape from her depression.

The Scottish film *Wilbur Wants to Kill Himself* (2002) is educational only as far as it allows the viewer to witness the various stereotypes and misconceptions possible in a movie. Wilbur is a depressed and angry man who curses children, rejects women, and cheats with his brother's wife even though his brother is the person who repeatedly keeps Wilbur from killing himself. The brother is depicted in the role of protector, frequently checking up on Wilbur, supporting him, and removing sharp objects from his home. Wilbur's persistent suicide attempts include pills, gas from the oven, hanging, drowning, cutting his wrists in the bathtub, and standing at the edge of the roof of a building. Wilbur's determination to commit suicide ends once his love for his brother's wife becomes mutual. This perpetuates the misconception that love conquers mental illness. Equally disturbing is the film's blatant stereotypes of two psychologists leading a group; one smokes cigarettes during sessions and comments that the patients would be better off without group therapy; the other violates boundaries with a patient, licking his ear, going out on a date, engaging in sexual activity in a hospital closet, and violating confidentiality.

Another film about a character repeatedly attempting suicide, and failing, can be found in *The Face* (1999, South Korea). The protagonist is a diagnostic quandary – she lives a completely isolated life, rarely leaves her house, and has no friends, and her only social contact is her younger sister who berates her and abuses her. She is socially inept and spends her life sewing, until her mother dies suddenly, after which she strangles her younger sister to death. This character loses touch with reality, suggesting a link between dissociation and suicide attempts. The film ends with the protagonist escaping from life by swimming away on an inflatable tube in the ocean; this is simultaneously a suicide attempt (like the protagonist in Kate Chopin's *The Awakening*) and the realization of her ultimate dream (to learn to swim). The viewer may also be reminded of another attempted suicide by drowning in *The Piano* (1993).

A classic film, *Diary of a Country Priest* (1951, Italy), directed by Robert Bresson, chronicles the life of a young priest who has somatic depression. This is apparent from the opening shot which depicts him as tired, wiping his forehead, and behind the bars of a gate as if locked in his own prison. He is isolated and displays sadness, low appetite, and a variety of somatic symptoms such as light-headedness, sweating, and an upset stomach. He is quick to self-criticize, usually because he believes he has not prayed enough (which might be considered **scrupulosity**). He eventually receives a diagnosis of stomach cancer and continues to deteriorate.

South Korea has Asia's highest rate of suicide, but Japan also has an alarmingly high rate of suicide, and *A Step Forward* (2019, Japan) introduces the viewer to Sandanbeki Cliff, a popular Japanese suicide location. There is a small church near the cliff, where a priest runs a suicide hotline. He offers housing and employment to people who feel they have no other options, and in doing so he saves lives. The chief cook in the priest's restaurant is a man who was saved from suicide.

February's Dog (2022, Canada) depicts the anxiety, depression, and isolation that results when two men are laid off from their oil field jobs with no advance notice. The stress of unemployment is exacerbated by alcohol abuse, marital stress, and threats of divorce.

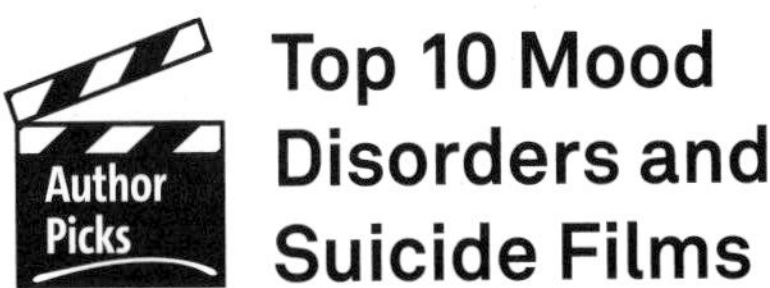

Top 10 Mood Disorders and Suicide Films

Bipolar Disorder

Michael Clayton (2007)
Silver Linings Playbook (2012)
Touched With Fire (2015)

Depression

Scent of a Woman (1992)
Melancholia (2011)
The Beaver (2011)
Manchester by the Sea (2016)

Suicide

The Hours (2002)
House of Sand and Fog (2003)
Boy Interrupted (2009)

Chapter 5

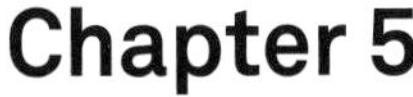

Anxiety and Obsessive-Compulsive Disorders

Sometimes I truly fear that I ... am losing my mind.
And if I did it ... it would be like flying blind ...

Howard Hughes in *The Aviator* (2004)

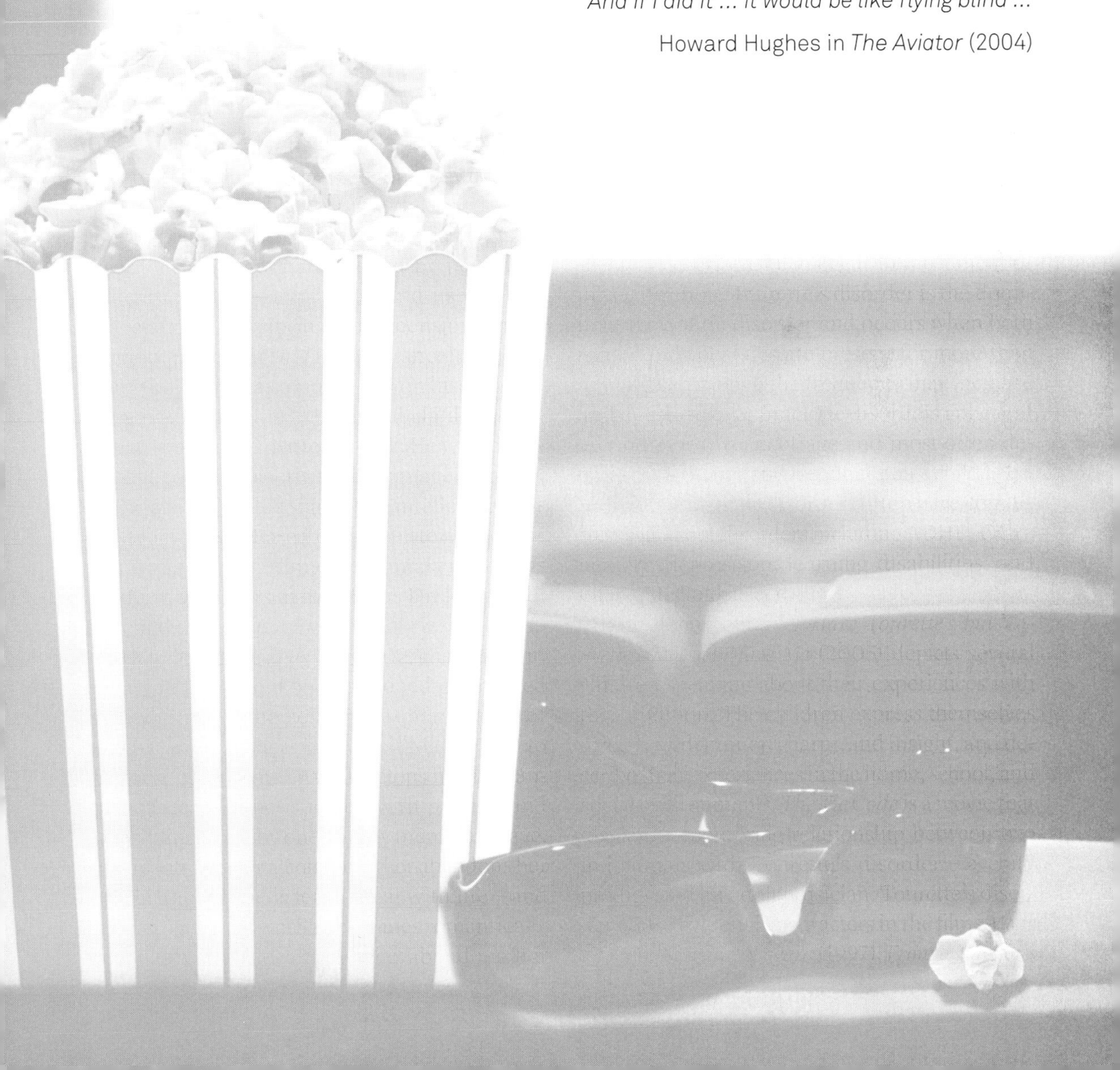

Anxiety Disorders

Anxiety, a normal reaction to a situation or stressor, is a motivator for performance and can be a healthy warning signal of danger or something that needs attention. The DSM-5 distinguishes anxiety from fear noting that "*Fear* is the emotional response to real or perceived imminent threat, whereas *anxiety* is anticipation of future threat" (APA, 2013, p. 189). Existentialist writers and mental health specialists agree that anxiety is an expected part of the human condition.

There are a variety of theoretical explanations for anxiety. Richard Lazarus, a well-known psychologist, described anxiety as a negative emotion that occurs when facing an uncertain, existential threat (Lazarus, 1999). Psychoanalysts view anxiety as a warning signal that danger is present and that overwhelming emotions are imminent, giving rise to unmanageable helplessness. Cognitive behaviorists associate persistent anxiety with a negative self-view, along with a keen sense of desperation and vulnerability.

When anxiety significantly interferes with school, work, or social interactions, an underlying psychiatric disorder may be present. The DSM-IV-TR included OCD, panic disorders, phobias, and PTSD as subcategories under the broad rubric of anxiety disorders (APA, 2000). In contrast, the DSM-5 privileges OCD and trauma- and stressor-related disorders as major categories separate and apart from anxiety disorders. The commonality of all anxiety disorders is an abnormal or exaggerated anxiety response that negatively affects physical health, psychological well-being, and cognitive and social functioning. Stress exacerbates the symptoms. Untreated, anxiety disorders can result in physical deterioration, despair, extreme fear, broken relationships, and unemployment. Suicide may be the ultimate outcome.

The subcategories of anxiety disorder included in the DSM-5 are **separation anxiety disorder**, **selective mutism**, **specific phobias**, **social anxiety disorder**, **panic disorder**, **agoraphobia**, and **generalized anxiety disorder**. As with other disorders, there are specific diagnoses to cover anxiety that results from substance- or medication-induced disorders or medical conditions, and there is the option of coding the disorder as specified or unspecified.

The subcategories of OCD include **OCD**, **body dysmorphic disorder**, **hoarding disorder**, **trichotillomania** (hair-pulling disorder), **excoriation** (skin-picking) disorder, and OCD that relates to substances or medications or due to another medical condition.

Obsessive-Compulsive Disorder

People with **obsessive-compulsive disorder** (OCD) are distressed by recurring thoughts and/or irrational behaviors that can be so time consuming that they interfere with work and social relationships. In severe cases of OCD, these thoughts and behaviors dominate virtually every minute of every day.

Obsessions are intrusive, inappropriate, recurrent and persistent thoughts, impulses, or images that cause marked anxiety or distress. Obsessions are of greater magnitude than the everyday worry that is part of almost all our lives. Those with OCD repeatedly try to suppress these thoughts, but the very act of suppression serves to increase their intensity. These recurrent thoughts are disagreeable and alien to the sense of self (i.e., ego-dystonic). Common obsessional themes include harming others (especially children or helpless individuals), contamination with germs or feces, exposure to toxins or infectious diseases such as AIDS, blasphemous thoughts, and sexual misbehavior. Obsessions can also coexist with other disorders such as PTSD.

Compulsions are repetitive behaviors or mental acts carried out to reduce discomfort associated with obsessions. Sometimes there is a logical connection between the compulsion and the obsession (e.g., repeated handwashing *may* help prevent contamination from germs). However, in other cases there is no logical connection between the two (e.g., the patient who feels

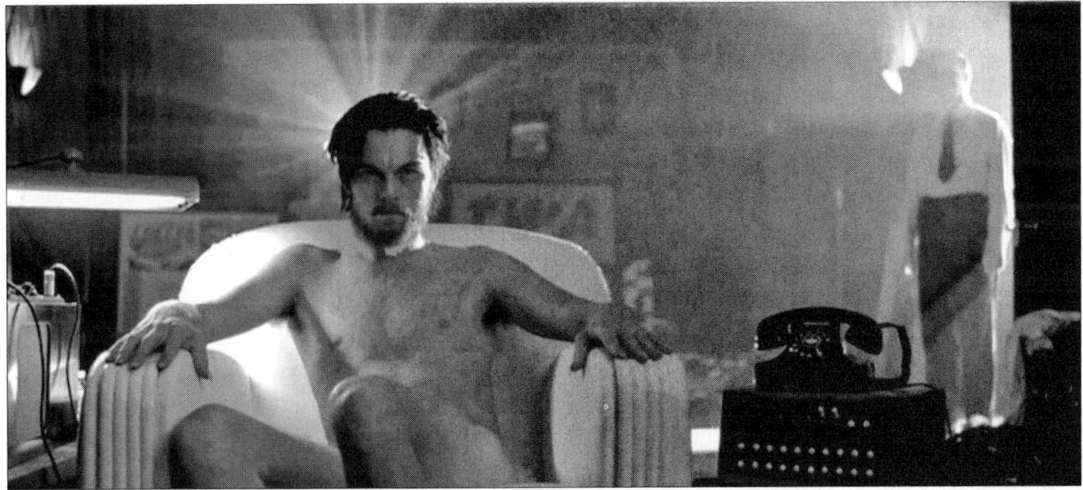

Figure 20. *The Aviator* (2004, Forward Pass, Appian Way, IMF Internationale Medien un Film GmbH, Initial Entertainment Group, Warner Brothers, Miramax). Produced by Sandy Climan, Charles Evans Jr., Grahma King, Michael Mann, et al. Directed by Martin Scorsese.

a compulsive need to sing the first few lines of a popular commercial before pulling away from every stoplight knows there is no meaningful connection between the behavior and the likelihood of an accident).

"I want ten chocolate chip cookies. Medium chips. None too close to the outside."

Howard Hughes (Leonardo DiCaprio) in *The Aviator* (2004), displaying OCD behavior

The Aviator and OCD

The Aviator (2004), an award-winning film directed by Martin Scorsese and starring Leonardo DiCaprio, illustrates many factors that may contribute to the development of OCD – overprotective parents, fear of germs, impulsivity, need for immediate gratification, and the premature death of both parents. Based upon the real life of the tycoon Howard Hughes Jr. (1905–1976) from age 24 to 42, the film depicts his psychosocial and physical deterioration. The underlying effect of his addiction to codeine is not as clearly portrayed, but the use of alcohol can be clearly seen. Like symptoms of many people with OCD, Hughes's obsessions and compulsions develop over time. The film also shows how stress can exacerbate one's symptoms. Leonardo DiCaprio prepared for his marvelous portrayal of Hughes by spending time interacting with patients with OCD. Figure 20 captures Hughes' physical and mental state at the end of his life, a time when he was clearly debilitated and disabled by his illness.

Matchstick Men (2003) does an outstanding job of highlighting the psychological consequences of OCD. Roy Waller, played by Nicholas Cage, is a successful con artist who can use his attention to detail to execute complicated bait-and-switch schemes. When his life is disrupted by the appearance of his estranged teenage daughter (whom he has never seen), he is no longer able to maintain control over his illness or his life. His symptoms erupt, and he deteriorates. The viewer can not only observe the numerous odd, incapacitating behaviors of a patient with OCD, but also his therapy sessions in which he vividly explains internal conflicts typical of OCD. Figure 21 illustrates Roy Waller's obsessive need to take a placebo medication that he is convinced is necessary to control his symptoms.

In another popular film, *As Good as It Gets* (1997), Melvin Udall, a misogynist and a homophobe played by Jack Nicholson, has a pronounced obsession with cleanliness. He eats at

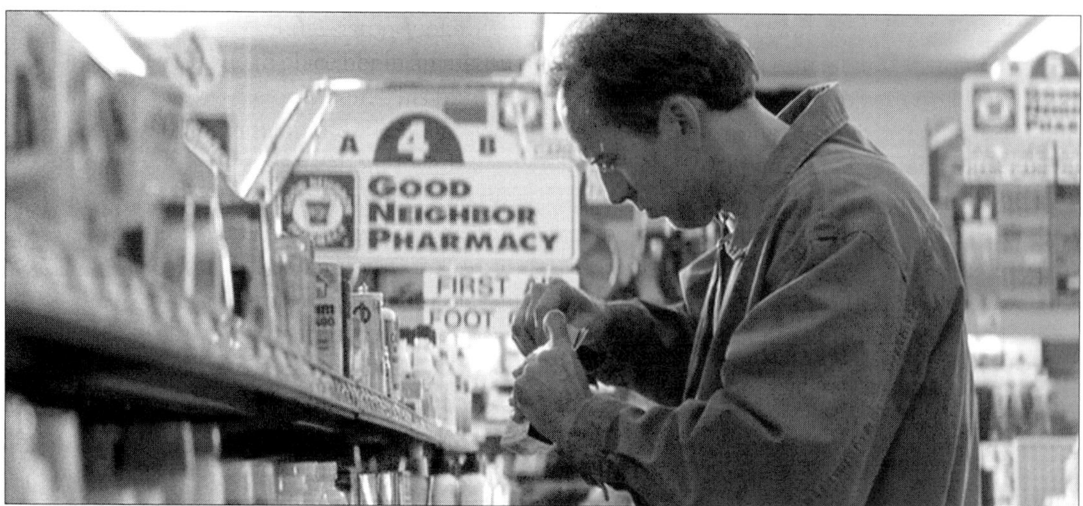

Figure 21. *Matchstick Men* (2003, Warner Bros.). Produced by Sean Bailey, Ted Griffin, Jack Rapke, Ridley Scott, and Steve Starkey. Directed by Ridley Scott.

the same restaurant every day, sits at the same table, insists on the same waitress (Helen Hunt), and always orders the same meal. Melvin always brings his own paper-wrapped plastic utensils to this restaurant, so he does not have to risk contamination from dirty silverware. Whenever anything disrupts this well-established routine, Melvin becomes anxious and belligerent. He wipes off door handles before opening doors, and he carefully avoids stepping on cracks as he walks to his therapist's office. Melvin's obsessions are his repetitive thoughts about germs and disease; his compulsions are the ritualistic behaviors he engages in because of his thoughts. Patients with OCD frequently have multiple obsessions, and the film *As Good as It Gets* provides a realistic presentation of the disorder (with the possible exception that a patient with an obsession about cleanliness as severe as that present in Nicholson's character would be unlikely to be willing to touch a small dog). Some clinicians argue that Melvin also would meet the DSM-5 criteria for a dual-diagnosis of OCD and **obsessive-compulsive personality disorder** (OCPD) due to his pervasive rigidity, interpersonal control, and inflexibility.

It is rare to find a film that depicts OCD patients who are compulsive handwashers. Two exceptions can be found in a short film and a feature-length film, *Waiting for Ronald* and *Phoebe in Wonderland*. *Waiting for Ronald* (2003) is a short film about a man, Ronald, leaving a supervised residence to take a bus to live in the community with his friend, Edgar. Both men have developmental disabilities. Edgar has OCD and he is a compulsive handwasher. He is very precise in the way he places his hat, fixes the folds in the hat, and places objects in his bag. He arrives early at the bus stop, and since Ronald misses the first bus, Edgar must wait longer than he had anticipated. Edgar has a strong need to use the restroom, which he finally does, knowing he might miss Ronald's arrival. Edgar begins to wash his hands and continues, even though he has heard the bus arrive. He wants to stop washing but cannot; his anguish is palpable. He winces and struggles, moaning in mental pain. He washes his hands harder, crying, trying to push himself away from the sink. The viewer can clearly see the pain and suffering the handwashing causes him. Edgar coaches himself over and over (using the words and name of his therapist): "You can do it. Joe says you can do it ... just breathe." Eventually, he slowly pulls his hands away from the sink one hand at a time.

Phoebe in Wonderland (2008) is a feature film that portrays a child with OCD. Phoebe displays repetitive handwashing, to the point that her hands bleed. The impact of her disorder is clear when her obsessive-compulsive behavior causes her to run late for an audition and to be late for a family dinner. She uses elaborate rituals; for example, she employs a particular jumping pattern while clapping a certain number of times to win a particular role; as is common in individuals with OCD, she gets frustrated when she is interrupted, and she explains that she cannot avoid engaging in her behavior. Phoebe quickly generates rituals when she becomes afraid, such as jumping up and down repeatedly to the extent that she has cuts and burn marks on knees. Other OCD behaviors include repeating what is said to her and spiting in the face of other children who provoke her. She is also diagnosed with Tourette's disorder.

> **"All the answers are in a bottle. I've seen that solution! I've seen it all around me and that is a life of side effects and dull minds. Your profession just doesn't like kids to be kids."**
>
> **Felicity Huffman, as Phoebe's mother, challenging the psychiatrist, in *Phoebe in Wonderland* (2008)**

The comedy *What About Bob?* (1991) stars Bill Murray as a patient with multiple problems, including overwhelming anxiety when he cannot be close to his therapist, played by Richard Dreyfuss. Bob would be diagnosed with both OCD and dependent personality disorder.

Body dysmorphic disorder, formerly noted as a somatoform disorder in DSM-IV, refers to a preoccupation with a perceived physical imperfection that is not observable, or which appears slight to others. Individuals with this problem may spend hours each day looking into a mirror and brooding about the perceived defect or flaw.

In 1987, Steve Martin played the role of a modern-day Cyrano de Bergerac in the film *Roxanne*. However, in this film, his nose is truly of grotesque proportions, and he would not qualify for the diagnosis of body dysmorphic disorder (which requires an *imagined* defect in appearance). In the French film version of *Cyrano de Bergerac* (1990), Depardieu's nose is elongated but not grotesque, and one suspects that his concerns are at least as much psychological as real.

The artistically eccentric Peter Greenaway directed the film *The Belly of an Architect* (1987) in which the viewer is introduced to Stourley Kracklite (Brian Dennehy) who is a prominent American architect putting on an exhibition in Rome. Kracklite is too preoccupied with himself to care much about his wife's flirtations with a younger man, and he becomes obsessed with his stomach. This begins to occupy all his attention. His doctor states it is nothing more than gas and egotism. Kracklite examines other options – dyspepsia, fatigue, overexcitement, lack of exercise, too much coffee, too much constipation – but his stomach obsession continues. He makes photocopies of a statue of Augustus, obsesses over the statue's stomach region, and compares it with his own. In a memorable scene, Kracklite's obsession with his stomach extends to his covering his entire room including the floor with photographs of bellies. The film presents interesting differential diagnosis challenges involving somatoform disorders, OCD, and delusional disorder. Support for a diagnosis of hypochondriasis can be found in his unshakable belief that his body is being consumed by a tumor. There are other psychological elements contributing to his disorder: fear of being embarrassed, fear of death, isolation, psychological stress, and narcissistic grandiosity and self-preoccupation.

> **"The most important words in the English language are not 'I love you' but 'It's benign.'"**
>
> **Woody Allen's character obsesses over his health, in *Deconstructing Harry* (1997)**

Compulsive hoarding was not an official DSM-IV-TR diagnosis; however, hoarding disorder is now recognized as a bona fide condition in the DSM-5. Hoarding disorder is commonly associated with OCD; the term refers to the collecting and saving of excessive quantities of possessions (e.g., newspapers, pets, sticks) that are of little use or value; in severe cases, safety and health can be at risk. Hoarding is portrayed briefly in Juliette Binoche's character in *Bee Season* (2005) and in the character of Harvey Pekar, the comic strip artist portrayed in *American Splendor* (2003) (see the section Depressive Disorders, in Chapter 4). In *Winter Passing* (2005), Ed Harris portrays an alcoholic who is a disheveled mess, partly as a reaction to his wife's recent suicide. He lives in a home filled with trash. He is a compulsive hoarder, and the numerous stacks of books in his home serve as a symbolic boundary outlining the entire house, including the stairs and each room, making it challenging to maneuver. It is estimated that the prevalence of hoarding disorder in the United States and Europe is 2–6%, with a greater prevalence among males and in older adults (American Psychiatric Association, 2013).

Animal hoarding is a special case of hoarding disorder; people diagnosed as animal hoarders typically fail to provide adequate sanitation or nutrition for the animals in their homes, and the animals sometimes die because of overcrowding or starvation. *Cat Ladies* (2009) is a documentary film that depicts four women whose lives revolve around the animals they own.

Trichotillomania (hair-pulling disorder) refers to pulling out one's hair to such an extent that it results in noticeable hair loss. There is an increase in tension prior to pulling the hair, and pleasure or relief upon pulling the hair out. Trichotillomania is rarely depicted or even referred to in movies, and it is one of the least represented psychological disorders in film. An exception is the brief portrayal of the disorder in *Dirty, Filthy Love* (2004, UK), a film about a man with OCD. In attempting to manage his condition through treatment, self-help, and support groups, the protagonist meets a woman who has been diagnosed with OCD, but who also displays behaviors associated with a diagnosis of trichotillomania. The viewer observes her pulling out a couple of hairs. She later gets in a fight, and her wig is pulled off exposing the bald patches typical for those suffering from this condition. In *The Internship* (2013), one character working at Google is a young man with trichotillomania who pulls out his hair when he becomes stressed. By the end of the various team challenge tasks, his eyebrows have to be painted on.

Excoriation disorder (skin picking) is portrayed briefly in several films. Nina, the ballet dancer who portrays both the white and black swans in *Black Swan* (2010), exhibits criteria for several DSM-5 disorders, including skin picking and scratching. The excoriation relates to her competitiveness and her difficulty managing stress, and this condition coincides with other OCD phenomena such as perfectionism, rigidity, anxiety, and ritualistic behavior. The film *Personal Velocity* (2002) depicts an adolescent boy who pricks the skin on his fingers, arms, and other areas of his body. Many of the areas are infected. The boy appears to have been severely abused and is running away by hitchhiking; he presents as severely withdrawn.

Panic Attacks

Panic Attacks

Intense, irrational fears, and very distressing physical reactions are the primary symptoms of **panic attacks**. Some people fear losing control, while many others fear dying. Panic attacks peak within minutes, and the DSM-5 diagnosis requires four or more of the following symptoms: palpitations, sweating, trembling, shortness of breath, choking, chest pain, nausea, dizziness, chills or heat sensations, numbness, or tingling, derealization, fear of going crazy, or fear of dying. Panic attacks are most found in the various anxiety disorders; however, they can be associated with any number of other disorders (e.g., depression, PTSD, substance use disorders), and when they are, panic attacks are coded as a DSM-5 specifier for the disorder (e.g., major depressive disorder with panic attacks). Note that a panic attack itself is *not* a mental disorder.

Even though these fears are recognized as illogical, they *feel* very real. Events associated with loss of control such as being in an enclosed space or being raped or abused can also be antecedents to the attacks. Patients usually vividly recall their first panic attack.

In *Dirty, Filthy Love* (2004), Mark's anxiety often leads to panic attacks. In *Matchstick Men*

(2003), Roy has several panic attacks throughout the film. In *Something's Gotta Give* (2003), Jack Nicholson's character, Harry Sanborn, experiences panic attacks on two separate occasions. This film makes the point that panic can often present with symptoms like those accompanying a heart attack; the cause of Harry's panic is relational stress with the main female character, Erica Barry, played by Diane Keaton. In the film *The Departed* (2006), Billy Costigan (Leonardo DiCaprio), experiences panic attacks that contribute to the suspense of the movie; his medication (lorazepam) is discussed as an anxiety treatment. Panic attacks are also depicted in the Australian clay animation, *Mary and Max* (2009) about two overseas pen pals, in which one character, Max, experiences panic attacks when he receives a letter from Mary, as it triggers deep emotions and memories.

In *Broken English* (2007), Parker Posey portrays an event planner who sits around much of the day bored at her computer. When she begins to date and moves toward a relationship commitment, she begins to experience panic attacks in public. She immediately escapes from the situation back to the comfort of her home. She later faces her anxiety directly, symbolized in her traveling to another country where the man she had been trying to avoid lives; she initially travels with a supportive friend, but when the friend leaves, she is forced to confront her anxiety on her own.

Panic Disorder, Agoraphobia, Specific Phobias, Social Anxiety Disorder, Generalized Anxiety Disorder, and Selective Mutism

Panic Disorder

A **panic disorder** is diagnosed when panic attacks become regular, but are still unpredictable events *and* the individual has at least 1 month of concern or worry that they will have additional panic attacks or feel that they are "going crazy," losing control, or having a heart attack. It is the latter set of criteria that are most challenging when attempting to diagnose cinematic movie characters, as films often do not reveal the internal dialogue of the characters.

Panic attacks seem to come out of nowhere. The fact that they occur anywhere and at any time is one of the reasons that a panic disorder is such a debilitating condition. Some people will have daily panic episodes, while others may be able to go for weeks or months without experiencing panic. Misdiagnosis often leads to delays in treating panic disorder, which in turn exacerbates the anxiety disorder. In the true story *Nobody's Child* (1986), patient rights' advocate Marie Balter (Marlo Thomas) is misdiagnosed as having schizophrenia and spends more than 15 years in a state psychiatric institution. She suffers from depression and panic disorder. Following her release, she earns a baccalaureate and master's degree and returns to the state hospital as an administrator.

Robert De Niro plays a mob boss with panic disorder who meets with a psychiatrist, played by Billy Crystal, in both *Analyze This* (1999) and *Analyze That* (2002). Paul Vitti (De Niro) believes he is suffering a heart attack, but Dr. Ben Sobel (Crystal) explains the crucial difference between a panic attack and a heart attack and eventually helps Vitti get in touch with the deep pain and suffering that trigger his attacks. Although Vitti resolves some prominent issues in his life, this therapeutic approach risks misleading the viewer into believing this is the typical treatment for panic disorder; in fact, empirically validated treatments such as medications, cognitive behavior therapy, and exposure therapy are much less dramatic, and require much more work on the part of the patient.

Another hit man who suffers from panic disorder is Pierce Brosnan's character in *The Matador* (2005). In *Panic Room* (2002), Meg (Jodie Foster) and her young daughter, Sarah, move into an extravagant mansion on the Upper West side of Manhattan, and while spending their first night in their new home, three thieves, expecting an empty house, break in hoping to steal millions of dollars. Meg and Sarah find refuge in the steel-plated, impervious "panic room" which holds both the money and their safety. The viewer sees Meg experiencing symptoms of a panic disorder as she has trouble breathing. Her face expresses fear when she is enclosed in the panic room for the first time in a nonthreatening situation, and her daughter asks, "Mom you're not gonna wig out, are you?" When confronted with a dangerous situation, Meg shows resilience, and her panic is justified. It is interesting to note that the stress of the situation triggers Sarah's anxiety and causes a hypoglycemic response so severe her face changes color.

In *Lady in a Cage* (1964), Olivia de Havilland stars as Mrs. Hilyard, an upper-class woman who is trapped inside her home elevator when the electricity in her house goes out. In making a call for help, she attracts thieves who rob her and try to hurt her. The film melodramatically and metaphorically illustrates claustrophobia and panic attacks. Panic attacks are also frequently depicted in a realistic way but with only a minor role in the overall story, as in *Das Experiment* (2001), *My First Mister* (2001), *Monster's Ball* (2001), and *Hannah and Her Sisters* (1986).

Agoraphobia

Agoraphobia is diagnosed when there is marked fear or anxiety in two or more of five specific situations: (l) using public transportation; (2) being in open spaces; (3) being in enclosed spaces; (4) standing in line or being in a crowd; and (5) being outside of the home alone (American Psychiatric Association, 2013). Although the word "agoraphobia" comes from the Greek word for fear of the marketplace, the idea that people with agoraphobia only fear open places is incorrect: The person may associate any number of situations or places with fear and anxiety. In the film *Matchstick Men* (2003), it is unclear if Roy is afraid of panic or simply afraid of situations and places. If it is the latter, then it is more likely he is experiencing **situational** panic due to his fear of contamination (relating to his OCD), and this is what causes him to avoid public places – nevertheless, these symptoms would not be sufficient to justify a diagnosis of agoraphobia.

Drew Barrymore and Jessica Lange portray the infamous mother and daughter, Edie and Edith Beales, in *Grey Gardens* (2009). Edith Beales (Jessica Lange) was a first cousin to Jacqueline Kennedy Onassis, and in the film displays dependent personality and extreme symptoms of agoraphobia. The extreme avoidance and pathology of the characters results in the deterioration of the mansion they are living in, which becomes nothing but a cesspool of filth, cat urine, and dilapidation. Agoraphobia would be diagnosed if a fear of panic attacks were also present; the viewer does learn that she just wants to be at home, as it is the only place she feels she can be herself, and her behavior of never leaving her house and refusing to sell it are further evidence supporting the diagnosis of agoraphobia. In real life, President John F. Kennedy actually paid for the home to be revamped.

Columbus Circle (2012) is set up as a murder mystery and depicts a woman with agoraphobia who has not left her apartment in many years. She rarely interacts with others and has a manager shop for her. She is reticent to speak with the detective investigating the mystery, displays rigid behavior, and is meticulous about keeping her apartment a particular way. She is afraid to leave her apartment, but when she witnesses domestic abuse outside her door, she finally breaks "the plane" of her doorway to help the victim. This new friend later helps her step fully out of the doorway and to then take small steps down the hall. She experiences physiological and psychological anxiety symptoms – including an ardent desire to avoid being outside her home – with this exposure to her fear.

Sean Connery's character William Forrester in *Finding Forrester* (2000) could be diagnosed with agoraphobia (he also has characteristics of avoidant personality disorder, a clinical problem with features that overlap with anxiety disorders). Forrester does not leave his apartment (in part out of a fear he will have a panic attack in public), is socially awkward, and experiences panic when he is required to go into a public place. He does what many people with agoraphobia do – he has his groceries delivered so he does not have to leave his apartment. The film captures the subjective experience associated with Forrester's panic attacks when the camera shows his "spinning" feeling, and sound is blurred. In the throes of his anxiety, Forrester wanders off and gets lost. At the end of the film, the viewer sees the potential for successful treatment of agoraphobia when Forrester is shown riding his bike on busy and crowded streets.

One of the most interesting cinematic portrayals of agoraphobia is found in Robert Taicher's movie *Inside Out* (1986). In this film, Elliott Gould plays Jimmy Morgan, a New York businessman with marked agoraphobia who has not left his house for 10 years. He has food delivered to him, arranges for call girls to come to his apartment for anonymous sex, places bets over the phone, and almost never ventures out of his house until forced to by circumstances beyond his control. Sigourney Weaver plays the role of Helen Hudson, an agoraphobic psychologist, in the murder mystery *Copycat* (1995). An agoraphobia mother is forced to confront her fears in *The Falling* (2014, UK) when she must leave her home to rescue her daughter.

Amy Adams plays Dr. Anna Fox, an agoraphobic child psychologist, in *The Woman in the Window* (2021), a Netflix movie. The film was panned by reviewers, but I found it modestly engaging, and an interesting portrayal of an impaired and suicidal professional who treats her anxiety with psychotropic medications mixed with red wine. Dr. Fox witnesses a murder, and then the plot becomes *very* complicated. The agoraphobic psychologist overcomes her disorder after killing the murderer by pushing him through a glass ceiling at the top of her apartment building.

Specific Phobias

Fears are labeled as **phobias** only when specific conditions are met. Marked anxiety must be present in the presence of a specific phobic stimulus and must routinely occur with exposure to the stimulus. In addition, the phobic individual must be aware that the magnitude of the fear response is excessive. Most people with specific phobias will avoid the stimulus situations that leave them fearful, to avoid the extreme distress they experience in these situations. Successful treatment of phobias involves exposing the person to the phobic object in a safe and controlled environment. Over time and with continual exposure, the person becomes comfortable with the object. However, the fear never truly leaves, and at times of extreme stress, the original fear and anxiety around the object can reappear.

Tom Hanks' character Dr. Robert Langdon in *The Da Vinci Code* (2006) is afraid to go into small, enclosed spaces such as an elevator or the back of a locked truck. He experiences shortness of breath and becomes hyper focused (intense mental concentration focusing on a narrow subject). Claustrophobia is also depicted in producer M. Night Shyamalan's *Devil* (2010) in which five people are trapped in an elevator in a Philadelphia skyscraper, along with the devil. A guard in the film displays this specific phobia, and the film deliberately provokes anxiety in the viewer since it is filmed in such a small space. Mel Brooks' character in *High Anxiety* (1977) suffers from severe acrophobia which generalizes to a fear of planes, escalators, elevators, higher numbered floors in hotels, and any high places where he can look down. He experiences dizziness, nausea, and vertigo in these situations.

Specific fears are sometimes justified. Spiders can bite us; people do fall from high spaces; and even small cats can scratch us. Specific phobia occurs when there is excessive or unreasonable fear of an object or situation, and the anxiety-provoking stimulus is avoided. Various subtypes of this disorder include fear of animals (e.g., dogs and insects), the natural environment (e.g., storms and water), blood-injection injury (e.g., medical procedures), locations (e.g., bridges, elevators), or other miscellaneous stimuli (e.g., situations that might lead to choking). Specific phobias will occasionally remit spontaneously without treatment, but this is rare. A fear of flying is depicted in Rachel McAdams's character in the Wes Craven thriller *Red Eye* (2005).

Many specific phobias are triggered by a specific traumatic event (at least traumatic to the individual experiencing the event). This was clearly the situation in *Vertigo* (1958), a classic Alfred Hitchcock film that stars Jimmy Stewart as John Ferguson, a San Francisco police detective, who is paralyzed by his fear of heights. The phobia has a traumatic etiology: While chasing a criminal across a rooftop, John almost falls to his death. A fellow officer, trying to aid John, is killed when he plunges to the street below. John, overcome with guilt, develops **acrophobia**, a debilitating fear of heights. The term "vertigo" refers to either marked dizziness or a confused, disoriented state of mind. Both meanings apply in this complex and engrossing film. At one point in the film, John designs his own behavior modification program, stating, "I have a theory that I can work up to heights a little bit at a time." He puts a stepladder near the window, stands on the first step, waits, gets down, stands on the second step, waits, goes to the third step, becomes frightened and dizzy, and then falls to the floor.

In *Batman Begins* (2005), 8-year-old Bruce Wayne (Christian Bale) develops a bat phobia after falling into a cave and encountering a swarm of bats. After Bruce urges his parents to leave an opera featuring actors dressed as bat-like creatures, his parents are murdered in front of him. He blames himself for his parents' murder by reasoning that they would not have left the theater if he had not been afraid of bats. In response to these traumatic events, he gradually exposes himself to the feared stimulus and eventually transforms himself into a superhero with a bat-like appearance. By becoming Batman, he further reduces his anxiety and conquers his fear.

Arachnophobia (1990) builds on the widespread fear of spiders; one of the lead characters is Dr. Ross Jennings, played by Jeff Daniels, who has an intense and debilitating fear of spiders. Claustrophobia also is evident in Dakota Fanning's character in *War of the Worlds* (2005). Her father repeatedly teaches her to use coping skills involving an integration of safety reminders, closing her eyes, positioning her arms in a self-soothing way, imagination, and self-talk.

Fall (2022) is a film about two friends, one of whom, Becky, has spent the past year in a drunken stupor after losing her husband in a climbing accident. A former friend joins her and

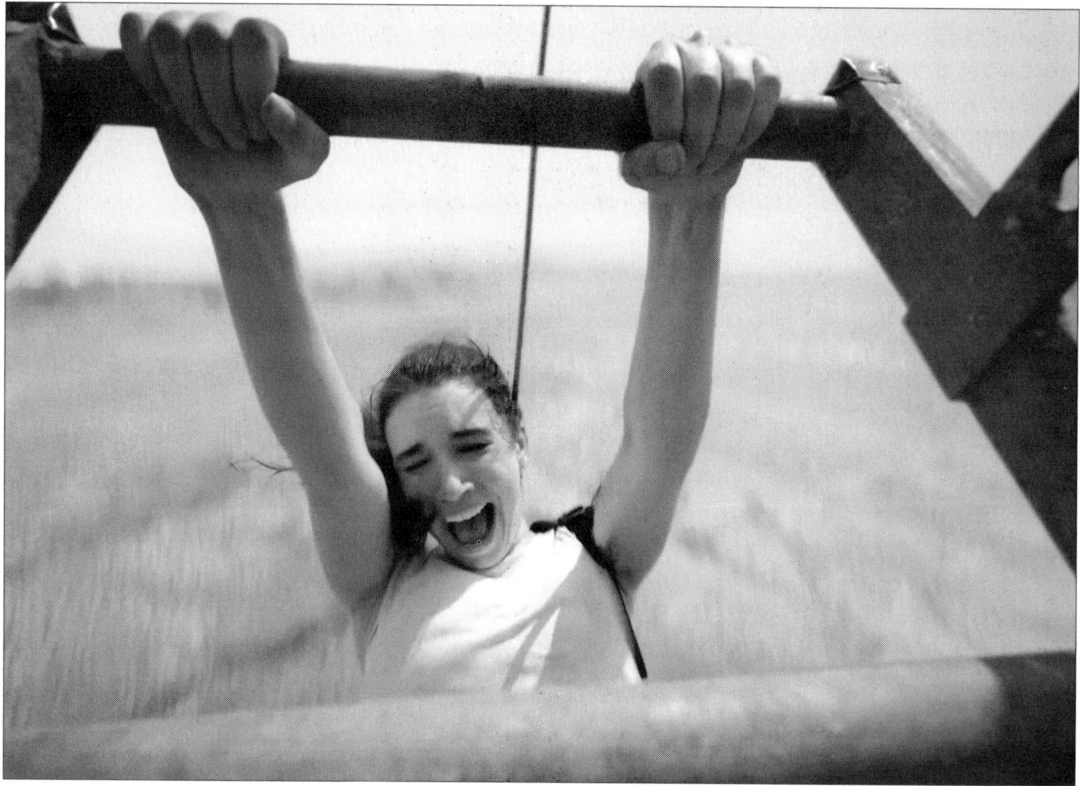

Figure 22. *Fall* (2022, Tea Shop Productions; Capstone Studios). Produced by Dan Asma, David Haring, James Harris, Brianna Lee Johnson, et al. Directed by Scott Mann.

encourages Becky to confront and overcome her fear of climbing by taking on an isolated 2,000-foot (610-m) television tower. Unfortunately, after reaching the top, the old and decaying ladder that got them there falls apart and topples down, leaving the two girls trapped without smartphone reception or water (Figure 22). Vultures attack the girls to get at bloody wounds that resulted from earlier injuries; after her friend dies, Becky manages to live by capturing one of the vultures and drinking its blood. She is eventually rescued after her father notifies emergency crews about his missing daughter. The film is mildly engaging but shouldn't be watched by anyone with a genuine fear of heights.

Social Anxiety Disorder

Intense and persistent fears of criticism and rejection characterize social anxiety disorders, which are also known as social phobias. People with social anxiety disorders experience anxiety in response to the possibility or the thought of negative evaluation or scrutiny, and consequently they avoid situations in which they are likely to be observed by others. The disorder can take many different forms and occurs in situations that require public speaking, public performance, test taking, or social skills. Some male patients with social phobias are unable to urinate in public places (also called **paruresis**), as shown briefly in *Roger Dodger* (2002); other patients are unable to eat in public for fear they will make a mistake and be ridiculed. The disorder is related to common phenomena such as performance anxiety, stage fright, and shyness. The specifier **performance only** is used if the debilitating fear is restricted to public speaking or performing in public.

The onset of social phobias typically occurs in childhood or adolescence, and the clinical course, if left untreated, is usually chronic, unremitting, and associated with significant impairment. Few people with social anxiety seek professional help. The symptoms of social phobia include tachycardia, trembling, sweating, blushing, dizziness, and hyperventilation, and they occur in anticipation of or during a social interaction. Even more distressing is the sensation of impending doom that frequently occurs. Finally, patients feel an overwhelming need to escape from the social situation that is causing their distress. In *The 40 Year Old Virgin* (2005), Andy Stitzer (Steve Carell) avoids dating and sexual relationships due to anxiety. The film's premise is that Andy is a virgin due to intense fear of criticism or rejection.

Woody Allen's character in *Play It Again, Sam* (1972) is an exaggerated portrayal of someone with social anxiety (related to dating) and other neuroses. His portrayal personifies the worst-case-scenario thinking that individuals may engage prior to and even during a date. His character bumbles about and knocks things over, all in chaotic, comical movements. Any person nervous about an upcoming date can watch this portrayal and think, "At least I won't be that bad!" It is important to remember that shyness, performance anxiety, stage fright, and anticipatory anxiety are *normal* anxiety experiences in stressful and/or social situations.

Anticipatory anxiety about social situations often sets up a self-fulfilling prophecy. The phobic individual worries excessively about the performance demands of an upcoming event, loses sleep worrying about the situation, becomes tremendously anxious just before the event, and in fact performs poorly in the actual situation because of the elevated levels of anxiety. This deficient performance then confirms people's beliefs about their inability to perform in these situations, and their fear is exacerbated, causing them to perform even more poorly in similar situations in the future.

Social phobias are portrayed or implied in numerous films. In *Coyote Ugly* (2000), a young woman, Violet, moves to New York City to try to make it as a songwriter. Her social anxiety disorder keeps her from reaching her full potential, so she takes a job as a "coyote" bartender at a wild nightclub. At this bar she begins to perform in front of large groups, deliberately "exposing" herself to those situations that she fears; moreover, her boyfriend helps to desensitize her by having her sing in the dark. It is this exposure that helps her manage and work through her anxiety symptoms. In the film's climax, she begins to get stage fright while performing and attempts to leave the stage; however, when the lights are turned off, she can perform, and she continues performing when the lights come back on. Violet believes the etiology of her social phobia is genetic; her mother also went to New York City to be a singer but left because of her own social phobia, and Violet believes she is carrying a "gene" for her inability to sing in front of others and her other avoidance symptoms. After she can perform, Violet learns it was her father who encouraged her mother to move home, and her mother never had a social phobia.

The painfully shy woman is a common film motif also found in *Amélie* (2001), *Lonely Hearts* (1981), *Rocky* (1976), *The Fisher King* (1991), and *I've Heard the Mermaids Singing* (1987). Shy and socially unskilled men are portrayed in *Bubble* (2005), *The Shape of Things* (2003), *Dummy* (2002), *Marty* (1955), *Untamed Heart* (1993), *Awakenings* (1990), *Goodbye, Mr. Chips* (1939), *Howard's End* (1992), *The Remains of the Day* (1993), and all of the Charlie Chaplin films in which he played the Little Tramp. The ways in which two shy adolescents come to grips with their emerging sexuality and a racist society are portrayed in a wonderful Australian film, *Flirting* (1990).

Generalized Anxiety Disorder

Some people are characterologically anxious; they walk around with a sense of apprehension and experience physiological arousal in a variety of different situations. They display what is sometimes called **free-floating anxiety**. Their condition can be quite debilitating. These individuals frequently receive a diagnosis of **generalized anxiety disorder**; the diagnosis requires that worry and anxiety be present more days than not.

The DSM-5 diagnosis of generalized anxiety disorder requires the presence of excessive anxiety or worry that occurs more days than not for at least 6 months. In addition, at least three of the following six symptoms must be present: restlessness, fatigue, difficulty concentrating, irritability, muscle tension, or sleep disturbance.

Anxiety symptoms associated with generalized anxiety disorder include the same physiological, cognitive, and behavioral symptoms associated with other anxiety disorders, but the symptoms are chronic. The individual with this disorder may have multiple somatic complaints such as tachycardia, a dry mouth, and gastrointestinal distress. They will worry constantly about the multiple things that can go wrong in life and may be irritable and short-tempered because of anxiety. The lifetime morbid risk for generalized anxiety disorder is about 9% in a White, US population. There are lower risks for African-Americans, Hispanics, and Asians; however, across categories, relatively few individuals with generalized anxiety disorder will seek out treatment (Asnaani et al., 2010). Onset of symptoms typically occurs in childhood or adolescence, and females are about twice as likely as males to experience the disorder.

In *Greenberg* (2010), Ben Stiller portrays Roger Greenberg, a selfish man who is consistently neurotic. His generalized anxiety disorder leads him to be anxious in a variety of everyday situations, and it dampens his life ambitions (e.g., his goal in life is to do nothing). He uses alcohol to cope with his anxiety. He is hospitalized for "mental problems," and he has a history of suicide attempts. He experiences intense anxiety. While his primary diagnosis is generalized anxiety disorder, a mental health professional treating Roger would need to differentiate generalized anxiety disorder from his symptoms of depression and social phobia, as well as interrelated personality factors such as OCPD.

Nicholas Cage plays two twin brothers, Charlie and Donald, in *Adaptation* (2002). Both brothers are screenwriters, but one is much more neurotic than the other. No makeup or artistic tricks are used to differentiate the two twins; instead, Cage's talent alone is sufficient to portray both the worried and neurotic Charlie and the easy-going Donald. This provides a nice contrast for people studying anxiety. Charlie anxiously struggles with writer's block and is plagued with self-doubt and preoccupation with himself, both hallmark symptoms of generalized anxiety disorder. In another scene, Charlie is too anxious to approach an attractive woman played by Meryl Streep. The viewer learns about Charlie's anxiety, worry, and rumination not only through cinematic close-ups displaying his anxiety symptoms (e.g., sweating), but also through the voice-over indicating his thought processes. A major theme of this film speaks to how people try to "adapt" to circumstances, problems, and, in this case, anxiety.

"I check my answering machine nine times every day and I can't sleep at night because I feel that there is so much to do and fix and change in the world, and I wonder every day if I am making a difference and if I will ever express the greatness within me, or if I will remain forever paralyzed by muddled madness inside my head. I've wept on every birthday ... and I feel that life is terribly unfair and sometimes beautiful and wonderful and extraordinary but also numbing and horrifying and insurmountable and I hate myself a lot of the time. The rest of the time I adore myself and I adore my life in this city and in this world we live in. This huge and wondrous, bewildering, brilliant, horrible world."

Jessica Stein describing the ways her anxiety disorder has limited her life, in *Kissing Jessica Stein* (2002)

Kissing Jessica Stein (2002) explores sexuality and relationships through the character of a New York journalist, Jessica Stein, who is tired of the dating scene and its limited offerings. She places an ad for "women seeking women" and meets a woman who turns out to be a great match. As their relationship develops, Jessica must battle her own neuroses about a lesbian relationship as well as her feelings for an ex-boyfriend who is still in love with her. Jessica experiences generalized anxiety as a worrier and classic neurotic. She is nervous and rigid, and very anxious about anything new or different. She does not have the self-confidence necessary to defend herself when she is criticized in public. She rarely stands up for herself and is unable to be honest to family or friends about her female lover. Jessica describes her experiences with panic attacks and mentions various other anxiety symptoms. She stumbles over her words and tries to control situations in which she becomes nervous. After reading a book about lesbians she realizes she is afraid of both sexuality and sensuality. Her anxiety is particularly noticeable at the dinner table prior to a family member's wedding; she is preoccupied with what people think of her and is unable to be honest, covering up the truth with repeated lies. This film emphasizes honesty, individuality, and the potential for change.

Most Woody Allen comedies will include at least one character with an anxiety disorder, and many depict characters with generalized anxiety disorder (usually played by Woody Allen himself). Indeed, neurotic, insecure, and self-absorbed characters, and the existential anxiety produced by the need to cope with a complex and impersonal world form the basis for much of Allen's humor. *Annie Hall* (1977) and *Manhattan* (1979) are the Woody Allen films that best illustrate generalized anxiety disorder.

Mel Brooks' classic film *High Anxiety* (1977) makes fun of numerous movies with Hitchcock-like psychological motifs. Mel Brooks plays Dr. Richard H. Thorndyke, an anxiety-ridden psychiatrist, who takes over a prestigious mental institution, "The Psycho-Neurotic Institute for the Very Very Nervous." Thorndyke must battle an unethical and murderous staff to save his patients and himself. Meanwhile he struggles with his own generalized anxiety and phobias.

Selective Mutism

Selective mutism involves the failure to speak in specific social situations in which one is expected to speak, and this interferes with educational, social, or occupational functioning. This condition is seldom depicted in movies. In *Disco Pigs* (2001), the character of Runt, one of two dizygotic twins, has a period of mutism when sent to a psychiatric institution. Other diagnoses would need to be ruled out to determine if selective mutism is the primary diagnosis for Runt.

When mutism is portrayed in films, it is customary to portray mutism as the result of trauma. In *My House in Umbria* (2003, UK/Italy), the mutism of a little girl is due to a traumatic reaction to a train crash. Similarly, in *Henry Poole Is Here* (2008), a young girl becomes mute for a year after being abandoned by her father. In these instances, acute stress disorder and PTSD would need to be ruled out as diagnoses.

International Films: Anxiety and Obsessive-Compulsive Disorders

An excellent portrayal of OCD is seen in *Dirty, Filthy Love* (2004, UK). This short but powerful film begins with a successful architect, Mark Furness (Michael Sheen), taking a leave of absence from work due to his OCD. His wife leaves him because she can no longer deal with his odd behaviors. During periods of stress, his OCD symptoms are exacerbated, and his tics (from Tourette's disorder) worsen. This film depicts a warm and sensitive person who is trying to cope with the challenges and consequences of mental illness. Many typical compulsions are displayed, such as climbing the stairs by walking up four stairs and down two, flicking lights on and off, and touching walls going up and down the stairs. Throughout the film, rituals dominate every aspect of Mark's life. Seeing Mark find acceptance in a support group allows the viewer to glimpse the variety of behaviors associated with OCD and the spectrum of behavioral interventions used in treating anxiety disorders. As Mark becomes increasingly ill, the destructive nature of mental illness is portrayed.

In the comedy, *Nothing* (2003, Canada), two roommates, Dave and Andrew, struggle with the stress and demands of everyday life. Andrew has one or more anxiety disorders, panic disorder, and agoraphobia. He refuses to leave the house and has avoided going outside since his teen years. He has arranged to work as a travel agent so he can stay at home. He reacts to situations with anxiety and distress, always thinks the worst in any situation, catastrophizes, jumps to conclusions, and is exceedingly fearful. Dave and Andrew discover that they can make something disappear by hating it. The problem is if they go too far with this ability, they are unable to make things reappear again.

The Norwegian film *Elling* (2001) presents an honest and fair portrayal of what it is like to cope with the debilitating effects of mental illness. A small, feeble man named Elling is taken to a psychiatric hospital after his mother, who was his caregiver for 40 years, dies. It is there that Elling meets another eccentric, Kjell, who has sexual obsessions about women and problems with anger management. The two men are discharged together and placed in supportive housing under the guidance of a social worker. The film is about their return to the reality of everyday living. Each man must prove he can live on his own.

Elling states he has two enemies: dizziness and anxiety; "they follow me everywhere." He refuses to leave his house and believes he is unable to answer the phone (even when it is only the social worker checking in). He has learned to be completely dependent on his mother and the hospital staff, so it is a great achievement when he can walk to the end of the block to go to a store. Further challenges are met when Elling begins to talk on the phone, eat at a restaurant, and go on vacation. Elling takes another big risk in battling his anxiety by going to a public poetry reading; arriving several hours early, he befriends an isolated, famous poet. Elling is rigid in his behavior, worries constantly, and is terrified of losing his only friend Kjell to Kjell's new girlfriend. Elling expresses this fear in jealous passive aggressiveness whenever he feels he has been left out or abandoned. His friendship with Kjell develops and deepens as they sacrifice for one another and stick together through the tough times. "Hard work pays off" is a theme applied to the psychological challenges Elling and Kjell face. Rather than avoiding their fears, they face them and, in turn, find freedom - freedom from dependency, from the hospital, and from isolation.

The interaction between the social worker, Frank, and Elling is noteworthy and inspirational. Frank sets firm boundaries and gives clear directives to Elling, taking a "tough love" approach that emphasizes that Elling must take chances to challenge himself, or he will lose his new residence. Frank is accepting and understanding of Elling's eccentric ideas, and tolerant at the film's end when he walks into the home and finds Elling lying on the couch, drunk, and having thrown up on himself. Elling awakens and believes he is sure to lose his house and his freedom; instead, the opposite happens because this all-too-human behavior confirms in Frank's mind Elling's readiness to live on his own in the outside world.

The protagonist in *She's One of Us* (2003, France) clearly struggles with social anxiety. She is socially awkward, frequently displays inappropriate affect, and misperceives social situations. In interactions, she pauses, looks away, hesitates and shakes; heavy breathing can be heard off-camera to simulate her anxiety. She is eager to please and to seek reassurance.

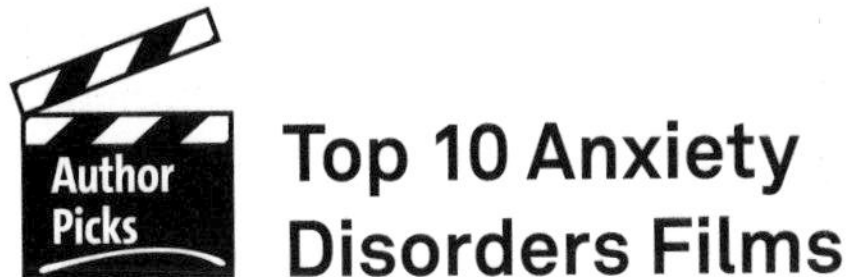

Top 10 Anxiety Disorders Films

Obsessive-Compulsive Disorders

As Good as It Gets (1997)
Matchstick Men (2003)
The Aviator (2004)
Dirty, Filthy Love (2004)
Phoebe in Wonderland (2008)

Anxiety Disorders

Vertigo (1958)
Play It Again, Sam (1972)
Elling (2001)
Adaptation (2002)
Batman Begins (2005)

Chapter 6

Trauma- and Stressor-Related Disorders

I've been on edge ... mood swings ... that sort of thing.

An inarticulate soldier describing his PTSD symptoms, in *The Dry Land* (2010)

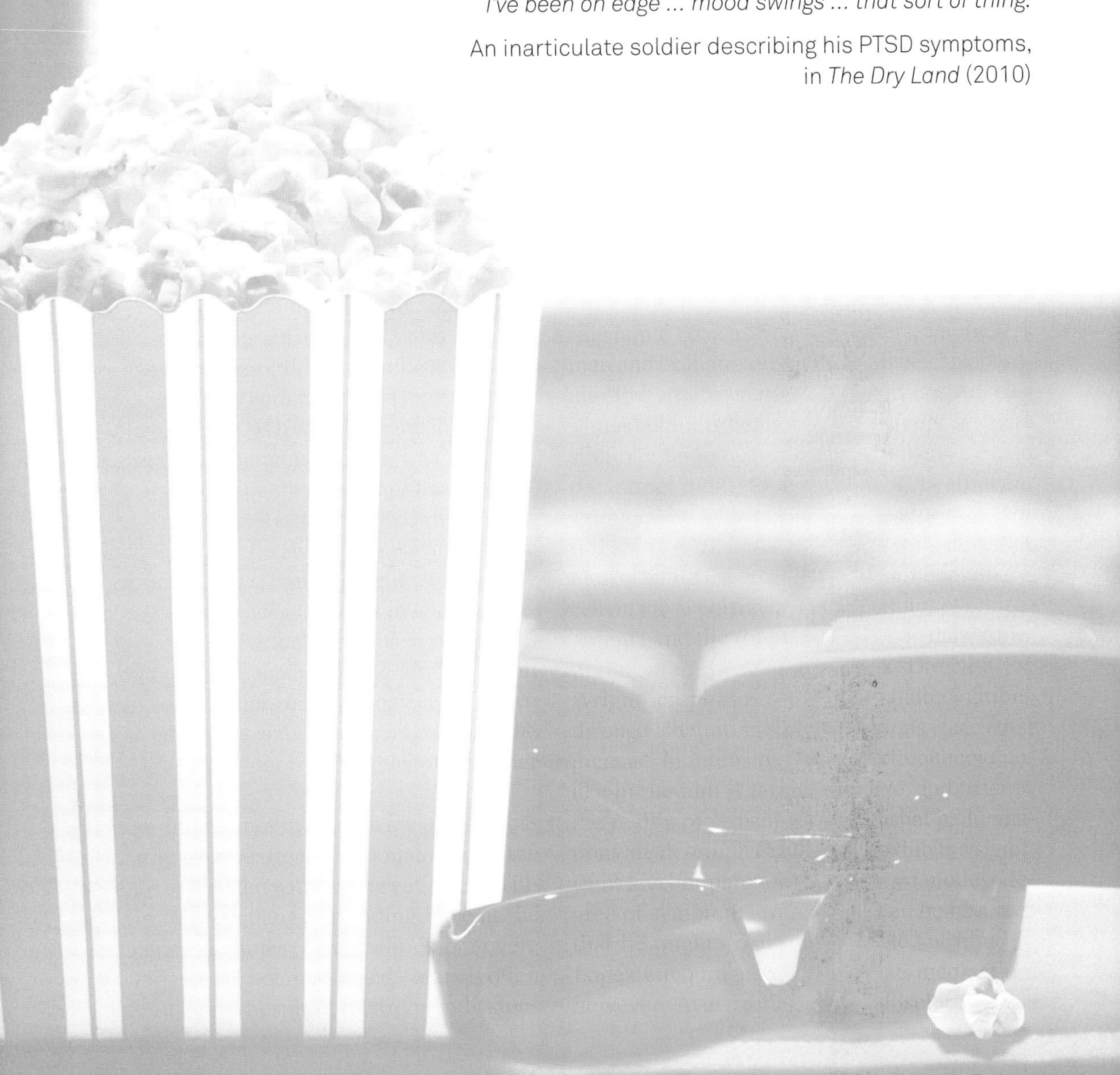

Trauma- and Stressor-Related Disorders

The DSM-5 now includes a separate chapter for those disorders that originate after exposure to a traumatic or stressful event. The diagnoses included in this chapter are **reactive attachment disorder**, **disinhibited social engagement disorder**, **PTSD**, **acute stress disorder**, and **adjustment disorders**. This chapter will make it clear that there is wide individual variability in the ways in which people respond to stress: Some people will react with anhedonia and dysphoria; others with anger or aggression; still others with dissociative symptoms. Reactive attachment disorder and disinhibited social engagement disorder are both disorders of childhood that result from social neglect. The former is expressed as an internalizing disorder (e.g., depression, withdrawal), while the latter is expressed as an externalizing disorder (e.g., disinhibition). PTSD, acute stress disorder, and adjustment disorders are described below.

Posttraumatic Stress Disorder

PTSD occurs after exposure to traumatic events. The individual with a PTSD must have personally witnessed or experienced some event that involved actual or threatened death or serious injury and must have responded with fear, helplessness, or horror. The traumatic event is then re-experienced by the individual in the form of nightmares, recurrent recollections, and flashbacks, or as physiological distress. The PTSD victim works hard to avoid these recurrent experiences. In addition, the individual usually experiences sleep disturbance, irritability, difficulty concentrating, hypervigilance, or an exaggerated startle response.

Kertesz et al. (2005) have published a now dated but still valuable list of films that can be used to sensitize primary care physicians to PTSD. They note,

> One of the main barriers to the identification of PTSD by physicians is their lack of a point of reference with regard to this disorder. Unless they have personally experienced trauma, they are often unable to fully appreciate the psychological impact of this disorder. A case in point is the fact that many of the more than 20 million people who emigrate to the USA each year come from war-torn nations where they may have experienced violence in their home and community. A substantial percentage of these refugees have experienced or witnessed numerous catastrophes and atrocities, such as famine, war, rape and repression, over an extended period of time. PTSD also frequently occurs because of more commonplace events that are outside the experience of many healthcare professionals, such as robberies and motor-vehicle accidents. Film clips can provide a means for physicians to begin to realize and visualize the magnitude of the emotional trauma for the individual and may ultimately assist in facilitating better diagnosis and treatment of this disorder. (p. 75)

Shen (2015) made similar points, noting that counselors are often called upon to treat clients from diverse, multicultural backgrounds, when they have little experience with these cultural groups. Shen argues that exposing these students to varied cultural norms and mores via films is the best practical option for students with limited multicultural experience.

Although forcibly displaced people have a high prevalence of mental illness, they seldom utilize mental health services. Denkinger et al. (2022) studied 134 people with such a history. They showed these individuals a short educational film titled *Coping with Flight and Trauma*, and concluded,

> Self-stigma was shown to be a robust and persistent issue, which tends to be underestimated by individuals not affected by mental illness. Low-threshold psychoeducational online interventions may be a promising tool to reduce barriers to accessing mental health services for forcibly displaced people. (Denkinger et al., 2022)

Military combat is a common cause of PTSD, but the disorder can also occur in response to earthquakes, fires or floods, mugging, rape, the witnessing of violence, or any of a variety of other traumatic situations. Often, innocuous stimuli will cause an individual to relive the anxiety-producing experience: for example, hearing a car backfire may trigger a terrifying war memory of combat for a war veteran. "According to the National Center for Posttraumatic Stress Disorder (PTSD), approximately 11% to 20% of veterans who served in Operations Iraqi Freedom and Enduring Freedom, 12% who served in the Gulf War, and 15% who served in Vietnam have been diagnosed with PTSD" (Vassar et al., 2020, p. 579). These authors argue that "popular American war movies emphasize a distorted and inaccurate portrayal of PTSD, its features, and outcomes" (p. 579), and they share the Entertainment Industries Council recommendations for mental health challenges for veteran characters in films.

The Dry Land and Posttraumatic Stress Disorder

The Dry Land (2010) offers students a compelling and realistic introduction to the symptoms of PTSD. The film revolves around the experiences of James, an Iraq war veteran, who returns to a small West Texas town, and the friends, family, and life he led there, only to discover that you cannot go home again. He has changed because of his combat experiences: He is irritable, labile, and anxious, and he seriously considers suicide with a gun he keeps in his trailer closet. He drinks heavily when he is out with his friends, and his suicidal ideation is most apparent when he is intoxicated. Simple events like seeing someone shooting a rabbit, something that would have seemed perfectly normal at one time, now trouble him deeply and led to a fistfight with the shooter. His marriage is on the rocks, and his wife, fearing for her own safety, leaves him to stay with her parents. James is only comfortable with his former combat buddies, and he traveled several days to visit one of these friends who had been hospitalized because of his Iraq injuries (Figure 23).

What we now call "posttraumatic stress disorder" was referred to as "battle fatigue" or "combat neurosis" in previous wars. *Patton* (1970) depicts George C. Scott in the title role of the film slapping a soldier with PTSD whom he accuses of being a "dirty coward." The horrors of war are also vividly depicted in older, classic films such as *All Quiet on the Western Front* (1930) and *Paths of Glory* (1957).

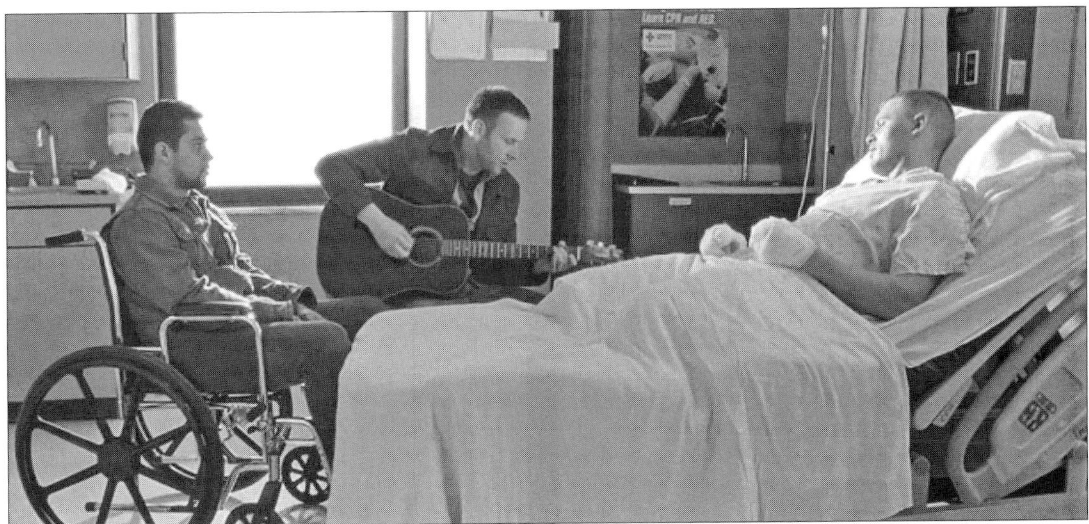

Figure 23. *The Dry Land* (2010, Maya Entertainment). Produced by Heather Rae. Directed by Ryan Piers Williams.

Patton: "What's the matter with you?"
Soldier: "I ... I guess I ... I can't take it, sir."
Patton: "What did you say?"
Soldier: "It's my nerves, sir. I ... I ... I just can't stand the shelling anymore."
Patton: "Your nerves? Well, hell, you're just a God-damned coward."
[Soldier starts sniveling]
Patton: "Shut up! I won't have a yellow bastard sitting here crying in front of these brave men who have been wounded in battle! ... . You're going back to the front, my friend. You may get shot, and you may get killed, but you're going up to the fighting. Either that, or I'm going to stand you up in front of a firing squad. I ought to shoot you myself, you god-damned ... bastard! Get him out of here!"

General George S. Patton slapping and denigrating a soldier coping with PTSD, in the film *Patton*, which would have then likely been called "combat exhaustion."

In war films such as the award-winning *Saving Private Ryan* (1998), even though PTSD is not portrayed per se, it would be easy to understand how one could develop it, as the viewer observes the ubiquitous trauma the soldiers experience. *Gran Torino* (2008) depicts the adjustment problems of Clint Eastwood playing the role of Walt Kowalski, a decorated but racist and embittered Korean war veteran. The award-winning film, *In the Valley of Elah* (2007) is based on the July 13, 2003, murder of Richard Davis, a 23-year-old army soldier who had just returned to Fort Benning, Georgia, when he was declared AWOL. The young veteran's charred remains were discovered in the woods 4 months later. Hank Deerfield (Tommy Lee Jones), father of the murdered soldier and a retired army investigator, uncovers the events surrounding his son's murder.

"Every man I kill, the farther away from home I feel."

Capt. John H. Miller (Tom Hanks), in *Saving Private Ryan* (1998)

Waltz With Bashir (2009) is an acclaimed, animated documentary inspired by actual events. Ari Folman, an Israeli veteran of the first Lebanon war, is unable to remember much of what happened when he was engaged in war. His memory is mostly full of gaps as he tries to figure out what happened on the day of a massacre for which he has one distinct memory. He asks questions and confronts his past to deal with his trauma. As students consider the PTSD criteria Ari meets, they might need to extrapolate from statements and scenes to fill in gaps where there is a lack of clarity. In an interview about the film, the director shared the experience of finding that the making of the film was therapeutic and healing for him because it helped him directly confront the trauma and reality of war (Guillen, 2009).

Many victims of combat or natural disasters experience **survivor guilt**. Some might feel guilty when they realize that their lives were spared while those of more worthy individuals (e.g., children, young parents) were taken. Consider Tom Cruise's character Ron Kovic, who would meet the criteria for PTSD, in *Born on the Fourth of July* (1989). Kovic's guilt about the death of his buddy "Wilson" is an example of survivor guilt. A brother meets the criteria for PTSD and experiences considerable survivor guilt after his brother dies during a storm in *Ordinary People* (1980). Two high school students experience survivor guilt after a school shooting in which many of their classmates died in *The Fallout* (2021).

In the fictitious film *Reign Over Me* (2007), Adam Sandler plays the role of a dentist coping with PTSD and survivor guilt after the death of his wife and three daughters who were passengers on one of the planes involved in the 9/11 destruction of the World Trade Center. Refusing to acknowledge his past or the tragedy, the character Charlie Fineman enters extreme isolation, regressing to a child-like existence in which he spends his time playing video games, listening to loud music, riding around on a scooter, watching movies, and pounding on his drums. He gets considerable emotional support because of the efforts of an old friend, another dentist played by Don Cheadle. However, the film is clumsy in dealing with this delicate subject and teaches the viewer little about the sequelae associated with something as traumatic as the loss of one's entire family.

Suicide and suicide attempts are common in patients with PTSD. In addition, it is essential to assess for comorbidity (especially substance abuse) in cases of PTSD. Nearly all PTSD patients who are suicidal will be found to have a concomitant psychiatric condition.

The movie *Fearless* (1993) provides an interesting picture of an unusual reaction to trauma. Max Klein (Jeff Bridges) is one of a small group of survivors of a devastating plane crash. He assists several other passengers and is celebrated as a hero and a saint. He becomes convinced he is invulnerable and grows increasingly impatient with the banal concerns of his wife and child. After a near-death experience precipitated by an allergic reaction to strawberries, he returns to normal and reestablishes a loving relationship with his wife and son. The movie includes an interesting segment in which a psychiatrist (who is employed by the airline because he has authored a best-selling book about PTSD) leads a discussion group for survivors of the crash.

Unbreakable (2000), directed by M. Night Shyamalan, has a similar theme and a surprise ending, and it is reminiscent of Shyamalan's earlier movie, *The Sixth Sense* (1999). Bruce Willis is the sole survivor of a train wreck that kills 131 of the other passengers. He later meets a mysterious man (Samuel L. Jackson) who tells him that he is one of a rare group of "unbreakable" people who never get sick and can survive accidents that kill mere mortals. Shapiro et al. (2018) use this film to teach medical students and psychiatric residents about PTSD.

Kevin Spacey's portrayal of Prot, a man who claims to be from another planet, presents a diagnostic enigma in *K-Pax* (2001). One way to view the film (another way is discussed in Chapter 3) is to assume that this character has PTSD. The viewer learns through flashbacks that Prot is Robert Porter, a man who had experienced trauma when he returned home to find his wife and daughter murdered and the killer still in the house. Prot/Porter re-experiences the trauma under hypnosis and displays significant physiological arousal (e.g., a racing heart rate, elevated blood pressure) when his psychiatrist (Jeff Bridges) forces him to recall the traumatic incident. Porter engaged in extensive avoidance following the trauma – denial, estrangement from his hometown, inability to recall information, and a restricted range of affect.

In *The Fisher King* (1991), Robin Williams plays a former college professor who becomes homeless and psychotic after witnessing his wife being gunned down in a restaurant. However, the active, well-formed, and specific hallucinations Williams experiences (e.g., a red knight riding a horse in Central Park with flames shooting out of his head) would be very unlikely to occur because of a traumatic experience. The character Jeff Bridges plays in the same film, a disc jockey who withdraws from life and abuses alcohol and drugs after a traumatic event, presents a far more realistic portrayal of PTSD. Although *The Fisher King* is imprecise and confusing in the way it links trauma to psychosis, it is true that PTSD is common among people who are homeless.

The stressors experienced by homeless people are illustrated in the films *Ironweed* (1987) and *The Saint of Fort Washington* (1993). *Ironweed* (1987) is a compelling film in which Jack Nicholson plays an alcoholic whose drinking is related to his guilt about dropping and killing his infant son. Many of the symptoms of PTSD have become obliterated by Nicholson's alcoholism, which has become the dominant theme in his life. *Ironweed* illustrates how alcohol abuse can develop as a secondary problem in response to trauma and can become the primary psychological problem as abuse progresses to addiction.

Dozens of movies have been made about the Vietnam War, and many of these (as well as other war movies) illustrate either acute stress disorders or, more commonly in those that follow the hero home after the war, PTSD. Some of the most powerful of these films are *Coming Home* (1978); *The Deer Hunter* (1978); *Apocalypse*

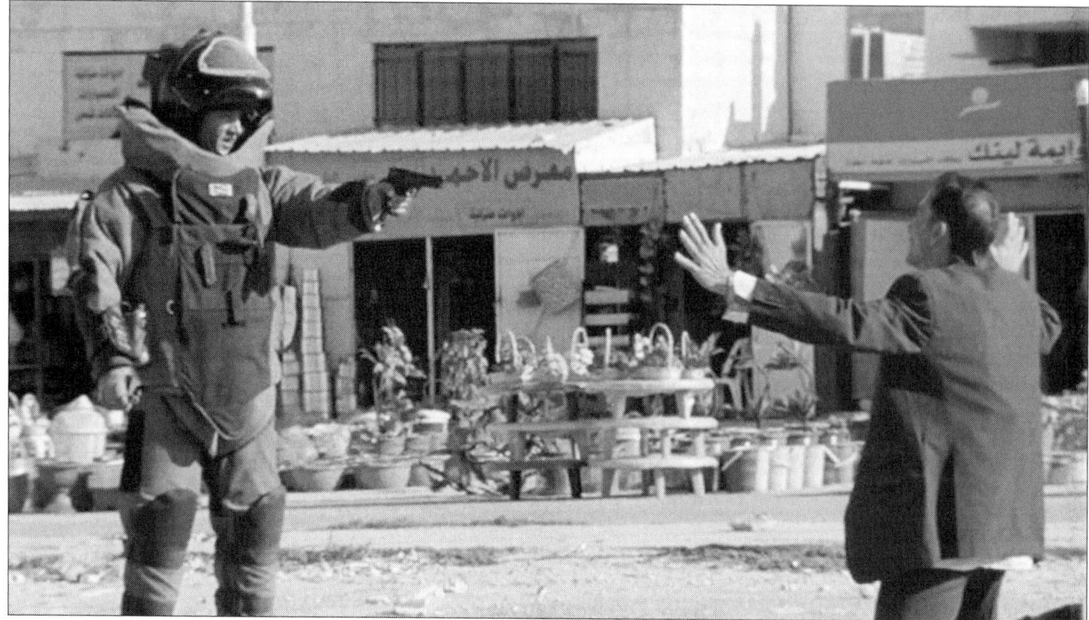

Figure 24. *The Hurt Locker* (2008, Voltage Pictures, First Light Production, Kingsgate Films). Produced by Katheryn-Bigelow, Mark Boal, Nicholas Chartier, Jenn Lee, et al. Directed by Kathryn Bigelow.

Now (1979); *The Killing Fields* (1984); *Rambo: First Blood* (1982) and the numerous *Rambo* sequels; Oliver Stone's trilogy *Platoon* (1986), *Born on the Fourth of July* (1989), and *Heaven and Earth* (1993); *Full Metal Jacket* (1987); *Good Morning, Vietnam* (1987); *Hamburger Hill* (1987); *We Were Soldiers* (2002); and *The Hurt Locker* (2008), in which a soldier assigned to a bomb disposal unit finds readjustment to civilian life almost impossible. *The Hurt Locker* is especially effective in dramatizing the stress associated with making quick life or death decisions in combat situations (Figure 24). The film *Heaven and Earth* (1993) addresses multiple traumas, including those associated with rape, torture, war, and suicide.

All Quiet on the Western Front (*Im Westen Nichts Neues;* 2022, Germany) is a film with English subtitles that depicts the futility and stupidity of war. In this case, it is World War I, and the Germans are fighting the French, but the message generalizes to all wars, all times. Of course, this is a remake of a classic 1930 film.

Dog (2022) depicts an Army Ranger veteran who finds his relationship with a combat-trained dog he is taking to a friend's funeral helps him deal with his personal demons. Both the man and the dog were scarred by their combat experiences.

Hediger et al. (2021) conducted an extensive meta-analysis examining the effectiveness of animal-assisted interventions (AAI) for children and adults with PTSD symptoms. They found that AAI was superior to a waitlist control, and there were clear benefits from interacting with service dogs. AAI "led to comparable effects in reducing depression as standard PTSD psychotherapy," and getting a service dog also helped alleviate the symptoms of PTSD.

In the original version of *The Manchurian Candidate* (1962), Frank Sinatra plays a brainwashed trauma victim who has recurring nightmares. He wakes up screaming with extensive sweating and a recollection of traumatic dreams that seem real. In a recent remake of *The Manchurian Candidate* (2004), director Jonathan Demme updates the film by including contemporary politics and more recent wartime experiences. Denzel Washington plays a major who returns from the Gulf War with PTSD, paranoia, nightmares, and memories he cannot understand. He displays flat affect when he describes events surrounding the war, and he experiences intrusive memories. He becomes obsessed with trying to uncover the truth about what happened to him and his men. He hallucinates blood oozing from the forehead of a woman and has a flashback to a time when he was seeing a hypnotist; this symbolizes a real memory coming back and triggers a panic attack. He slowly begins to put together the sinister pieces of a political plot that involved extensive trauma and torture as well as physical and psychological abuse and brainwashing. PTSD symptoms are also displayed by Nicole Kidman's character in *The Human Stain* (2003), and by other actors in *Open Hearts* (2002), *The Princess and the Warrior* (2000), and *The Pawnbroker* (1965). The last of these films portrays a defeated concentration camp survivor who has become numb and indifferent in response to wartime experiences that included seeing his wife raped and his children killed.

The film *Mystic River* (2003) portrays multiple characters who experience PTSD, most notably the character of David Boyle (Tim Robbins), who was sexually abused as a young boy, and Jimmy Markum (Sean Penn), whose daughter is murdered. In *Shutter Island* (2010), Leonardo DiCaprio plays the role of Teddy Daniels, a federal Marshall who was initially traumatized by his experiences liberating a Nazi concentration camp in World War II, and later by seeing his wife burn to death in a fire. *The Brave One* (2007), starring Jodie Foster, deals with the trauma that results when a woman is molested in Central Park and sees her boyfriend being killed.

School shootings almost always result in PTSD for the children who survive the shooting, and often for their parents. Examples include *Elephant* (2003), *We Need to Talk About Kevin* (2011), *Mass* (2021), and *The Fallout* (2021). *Mass* is especially powerful in depicting what it must feel like to be a parent – on either side – who must make sense of the loss of a child after a school shooting. I will discuss these films in more detail in Chapter 15.

"I feel mad because I had no idea one guy with a gun could fuck up my life so hard in six minutes. Fuck up so many lives! Then I think I should be grateful to be alive. I feel like, I don't know, maybe there's some weird fucked up reason why I made it, and other people didn't. Um, but then when you sit back and you think about it, you realize, 'No! There isn't. There's no fucking reason.' None of us should have died."

Vada Cavell experiences survivor's guilt after a school shooting in *The Fallout* (2021)

EMDR: A Documentary Film (2011) presents a series of case histories of people who have benefited from eye movement desensitization and reprocessing (EMDR), a popular but still controversial treatment for PTSD. Another documentary, *The Invisible War* (2012), documents an epidemic of rape in the military and the ways in which victims are affected by rape (often experiencing PTSD symptoms every bit as serious as those experienced by combat veterans).

Acute Stress Disorder

Acute stress disorder results from exposure to threatened death, serious injury, or sexual trauma; it requires at least nine of 14 symptoms be present (e.g., recurrent intrusive memories or dreams, dissociative symptoms, avoidance, sleep disturbance). Acute stress disorder is in many ways like PTSD. However, acute stress disorder occurs between 3 days and 1 month following a traumatic event and may resolve quickly, or develop into PTSD. In contrast, the symptoms of PTSD must last more than a month, and the onset of symptoms may occur months or even years after exposure to trauma.

According to the DSM-5, acute stress disorder occurs in less than 20% of cases in which the traumatic event did not involve interpersonal assault; however, much higher rates are reported following interpersonal traumatic events such as rape or witnessing public bombings like those that occurred in 2013 during the Boston Marathon. The risk for acute stress disorder is greater for woman, and there is wide variability across cultures in how people respond to acute stress situations.

Brothers (2009) is a compelling film that offers a rare cinematic depiction of the symptoms of acute stress disorder as they develop into PTSD. The film contrasts the lives of two brothers, Capt. Sam Cahill (Toby Maguire) and Tommy Cahill (Jake Gyllenhaal). Sam is happily married to Grace Cahill (Natalie Portman), and can be described as a man of strong character, involved with his family, responsible, and a hard-working leader. Tommy, on the other hand, is volatile, angry, lacks self-control, has family problems, drinks too much, and cannot sustain a long-term relationship. Their father makes the distinction that Sam is perseverant (there is "no quit in him") while Tommy is a "quitter" who easily gives up. A surprising yet realistic role reversal takes place. Sam goes to war and is captured and tortured for months in Afghanistan and then forced to do the unthinkable – to beat another soldier to death with a lead pipe. He escapes and returns home, hardened, unemotional, and profoundly affected by the traumatic experiences. Tommy, on the other hand, steps up to help his brother's family (his sister-in-law Grace and her two girls). Tommy takes on responsibilities such as remodeling the kitchen, providing genuine care for his nieces, and participating in family gatherings; these acts pave the way for him to then express kindness to a woman he had previously robbed. Meanwhile, Sam's acute stress disorder worsens as he cannot share any of his internal experience with his family, and his mental suffering worsens greatly. He projects his pain onto his wife, brother, and daughters. Sam becomes easily irritated and difficult to be around; his daughters pick up on this behavior and even share that they would rather have "Uncle Tommy" around than their dad. Sam's full-blown PTSD becomes so serious that the only thing Sam can imagine doing to cope, is to leave his family and return to combat or commit suicide. Then, a turning point emerges when Tommy repeatedly and lovingly reminds him: "You're my brother. You're my family." This breaks through Sam's hardened shell, and he agrees to inpatient treatment. During a hospital visit by his wife, Sam finally shares his horrible secret: "I have seen the end of war. The question is: Can I live again?"

Brothers is directed by Jim Sheridan who tends to make films that deal with redemption within the complexities of family life (e.g., *In America* [2002]). He explains that this film, although about war trauma, also is about how a family can put Humpty Dumpty back together again. Indeed, PTSD victims often are shattered.

Martha Marcy May Marlene (2011), directed by Sean Durkin, depicts a young woman, Martha, who has escaped from a cult after being indoctrinated for 2 years. The film shows both the present-day coping (acute stress disorder) and flashbacks depicting the cult's abusive practices – drugging, manipulation, subtle inconsistencies, distortion of the word *family,* and use of women to recruit new members into a self-sustaining farming commune. After Martha escapes from the cult through the woods, she calls her estranged sister and finds solace at her sister's remote retreat home. Martha begins to experience memory flashes, paranoia, and blunted affect. She becomes isolated, refuses to share details of her past experiences, and manifests inappropriate behavior. At a party, her paranoia peaks and she loses control. She is haunted by her traumatic past, frequently thinking people she meets are cult members trying to recapture her. This film offers a good portrayal of acute stress disorder that is likely to turn into PTSD about a month post trauma. The related short film, *Mary Last Seen* (2010), also by Durkin, depicts manipulative tactics to indoctrinate a girl into a cult.

In the small, but powerful movie *Grace Is Gone* (2008), Stanley Philips (John Cusack) is unable to accept and process his wife's death in Iraq. Instead, he drives his daughters from the upper Midwest to a Disneyland-like park for a brief vacation. Marisa Tomei's character in the film *In the Bedroom* (2001) experiences a traumatic event when her boyfriend is murdered by her estranged husband. In a subsequent scene, she is shown as depressed and expressionless. Acute stress disorder is also present in Roman Polanski's *Death and the Maiden* (1994), and in the TV movie *My House in Umbria* (2003, UK/Italy).

Testament (1983) stars Jane Alexander and provides an understated portrayal of the human cost of nuclear war; Kyle Fitzpatrick (2020) has described how his Latina mother used this film – along with others – to cope with loneliness, an alien environment (living in Fort Knox), and her husband's protracted absence from the home.

> An hour into *Testament*, Carol's children start to die. In one scene, she fills the bathroom sink with water in the middle of the night. She carries in her youngest son, naked, and rests him on the counter. She dabs him with a wet washcloth, cleaning him while humming and whispering gently. He slumps against the wall, barely able to lift his arms. When the bathing is done, she wraps him in a clean white towel, swaddling him, smiling at him, before lifting him to her shoulder. She stops, facing the mirror, caught by something she sees: a red stain spreading across the towel, blood coming out of her son's bottom. It's a quiet moment. It's a horrible moment. It's a moment that no parent wants to experience. ... The movie uses the home as a backdrop for tragedy and disaster. Whether it's running out of food or losing track of the days, explaining sex to your tween daughter who will never experience the act, or digging graves in your backyard next to the swing set, the horrors of disaster happen in the domestic domain. (Fitzpatrick, 2020)

Vassar et al. (2020) have argued that "popular American war movies emphasize a distorted and inaccurate portrayal of PTSD, its features, and outcomes" (p. 579), and they share the Entertainment Industries Council recommendations for mental health challenges for veteran characters in films. They go one to state that "these recommendations advocate for character portrayals that showcase positive help seeking behaviors and reduce misperceptions and stigma surrounding Veteran's issues and mental health" (p. 580).

Adjustment Disorders

An adjustment disorder is diagnosed when a person develops significant emotional or behavioral symptoms in response to a particular psychosocial stressor, and the response exceeds what would typically be expected in such a situation. Social, academic, or occupational functioning may be affected. Adjustment disorders are usually associated with depression, anxiety, disturbance of conduct, or some mixture of each.

The adjustment disorder displayed by Terry Ann Wolfmeyer (Joan Allen) in *The Upside of Anger* (2005) includes a mixture of disturbance of conduct and emotions. We see this in her reaction when she learns her husband has been having an affair, and she becomes convinced that he has gone off to Sweden to be with a younger woman. Terry becomes incredibly bitter, irritable, lonely, and explosive. She begins to drink alcohol regularly and becomes increasingly angry and cynical, particularly when interacting with her daughters.

It is not difficult to find other films portraying adjustment disorders – numerous movies exhibit characters facing a stressor, conflict, or challenge, and frequently this affects an area of their functioning in a significant way. Many films depicting relationship stress or those addressing problems with work include characters with adjustment disorder symptoms, such as the anxiety displayed by Harry Sanborn (Jack Nicholson) in *Something's Gotta Give* (2003) and the disturbance of conduct exhibited by Tommy Rowland (Matt Dillon) in *Beautiful Girls* (1996). The protagonist in *Meet Bill* (2007), played by Aaron Eckhart, is a man languishing in several areas of his life. He struggles to cope with his wife's infidelity, and this leads to numerous changes in his life; while at first it disturbs his functioning, he eventually finds ways to make meaning out of the stress he is experiencing. A similar theme (adjusting to infidelity) can be found in *Tennis, Anyone ...?* (2005).

Films that integrate several vignettes or stories are almost certain to have at least one character with an adjustment disorder. Some good examples include *Lantana* (2001), *The Last Kiss* (2006), and *13 Conversations About One Thing* (2001).

Persistent Complex Bereavement Disorder

Persistent complex bereavement disorder, a controversial diagnosis, is noted as a "condition for further study" in DSM-5, and at the same time, it can be diagnosed under the coding for other specified trauma- and stressor-related disorder. This means that grief symptoms following the death of a loved one cause clinically significant distress or impairment in social, occupational, or other important areas of functioning. DSM-5 suggests that this "disorder" occurs if the symptoms last longer than 12 months after the death of a loved one for adults and longer than 6 months after the death for children. The individual may have a reactive distress to the death (e.g., difficulty with positive reminiscing, accepting, and believing the death) and social-identity disruption (e.g., a desire to die to be with the deceased, feeling life is meaningless). One of the controversies with the DSM-5 involved the decision to remove the DSM-IV **bereavement exclusion**, which stated that major depressive disorder could not be diagnosed in anyone who had experienced a recent loss of a loved one; this change ostensibly helps clinicians avoid overlooking cases of major depressive disorder that could be helped by aggressive treatment. However, many mental health providers feel that grief and bereavement are existential challenges all of us will face at some point, and they believe it is inappropriate to pathologize those emotions that are quite naturally associated with loss. These clinicians emphasize that the experience of bereavement symptoms and suffering is normal, especially following the loss of someone close to oneself. Indeed, to *not* experience these symptoms after the loss of someone you deeply love would be pathological.

Two poignant films about bereavement of parents following the loss of a child are the independent film *Morning* (2010) and the popular film *Rabbit Hole* (2010), the latter starring Nicole Kidman and Aaron Eckhart. Each film shows unproductive and unhealthy coping and a significant impact of loss on marital relationships. Grief counselors and support groups are depicted in both films. *Morning* offers a melodramatic illustration of coping; for example, the husband regresses to childlike behavior as he makes a mess of the house, hits the tops of indoor flowers with his golf club, and runs around the house as if playing "cowboys and Indians," while the wife dissociates while putting on makeup at a department story and runs to the bathroom to vomit. Whenever she is reminded of her son, she screams - wherever she is. Although we would caution against giving *any* of these characters this diagnosis, we include these films because of their compelling portrayal of bereavement. In addition, they would not meet DSM-5 criteria, because the films do not depict the characters' lives post–12 months from the death of each child. A third movie depicting bereaved parents following the loss of a child is Lars von Trier's *Antichrist* (2009), a film that takes disturbing content (i.e., the recent, untimely death of a child) and devastated parents to a new level, in which the parents deal with their grief by beginning to torture one another. Each of the characters in these films should be monitored over the months and years for not only complicated bereavement but also depression and conditions relating to stress and trauma.

Mother: "You're not right about everything, you know? What if there is a God?"
Becca: "Then I'd say he's a sadistic prick."
Mother: "All right, Becca, that's enough."
Becca: "'Worship me and I'll treat you like shit.' No wonder you like him. He sounds just like Dad."

Nicole Kidman's character pushes back, in *Rabbit Hole*, when her mother encourages her to go to church after losing a child.

In *Mother Ghost* (2002), a man begins to have significant conflicts with his wife, ignores his son, numbs his pain by getting drunk, and is unable to sleep. At the same time, his deceased mother's jewelry begins to appear. The reactions to deaths in both *Truly, Madly, Deeply* (1991) and *In the Bedroom* (2001) seem to go beyond healthy bereavement and consequently would warrant a diagnosis, though by the end of each film, the viewer gets the sense that the characters have found healing and have learned to cope with their losses. Sandy Edwards (Toni Collette) in *Japanese Story* (2003) and a young girl in *Ponette* (1996) both experience protracted bereavement.

In each of the following three films the bereaved character copes by immediately going on a journey in reaction to their pain: Jack Nicholson as Warren loses his wife of many years in *About Schmidt* (2002), a young woman loses her beloved father in *Searching for Paradise* (2002), and another young woman loses her boyfriend to suicide in *Movern Callor* (2002).

International Films: Trauma- and Stressor-Related Disorders

Enduring Love (2004, UK) is a film about a freak hot air balloon accident in which several men attempt to save a young boy by grabbing onto the out-of-control balloon. As the balloon rises higher and higher, each man saves himself by letting go soon enough, except for one who eventually dies. This traumatic incident leads the boy to develop symptoms of acute stress disorder and to vacillate from avoidance to rumination and from detachment to agitation in his relationships. His emotional distress is palpable as he displays inappropriate affect and struggles with guilt and anger.

In the Australian film *Walking on Water* (2002), an assisted-suicide plan for a man dying of AIDS goes awry, and a friend forcefully suffocates the dying man. The friend is plagued by intrusive images and memories of the suffocation; he tries hard to avoid his memories, acts out in self-destructive ways, and displays considerable irritability and interpersonal conflict. He is suffering from **acute stress disorder.**

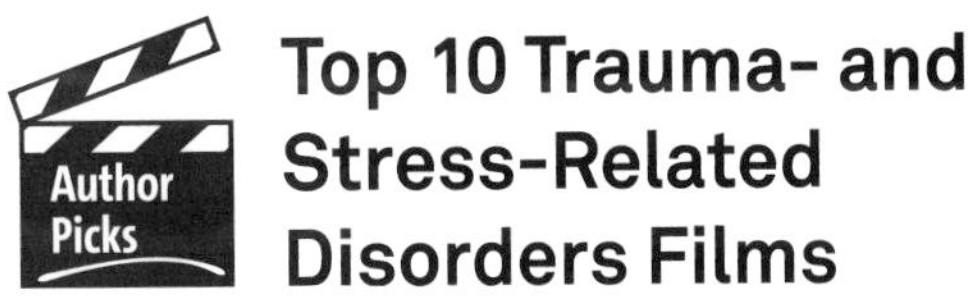

Top 10 Trauma- and Stress-Related Disorders Films

The Deer Hunter (1978)
Testament (1983)
Mystic River (2003)
A History of Violence (2005)
Reign Over Me (2007)
Waltz With Bashir (2009)
Brothers (2009)
Rabbit Hole (2010)
Martha Marcy May Marlene (2011)
The Dry Land (2012)

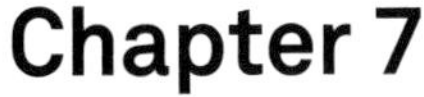

Chapter 7

Dissociative Disorders

Matricide is probably the most unbearable crime of all ... so he had to erase the crime, at least in his own mind.

A police psychiatrist attempts to explain Norman Bates's behavior, in *Psycho* (1960)

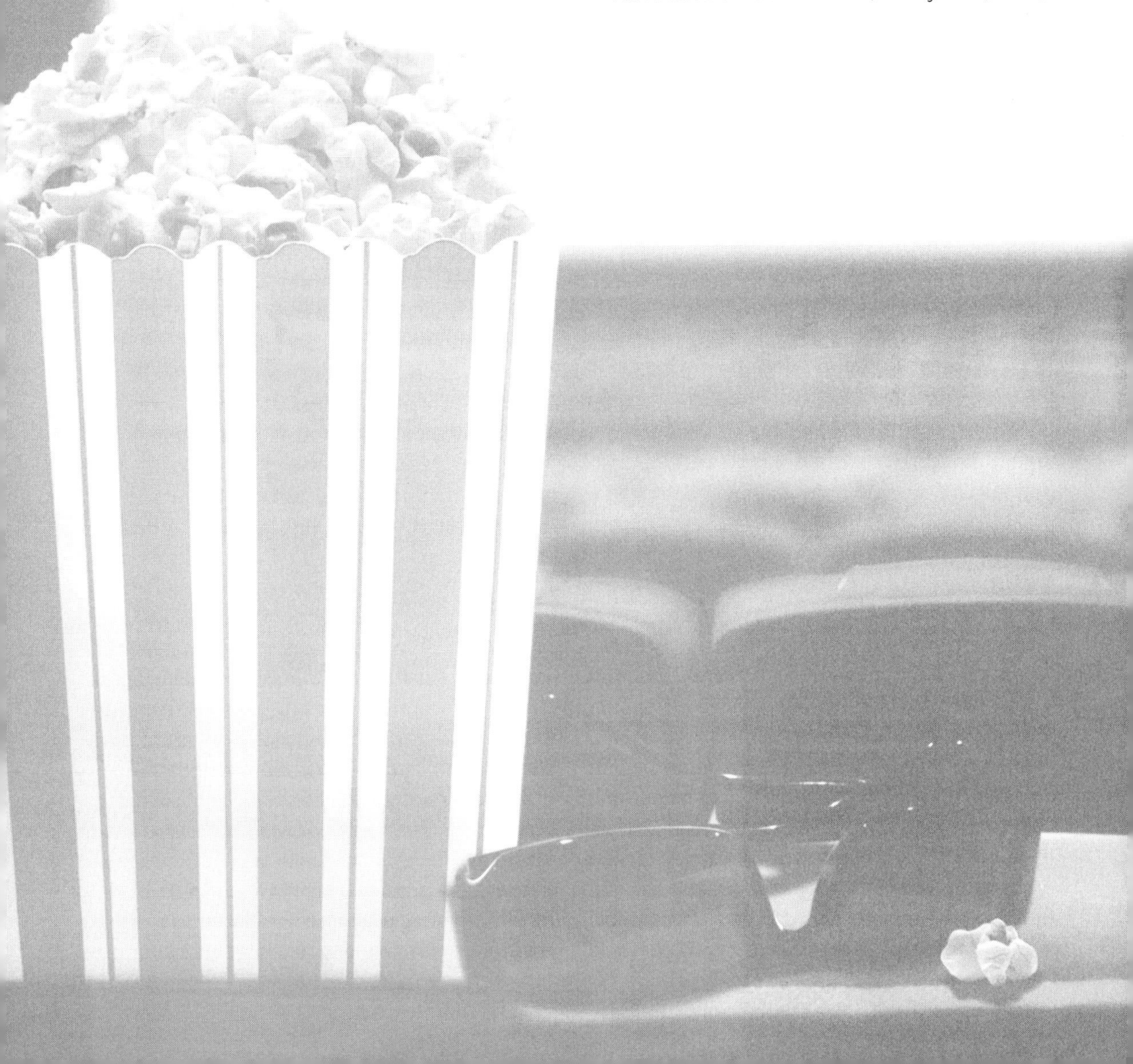

Dissociation and Films

Alteration in consciousness can occur under many different conditions. With alcohol intoxication, there is a clouding of consciousness, with attenuated awareness of sensory stimuli and diminished attention to the environment and self. Some drugs produce a dream-like state in which the individual is conscious but inattentive. Heightened states of attention, concentration, and absorption brought about through hypnosis, meditation, or relaxation are further examples of alterations in consciousness.

Dissociation involves an unwelcome shift in consciousness that is accompanied by the sense that one's core identity has changed. In dissociation, events and information that would ordinarily be connected or integrated are divided from one another. Dissociation is often viewed as a normal defense mechanism that can be used in frightening, stressful, or painful situations to cope with stress. It allows an individual to detach from overwhelming fear, pain, and helplessness generated by trauma.

Dissociation can be viewed on a continuum from minor dissociative experiences of everyday life (i.e., daydreaming) to major forms of psychopathology, such as multiple personality disorder (Allen & Smith, 1993; Bernstein & Putnam, 1986). Most people have minor dissociative experiences, such as driving a car over a familiar route and suddenly realizing that they do not remember what happened during all or part of the trip. In some cultures, dissociative states, such as trances, are common and accepted cultural activities or a routine part of religious experience. The development of extreme dissociative behavior patterns has been linked to trauma. For example, in *Sybil* (1976), the lead character's development of 16 different personalities was the result of repeated physical and psychological abuse she experienced at the hands of a deranged and delusional mother.

Numerous films depict characters experiencing a traumatic event and many depict the lead character dissociating from the traumatic experience to cope. However, it is unlikely that any of the characters in the following five examples would be given a dissociative disorder diagnosis, as there is not enough evidence in the film to meet all of the diagnostic criteria. In *Lilya 4-Ever* (2002), a young girl is prostituted against her will in a foreign country, and she is neglected and abused; she dissociates during sexual intercourse with a paying customer. In *The Princess and the Warrior* (2001), a man is trapped in a bathroom stall while his wife is killed; his various traumatic reactions include freezing, dissociating from reality, feeling tense and shaky, and experiencing flashbacks. In *Natural Born Killers* (1994), Woody Harrelson and Juliette Lewis play characters who are both victims and perpetrators of various violent and traumatic events; in the film, dissociative numbing, dissociative perceptual distortion, dissociative time distortion, and dissociative derealization are depicted. *Swimming Pool* (2002) portrays a young woman exhibiting dissociative amnesia in her inability to remember killing a man. One dissociative episode occurs when she thinks she is seeing her mother; she screams when she is told her mother is not there, and then she faints. In the independent film *Searching for Paradise* (2002), a woman, in the middle of sex with a "fantasy-come-true" man, suddenly stops and states she feels betrayed by her partner; this is a dissociative experience in which she is confusing her father who had left her and this fantasy man who has become real.

Another dissociative experience often present in traumatic situations is **derealization** or **depersonalization**. In derealization, a person feels detached from familiar people or places that seem unreal and unrecognizable. The size or shape of objects may be perceived as altered or strange, and people may seem mechanical. During the 1989 San Francisco Bay Area earthquake, 40% of 101 persons interviewed afterward reported feeling as though their surroundings were unreal (Cardeña & Spiegel, 1993). David Lynch's films seem to induce a derealization state for both his characters and his viewers, his characters' identities are often confused, and locations seem unreal. The films *Lost Highway* (1997) and *Mulholland Drive* (2001) are particularly good examples of this kind of derealization.

Depersonalization is related and occurs when someone feels that they are "outside their body," observing themselves behave and think as though they were watching a third party interacting with the world. In DSM-5, derealization and depersonalization are linked as a single syndrome.

Dissociative Disorders in Films

There is controversy in the mental health community about the categorization of dissociative experiences as psychiatric disorders. Dissociation, by itself, does not necessarily lead to impairment and is not clear evidence of psychopathology. However, if dissociative states lead to distress and impairment in psychological, interpersonal, social, or vocational functioning, then they should be evaluated as psychiatric problems. Because dissociative symptoms such as amnesia and depersonalization can be present in other psychiatric disorders such as PTSD and schizophrenia, no other psychiatric disorders can be present if a person's symptoms are to be diagnosed as a dissociative disorder. In addition, the disorder cannot be caused by a traumatic brain injury; this is the reason films such as *Memento* (2000) are discussed in Chapter 12, Neurocognitive Disorders. There are **three primary dissociative disorders**: *dissociative identity disorder, dissociative amnesia,* and *depersonalization/derealization disorder.*

Dissociative Identity Disorder

Dissociative identity disorder (DID), formerly called "multiple personality disorder," is an extremely rare condition characterized by disturbances in memory and identity along with a marked discontinuity in one's sense of self. The essential feature is the presence of two or more distinct identities, or **alters** (personality states), that assume control over behavior. Amnesia is present in one or more of the personalities. Usually, the more passive the personality, the greater the amnesia. DID is usually believed to be a posttraumatic condition that emerges after overwhelming traumatic childhood experiences.

The symptoms of DID are associated with many other psychiatric states such as anxiety symptoms (phobia, panic attacks, and obsessive-compulsive behaviors), mood symptoms (manic and depressive), other dissociative symptoms (amnesias, fugues, and depersonalization), somatic symptoms (conversion), sexual dysfunctions, suicide attempts, self-mutilations, substance abuse, eating disorders, sleep disturbance, symptoms of schizophrenia, symptoms of PTSD, and borderline personality disorder. Since many symptoms of PTSD occur in DID, some argue that these two are variants of the same disorder (Piper & Merskey, 2004).

The DSM-5 cites a study suggesting a 12-month prevalence for DID of 1.5% among adult Americans with males slightly more likely to develop the condition than females (Huntjens et al., 2019). However, many mental health professionals challenge the very existence of DID, and they would be very dubious about a prevalence as high as that suggested by the DSM-5 (Lilienfeld & Berg, 2012; Nathan, 2011). Debbie Nathan's book *Sybil Exposed: The Extraordinary Story Behind the Famous Multiple Personality Case*, suggests that the Sybil story is "scant[ly] more than an elaborate fabrication, an intricate web of lies spun by an ambitious psychiatrist and eager journalist" (Lilienfeld & Berg, 2012). In their review of this book, the late Scott Lilienfeld and Joanna Berg (2012) note that,

> Prior to the publication of *Sybil*, DID was presumed to be an exceedingly rare condition, even a psychiatric curiosity. As of 1970, there were fewer than 80 documented cases of DID in the world literature .... Yet not long after Sybil's story appeared in print and on the small screen, the number of DID cases skyrocketed. By 1986, there were approximately 6,000 reported cases of DID; by 1998, this number had mushroomed to 40,000. Today, some DID experts place the prevalence of DID at several million individuals in the United States alone;

> psychiatrist Colin Ross (1991) contends that DID is at least as common as schizophrenia.
>
> Sybil's influence did not end there. As Spanos (1994) observed, prior to the publication of *Sybil*, few if any individuals with DID reported a history of child abuse. Following *Sybil*, severe abuse became a virtually ubiquitous fixture of DID's clinical portrait, so much so that some experts regarded it as a *sine qua non* for the condition's emergence. Furthermore, before *Sybil*, most individuals with DID reported only one alter (the so-called split personality); following *Sybil*, most reported multiple alters (Lilienfeld et al., 1999). ... From its inception, the DID epidemic [...] was dogged by a vexing question. Are the alters in DID discovered, as DID advocates insist, or are they created? (Lilienfeld & Berg, 2012)

There is no evidence of spontaneous remission or integration of personality alters without mental health treatment. Therapy is long-term and requires the establishment of a strong therapeutic relationship with the individual. Hypnosis may be used at varying stages of treatment. Through the support of the relationship, the original traumas are accessed and examined, and the psychological pain is soothed and viewed from an adult perspective. At this point in therapy, internal conflict can be addressed and resolved.

Psycho and Psychopathology

In the latter half of the 1900s, films began depicting the psychological complexities of human personality. *Psycho*, Alfred Hitchcock's 1960 film, describes a young man who assumed the personality of his mother after he murdered her and her lover. This film is regarded by many as Hitchcock's finest film. It is a superb movie; unfortunately, it also contributes to the negative stereotype of people with mental illnesses.

The film begins in a hotel room in Phoenix, with Marion Crane, played by Janet Leigh, who is scantily dressed. She is discussing her future with her lover, Sam Loomis, played by John Gavin. Marion wants to get married, but Sam is unable to make a commitment because of previous financial commitments to his ex-wife. After the afternoon rendezvous, she returns to work, where she steals $40,000. The next morning, she heads toward Sam's hometown with the money.

During a rainstorm, she seeks shelter at the Bates Motel, only 15 miles from Sam's home. Norman Bates, played by Anthony Perkins, invites her to dinner at his home behind the motel. Marion hears Norman's mother yelling at him for wanting to bring a girl to dinner. Norman fixes sandwiches for Marion and apologizes for his mother's behavior. They talk in a room adjacent to the office, and Norman shows off his taxidermy collection. Norman later watches her undress through a peephole separating her room from the office. That night Marion is brutally murdered by someone who appears to be Norman's mother. The murder scene occurs in a shower, and this scene (with its dramatic, nondiegetic music) is one of the most famous scenes in film history.

Norman cleans up the blood from the shower and puts Marion's body in the trunk of her new car (and unknowingly hides the stolen $40,000 there as well). He then drives the car to an isolated area, where he can sink the car and its contents into a swamp.

"I'll just sit here and be quiet, just in case they do suspect me. They're probably watching me. Well, let them. Let them see what kind of a person I am. I'm not even going to swat that fly. I hope they are watching. They'll see. They'll see and they'll know, and they'll say, 'Why, she wouldn't even harm a fly.'"

Norman Bates sits in his cell, smiling and thinking about the future, in *Psycho* (1960)

Instead of telling the police about the stolen money, Marion's boss hires a private detective, Milton Arbogast, to track Marion and recover the money. He traces her to the Bates Motel after following Marion's sister, Lila, to Sam's. Neither Lila nor Sam knows anything about the stolen money. Mr. Arbogast is killed when he visits the

Bates home to investigate his hunch that Norman Bates is somehow involved in the disappearance of Marion.

Lila and Sam then contact the local sheriff, who is willing to investigate Marion's disappearance if an official missing person's report is made. He also informs Sam and Lila that Norman's mother has been dead for 10 years and that she killed herself after poisoning her lover.

Lila and Sam return to the motel to solve the case. In a very suspenseful ending, they find that Norman Bates had exhumed his mother's grave, mummified her corpse, and kept her body with him in the house for the past 10 years. Bates had always been a disturbed child, and, after he killed his mother and her lover, he coped with his guilt by assuming her identity. By the end of the movie, Norman has totally assumed the alter ego of his mother, as can be seen when he attempts to kill Lila dressed in his mother's clothes (see Figure 25).

Gus Van Sant remade *Psycho* in 1998, this time in color. Van Sant's version is faithful to the original script and pays homage to Hitchcock, but the remake lacks the power and fascination of the original.

The movie *Hitchcock* (2012) portrays the challenges Hitchcock confronted in producing the film (e.g., he was personally required to underwrite the costs of production). Marlene Eisenberg and Michael Blank reviewed this film for *PsycCRITIQUES* and identified three dominant themes: Hitchcock had a domineering mother and an abusive father; he developed a "megalomaniacal obsession with rigidity and control"; and he was misogynistic, although he had a long-term and stable relationship with his wife and creative partner, Alma Hitchcock (Eisenberg & Blank, 2013).

Ktarzyna Szmigiero (2022) has analyzed the portrayal of mental illness in all of Hitchcock's films. She notes,

> Some critics believe [Hitchcock's fascination with mental illness] reflects the director's own mental health issues. Yet, it is more likely that Hitchcock was inspired by the Gothic tradition and the legacy of Edgar Allan Poe as well as the popularity of psychoanalysis in post war U.S. culture. (Szmigiero, 2022)

Peacock

Cillian Murphy offers an extraordinary performance as both the male and female personalities of the same character in *Peacock* (2010), a film that clearly focuses on depicting DID. The film offers an in-depth character analysis, accurate depiction of a dissociative disorder, and realistic psychopathology origins. Unfortunately, this otherwise great portrayal of DID is marred by the significant violence of the protagonist, hence perpetrating the misconception that all people with mental illness are violent. This stereotype is rampant in most films attempting to portray DID.

The protagonist in *Peacock* is John, a passive, taciturn, and socially awkward man. He is a

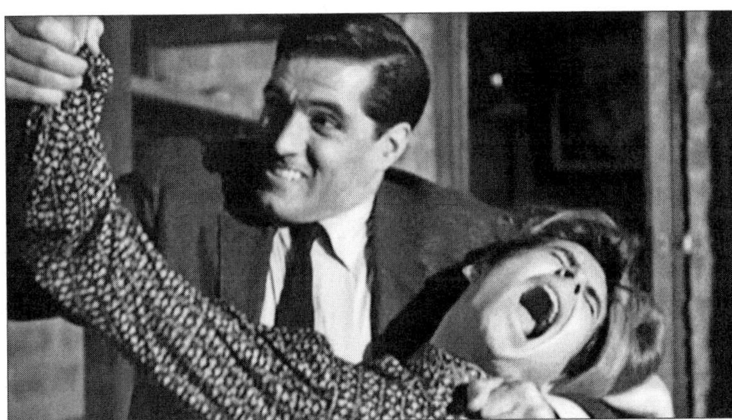

Figure 25.
Psycho (1960, Shamley Productions). Produced by Alfred Hitchcock. Directed by Alfred Hitchcock.

compliant and hard worker who isolates himself at work and at home. The viewer learns that after John's mother died over a year ago, a new personality called Emma emerged; Emma is sweet and quiet, but thoughtful. Emma writes love notes to John and prepares his food. Following a random incident of a train going off the track and ending up in his front yard, John and his house are thrust into the public eye, as townspeople and political figures attempt to learn more and even take advantage of the situation. As a result, John becomes more controlling, irritable, and impulsive, and he begins to unravel. Interestingly, Emma develops in a positive way: She becomes more altruistic and caring while maintaining insight. Both personalities know of the other's existence but are not necessarily aware of everything the other says and does.

DID is associated with trauma, abuse, neglect, and other overwhelming experiences. In *Peacock*, significant abuse is indeed alluded to, but it is not depicted in the film. The viewer learns that John's mother forced John to have sex with a call girl named Maggie (Ellen Page) who became pregnant. His mother then gave Maggie monthly child support.

The interior of the home is eerie and dark, and the identity switch from John to Emma occurs in John's mother's room where he puts on extensive makeup and dresses up in dainty clothes. In one scene, Maggie comments that she thought Emma was the mother due to the similar appearance. As the film progresses, the Emma alter appears to have taken substantial control of John and becomes protective, generous, and supportive of Maggie and her son. She encourages them to safely leave the town of Peacock, Nebraska. At one point Emma takes a photo of the son playing, which appears to replace the painful childhood memories. To outsmart Emma, John kills a vagabond and burns the body and a motel room to fake his own death.

Cillian Murphy engaged in extensive analysis of DID to play the roles of John and Emma. He reported that he studied the origins, pathogenesis, and diagnosis of DID to fully capture the complexities and subtleties of this interesting condition. Reviewing this film, Cardeña and Reijman (2010) noted, "sometimes a house or a self must be split asunder to reveal its rotten foundations."

Fight Club, *Identity*, and *Secret Window*

None of these three popular, contemporary film examples of DID is especially helpful in portraying important and accurate psychopathology information of this disorder, and they are not as educational as *The Three Faces of Eve* (1957) and *Sybil* (1976) (to be discussed in the section on Sybil). In their defense, these films do not pretend to educate viewers about DID; instead, the condition is used as an important plot device to enhance excitement, intrigue, fascination, and entertainment. Each of the three films is unique in its cinematic approach and has something to offer the viewer interested in dissociative disorders, and therefore each is worth seeing.

David Fincher's fast-paced, visceral *Fight Club* (1999) begins with the narrator, Jack (brilliantly played by Edward Norton), struggling with insomnia and depression. Jack begins to deteriorate as he is entrenched in an unsatisfying consumerist lifestyle, feels apathetic at work, and becomes addicted to attending different support group meetings each day just for emotional release. The culmination of his deterioration happens early in the film when he meets Tyler Durden (Brad Pitt), although he (and the viewer) do not realize Tyler is Jack's alter ego for much of the film. Tyler is everything Jack is not: flamboyant, exciting, seductive, unconventional, and self-empowering. The dramatically different personality types are illustrated in Figure 26. The two (both are just Jack) fight one another (he fights himself) and begin a "fight club" that attracts other disenfranchised men wanting a release. It is interesting to note that there are many clues to Jack's DID in the film, including one-frame cinematic flashes of Tyler Durden until the full alter develops, illustrating Jack's full dissociation. Some mental health professionals argue that the identities of DID typically are not aware of one another; this is the case in *Fight Club*.

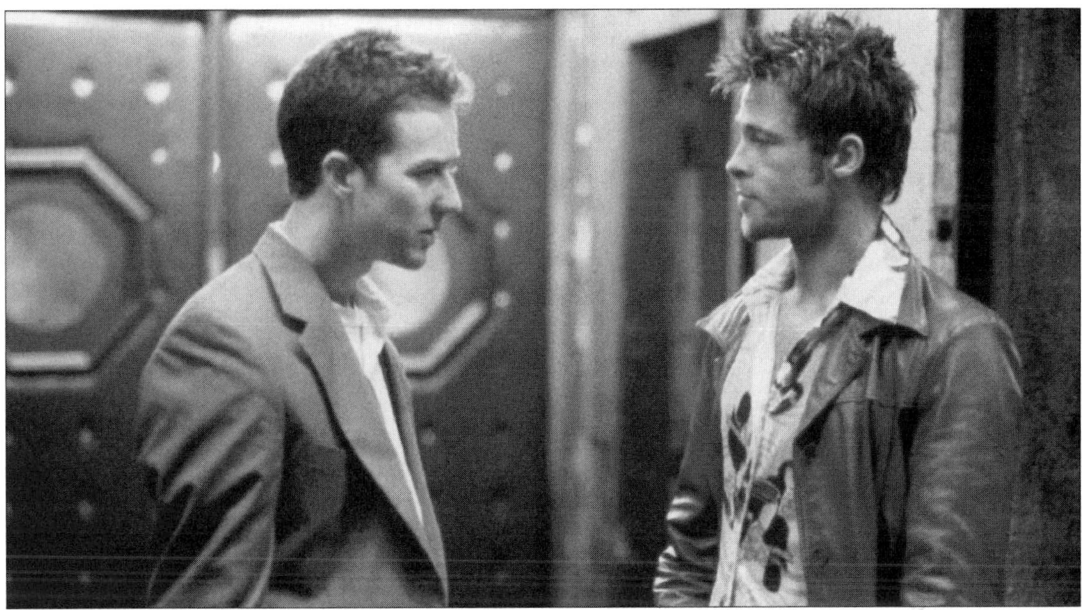

Figure 26. *Fight Club* (1999, Fox 2000 Pictures, New Regency Productions, Linson Films, Atman Entertainment, Knickerbocker Films, Taurus Film). Produced by Ross Grayson Bell, Ceán Chaffin, John S. Dorsey, Art Linson, and Arnon Milchan. Directed by David Fincher.

Identity (2003) takes a different approach to DID. The viewer sees two stories: One story depicts 10 characters stranded at an isolated motel trying to hide from and elude a mysterious serial killer on the loose in the area; the other story portrays a convicted serial killer, Malcolm Rivers, on the night of his final hearing before having the death penalty carried out. The viewer later learns these two stories are integrated in that Malcolm has DID and that the 10 characters represent Malcolm's alters whom he is trying to kill off to achieve integration.

Secret Window (2004) manipulates the viewer, and it is not until the conclusion of the film that the protagonist's DID is revealed. Johnny Depp plays Mort, a man who experiences the trauma of seeing his wife cheating on him in a motel room. Mort confines and isolates himself in the woods to write his next novel and subsequently begins to deteriorate (this is a direct parallel with Jack Nicholson's famous and more dramatic character in *The Shining* [1980]). Coinciding with his deterioration (which takes the form of angst about his deteriorating marriage, anger toward his wife's boyfriend, an inability to quit smoking, alcohol abuse, and writer's block), are Mort's provocative encounters with Shooter (John Turturro) who wants amends, claiming Mort has stolen his story. These interactions become more dangerous and threatening, and Shooter kills various people and Mort's dog. Toward the end, a frustrated Mort throws an ashtray against the wall – the wall and house begin to crack, and he hallucinates the crack spreading around the house; this scene is a metaphor for his own fragility and continuing decompensation. We then see Mort talking to himself and begin to hear his inner voice, which then shows up visually and multiplies. Mort had been so afraid of the Shooter part of his personality that he developed it as an alter and suppressed it from his conscious awareness.

In many ways, *Secret Window* (2004) echoes Stanley Kubrick's *The Shining*, a classic film based on a novel of the same name by Stephen King. The film portrays Jack Torrance (Jack Nicholson) as a recovering alcoholic writer who becomes a winter caretaker at an isolated resort in Colorado. He is accompanied by his wife, Wendy (Shelly Duvall) and his son Danny. The film allows us to track Torrance's slow descent into insanity, and he eventually attempts to kill both his wife and son (using an axe and perpetuating the myth that people with mental illness are axe murders). Nicholson's "here's Johnny" line was improvised, but it has become iconic and one of the most memorable lines in film history. Another scene in which Torrance sits at a typewriter, endlessly typing "All work and no play makes Jack a dull boy" is especially memorable. Torrance's diagnosis is never clear, but he is clearly psychotic.

The Three Faces of Eve

In *The Three Faces of Eve* (1957), narrator Alistair Cooke prepares the viewer for a true story about a woman with multiple personality disorder (i.e., DID). This black-and-white film takes place in 1951 in a small Georgia town. Joanne Woodward introduces the viewer to Eve White, a quiet, passive, modest homemaker who begins having severe headaches, followed by "spells." She cannot remember what she does during these spells. Mrs. White is married to a rigid, dull, unimaginative man named Ralph, who is frustrated with the changes in his wife's behavior. Their unhappy marriage is even more stressed by these unexplained events.

During these spells, Eve Black, the second personality, comes out. Eve Black is a seductive, sexually promiscuous single woman, who buys flashy and provocative clothes, smokes, drinks, and frequents nightclubs. Eve White, who is unaware of Eve Black's existence, is afraid she is going crazy because of her unexplained periods of amnesia and hearing voices. Eve Black, on the other hand, knows of Eve White, dislikes her husband and their child, Bonnie, and delights in having Eve White feel the hangover following Eve Black's night of carousing. Eve White and her husband seek psychiatric treatment from Dr. Curtis Luther, played by Lee J. Cobb, for her headaches and spells.

It is well over a year before Dr. Luther can identify the existence of Eve Black. Following an incident in which Eve Black attempts to strangle Bonnie, Eve White is admitted to the hospital. She vows not to be reunited with her daughter until she is well. While Eve is in the hospital, Dr. Luther can establish a therapeutic relationship with both personalities and attempts to integrate them into one. The diagnosis of multiple personality disorder is explained to Eve White and her spouse, who both attempt to understand the problem. Ralph is never able to understand the disorder and eventually divorces Eve.

As Eve White struggles to work during the day, Eve Black parties at night. They both continue to be treated by Dr. Luther. Eventually, a third personality, Jane, emerges who is aware of both Eve White and Eve Black, even though neither is aware of her. Following a visit with her daughter, Bonnie, at her parents' home, Jane begins to have memories of playing under the porch as a child. Gradually, using hypnosis, Dr. Luther can help Eve recall the trauma that precipitated her personalities splitting (being forced to kiss her dead grandmother's corpse). After reliving the memory, only Jane remains.

Sybil

The film *Sybil* (1976), based upon a true story, stars Sally Field as Sybil and Joanne Woodward as Dr. Cornelia Wilbur. It is interesting to note that Woodward, who received an Academy Award in 1957 for her lead role in *The Three Faces of Eve,* returned almost 2 decades later to play the psychiatrist treating Sybil. The viewer is introduced to Sybil, a distressed young woman who is working as a preschool teacher while attending art school. As Sybil is talking with the children, the creaking sound of a swing stirs traumatic childhood memories. Sybil unsuccessfully attempts to attend to her assigned task of organizing the children into a game of follow-the-leader. In the next scene, Sybil is standing in the middle of a fountain, obviously confused. Her supervisor is scolding her for leading the children the wrong way. Sybil returns to her apartment, where she curls into a fetal position, trying to escape her tormenting memories. In desperation, she breaks her apartment window, which seems to give her some psychological relief. Because of her cut wrist, she ends up in an emergency room. Due to her confusion, she is referred to a psychiatrist, Dr. Wilbur, who evaluates her and begins treatment that lasts for 11 years.

This episode represents one of many in which Sybil is initially overwhelmed with flashbacks of traumatic childhood events that lead to periods of irrational behavior followed by a climactic event, such as breaking a window and injuring herself. The viewer gradually realizes that as Sybil recalls traumatic memories, one of her 16 other personalities, or **alters**, gains control and triggers irrational behavior. Each of the other alters represents a part of Sybil and serves a particular purpose. For example, Vanessa is musical and enjoys playing the music Sybil once played. Vicki is very much in charge of life and is fearless. Peggy is a child who feels the terror and anger of childhood trauma. Marsha represents her despair and is often suicidal.

Through interaction with the different personalities and the use of hypnosis, Dr. Wilbur gradually pieces together Sybil's traumatic past. The goal of therapy is to integrate the personalities by helping the alters remember the past, experience the emotions associated with the traumatic events, and develop an adult perspective on the trauma. Patiently, Dr. Wilbur develops a warm, therapeutic relationship with all the alters who can share their experiences. Dr. Wilbur, in turn, can help Sybil remember parts of her life that were previously shut off. Gradually, as the repeated abuse of her childhood is relived, Sybil can remember her childhood experiences and integrate them into her whole personality.

Frankie & Alice

Frankie & Alice (2010) stars Halle Berry as Francine (Frankie) Murdoch, a woman with DID. Frankie works in a strip club, and she has multiple problems in her life that bring her to a psychiatric hospital where she meets Dr. Joseph Oswald (Dr. Oz) who diagnoses three distinct personalities: Frankie, a right-handed 32-year-old Black woman; Alice, a left-handed Southern White woman of indeterminate age; and "Genius," a very bright but very frightened young child. Interestingly, the personality of Alice is quite racist. Dr. Oz uses hypnosis to treat and eventually integrate the three distinct personalities. The movie is based on a true story. Although we appreciate and admire Halle Berry, the film is ultimately disappointing and teaches little about DID.

Frankie Murdoch: "Multiple personality, huh? But who are they?"
Oz: "Well, they're you. Your aspects of you. Your subconscious."
Frankie Murdoch: "Okay, but why?"
Oz: "That's what we'll have to find out."
Frankie Murdoch: "So, what you're saying is, I got all these different ... people living inside of me, right? But I don't know who they are."
Oz: "Well, we all have different personalities and different selves. 'Do I contradict myself? Very well, then I contradict myself. I am large, I contain multitudes.' It's Whitman."

Dr. Oz describes dissociative identity disorder in *Frankie & Alice* (2010)

Other Dissociative Identity Disorder Films

The film *Primal Fear* (1996) should be seen to provide a certain degree of skeptical balance, as it portrays a man (Edward Norton) who feigns DID to evade murder charges. This film reminds clinicians of the potential for malingering in suspected cases of multiple personality disorder.

"Well... good for you, Marty. I was going to let it go at that. You was looking so happy just now. I was thinking, hmmm God. But to tell you the truth, I'm glad you figured it out, because I have been dying to tell you. I just didn't know who you'd wanna hear it from, you know? Aaron or Roy... or Roy or Aaron. Well, I'll let you in on a little secret. A sort of a client-attorney-privilege type of a secret, you know what I mean? It don't matter who you hear it from. It's the same story."

Roy (Ed Norton) responds to his attorney, Martin Vail (Richard Gere), in *Primal Fear* (1996)

In *X-Men: The Last Stand* (2006), superheroine mutant Jean Grey is portrayed as someone with a dissociative identity disorder. She quickly becomes a danger to herself and others and, as is painfully common in most films depicting "split personalities," the alter becomes dangerous, murderous, out-of-control, and perpetrates the misconception that people with mental illness are violent. Actress Famke Janssen, who researched DID to make her character more realistic, plays the part. The movie is an allegory in which society's need to control and limit the mutant's powers parallels society's inevitable attempts to make "them" more like "us."

DIDs are also illustrated in *Raising Cain* (1992) and *Voices Within: The Lives of Truddi Chase* (1990), a made-for-TV movie based on the bestselling book *When Rabbit Howls.*

The movie *Birdy* (1984) stars Matthew Modine and Nicholas Cage playing the roles of Birdy and Al, two Vietnam veterans who have been traumatized by the war. Birdy has always been obsessed with birds, and he is passionate in his attempts to fly; after Vietnam, he is hospitalized because of his mutism and his belief that he is in fact a bird. With help from Al, Birdy recovers, begins to speak, and the two men escape from the military hospital where they have been confined. It is not at all clear whether Birdy's condition is best conceptualized as a DID or a delusional disorder; however, it is apparent that Birdy has become amnestic for much of what happened to him while in Vietnam.

In *Me, Myself & Irene* (2000), Jim Carrey plays Charlie, a state trooper, and a cuckold with a double identity as Hank. Charlie is insecure, hesitant, and bumbling; Hank is confidant, self-assured, and quite a ladies' man. Despite occasional funny moments, the movie disappoints and gets laughs at the expense of people with mental illness. For example, when someone incapacitates Hank with a Taser and shouts to his friends "Let's kick the shit out of this bastard," Irene (Renée Zellweger) comes to Hank's rescue, shouting, "Wait, he's a schizo!" Most audiences laugh at both lines.

M. Night Shyamalan's *Split* (2016) portrays a man with 24 personalities. The movie is unrealistic and promotes harmful stereotypes about mental illness. In one scene, one of the alters injects insulin because he is diabetic – but this simple act would have surely resulted in hypoglycemic coma and killed the other 23 personalities! Insulin poisoning is "a common mode of suicide in nondiabetics, especially medical and paramedical personnel and relatives of diabetic patients" (Gundgurthi et al., 2012). Reviewing the film in *PsycCRITIQUES*, Brand and Pasko (2017) note,

> By portraying people with dissociative identity disorder (DID) as predators who are extremely violent, this movie reinforces fears about people with mental illness. Although the filmmaker accurately conveys that DID results from severe childhood abuse, most of his portrayal about DID and its treatment is far afield from reality. This film exploits people who have a serious mental illness and who are much more likely to be victimized rather than to victimize others.

A 2010 documentary film, *The Woman With 15 Personalities*, introduces viewers to Paula, a woman with 14 alters. They include the following: Jonathan, a 12-year-old boy, Miss V, a 25-year-old teacher who is self-assured and confident, and two alters that Paula fears – Teddy Claire, an angry woman who cuts herself and who has attempted suicide twice, and "Freedom," a sexually liberated woman who has slept with three men at one time and engaged in other sexual behaviors that frighten Paula, who is quite conservative. Each alter has a distinct handwriting style (e.g., Mariah writes in a childlike scrawl). Part of the film is devoted to an electroencephalogram (EEG) session in which different alters display different EEG patterns; for example, Miss V. shows a 10-beat reduction in heart rate when she emerges. Paula is attempting to integrate the various alters but acknowledges that she will miss them when they are no longer a part of her life.

Dissociative Amnesia

Dissociative amnesias are characterized by an inability to recall important personal information, usually of a traumatic or stressful nature (e.g., the death of a child). Affected individuals can usually remember events up to the time of the trauma but have memory loss for events that occur after the event. Even though significant personal information is lost with dissociative amnesias, cognitive abilities and the ability to learn new information remain intact. This memory impairment is reversible. In the classic disorder, the person is quickly brought to a mental health provider because of the overt, dramatic change in memory. Persons with amnesia may have intense emotional reactions to stimuli without knowing the reasons for the reaction or the significance of it.

Even though filmmakers do not typically focus on the psychological etiology of amnesia, they have often used amnesia as a central theme. One example is the 1940 Academy Award-winning satire, *The Great Dictator,* starring Charles Chaplin, Paulette Goddard, and Jack Oakie. Chaplin plays a dual role as a Jewish barber and Adenoid Hynkel, dictator of Tomania. This spoof of Adolf Hitler begins when Chaplin plays a Jewish barber in a "Tomanian" ghetto who is recovering from amnesia and wakes up to find himself living under the thumb of Hynkel (also played by Chaplin). He escapes to Austria with a Jewish laundress, played by Paulette Goddard, who is in love with him. In Austria, he is mistaken for Hynkel, who had recently assumed control of the country. Chaplin then assumes the role of the dictator.

Amnesia is also portrayed in the excellent film *Sullivan's Travels* (1941) starring Joel McCrea and Veronica Lake and directed by Preston Sturges. The main character becomes amnestic when he is hit over the head and ends up being sentenced to 6 years on a chain gang. An example of traumatic amnesia triggered by a murder can be found in the film *Dead Again* (1991).

Amnesia allows a spoiled, self-centered, rich woman to experience life at the other end of the social ladder in the comedy *Overboard* (1987), directed by Garry Marshall. Dissociative amnesia is also illustrated in the classic films *Spellbound* (1945) and *Suddenly, Last Summer* (1959).

The Jim Carrey and Kate Winslet characters in *Eternal Sunshine of the Spotless Mind* (2004) have some form of dissociative amnesia, as they are unable to remember certain events and people, particularly those related to a former significant other. However, because the memories are intentionally eliminated with the help of a specialist who erases traumatic memories with sophisticated technology, the diagnosis would not apply.

Hollywood movies have reaped some financial gain with action films using amnesia as a plot device, such as the successful *The Bourne Identity* (2002) and the unsuccessful *Paycheck* (2003). In the former, Jason Bourne, a CIA assassin, loses his memory after a failed spy mission, and he is left to try to uncover who he was before he is killed.

The Forgotten (2004) stars Julianne Moore as Telly Paretta, a mother grieving over the loss of her 9-year-old son, who was killed in an airplane accident. The plot thickens when Telly's husband and her therapist tell her that she never had a son, and that she created all the memories she has of her son as a response to a miscarriage. The movie is spoiled by a silly ending that negates the value of what could otherwise have been a meaningful psychological exploration.

In *50 First Dates* (2004), Adam Sandler plays the role of Henry Roth, a happy veterinarian living in Hawaii. Henry falls in love with Lucy (Drew Barrymore), a woman who suffers from **anterograde amnesia** because of a motor vehicle accident. Henry arranges to meet Lucy each day, and eventually marries her.

Mirage

In the film *Mirage* (1965), David Stillwell, played by Gregory Peck, develops amnesia after witnessing the accidental death of his boss and mentor, Calvin Clark. Stillwell, a scientist, has just discovered a method for neutralizing the effects of nuclear fallout. Believing that his mentor was working for world peace, Stillwell shares the information with him. When Stillwell realizes that his formula would end up being used to produce nuclear weapons, he sets the formula on fire in front of an open window. To save the piece of paper, Calvin lunges toward Stillwell and falls to his death from the 27th floor. Stillwell observes the fall, is horrified, and then calmly picks up his empty briefcase and leaves the office. He has developed amnesia. The lights in the office building go out.

The audience has none of this information until the end of the film. The film opens during a blackout in an office building in New York City. David Stillwell is a very calm, rational individual who leads a woman, Sheila, played by Diane Baker, down the darkened stairs. He does not recognize Sheila, but she recognizes him. Upon returning to his apartment, he is greeted by a man who attempts to kill him. Stillwell overpowers the intruder and leaves him unconscious in the service quarters. Gradually, Stillwell begins to realize that he has lost his memory, but he becomes convinced that he has been in an amnestic state for 2 years instead of 2 days. He seeks help from a psychiatrist, who questions his amnesia and throws him out of the office.

In this Hitchcock-style thriller, Stillwell's belief that he had been an accountant in New York is reinforced by his enemy, the Major, who hires thugs to follow Stillwell and get the formula. Stillwell next employs Detective Ted Caselle, played by Walter Matthau, to discover his identity and figure out who is trying to kill him. Caselle attempts to fit the pieces together but is killed in the process. A romance is rekindled between Sheila and Stillwell, who had previously been lovers.

Following the detective's death, Stillwell desperately contacts the same psychiatrist, who is again skeptical of Stillwell's amnesia. By now, Stillwell's memory is beginning to return, and he realizes that his memory loss has been present for only 2 days. The psychiatrist asks some questions that provoke the retrieval of more memories. Gradually, the amnesia for his mentor's death lifts, and he can face the horror of the event.

Dissociative fugue, emphasized as a separate, distinct diagnosis in DSM-IV, is now only a specifier under dissociative amnesia, in DSM-5 (e.g., **dissociative amnesia with dissociative fugue** [F44.1]). Fugue states are characterized by sudden, unexpected travel away from home or one's customary place of work, an inability to recall one's past, and confusion about personal identity, or the assumption of a partial or completely new identity (e.g., a person whose business is failing may show up in a new city with a new identity and no memory of previous problems). With the onset of fugue, a person begins a new autobiographical memory that replaces the original one. These individuals appear normal and will not reveal any evidence of dissociative symptoms unless asked. When the fugue resolves, the original memories are recovered, but the fugue memories are lost. The individual then has a permanent void in personality history. Even though the prevalence of dissociative fugue has been reported to be only 0.2% of the general population, it may be more common in times of war, natural disaster, and dislocation (Fullerton et al., 2004).

Some patients with dissociative fugue disorders will travel short distances over brief periods; others may travel far and remain in a fugue state for months or years. The acclaimed and thought-provoking Wim Wenders film, *Paris, Texas* (1984) introduces the character of Travis Clay Henderson, an individual suffering from dissociative fugue. He has been lost for 4 years and is found wandering in the desert. Eventually, he (partially) puts the pieces of his shattered life back together.

Renée Zellweger's character in *Nurse Betty* (2000) witnesses her husband's murder and shortly thereafter becomes convinced she is the former fiancée of her soap opera idol, and she travels across the country to find him. This character provides a fascinating springboard for a discussion of the differentiation between delusional disorder and other potential diagnoses. Jim Carrey's lead role in *The Majestic* (2001) would be another example of dissociative fugue had the experience not been caused by a head injury from an automobile accident; Carrey's character has amnesia, has traveled away from home, and readily takes on the identity of a missing-in-action soldier in a small town.

Amnesia and identity are central themes in *Identity Unknown* (1945), starring Richard Arlen and Cheryl Walker. In this film, a soldier develops amnesia during World War II and works to recover his identity.

Unknown White Male

The best film to date to examine the life of someone experiencing a fugue state is *Unknown White Male* (2005). This documentary, directed by Rupert Murray, is based on the real-life experience of Doug Bruce, a man who without reason developed a profound **retrograde amnesia** for everything that had happened to him before July 3, 2003. Bruce is disoriented when he discovers himself on a subway bound for Coney Island with no recollection of any of the previous 37 years of his life. He is taken to a Coney Island hospital where he is examined for neurological injuries and then taken to a psychiatric ward where he is given a wristband that reads "Unknown White Male."

> **"There are aspects of his experience I do envy. Everything is new to him. To eat chocolate mousse for the first time and to have the language to describe it ... that is an experience we won't have. To wipe the slate clean is desirable in a way. The first film he saw at the cinema was a restored print of *Taxi Driver*. Someone gave him a list of 50 films he had to see, and he's become a real movie buff [because] he's never seen a bad one."**
>
> ***Unknown White Male* (2005) director Rupert Murray**

The film underscores the fascinating complexity of what we unthinkingly call memory. Bruce cannot remember his own name, but he remembers how to *sign* his name (although the signature is illegible). He goes to the beach and remembers how to swim – but he does not *know* that he remembers until he is in the water. He is unable to recall the names of his parents, but he can still speak French. He does not remember that he once liked the Rolling Stones, but he enjoys their music when it is played for him. (Signing his name, swimming, typing, playing a musical instrument, and riding a bike are all examples of **procedural memory**.)

Unlike many individuals who experience fugue states, Bruce is frustrated and deeply troubled by his loss of memory. He has a girlfriend's phone number in his pocket, and she agrees to take him from the hospital and help him reestablish his past life. The cause of Bruce's memory loss was never determined. The film underscores the intimate and profound link between memory and one's sense of self, and illustrates what it is like for someone to genuinely experience what Buddhists call beginner's mind.

K-Pax

Kevin Spacey as both Robert Porter and Prot in *K-Pax* (2001) is a diagnostic quandary. In addition to hypothetical diagnoses of schizophrenia and PTSD, a valid and highly arguable case can be made for dissociative amnesia with a dissociative fugue specifier.

From this vantage point, a man named Robert Porter experiences a highly traumatic event. Upon returning from work one day, he finds his wife and child murdered with the perpetrator still in his house; Porter quickly kills the man, cleans up, and jumps into a nearby river. He then travels from his home in New Mexico to New York City under a completely new identity as Prot, a highly spiritual person with a vast knowledge of planetary rotations. Porter interacts with other people comfortably with this new identity and claims no knowledge of any other history. Under clinical hypnosis (age regression), the amnesia is lifted, and he painfully faces his past trauma.

Depersonalization/Derealization Disorder

Depersonalization/derealization disorder is diagnosed when there is evidence of persistent or recurrent feelings of detachment from one's mental processes or body. In depersonalization, there is an alteration in the perception of self and often a sense that one is living out a dream. The person feels like an outsider looking in but continues to relate to reality during the experience. Transient experiences of depersonalization are common in adolescents and decline with age in normal individuals (Putnam, 1985). During a traumatic event such as rape, depersonalization is sometimes experienced by women who report they were floating above their own bodies during the assault (Classen et al., 1993).

Closely related to depersonalization experiences are **out-of-body experiences** in which the individual has the distinct feeling that they are leaving their body. Often these individuals can describe scenes as if viewed from above and report a sense of being isolated and detached from their bodies.

In derealization, the external environment seems unreal, and there is a sense of detachment from one's surroundings; individuals experiencing derealization often feel like they are caught in a dream or that they exist in an unnatural environment. These patients frequently have a distorted sense of time, and time may seem to move very rapidly or very slowly.

Since depersonalization and derealization occur as a symptom in a variety of disorders, some authorities have questioned whether these two phenomena constitute a distinct disorder. The cause of depersonalization/derealization is unknown. Some authorities speculate that the phenomenon is related to a neurobiological disturbance produced by temporal lobe dysfunction. Others claim that depersonalization is an adaptation to overwhelming trauma. Still other authorities argue that depersonalization is a defense against painful and conflictual stimuli, or that it is a split between the observing and participating selves, that allows the person to become detached from self (Steinberg, 1991).

Transient depersonalization/derealization is common in the general population, and about half of adults will have this experience at some point. However, it is far less common for people to meet the full criteria for this diagnosis. DSM-5 estimates the 12-month prevalence of dissociative identity disorder in the United States is around 1.5%, with prevalence slightly greater for males (American Psychiatric Association, 2013).

"I just wanted to let you know that if you lost all your limbs, we'd still be together forever. I mean I really hope that doesn't happen because I think your limbs are pretty great. And when I said your name, it would always sound safe. I'm not sure about the perfume and the cologne thing but I could try ... And if you like this shirt, I wouldn't take it off for a month. And I would be more than willing to paint your grandmother's toenails, so your grandfather doesn't have to do it anymore. You don't have to save me, Sara. But I am going to love you for the rest of my life, so things would be a lot better for me if you were around."

Matthew admits his love for Sara, in *Numb* (2007)

Numb (2007) is one of the few films in which a leading character is explicitly diagnosed with depersonalization disorder (a term likely to be very unfamiliar to most viewers). The movie stars Matthew Perry as Hudson, a screenwriter who developed his profound sense of detachment after taking 12 hits from a bong in 12 minutes (it is important to note that if depersonalization symptoms occur exclusively as a direct effect of a substance, then the diagnosis of depersonalization disorder would not be given). He feels chronically detached, much as though he were watching himself in a film. He has no interest in himself, others, or anything that is happening around him. He spends his days and most of his nights watching the golf channel or very long-running movies (e.g., *Star Wars*). His neurological exam is normal, but he tells the doctor "Stab me with a fork and I wouldn't feel it." He is treated with clonazepam but finds the medication dramatically diminishes his libido (a genuine potential side effect of the drug). He engages in extensive "doctor shopping," seeing one therapist after another. One psychiatrist is only interested in pharmacological management of Matthew's problems ("Fuck talking ... take drugs!"). However, Matthew can overcome his malady only when he becomes genuinely interested in a new woman in his life, Sara (Lynn Collins). The film perpetuates the misconception that love is sufficient to conquer mental illness. While it is questionable whether Hudson has either depression or depersonalization (since depersonalization is being used as a convenient plot device), it makes for interesting discussions on differential diagnosis.

The Butterfly Effect

It might be a stretch to place the film *The Butterfly Effect* (2004) under this diagnostic category; however, while it does not seem to fit any category neatly, it can inform us about depersonalization. Evan, a 20-year-old college student, experiences frequent blackouts during highly emotional or stressful times. When he reflects on his amnestic blackouts and reads his copious journal entries about a given memory, he is transported to the actual past memory. He is then able to change the memory with various ensuing consequences on his and others' lives in the present.

Each of the memories he engages can be seen as his detachment from his body; he enters the memory, relives it, and changes it while maintaining reality testing to his world and the new world (due to the changed memory) around him. This process causes him significant personal and social distress as he realizes each of these detachment episodes has a profound effect on his own life and on the lives of the people he loves.

Other Examples of Dissociative Disorders in Films

Dissociative disorders are among the most fascinating forms of mental illness, and it is not surprising that relative to their prevalence, they are portrayed often in films. In addition to the clinical examples cited, film history is replete with examples of quasidissociative conditions in which one character exchanges personalities (or sometimes even bodies) with another. The classic example is Bergman's *Persona* (1966, Sweden), in which two characters gradually exchange personalities. A similar theme is found in the Robert Altman film, *3 Women* (1977), in which two of the women appear to exchange personalities.

In the mock-documentary-comedy, *Zelig* (1983), Woody Allen plays a human chameleon whose personality changes to match whatever situation he is in – if he is around black musicians, he talks and acts like black musicians; if he is around politicians, he becomes a politician. Ronald Coleman finds himself merging his own personality with that of Othello in *A Double Life* (1947). The comedy *Prelude to a Kiss* (1992) is about an old man and a young bride who mysteriously exchange bodies after kissing on the bride's wedding day. The film raises interesting questions about what it is that one person loves in another: Is it a physical body or a set of personality characteristics, such as wit, charm, and grace? The means through which the transformation is effected are never specified in *Prelude to a Kiss*. In contrast, it is clear in *Black Friday*, a 1940 horror film in which Boris Karloff transplants the brain of a criminal into the body of a college professor.

The theme of contrasting personalities in the same person is seen in those films in which someone presumed to be dead returns to their old social roles, usually as a vastly improved human being. We see this in *Sommersby* (1993) and *The Return of Martin Guerre* (1982). The dramatic force of both films is heightened by the sexual excitement both women feel as they go to bed with a man who may or may not be the husband who left them years earlier.

Dissociation is also used in many films that contrast the forces of good and evil inherent in us all. Oftentimes, evil is inherent in a twin. For example, the personalities of good and evil twins are juxtaposed in *The Dark Mirror* (1946) and in Brian De Palma's *Sisters* (1973). The latter film adds an interesting twist by making the two women Siamese twins who were separated as children.

Films have often presented the duality of the human personality, usually depicting a struggle between good and evil. In 1920, *Dr. Jekyll and Mr. Hyde* was first introduced as a silent film, starring John Barrymore and Martha Robinson. The

1931 remake, directed by Rouben Mamoulian, was the first sound version of this Robert Louis Stevenson classic. In the remake, Dr. Harry Jekyll (played by Fredric March, who won an Academy Award for his performance) represents all that is good and kind. He is a well-respected physician who devotes endless hours to hospital charity work. His innate curiosity and his own socially unacceptable feelings have led him to speculate about good and evil within humans. He believes that the evil of humans can be captured and isolated. As the film opens, he is engaged to Muriel, played by Miriam Hopkins, with whom he is deeply in love. According to the custom of the time, Muriel's father has set a marriage date that is far in the future, but too far to suit Harry. The audience gets a glimpse of Dr. Jekyll's underlying impulsiveness, his impatience, and the sexuality that he is trying hard to repress.

When Muriel's father takes her away for an extended trip, Dr. Jekyll tests his theory about inherent evils. He mixes and swallows a potion that he believes can isolate the evils of human beings. He then becomes the evil Mr. Hyde, who seduces, abuses, and finally kills a woman who is his social inferior. Eventually, he can no longer control the "coming out" of the alter personality (Mr. Hyde), and he confides his mistake to his future father-in-law. After attacking his fiancée, Dr. Jekyll is caught and killed.

Dr. Jekyll and Mr. Hyde was remade in 1941, this time starring Spencer Tracy and Ingrid Bergman. It was filmed again in 1968, with Jack Palance, and given the full title *The Strange Case of Dr. Jekyll and Mr. Hyde*. One of the best adaptations of the Dr. Jekyll and Mr. Hyde story is in the more recent *Mary Reilly* (1996), starring John Malkovich and Julia Roberts. A different twist on the same theme is found in *Steppenwolf* (1974), an adaptation of the Hermann Hesse novel, illustrating the problem of a single individual grappling with these two competing aspects of self.

Additional film examples of depersonalization disorder are found in the fascinating movie *Tarnation* (2003), as well as *Dead of Night* (1945), *Altered States* (1980), and Martin Scorsese's *The Last Temptation of Christ* (1988).

International Films: Dissociative Disorders

Persona (1966, Sweden), the complex Ingmar Bergman film regarded by critics as one of the greatest films ever made, deals with a famous actress, Elisabeth Vogler (Liv Ullmann), who suddenly, and seemingly without reason, stops talking. Her doctor can find nothing wrong with her and is at a loss to explain her patient's symptoms. However, she prescribes rest and constant attention, and Elisabeth spends the summer at a house on the coast in the care of a full-time nurse, Alma (Bibi Andersson). Although Elisabeth almost never speaks, we know that she retains the capacity for speech. At one point, when Alma appears to be about to throw boiling water on Elisabeth, the actress shouts, "Don't!"

Although the conversion disorder portrayed in the film is fascinating, the more interesting element is the merging of the personalities of the two women. There are several interesting dream sequences, and one scene presents a face on the screen that is a composite of Elisabeth and Alma (one half of each woman's face is shown). In selecting the title for the film, Bergman was thinking both about the masks worn by Greek actors in classical theater and of Carl Jung who used the term to refer to those parts of our personality that we show to the outer world. Perhaps Elisabeth quit speaking because she had resolved to stop acting and wear no more masks. The ending of the film is unclear, but Elisabeth returns to acting, Alma returns to nursing, and the personalities of the two women do not remain merged.

Interpersonalities (2008, Canada) is a short thriller-mystery that unfolds like a puzzle for the viewer. A young boy is depicted talking with a psychiatrist, then the viewer sees different characters suddenly pop into and out of the scene; these are the other personalities or alters. Those alters that are present at any given time can communicate with one another. The film portrays the killing of one alter, and the reluctance of an alter not wanting to kill another. In one scene, an alter suggests shifting the approach to "focus on the strengths," but the psychiatrist replies that is too dangerous and that one alter must eliminate the other.

The Falling (2014, UK) is an interesting film that illustrates mass hysteria and the contagion effect. The film takes place in a Catholic girls' school. One student, Abby, gets pregnant and subsequently dies. Her death triggers episodes of fainting that occur throughout the school, spreading from one student to another. The fainting is related to the practice of having a girl close her eyes while another girl slides a wet finger back and forth between the first girl's lips, simulating fellatio. The girls are hospitalized and treated with tranquilizers, but all medical tests are negative. The school is eventually closed. Lydia, the protagonist, has an agoraphobic mother, a cosmetologist who practices out of her home and has not left her house in years. There is considerable sexual tension throughout the film, and Lydia eventually becomes involved in an incestuous tryst with her brother. The film is likely loosely based on a similar episode of mass hysteria that occurred at Hilda Girls' School in Blackburn, England in 1965. It is interesting that there is a dramatic difference between top critics' ratings and audience ratings on the website Rotten Tomatoes (73% vs. 35%). Anyone interested in the history of hysteria will profit by reading a fascinating overview by Carol North (2015).

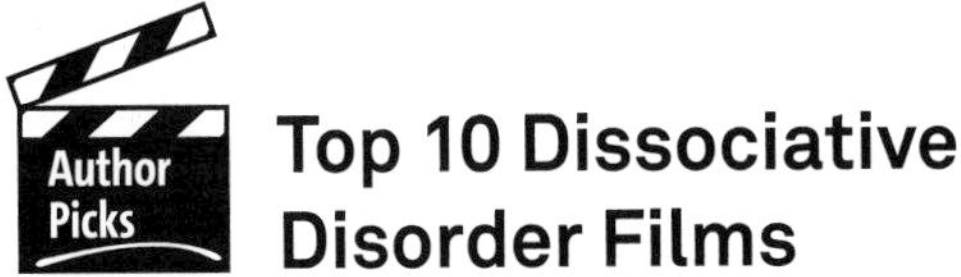

Top 10 Dissociative Disorder Films

The Three Faces of Eve (1957)
Psycho (1960)
Sybil (1976)
Paris, Texas (1984)
Birdy (1984)
Primal Fear (1996)
Fight Club (1999)
Unknown White Male (2005)
Peacock (2010)
Shutter Island (2010)

Chapter 8

Sleep–Wake, Eating, and Somatic Symptom Disorders

Are you happy or are you pretending to be happy?

A question put to Hunter in *Swallow* (2019)

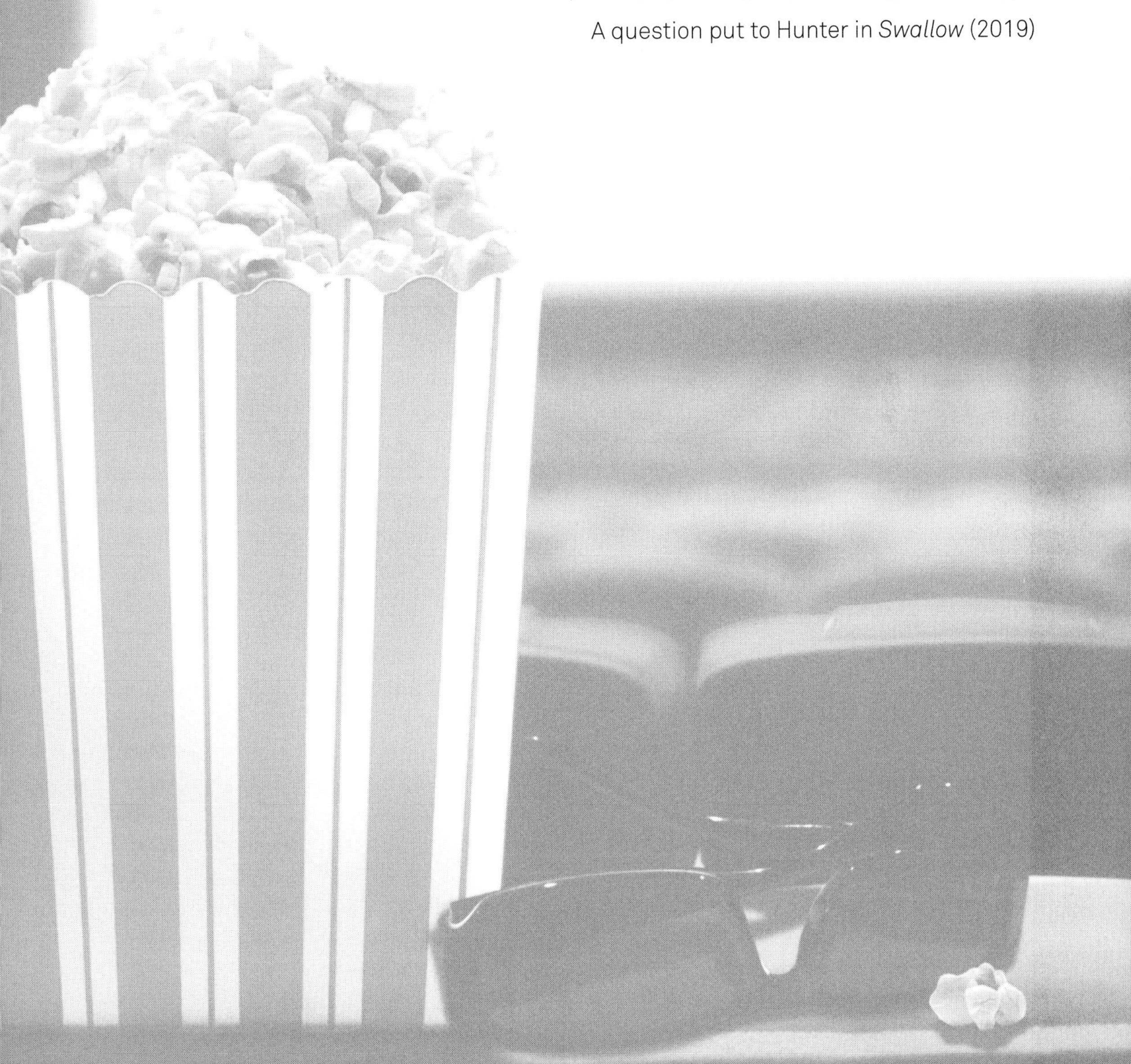

Sleep–Wake Disorders

The DSM-5 lists 10 categories of sleep-wake disorders: **insomnia disorder, hypersomnolence disorder, narcolepsy, breathing-related sleep disorder, circadian rhythm sleep-wake disorder, non-rapid eye movement (NREM) sleep arousal disorder, nightmare disorder, rapid eye movement (REM) sleep behavior disorder, restless legs syndrome**, and **substance/medication-induced sleep disorder**. The common denominator for each of these disorders is patient dissatisfaction with their sleeping habits, and daytime fatigue or impairment. Due to the complexity and extent of sleep disorders, we will focus on insomnia in this chapter, the most common sleep complaint found in clinical settings.

Sleep researchers recognize five **sleep stages**: Stages 1 through 4 (NREM sleep), and rapid eye movement (REM) sleep. Each of the first four stages of sleep gets progressively deeper, and each has distinct differences on an EEG. Stage 1 is a transition stage from wakefulness (light sleep), Stage 2 occupies about 50% of the time spent asleep, and Stages 3 and 4 (slow-wave sleep) are the deepest levels of sleep. Stage 5, REM sleep, is where most dreams are reported; it occurs cyclically throughout the night, and alternates about every hour and a half with NREM sleep (the first four stages). Individuals with insomnia will typically have increases in Stage 1 sleep and decreases in Stages 3 and 4. In narcoleptic individuals, the onset of REM sleep is more rapid after sleep onset, and there is an increase in REMs.

Sleep laboratories are used to conduct sleep studies to ascertain accurate diagnoses. **Polysomnography** (PSG) is the most common sleep test and involves EEG and electrocardiographic (ECG) readings, respiration, leg movements, and other physiological activities during sleep. The PSG helps to diagnose different forms of sleep apnea (most often the cause of breathing-related sleep disorder). The **Multiple Sleep Latency Test** (MSLT) is used by sleep labs to diagnose narcolepsy. Referrals to sleep labs are usually done through physician prescription, which can often be encouraged by mental health professionals.

Film depictions of sleep disorders are rare. When depicted, they are usually either very brief or flawed. The film *Insomnia* is an exception.

Insomnia Disorder

Insomnia Disorder as Portrayed in *Insomnia*

Sleep disorders are rarely portrayed in films, particularly not to the extent they are highlighted in this film. *Insomnia* (2002), a remake of a well-done, 1997 Norwegian film of the same name, is deeply psychological with multiple layers of complexity. One of these layers is the deteriorating mental status of Al Pacino's character, Los Angeles police officer Detective Will Dormer. Director Christopher Nolan accurately depicts this deterioration, documenting both the realities and dangers of insomnia. This film provides a powerful illustration of the ways this disorder can devastate someone's life.

Dormer flies to Alaska to lead a murder investigation. He arrives in Alaska, already tired, at a time of year when the sun never sets ("white nights") so it never gets dark outside. (His travel to Alaska from California takes him across just one time zone, so he would not meet the criteria for circadian rhythm sleep-wake disorder). Throughout the investigation, Dormer lies in bed with his eyes open, struggling to get some sleep. Under internal pressure to sleep, Dormer employs various strategies, such as blocking all light coming into the room, drinking water, hiding the alarm clock, chewing gum, and turning the phone off. As his insomnia worsens, he sees flashes and trickles of light that become associated with flashes of memory. His vision becomes blurry; he nods off during conversation, often has an unkempt appearance, and frequently stares blankly into space. The longer Dormer goes without sleep, the more severe the consequences; his agitation develops into anger outbursts, he nearly runs a woman over with his car,

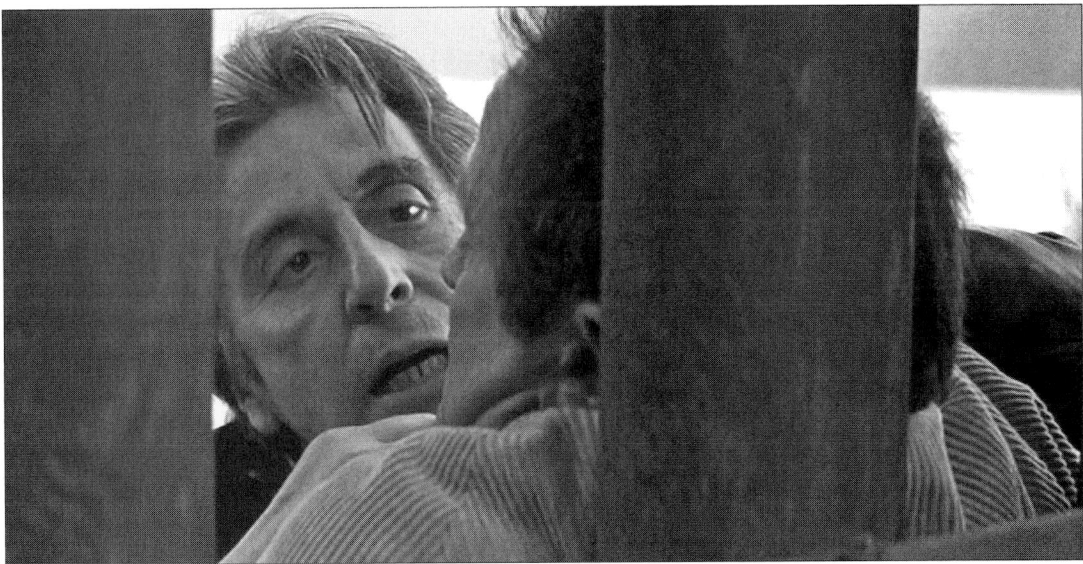

Figure 27. *Insomnia* (2002, Alcon Entertainment, Witt/Thomas Productions, Section Eight, Insomnia Productions, Summit Entertainment). Produced by George Clooney, Ben Cosgrove, Broderick Johnson, Paul J. Witt, et al. Directed by Christopher Nolan.

and he begins to hallucinate. Ultimately, Dormer goes 6 nights without sleep; his exhaustion and irritability are clearly depicted in Figure 27.

Dormer's insomnia symptoms are clearly exacerbated by the psychological pressure he is experiencing. Two major stressors include the pressures of the murder case, and his guilt about killing his partner and lying about it to protect himself in the upcoming Internal Affairs investigation. His current guilt triggers memories of other events in his life about which he feels guilty.

"A good cop can't sleep because a piece of the puzzle's missing, and a bad cop can't sleep because his conscience won't let him."

Ellie Burr to Will Dormer, in *Insomnia* (2002)

Insomnia is a powerful metaphor in the film. Director Christopher Nolan has discussed the challenges involved in making a film about insomnia that will not tire viewers; to avoid this problem, Nolan utilized various images in the film to symbolize the experience of insomnia. At the film's onset, the viewer is shown miles and miles of Alaskan glaciers – representing something of a dreamscape, followed by endless green trees covered by moving fog. Other examples of sleep-related imagery include empty streets with blinking traffic lights, flashes of light, tunnels and escape hatches, and things as mundane as trance-inducing windshield wipers. These all symbolize haziness, drifting, mental confusion, and disorientation.

Insomnia disorder can present in three ways: Some patients will experience tremendous difficulty falling asleep; others will find it difficult or impossible to sleep through the night; still others will be plagued by early morning awakenings and be unable to fall back asleep. The sleep disturbance must cause distress or impairment to qualify for the diagnosis, and it must be present at least three nights per week for at least 3 months. About a third of the adult population report experiencing the symptoms of insomnia, and 6–10% will meet the criteria for insomnia disorder. Insomnia disorder is about 44% more common in women than in men, and it is frequently comorbid with other conditions (most often major depressive disorder).

The effects of insomnia are graphically portrayed in *The Machinist* (2004). Christian Bale lost 60 pounds to play the role of the gaunt Trevor Reznik in this film. Trevor is a depressed and lonely man who has been unable to sleep for a significant period. He uses stimulants such as caffeine and nicotine, common among individuals who struggle with insomnia. Trevor is accused of using drugs, although this is never depicted or indicated. The insomnia clearly affects his daily functioning - he causes an accident, becomes paranoid that his coworkers are plotting against him, and at one point he throws himself in front of a moving car. He displays symptoms of both an amnestic disorder and a psychotic disorder (e.g., hallucinations, paranoia); however, his inability to sleep would need to be treated as the immediate clinical concern. Cinematically, the film's images become less distinct to the viewer because of the director's use of muted colors, distorted views through mirrors, and showing Trevor behind and beyond things in his environment.

In addition to the film *Insomnia*, Christopher Nolan created the remarkable film *Inception* (2010), an incredibly complex story that portrays characters in a dream within a dream within a dream (within a dream). It stars Leonardo DiCaprio, a thief who can infiltrate the dreams of high-powered individuals and steal secret information. He suffers from insomnia, and this is an important theme in the film. Nolan's most recent film, *Oppenheimer* (2023), depicts many of the mental health challenges Robert Oppenheimer confronted, including profound depression and an (aborted) attempt to poison a professor by injecting an apple with liquid cyanide. Oppenheimer had multiple affairs, and in the 20's he received a diagnosis of dementia praecox (what we today call schizophrenia). Oppenheimer was a life-long smoker who died of throat cancer in 1967 at age 62 (Werner, 2005).

Insomnia is one of the many symptoms experienced by Travis Bickle (Robert Di Niro) in *Taxi Driver* (1976). Because of his chronic insomnia, Bickle applies for and secures a job as a taxi driver; as his insomnia worsens, his psychiatric symptoms become more apparent.

The symptoms of insomnia are experienced by the two characters in *Lost in Translation* (2003), played by Bill Murray and Scarlett Johansson. Both characters are Americans who have traveled to Japan and experience apathy and loneliness in this unfamiliar setting. Both deal with their insomnia symptoms by going to the hotel bar and watching late-night television. Eventually they meet and build a friendship. One important scene depicts them lying awake in bed together at night; director Sofia Coppola is showing they are facing their symptoms (symbolized by being awake in bed) in a nonsexual, healthy way through communication.

Edward Norton's character in *Fight Club* (1999) suffers from serious insomnia. The insomnia may be a symptom caused by **circadian rhythm sleep-wake disorder** due to his work, which requires frequent travel. He states he feels as though he is never awake or asleep and that he loses weight because he cannot sleep. He exhibits blank stares, and his body language suggests that he is exhausted. It may be that jet lag exacerbates a preexisting problem with primary insomnia. His experience of sleeplessness triggers a break with reality leading to the development of DID. It is important to note that individuals with prolonged severe insomnia may experience dissociative symptoms or psychotic states, but there is no evidence it will cause DID.

"With insomnia, nothing's real. Everything's far away. Everything's a copy of a copy of a copy."

The narrator in *Fight Club* (1999)

In the movie *Return to Oz* (1985), based on the books *The Marvelous Land of Oz* and *Ozma of Oz* by L. Frank Baum, Fairuza Balk portrays Dorothy who is shown suffering from sleep problems. Aunt Em (Piper Laurie) decides to send Dorothy to a facility for treatment of insomnia where her tendency to repeatedly relate things to Oz is treated as a psychiatric symptom. The psychiatrist explains that ECT will be used to treat her insomnia and her "bad waking dreams" of Oz and its characters. Of course, there is virtually nothing accurate in the depiction here of insomnia treatment; however, the film provides an example of how filmmakers can create their own treatments to better fit their plotlines.

Hypersomnolence Disorder

Hypersomnolence disorder is diagnosed when a patient presents with a history of excessive sleepiness evidenced in prolonged, nonrestorative sleep or daytime sleep episodes that occur at least three times each week for at least 3 months, which causes significant distress or impairment. Like insomnia, hypersomnia can be a symptom of other disorders (e.g., major depressive disorder) or a separate entity itself. Although there are widespread individual differences in the amount of sleep people require, sleeping less than 7 hours each night suggests inadequate nocturnal sleep, while sleeping more than 9–10 hours suggests hypersomnolence.

In *American Splendor* (2003), Harvey Pekar's girlfriend moves in with him and sleeps all day. She has an agitated depression that manifests itself in irritability and in sleeping on the couch well into the middle of the day. This may reflect hypersomnia; the extended periods she spends in bed may also be a symptom of depression.

Narcolepsy

Narcolepsy is a devastating sleep disorder in which the individual experiences uncontrollable and unwanted daily sleep attacks. People with narcolepsy can fall asleep while talking, eating, or walking. The disorder is frequently accompanied by **cataplexy** (sudden loss of muscle tone without loss of consciousness). Narcolepsy most often occurs in obese individuals. A rare but accurate portrayal of narcolepsy occurs in the character of Mike Waters (River Phoenix) in *My Own Private Idaho* (1991).

The portrayal of narcolepsy in movies is often brief, unkind, and superficial, with the sole purpose of ridiculing the person with narcolepsy. This type of humor is highly predictable as it always involves a character falling asleep at an inopportune, unexpected, or embarrassing moment. Though the portrayals are not entirely inaccurate (since sleep attacks in narcolepsy are of rapid onset and can be triggered by intense emotion), they are grossly exaggerated and uniformly unflattering. Minor characters in *Moulin Rouge* (2001), *Deuce Bigalow: Male Gigolo* (1999), *Rat Race* (2001), and *Bandits* (2001) have narcolepsy. In *Rat Race*, Enrico Pollini (Rowan Atkinson, best known as Mr. Bean) falls asleep at a critical moment when he is about to win a race, and in *Bandits*, a bank manager falls asleep during a robbery due to the stress of the experience.

Nightmare Disorder

Nightmare disorder is a parasomnia in which an individual repeatedly awakens from sleep recalling a frightening dream. When waking, the individual quickly becomes alert and oriented. Themes of the nightmare usually involve threats to survival, security, or self-esteem. Four different specifiers are included in DSM-5: (a) during sleep onset; (b) with associated conditions (nonsleep disorder, associated other medical condition, or associated other sleep disorder); (c) acute, subacute, or persistent; and (d) severity (mild, moderate, or severe). About 6% of adults have nightmares that occur at least once a month.

Countless movies depict characters experiencing nightmares, yet only a handful of those characters would qualify for the diagnosis of nightmare disorder. Many filmmakers enjoy manipulating the plot in such a way that the viewer is never sure whether a film is a dream (or nightmare) or reality. This plot device is used in Cameron Crowe's *Vanilla Sky* (2001). Sometimes the character awakens from a nightmare the viewer may or may not have known was happening; other films leave the viewer confused as to what has been experienced or just occurred. David Lynch is famous for the use of this approach; the strategy can be seen in his films *Blue Velvet* (1986), *Lost Highway* (1997), and *Mulholland Drive* (2001). The last of these films is very confusing, and its second half is usually assumed to reflect a character's nightmare. In *Wristcutters: A Love Story* (2006), the two lead characters wake up in adjacent beds in a hospital room following suicide attempts, and it is assumed that everything the two had experienced together was only a linked nightmare.

Nightmares also are dramatically portrayed in two classic films: They are shown as a part of alcohol withdrawal in *The Lost Weekend* (1945), and the detective Scottie Ferguson (James Stewart) has vivid nightmares after the apparent bell tower suicide of Madeleine (Kim Novak) in Alfred Hitchcock's *Vertigo* (1958). The final scene in *Deliverance* (1972) shows the character of Ed (Jon Voight) waking from a nightmare in which he had seen his friend Drew's hand rising out of a lake. Michael Shannon plays the role of Curtis in *Take Shelter* (2011), a film that opens with Curtis having a dramatic nightmare about a coming storm during which his own dog attacks him. A few of the other films in which nightmares are portrayed include *David and Lisa* (1962), *Mysterious Skin* (2004), *The Pact of Silence* (2003), and Wim Wenders' *Land of Plenty* (2004, US/Germany).

Non-Rapid Eye Movement Sleep Arousal Disorders

Non-rapid eye movement (NREM) sleep arousal disorders usually occur during the first third of a major sleep episode, and they are accompanied by either sleepwalking or sleep terrors. **Sleepwalking** (somnambulism) involves repeated episodes of rising from bed and walking around during sleep. During these episodes, the person has a blank stare, is unresponsive to others, and can only be awakened with great difficulty. The person does not remember the episode, and there is no impairment in mental activity or behavior upon awakening. **Sleep terrors** are diagnosed when someone experiences recurrent episodes of abrupt awakening from sleep, often with a panicky scream. The person experiencing sleep terror disorder shows signs of significant distress (e.g., rapid breathing, sweating) and is disoriented and unresponsive to attempts to comfort them. The individual does not recall the dream itself or the experience of screaming.

Some films illustrate sleep terrors when a character screams in their sleep only to wake up unaware of what they were dreaming. This is depicted by an amnestic woman in *Dead Again* (1991), in an adolescent girl screaming during sleep while on an inpatient unit in *Manic* (2003), in a woman on a psychiatric unit of a woman's prison in *Gothika* (2003), and in a young boy who has been cloned partially with cells taken from a murderous child in *Godsend* (2004).

In *Secondhand Lions* (2003), Hub (Robert Duvall) sleepwalks each night and goes to stand near a pond; sometimes he acts out an imaginary battle. Garth (Michael Caine) warns others not to awaken the sleepwalker, particularly because Hub will fight in his sleep if he is disturbed. The film suggests that Hub is searching for a love who has died. A young adolescent, played by Haley Joel Osment, enjoys watching Hub but is anxious about his safety.

In *Donnie Darko* (2001), the lead character, Donnie (Jake Gyllenhaal), hallucinates and is discovered by his psychiatrist to be a sleepwalker, often following his hallucinations outside when sleeping or napping.

Waking Life (2001) blends animation and drama in a surrealist film with the feel of a lucid dream. The movie addresses existential themes and questions our own wakefulness during the day, utilizing the metaphor of humans as "sleepwalking" through the days often unaware of what is going on around them. The film explores dream states, reality, and the insights that can be reached with each. Many important questions and issues are raised for the viewer to reflect upon, with themes of "creating one's own life," reality versus illusion, lucid dreaming, free will versus determinism, mindfulness versus automatic pilot, destiny, and the experience of suffering in life. Similar themes are explored in the 2004 film *Sleepwalking*.

> **"The trick is to combine your waking rational abilities with the infinite possibilities of your dreams. Because, if you can do that, you can do anything."**
>
> **Guy Forsyth in *Waking Life* (2001)**

Feeding and Eating Disorders

There are two major categories of eating disorder: **anorexia** and **bulimia**. New diagnoses for DSM-5 include binge-eating disorder and avoidant/restrictive food intake disorder. Other problems with feeding and eating usually diagnosed in infancy or early childhood are **rumination disorder** and pica. For a graphic depiction of **pica**, see the film *The Princess and the Warrior* (2000), which portrays an adolescent psychiatric patient chewing and swallowing glass. A more recent film illustrating pica is *Swallow* (2019); although the official diagnosis given the protagonist is **pica**, there are clear elements of OCD present as the protagonist tries to assert herself and establish agency as she deals with an overbearing husband and his intrusive parents (see Figure 28).

Anorexia Nervosa

In anorexia, the individual refuses to maintain an appropriate body weight for their age and height and has an intense fear of gaining weight or becoming fat even though they are underweight. The anorectic patient also has a distorted perception of their weight and shape. Many symptoms are like those associated with starvation, such as amenorrhea, abdominal pain, and lethargy. Depression and obsessive-compulsive features associated with food are quite common co-occurring disorders. Anorexia

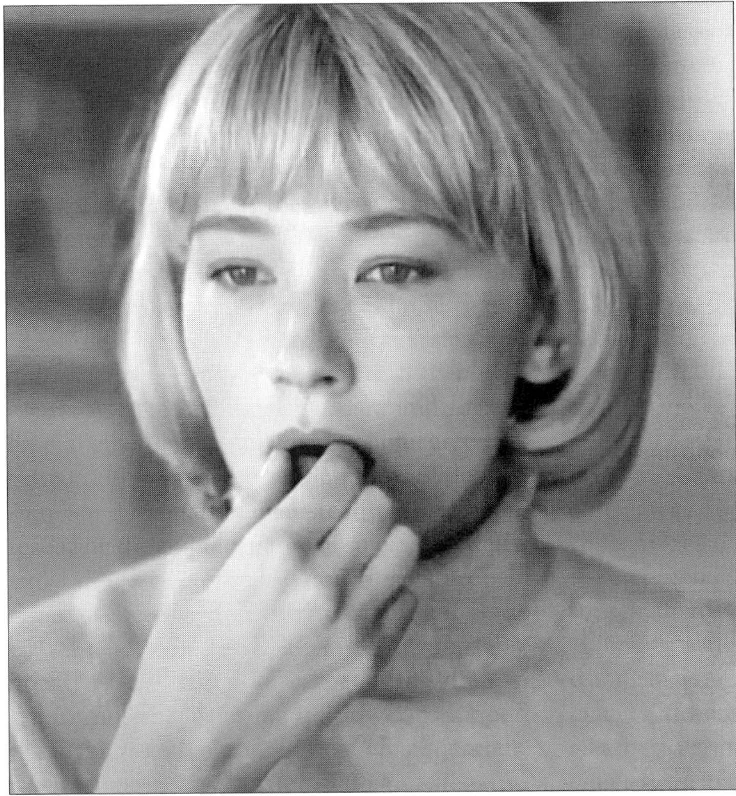

Figure 28.
Swallow (2019, Charades, Logical Pictures, Standalone Productions, Syncopated Film and The Population). Produced by Lauren Andrade, Mollye Asher, Carole Baraton, Haley Bennett, et al. Directed by Carlo Mirabella-Davis.

presents serious health risks and may lead to death by starvation, suicide, or electrolyte imbalance (more than 10% of anorectics are likely to die, making anorexia one of the most lethal psychological disorders). The DSM-5 includes three specifiers for anorexia nervosa: (a) restricting or binge-eating/purging type; (b) in partial or in full remission; and (c) severity (mild, moderate, severe, or extreme. The disorder is *far* more common among young females than among young males, with a female to male ratio of at least 10:1.

Thin (2006) is an HBO documentary that provides an inside look at the lives of women with eating disorders and their residential treatment from intake to discharge. Four women aged 15–30 and living in South Florida, suffer from anorexia or bulimia. The film depicts the young women in their counseling sessions, weighing in, during group activities, and socializing. Anxieties about weighing in, avoidance of food, medication misuse, and other issues common to those with eating disorders are portrayed. The film illustrates important themes related to the intense challenges of recovery, the significant cost of treatment, noncompliance, the sabotage of a fellow patient's treatment, and the high relapse rate.

To the Bone (2017) stars Keanu Reeves as Dr. William Beckham, a somewhat eccentric therapist treating a young woman (Lily Collins) for anorexia nervosa. The film is difficult to watch at times, but it presents an accurate and sympathetic portrayal of the disorder. It is highly recommended.

A fascinating twist on anorexia is found in *The Wonder* (2022), a film in which a 19th-century nurse saves the life of a young Catholic girl who is reported to have gone 4 months without eating, subsisting on "manna from God." This complex and engaging film is discussed more fully in the context of delusional disorders (Chapter 3). It is interesting to learn that Christian Saint Catherine of Siena, noted for her erotic mysticism, subsisted on water and vegetables, and died from starvation when she was 33 years old (*anorexia mirabilis*). At the time of her death, Catherine would eat nothing but a single consecrated host that was part of the daily Eucharist. Associated practices included lifelong virginity, hair shirts, binging and purging, and sleeping on a bed of thorns. The parallels between "holy fasting" and anorexia nervosa are clear (Bell, 2014; Forcen & Forcen, 2015).

Ellen: "I know I'm messed up, but you're supposed to teach me how not to be."
Dr. William Beckham: "You know how. Stop waiting for life to be easy. Stop hoping for somebody to save you. You don't need another person lying to you. Things don't all add up, but you are resilient. Face some hard facts and you could have an incredible life."
Ellen: "That's your pearl of wisdom? Grow a pair?"
Dr. William Beckham: "That's a more concise way of putting it. Yeah."

Keanu Reeves plays a therapist giving advice to his anorexic patient, in *To the Bone* (2017)

Big budget films rarely portray anorexia; however, the disorder is often portrayed accurately in television movies. A compelling examination of anorexia and its treatment is found in the film *The Best Little Girl in the World* (1981). Jennifer Jason Leigh dropped her weight down to 90 pounds for the role of Casey Powell in this movie. Other films depicting anorexia include *For the Love of Nancy* (1994), which stars Tracey Gold; *Dying to Be Perfect* (1996); *Dying to Dance* (2001); and *Hunger Point* (2003). Anorexia nervosa is common among professional dancers, especially ballerinas, and it is clearly present in the film *Black Swan* (2010).

Bulimia Nervosa

Bulimia is characterized by **binges**, which are self-indulgent and unrestrained eating episodes. In addition, some behavior is used to prevent weight gain, such as **purging** (self-induced vomiting), misuse of laxatives, diuretics, enemas, or medications, fasting, and/or excessive exercise. Bulimics are preoccupied with their body weight or shape. Depression, anxiety, substance abuse, and borderline personality are the most common co-occurring diagnoses.

In *Center Stage* (2000), one of the dancers, Maureen, suffers from bulimia. She has a very controlling mother who is trying to relive her life through her daughter. The mother talks about little other than dance opportunities for Maureen. Maureen was restricted as a child, and she was not allowed to play tennis or similar games with other children. To please a new boyfriend, she eats junk food and later purges to stay fit for the dance competitions. Elements of denial are evident when she is on a boat with her boyfriend who hears her purging; Maureen claims she is simply experiencing motion sickness. Her boyfriend later confronts her about "hurting her body." An element of insight emerges when Maureen sees another dancer fall and hurt herself, thus becoming unable to dance in the competition; she finds herself wishing she had been the one who was injured, because then the intense pressure both externally (her mother) and internally (herself) would have been gone.

In *Life Is Sweet* (1990), a rebellious adolescent girl, Nicola, is bulimic, binging and purging on chocolate bars hidden in her bedroom. She attempts to include the chocolate in her sex life by rubbing it over her body. She lives in a dysfunctional family obsessed with food, cooking, and the restaurant business. In *Girl, Interrupted* (1999), one of the characters hospitalized with Susanna Kaysen (Winona Ryder) has a serious eating disorder and self-mutilates; her rich, codependent father supports his daughter's eating disorder by bringing her baked chicken that she hides and hordes under her hospital bed. The film hints at an incestuous relationship between her and her father, and a pivotal moment occurs in the film when she commits suicide by hanging herself in her shower. *Requiem for a Dream* (2000) includes one character who is obsessed with food but needs to lose weight to appear on a television game show; her obsession with weight loss leads her to become addicted to diet pills.

In *Elephant* (2003), numerous characters are shown going through a typical day before a school tragedy occurs. Three adolescent girls, Brittany, Jordan, and Kelly, focus on the caloric contents of their lunch food. After eating, they walk into the bathroom together and, each using separate stalls, collectively purge. They do it quickly and without a word about the behavior – acting nonchalantly in the middle of their continuing conversation. They are depicted as attractive with slender bodies, and the three girls obviously want to maintain their appearance. Purging together provides social support for their aberrant behavior. *I Want Someone to Eat Cheese With* (2007) portrays an overweight man struggling with food; he frequently binges on snacks while sitting alone on the front of his car in an empty parking garage, he routinely breaks his diet, and he attends Overeaters Anonymous support group meetings.

Bulimia nervosa is much more common among young people than among older adults. Although 90% of people with bulimia are females, the prevalence seems to be rising in males. The film *Seabiscuit* (2003) displays a male horse-racing jockey (Tobey Maguire) who forces himself to throw up to maintain his low weight so he can ride faster. Ben Stiller's narcissistic, male-model character in *Zoolander* (2001) refers to purging after meals to lose weight, to look better, and keep his job.

Maggie: "What are you doing?"
Carol: "Donkey kicks. I've eaten everything in the place, and I'm trying to work it off before morning. I used to be bulimic. A year ago, I'd be in the bathroom throwing it all up. I'm much healthier now!"

Carol explains her vigorous exercise routine in Kenneth Branagh's film *Peter's Friends* (1992)

Bulimic themes are also evident in *Heathers* (1989), *Peter's Friends* (1992), the Korean film *301, 302* (1995), *Angus* (1995), *When Friendship Kills* (1996), and *Drop Dead Gorgeous* (1999).

Binge-Eating Disorder

Binge-eating disorder (BED) was listed in an appendix to DSM-IV; however, in DSM-5, it is identified as a bona fide, albeit controversial, disorder. BED involves eating an excessive quantity of food in a discrete period with the sense that one's eating is out of control and cannot be stopped. Three of five criteria must be present: (a) rapid eating; (b) discomfort from eating; (c) eating copious amounts of food even when not hungry; (d) eating alone because of embarrassment about one's eating habits; (e) feeling depressed, disgusted, or guilty after binge eating. In addition, binging must occur, on average, at least once a week for 3 months. In *Monster's Ball* (2001), the son of Halle Berry's character routinely binges on food he keeps hidden in his room. Binge-eating symptoms, along with symptoms of depression, can be found in the minimalist film *Visioneers* (2008), starring Zach Galifianakis.

Brendan Fraser won an Oscar for his performance in *The Whale* (2022) as Charlie, a 600-pound man coping with grief over the death of his lover and the fact that he is estranged from his teenage daughter, someone he left when she was a young child to be with his lover (Figure 29). Charlie's obesity required a fat suit and considerable skill from makeup artists, and Darren Aronofsky has been criticized for not choosing a man who was actually obese to play the role. Charlie is an online English professor who refuses to let his students see him on camera, believing they would find his obesity distracting. The film opens with Charlie masturbating to a homoerotic video, and it is clear that he has resigned himself to dying prematurely. Fraser's character would undoubtably meet DSM-5 criteria for binge-eating disorder.

Ellie: "Are you actually trying to parent me right now?"
Charlie: "No, I'm... Sorry. I just... I just thought that maybe we could spend some time with each other."
Ellie: "I'm not spending time with you. You're disgusting."
Charlie: "Well, I'm a lot bigger than I was since last time you saw me."
Ellie: "No, I'm not talking about what you look like. You'd be disgusting even if you weren't this fat. You'd still be that piece-of-shit dad who walked out on me when I was eight. All because he wanted to fuck one of his students."

Charlie tries to reestablish contact with the teenage daughter he left when she was eight in *The Whale* (2022).

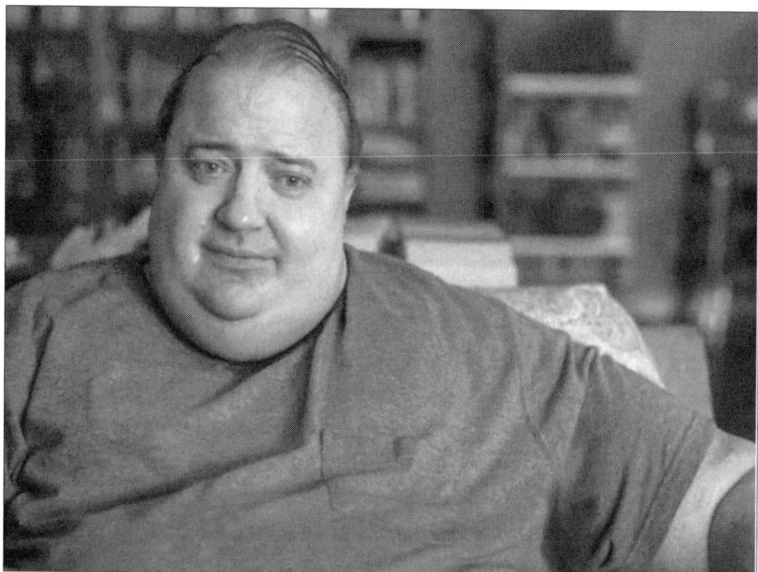

Figure 29.
The Whale (2022, A24 and Protozoa Pictures). Produced by Darren Aronofsky, Tyson Binder, Jeremy Dawson, Scott Franklin et al.). Directed by Darren Aronofsky.

Reviewing this film for *The Guardian*, Linda West (2023) wrote "people respond positively to *The Whale* because it confirms their biases about what fat people are like (gross, sad) and why fat people are fat (trauma, munchies) and allows them to feel benevolent yet superior. It's a basic dopamine hit, reifying thin people's place at the top of the social hierarchy." I found this criticism unfair, and I strongly recommend you see the film and form your own opinions.

Body Image and Eating Disorders

Body image is one of the most significant problems in both anorexia nervosa and bulimia nervosa. Many films, however, display characters struggling with their body image, though not all of them suffer from formal eating disorders. Often the use of a mirror or reflective surface shows characters viewing and assessing themselves, to convey a character's dissatisfaction with their body. Many times, the image in the reflection is shown as distorted, blurred, formless, or unclear to emphasize self-hate, self-deprecation, or self-distortion.

Girl (2003) and *I've Heard the Mermaids Singing* (1987) depict characters with problems with body image who stand in harsh self-judgment in front of a mirror. Toward the end of the acclaimed docudrama *What the Bleep Do We Know?!* (2004), the lead character (Marlee Matlin) stares in the mirror at her body, wearing only underwear, examining it with distaste, distortion, and rage. *What's Eating Gilbert Grape?* (1993) has a key character, Gilbert's mother, who weighs over 500 pounds and is too large to leave the house or even get off the sofa where she lives out her dreary existence. Gilbert (Johnny Depp) gives other children a "leg up" when they come to peer in the window at this morbidly obese woman.

Somatic Symptom Disorders

Somatic symptoms and related disorders is the subject of a new chapter in the DSM-5. This rubric encompasses several disorders that all involve significant distress or impairment because of preoccupation with somatic symptoms. Individuals with somatic symptom disorders commonly present in primary care settings rather than mental health settings. The diagnoses included in this section of the DSM-5 include **somatic symptom disorder**, **illness anxiety disorder**, **conversion disorder**, and **factitious disorder**.

Somatic Symptom Disorder

Somatic symptom disorder replaces the confusing term "somatoform disorder" in DSM-IV, although somatic symptom disorder is far less complex in that only one symptom that causes distress is needed for the diagnosis, as opposed to the previous condition in which multiple somatic complaints affecting multiple organ systems were needed for the diagnosis. Individuals with somatic symptom disorder have excessive thoughts, feelings, or behaviors associated with their somatic symptoms, and these are typically disproportionate, often requiring extensive time and energy. The previous DSM-IV condition, pain disorder, is now subsumed as a specifier (i.e., with predominant pain) under this condition.

Safe

The Todd Haynes film *Safe* (1995) focuses exclusively on a woman with a somatic symptom disorder. Carol White (Julianne Moore) slowly begins to deteriorate with unexplained symptoms related to chemical sensitivity. Doctors tell her that stress is the cause of her problem and advise her to learn to relax. However, it is difficult to see what is stressful in her life – she has a loving husband, beautiful home, good social life, and servants who to do the cooking and cleaning. Her bodily system becomes overloaded and overwhelmed by fumes, toxins, fragrances, and other "pollutants" – these come from traffic, her shampoo, her husband's cologne, and a new sofa. It is as if she is being attacked by plastics, ozone, chemicals, high-energy wires, pollution, additives, preservatives, and hamburger fumes. Carol continues to get physically sicker and sicker, leaving her physicians baffled. At one point, she was hospitalized due to extensive bleeding.

Carol makes the decision to travel to another part of the country to a specialized clinic that offers group therapy, seminars, and social activities for people suffering from similar anomalous problems. During a casual group session, the therapist asks probing questions of the patients (and metaphorically to society and the viewer): "Why did you get sick?" and "What's behind your sickness?" One character speaks of abuse experienced as a child, how she made herself sick to remember, and how she had not forgiven the perpetrator and took it out on herself. Other characters believed their illness was due to self-blame or anger, and in one man's case, a drug addiction. Upon hearing other characters speak of coming to terms with their inner self-hatred, Moore's character admits to also having a deep sense of self-hatred. However, despite all her treatment, she just gets worse. The treatment emphasizes simplistic themes of a need to love oneself more, that we all make ourselves sick, and the role of the mind. These factors can play a key role in the etiology and outcome of illness, and we know that thoughts and feelings affect the immune system; however, the approach in the film comes across as trite and misleading. The film is a dark comedy and a satirical social commentary. Todd Haynes cleverly uses the cinematic element of a subtle background hum to suggest to the viewer that we can never fully escape the impact of the environment.

Illness Anxiety Disorder

Patients with **illness anxiety disorder** are preoccupied with their health problems, even though their somatic symptoms are either nonexistent or minimal. These are anxious patients who repeatedly check their body for evidence of illness (or, more rarely, who avoid physicians or hospitals because of their anxiety about being diagnosed with a serious illness).

Patients who now receive a diagnosis of either somatic symptom disorder or illness anxiety disorder would have formerly been labeled as having **hypochondriasis**; however, DSM-5 avoids this term because it has become "loaded" and clearly stigmatizes individuals who are given this diagnosis. It is estimated that about 25% of patients formerly called hypochondriacs would be appropriately labeled as having illness anxiety disorder; the remaining 75% are more appropriately diagnosed with somatic symptom disorder – a far less stigmatizing label.

Patients with either somatic symptom disorder or illness anxiety disorder are often poor historians, and their complaints may vary from session to session. This problem is complicated by the fact that these patients easily become dissatisfied with their health care provider and may constantly be changing providers, sharing various parts of their story with each new provider. In addition, since most visits result in a prescription of some sort, these patients are often taking multiple medications, some of which produce side effects that result in general somatic distress. This pattern sets up a vicious cycle and makes diagnosis of the patient with a somatization disorder a challenging dilemma. Diagnosis is further complicated by the fact that some genuine medical conditions, such as multiple sclerosis, hyperparathyroidism, and systemic lupus erythematosus, can have vague symptoms that affect multiple organ systems.

The person with an illness anxiety disorder is preoccupied with thoughts of disease, infirmity, and death. This individual worries that simple, benign body sensations or symptoms may be indicative of a serious disease. In the extreme, such a person might interpret routine stomach pain as cancer of the bowel, headaches because of a brain tumor, and/or misplaced keys or glasses as an undeniable early indication of Alzheimer's. The preoccupations persist despite physical exams, lab tests, X-rays, and other examinations suggesting there is no illness present.

Some patients who have been labeled as hypochondriacs in the past are later found to have bona fide medical disorders. This is especially common with disorders that have vague symptoms and a slow progression (e.g., multiple sclerosis). In addition, patients who are initially believed to have hypochondriasis are sometimes later found to have somatic concerns related to anxiety, depression, or another psychiatric disorder.

In *2 Days in Paris* (2007), a relationship-oriented film directed by Julie Delpy, the male protagonist, Jack, has illness anxiety disorder. He is preoccupied with developing an illness, and he tries to control his environment in any way possible and avoids anything that might elicit symptoms. The viewer can clearly see how his somatic condition affects his relationships.

In *Dogville* (2003), one character is a doctor with illness anxiety disorder who misinterprets lumps and various other physical complaints; he is someone who needs the reassurance of others to tell him he is not dying. In *Something's Gotta Give* (2005), Jack Nicholson plays a 63-year-old man obsessed with dating younger women and develops illness anxiety symptoms after suffering his first heart attack; all subsequent episodes turn out to be panic attacks.

Bandits

In *Bandits* (2001), Billy Bob Thornton plays Terry Collins, a bank robber with illness anxiety disorder. Terry is convinced he has various illnesses despite his physician assuring him there is nothing wrong. While in prison, he ruminates about how helpful garlic is and becomes upset when it is banned from the prison cafeteria; in a subsequent scene, he incessantly screams in the prison yard about ringing in his ears. In his leisure time, he reads a medical dictionary and while driving listens to *Merck Manual* cassette tapes alphabetically defining diseases.

After escaping from prison and robbing a bank with his cohort in crime, Joe Blake (Bruce Willis), Terry's arm becomes numb, he complains of seeing spots, and makes weird noises with his throat. When challenged by his partner, he explains, "I have sanitation issues, Joe."

When stressed, Terry experiences a sneezing attack and a tic in his left eye. He then begins to talk rapidly and uses medical jargon. He also becomes preoccupied about one pupil being larger than the other. Each of his senses is affected in some way throughout the film. In addition, Terry suffers from food allergies, lactose intolerance, and various obscure phobias such as a fear of getting smaller, a fear of antique furniture, a fear of historic figures, and a fear of black-and-white movies. He experiences numbness in his arm, lips, and legs that leads him to collapse and flail about on the floor in one scene.

Hannah and Her Sisters

Hannah and Her Sisters (1986) is one of Woody Allen's funniest and most gratifying films. Allen plays Mickey, a neurotic television executive, who is a classic example of someone with an illness anxiety disorder. He is on his way to getting a blood test when the film opens, and we soon realize that he is preoccupied with doctors, hospitals, and his own fragile mortality. He works in a high-stress job, and early in the film he remarks, "Has anybody got a Tagamet? My ulcer is starting to kill me." (Director Woody Allen has a remarkable sense for the prevailing concerns and habits of the American public. A decade earlier, he had amused his viewers with a similar line about Valium.)

"This time I think I really have something ... It's not like that adenoidal thing, where I didn't realize I had them out."

Mickey Sachs (Woody Allen) discussing his hearing loss with his physician, in *Hannah and Her Sisters* (1986)

Mickey has experienced some hearing loss and is convinced that he has a brain tumor. He

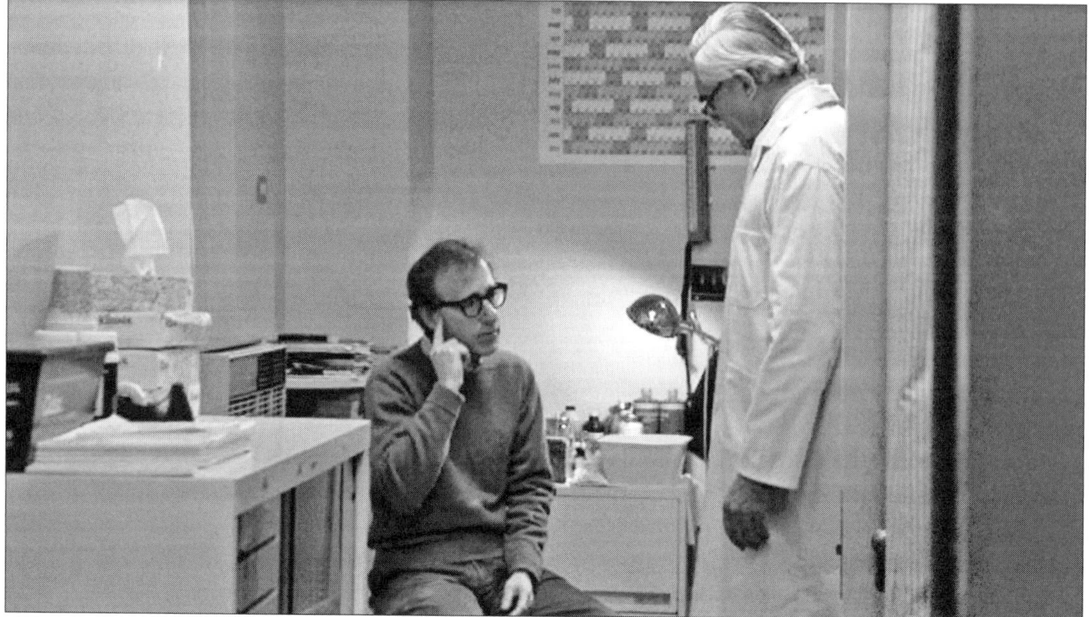

Figure 30. *Hanna and Her Sisters* (1986, Orion Pictures, Jack Rollins & Charles H. Joffe Productions). Produced by Robert Greenhut, Charles H. Joffe, Jack Rollins, and Gail Sicilia. Directed by Woody Allen.

suspects that his doctors have known this all along but "they don't tell you [these things] because sometimes the weaker ones will panic." He awakens in the middle of the night, terrified, crying out, "There's a tumor in my head the size of a basketball." He engages in an "organ recital" with each new physician (Figure 30), and with each new doctor and each new test, he grows more apprehensive. When his computed tomography scan turns out to be completely negative, he is at first elated and then plunges into despair as he realizes that this is just a temporary reprieve and, eventually, he must die.

Conversion Disorder

A **conversion disorder** exists when (1) patients experience significant distress or impairment from motor or sensory symptoms that appear to be neurological but for which no adequate neurological explanation can be determined, and (2) psychological factors have played a significant role in the etiology or maintenance of the disorder. In addition, the clinician must rule out malingering, before the diagnosis is made.

The very name "conversion disorder" is linked to a psychological theory that maintains that unconscious psychological distress can be "converted" into physical manifestations. Interestingly, symptoms are far more likely to occur on the left side of the body (presumably because most people are right-handed and unconsciously develop symptoms on the side that is less needed).

Conversion disorders are fascinating, in part because the underlying dynamics seem so transparent to an external observer. The soldier who cannot fire a rifle because his arm is paralyzed has found a convenient way of avoiding battle; the woman who becomes functionally blind after witnessing a car wreck in which her son was killed can never see anything this awful happen again. In actual practice, few cases of conversion disorder are this tidy.

Woody Allen's character, Val Wawman, in *Hollywood Ending* (2002) develops a clear example of hysterical blindness, a previously frequent but currently rare conversion disorder. Just prior to the first day of directing a new film (in which there is the added stress of his ex-wife being the coproducer with her new fiancé), he loses his sight. This would suggest a neurological condition, but an extensive medical examination fails to produce medical or physiological reasons for Wawman's blindness. He goes to see a psychologist who explains this is psychological in origin and supports this comment with individualized interpretations – Val's fears of failure, internal conflicts, and poor relationship with his son. Val also exhibits numerous hypochondriacal symptoms including his extreme fear of getting an illness and preoccupation with illness. He previously thought he had experienced many outlandish diseases (e.g., diseases that only trees can get, the plague, etc.), all due to his misinterpretation of bodily symptoms. Another case of hysterical blindness is portrayed in the 1939 film *The Secret of Dr. Kildare*. In this film, Dr. Kildare performs a sham operation to restore his patient's sight, raising interesting ethical questions that would not have been debated in the 1930s.

The film *Sorry, Wrong Number* (1948) stars Barbara Stanwyck as a bedridden heiress who is partially paralyzed, although her doctors cannot determine any neurological reason for her inability to walk. One evening, she happens to overhear two men planning a murder; later she realizes that she is the intended victim. Much of the suspense of the film revolves around the realization that she must get out of bed to save herself.

Thérèse: The Story of Saint Thérèse of Lisieux (2004), tells the story of Saint Thérèse who became a Carmelite nun at age 15 and died from tuberculosis when she was 24. Thérèse's mother died when Thérèse was only 4 years old, and she experienced marked periods of depression. She also appears to have multiple psychosomatic complaints including pounding headaches and stomach pains when she thinks about her sins. One evening she faints at the dinner table. She experiences restless sleep, and at one point she is delirious for 2 weeks. During the period of delirium, she does not eat, loses weight, cries out, and hallucinates. She coughs repeatedly and spits up blood when her father's health deteriorates. Her influence on the Catholic Church has been tremendous; her memoir, *Story of a Soul*, has been translated into over 60 languages and has sold over 100 million copies.

Agnes of God

The complex film *Agnes of God* (1985), stars Meg Tilly as a young nun (Sister Agnes), Anne Bancroft as the mother superior of the convent, and Jane Fonda as the psychiatrist sent to investigate the apparent murder of a newborn baby who was found wrapped in bloody sheets and stuffed in a wastebasket at the convent. The film juxtaposes reason and faith and quickly convinces the viewer that, although Sister Agnes is surely one of "God's innocents," she is just as surely the mother and the murderer of the child.

Fonda, playing the psychiatrist, uses hypnosis in treating Sister Agnes, and it turns out that her mother sexually molested her when she was a child. It also turns out that the mother was the sister of the mother superior. At the end of the film, the court finds Sister Agnes not guilty by reason of insanity, and she returns to the convent, where she will continue to receive psychiatric care.

Sister Agnes's confusion seems very real, and the label of insanity seems justified. A dissociative amnesia may have been present, and the viewer becomes convinced that Sister Agnes had repressed the memories of her rape and was genuinely amnestic for the incident in which she strangled the child with his umbilical cord. Agnes begins to experience stigmata, once in a convent room and once in a chapel while praying. **Stigmata** is the name given to bleeding in the hands and feet, from the sites that nails were driven into when Christ was crucified. It is a rare but well-documented phenomenon found in people with deep religious convictions. In the case of *Agnes of God*, the blood of Christ, the blood of the murdered infant, and the blood of Agnes all seem to comingle. The somatic element of the stigmata in this film is much more complex, powerful, and integrated into the story and personal life of Agnes than the stigmata depicted in the suspense film titled *Stigmata* (1999).

Factitious Disorder

Patients with somatic symptom disorder or illness anxiety disorder will often experience some amount of **secondary gain** because of their medical problems, such as extra care and attention from others, workers' compensation benefits, reduced expectations from family, or avoidance of difficult activities. It is important to be cognizant of normal secondary gain factors while separating a given somatoform disorder from both malingering and factitious disorder. In **malingering**, a person deliberately fakes their symptoms to achieve a clearly understood goal (e.g., one character in *Memento* [2000]). A death row inmate may feign symptoms of mental illness - for example, believing that the state cannot execute someone who is not mentally competent. Likewise, a small child may complain of stomach pain, remembering that the last time this occurred, he could stay home from school and eat ice cream.

In contrast to malingering, **factitious disorders**, a separate diagnostic category, involves feigning illness with the specific intent of assuming the sick role. Some patients with factitious disorders will present with psychological symptoms, while others will have physical symptoms. While the patient who is malingering reports symptoms for personal gain (e.g., insurance payment or disability benefits), the patient with a factitious disorder develops and reports their symptoms without any clear expectation of payment or benefit from the illness.

Factitious disorder imposed on another (previously called factitious disorder by proxy or **Munchausen syndrome by proxy**) occurs when symptoms are intentionally produced in another person, the classic example being the mother who makes her child sick so the child will assume a "sick role" and the mother can assume the role of a long-suffering and loving mother with a sick child. We see an example of factitious disorder imposed on another in Kevin Bacon's film *Loverboy* (2004), which stars Bacon's wife, Kyra Sedgwick, playing an enmeshed and overly protective mother (Emily), and the couple's real-life daughter, Sosie Bacon, who plays the role of Emily seen as a 10-year-old child in a series of flashbacks.

The term "psychosomatic" is often used as a derogatory term for people suffering with the disorders mentioned in this chapter. The term usually refers to physical disorders in which emotional processes play a role, indicating a mutual influence of physical and psychological factors; the generality of this concept can be applied to not only somatoform disorders but most medical and psychological conditions as well.

International Films: Sleep–Wake, Eating, and Somatic Symptom Disorders

Sleep Disorders

Control (2003, Hungary) is a comedy–drama filmed in a Budapest subway dealing with fictitious characters reflecting universal themes of good versus evil and feeling trapped in life. There are various odd characters in the film, one of whom is a worker with narcolepsy who falls asleep on the job when he gets angry or stressed. When conflicts arise between coworkers, he immediately falls asleep and experiences an utter sense of confusion upon awakening.

Nightmares in an adult that are related to childhood sexual abuse are portrayed in *Don't Tell* (2005, Italy/UK/France/Spain) and *The Celebration* (1998, Denmark/Sweden), and they play an especially important role in the former film. The seventh 1-hr film in renowned Polish director Krzysztof Kieslowski's 10-film series *The Decalogue* (1989, Poland) offers a good portrayal of sleep terrors. A child in the film has recurrent night terrors in which she screams in her sleep each night, is difficult to awaken, and is unable to recall her troubling dreams after she awakes. In the film, she is described as suffering from nightmares.

Eating Disorders

In the dark psychodrama *Primo Amore* (2004, Italy), a goldsmith, Vittorio, becomes obsessed with molding the perfect female body (paralleling his work of transforming metals into pure forms). He finds an already slender art school model, Sonia, and rigorously controls her diet to get her to lose more weight. Sonia, desperate to please him, is willing to submit to his delusional plans. His role can be seen as the extreme of a "controlling parent." Self-disgust, exhaustion from starvation, secrecy, and sneaking food are characteristic features found in the characters with eating disorders portrayed in this film. Vittorio's behavior is clearly abusive. While not a pure depiction of an eating disorder nor an accurate portrayal of all the dynamics that surround eating disorders, the film is nevertheless useful as a thematic illustration of this serious clinical problem.

Somatic Symptom Disorders

Gerard Depardieu stars in a French film, *The Pact of Silence* (2003, France), in which he plays a Jesuit priest who is also a physician trying to make sense out of a nun's spells during which she falls to the floor, experiences tremendous pain, and speaks incoherently. The psychosomatic episodes coincide with occasions when her twin sister, who is incarcerated, is in danger (e.g., when her prison cell is set afire by other inmates).

Georgette in *Amélie* (2001, France) would meet all of the criteria for somatic symptom disorder if she were to appear at a doctor's office. While operating a cigarette counter, she complains of various symptoms from sciatica to the discomfort of smoke getting in her eyes. One interesting quote used in the film describes Georgette precisely: "A woman without love wilts like a flower without the sun." When Georgette's mind is not occupied with love, she is preoccupied with enough symptoms to meet the criteria for somatization disorder, but when she has a love interest, she feels perfectly healthy and happy.

The Spanish film *Unconscious* (2004, Spain) is set in Barcelona in 1913 and satirizes psychoanalysis and psychoanalysts; for example, in one scene, a psychiatrist tries to hypnotize a patient using a swinging pocket watch, only to become hypnotized himself, eventually revealing his deepest secret (he is a transvestite). The film shows multiple examples of hypochondriasis and conversion disorder, and a character playing Sigmund Freud makes a brief appearance to promote his new book, *Totem and Taboo*.

Cultural differences in attitudes about illness are underscored in *The Farewell* (2019), a Chinese language film about a young Chinese American woman who returns to China to see her grandmother, who is dying from cancer, for the last time. The protagonist believes her grandmother has a right to know her diagnosis and prognosis; in contrast, her more traditional Chinese family, believes it is critical to withhold this information to protect the family's matriarch. *The Farewell* is a charming film that may leave you questioning your own beliefs and attitudes about end-of-life care.

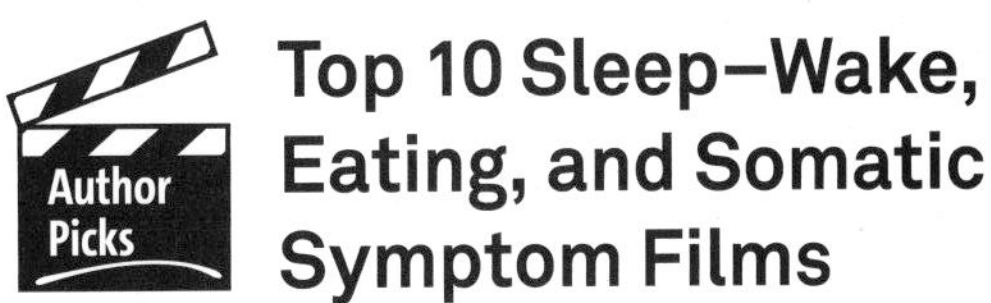

Top 10 Sleep–Wake, Eating, and Somatic Symptom Films

Sleep Disorders

Insomnia (2002)
The Machinist (2004)
Inception (2010)

Eating Disorders

Girl, Interrupted (1999)
Primo Amore (2004)
To the Bone (2017)
Swallow (2017)

Somatic Symptom Disorders

Agnes of God (1985)
Hannah and Her Sisters (1986)
Safe (1995)

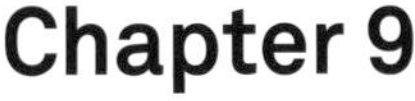

Chapter 9

Gender Dysphoria and Sexual Dysfunctions

I'm not like everybody else. I'm a hermaphrodite.

Teena Brandon's self-diagnosis
in *Boys Don't Cry* (1999)

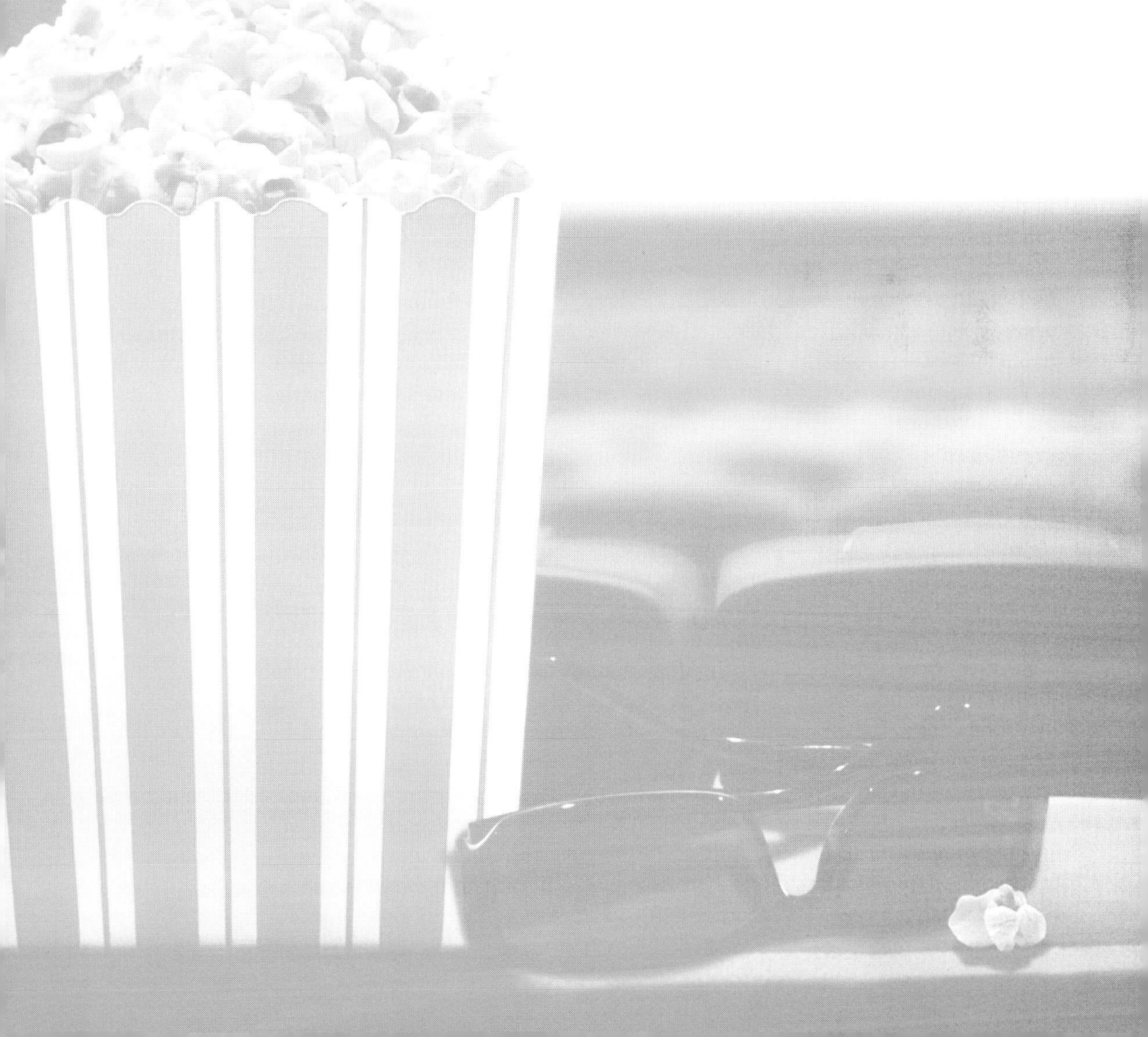

Gender Dysphoria

Sex and **sexual** refer to the biological indicators of male and female whereas **gender** refers to the individual's lived role as a boy or girl, man or woman. **Gender dysphoria** thus refers to the individual's cognitive-emotional discontent with their assigned gender as male or female. The DSM-5 refers to **gender dysphoria** rather than using the label "gender identity disorder"; the new terminology underscores the point that *the problem to be treated is not identity per se, but rather the discomfort and unhappiness that results from the lack of correspondence between anatomy and identity.* The term **transsexual** refers to an individual who is in process or has undergone a social transition from male to female or female to male. **Transgender** refers to the larger spectrum of individuals who identify with a gender different from their birth gender. Individuals who experience gender dysphoria are uncomfortable with their anatomic sex and often believe they are trapped in the wrong body. There is often an ardent desire to replace their genitals with the genitalia of the opposite sex; these urges can be intense enough to lead to self-castration in males. Separate but linked diagnoses are available for children and for adolescents and adults, and specifiers are given when there is a concomitant disorder of sex development (e.g., congenital adrenal hyperplasia). There is also a "post transition" specifier for those individuals who have undergone or who are preparing to undergo at least one relevant medical procedure (e.g., penectomy, mastectomy). People with marked gender dysphoria often suffer from concomitant depression, and suicide attempts are common. Before diagnosing someone with gender dysphoria, clinicians must rule out simple nonconformity to gender roles, transvestic disorder (discussed in Chapter 14), body dysmorphic disorder, and psychosis.

Other films focusing on gender dysphoria include *Normal* (2003), *Beautiful Boxer* (2005), and *Soldier's Girl* (2003). These three films, together with *Boys Don't Cry*, show the pain that a person with gender identity disorder faces and the struggles associated with sharing information about sexual identity with loved ones and society. In *Normal*, Roy (Tom Wilkinson) believes he was born in the wrong body, and he wants a sex change operation. His wife of 25 years (Jessica Lange) expresses a variety of reactions - denial, shock, anger, rejection, depression, and finally acceptance - as they work to keep their marriage intact. Roy desires to be accepted by his congregation, coworkers, boss, children, and society, but each presents a different struggle. *Soldier's Girl* is based on the tragic true story of Barry Winchell, a young man who enters the military and falls in love with a transsexual (a man who dressed as a woman in preparation for gender modification surgery). Likewise, *Beautiful Boxer* (2005) tells the true story of Parinaya Charoemphol, a Thai transgender kickboxer who took up the sport to earn money for gender reassignment surgery.

Transamerica (2005) is a touching film that stars Felicity Huffman as Bree, a presurgical male-to-female transsexual who is saving money and seeing a therapist in preparation for her upcoming operation. She receives a phone call from her son, Toby, a son she did not know she had (he was the byproduct of a casual college affair). Her therapist makes reuniting with her son a prerequisite for surgery, and this leads to a long road trip from New York to Phoenix, where Bree reunites with her dysfunctional family.

"Don't you find it odd that plastic surgery can cure a mental disorder?"

A fascinating comment explored in *Transamerica* (2005)

Interest in the phenomenon of transsexualism burgeoned in the United States and Europe 6 decades ago, after the 1951 gender modification surgery of Christine Jorgensen. (*The Christine Jorgensen Story*, a low-budget and insipid film, was released in 1970.) The mid-1980s witnessed a revival of interest, after widespread publicity and a television movie *(Second Serve)* about the sex reassignment of male surgeon

Richard Raskins into a female tennis star, Renee Richards. Other films that have explored transsexualism include *Myra Breckinridge* (1970) (starring film critic Rex Reed), *Dog Day Afternoon* (1975), *The World According to Garp* (1982), and *Come Back to the 5 & Dime, Jimmie Dean, Jimmie Dean* (1982). *The Crying Game* (1993) is a rich and nuanced film that explores a complex transsexual relationship; in one especially vivid scene, the protagonist throws up after discovering his transsexual lover is anatomically male.

Fergus: "Do they know?"
Dil: "Know what, honey?"
Fergus: "Know what I didn't know? And don't call me that."
Dil: "Can't help it! A girl has her feelings."
Fergus: "Thing is, Dil, you're not a girl."
Dil: "Details, baby, details."
Fergus: "So they do know?"
Dil: "Alright, they do."
Fergus: "Don't. I should've known, shouldn't I?"
Dil: "Probably."
Fergus: "Kind of wish I didn't."
Dil: "You can always pretend."
Fergus: "That's true. Your soldier knew, didn't he?"
Dil: "Absolutely."

A candid discussion of gender and sexual ethics in *The Crying Game* (1993)

Cowboys (2020) is a sensitive and highly recommended film about Josie Johnson, an 11-year-old child who identifies as a female-to-male boy (see Figure 31). "A tomboy is just another kind of girl, but I'm not a girl. I'm in the wrong body, Okay. I'm a boy!" Her Christian mother is adamant that "God made you a girl," but Josie is having none of it, rejecting the Barbie doll her mother wants to buy her, insisting on a toy gun instead. Josie and her father steal a horse and ride into the Montana wilderness. Their situation is complicated when Troy, a father with bipolar disorder, loses his medication and becomes manic. They are eventually caught, and

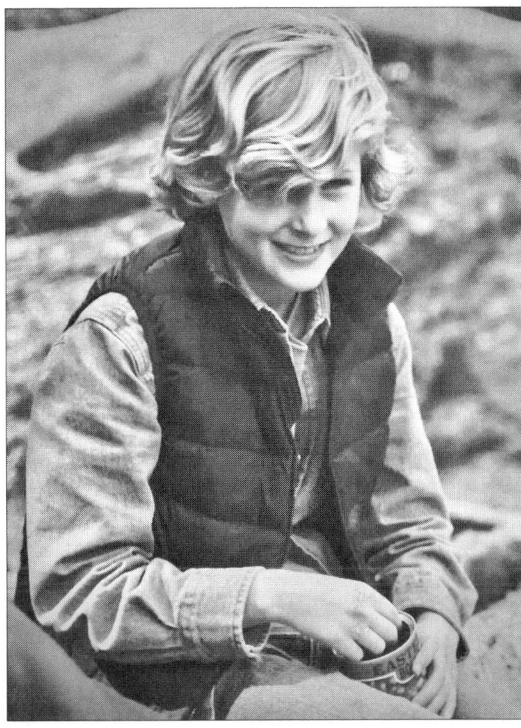

Figure 31. *Cowboys* (2020, Blue Finch Films, Front Row Filmed Entertainment, Samuel Goldwyn, Synapse, Vortex Media). Produced by Anil Baral, C. J. Barbato, Alex Dong, Gigi Graff, et al. Directed by Anna Kerrigan.

Troy is jailed for kidnapping. However, the mother comes to accept her daughter as trans, the family becomes reunited, and the film ends on an upbeat note.

The surgical treatment of transsexuals remains controversial, although tens of thousands of patients have undergone the procedure. Transsexualism occurs more often in biological males than in biological females, and many more males apply for sex reassignment surgery. Transsexuals can be heterosexual, homosexual, or asexual, both prior to and after their surgery. Many professionals who have worked with these patients have been struck by the fact that sexual behavior per se is often a secondary concern; the core issue is one of gender discontent, not sexual behavior.

There are several documentary films on gender dysphoria and gender identity, and a quick search on Netflix will reveal most of these.

Anyone wishing to learn more about affirmative care for trans individuals will benefit from reading a short book in the *Advances in Psychotherapy* book series titled *Affirmative Counseling with Transgender and Gender Diverse Clients* (dickey & Puckett, 2023).

The Range of Normal Sexual Behavior

Few areas of human behavior are as complex, varied, and interesting as sexual behavior. Both social scientists and the public are fascinated by the multitude of possibilities inherent in our sexuality. It is important to appreciate that the range of normal sexual behavior is exceptionally broad, and many behaviors that seem unusual or disturbing to some people do not qualify for a DSM-5 label. As a rule, remember that complex or elaborate sexual fantasies are commonplace and do not suggest that any type of psychological disturbance is present. A psychological problem exists when a person acts on their fantasies with unwilling partners or behaves in ways that distress other people.

Filmmakers have been quick to exploit our fascination with sexual behavior, and contemporary cinema is replete with examples of sexual psychopathology. A serious student can learn a great deal about abnormal psychology from selective viewing.

Sexual Dysfunctions

The human **sexual response cycle** includes the following four phases:

Desire: fantasies related to sex;
Excitement: arousal, sense of pleasure with physiological changes;
Orgasm: peaking of sexual pleasure with release of sexual tension;
Resolution: sense of muscular relaxation and general well-being.

There can be a sexual disorder at any level. For example, **erectile disorder** (impotence) is an excitement/arousal disorder while a male's **premature ejaculation** is an orgasm disorder. Another significant sexual dysfunction problem for women is **genito-pelvic pain/penetration disorder**; this diagnosis brings together disorders formerly labeled as **dyspareunia,** which is recurrent genital pain during sexual intercourse, and **vaginismus,** which is a recurrent involuntary spasm of the outer muscle area of the vagina that interferes with sexual intercourse. Approximately 15% of women in the United States report experiencing recurrent pain during intercourse.

Other DSM-5 diagnoses include delayed ejaculation, female orgasmic disorder, female sexual interest/arousal disorder, male hypoactive sexual desire disorder, and substance/medication-induced sexual dysfunction. Sexual dysfunctions can be lifelong, acquired, generalized or situational; these subtypes have important clinical implications and are indicated by a specifier included with the diagnosis.

There is a vivid portrayal of **premature ejaculation** in *The Squid and the Whale* (2005). Erectile dysfunction followed by premature ejaculation is depicted in *Boy A* (2007). *Y Tu Mamá También* (2001, Mexico) includes a memorable scene depicting premature ejaculation when a Mexican teenager has sex with an older traveling companion.

Erectile disorder is diagnosed when at least one of three symptoms are present on almost all occasions of sexual activity: Marked difficulty in **obtaining** an erection, marked difficulty **maintaining** an erection, and marked **decrease** in erectile rigidity during the sex act. These problems must have existed for at least 6 months and result in clinically significant distress, for an individual to be diagnosed using DSM-5 criteria.

Erectile disorder is much more common in older males: According to the DSM-5, only about 2% of men younger than 40–50 years have frequent problems with erections, but about half of all men 60 or older experience problems achieving or maintaining an erection.

The treatment of erectile dysfunction took a quantum leap forward in 1996 when Pfizer patented **sildenafil citrate** (Viagra) in the United States. Since that time, the US Food and Drug Administration (FDA) has approved four additional oral drugs to treat erectile dysfunction: Cialis, Levitra, Staxyn, and Stendra.

The films *Sex, Lies and Videotape* (1989), *Boxing Helena* (1993), *Noise* (2007), *The Hospital* (1971), *Italian for Beginners* (2001), and *Monster's Ball* (2001) each include at least one scene in which a man becomes impotent and has to face the consequences. Warren Beatty plays an impotent Clyde Barker in *Bonnie and Clyde* (1967), assuring Bonnie: "Ain't nothing wrong with me. ... I don't like boys." Peter O'Toole is impotent because of age and prostate cancer in *Venus* (2006). *Intimacy* (2000) depicts the frustration associated with premature ejaculation. John Voight plays Joe Buck in *Midnight Cowboy* (1969), a would be stud who is impotent the first time he is paid to perform, and William Hurt plays an impotent drug dealer in *The Big Chill* (1983). The sexually addicted protagonist in *Shame* (2011) also experiences erectile dysfunction when attempting to make love to anyone who is not a prostitute.

"Impotence is beautiful. Power to the impotent!"

Part of a soliloquy by a distraught physician played by George C. Scott in *The Hospital* (1971)

Antiwar films often portray characters that are impotent because of war. These include Ron Kovic (Tom Cruise) in Oliver Stone's *Born on the Fourth of July* (1989), and an earlier film, *Coming Home* (1978), in which John Voight plays a paraplegic Vietnam veteran who is impotent but still able to satisfy his partner (Jane Fonda) with cunnilingus in ways her Marine husband never could.

In Billy Wilder's *Some Like It Hot* (1959), Tony Curtis, playing Joe, pretends to be impotent to seduce Marilyn Monroe, playing the role of Sugar. Richard Burton plays an impotent college professor, George, in Mike Nichols' adaptation of Edward Albee's play *Who's Afraid of Virginia Woolf?* (1966).

Sugar: "Have you ever tried American girls?"
Joe: "Why?" (She takes a drumstick from him – and kisses him.)
Sugar: "Was it anything?"
Joe: "Thanks just the same." (He retrieves the drumstick and chews on it.)
Sugar: "You should see a doctor – a good doctor."
Joe: "I have. I spent six months in Vienna with Professor Freud, flat on my back." (He lies on the sofa.) "Then, there were the Mayo Brothers, injections, hypnosis, mineral baths. If I wasn't such a coward, I'll kill myself."
Sugar: "Don't say that!" (She rushes over to him.) "There must be some girl some place that could ..."
Joe: "If I ever found the girl that could, I'd marry her just like that."
Sugar: "Would you do me a favor?"
Joe: "Certainly, what is it?"
Sugar: "I may not be Dr. Freud or a Mayo brother, or one of those French upstairs girls, but could I take another crack at it?"
Joe: "All right, if you insist." (They kiss deeply, and the kiss is accompanied by a phallic image – his foot rises at the end of the sofa behind her.)
Sugar: "Anything this time?"
Joe: "I'm afraid not. Terribly sorry."
Sugar: "Would you like some more champagne? Maybe if we had some music? How do you dim these lights?"

Tony Curtis feigning impotence to seduce Marilyn Monroe in *Some Like it Hot* (1959)

The Oh in Ohio (2006) depicts a high school teacher who is frustrated by his wife's inability to achieve an orgasm and sexual satisfaction during their 10 years of marriage. He eventually has an affair with one of his students. His wife feels abandoned and becomes open to sexual exploration for the first time in her life, eventually having a satisfying sexual experience (an affair) with a character played by Danny DeVito, a swimming pool salesman. During a workshop on orgasm, one woman describes her vagina as a "velvet volcano." *Amy's Orgasm* (2001) is a film in which a confident, self-assured woman who writes self-help books about how women can manage fine without men falls in love with a "shock jock" radio announcer and finds sexual fulfillment.

Kinsey (2004) is an important film about a college professor, Alfred Kinsey (Liam Neeson), who helped reshape the way people viewed sexuality in the middle of the last century. Kinsey and colleagues published two landmark books based on interviews with tens of thousands of people across the country: *Sexual Behavior in the Human Male* (1948) and *Sexual Behavior in the Human Female* (1953). Many people criticized Kinsey's methodology and research, but his impact on society is undeniable. Kinsey contributed to normalizing homosexuality, premarital sex, and the use of multiple sexual positions; he also debunked numerous misconceptions (e.g., the belief that masturbation is harmful). The film portrays Kinsey training his team in conducting interviews that are objective and unbiased, reminding them that "maintaining a nonjudgmental attitude is harder than you think." A particularly striking scene occurs during Kinsey's straightforward teaching approach in his course on human sexuality where he displays slides of human genitalia. The film also depicts many of the shortcomings of this famous researcher, including his ritualistic compulsiveness (suggesting an obsessive-compulsive personality), barbiturate abuse, lack of personal sexual boundaries, and his superficiality in his interpersonal relations.

Good Luck to You, Leo Grande (2020) stars the ever-rewarding Emma Thompson and newcomer Daryl McCormack (see Figure 32). This is a charming film about Susan Robinson (aka "Nancy"), an aging religious studies schoolteacher who has never experience the joy of good sex. She was married for 31 years to an insipid and boring man who had died two years earlier. She has never had an orgasm. Hoping for some degree of sexual awakening before she is too old to enjoy it, she hires a male sex worker, Leo Grande, and they proceed to have hotel room sex several times before Susan's eventual orgasm. Embracing her sexuality isn't easy for Susan, who remarks "I'm just a seedy old pervert." She had experienced brief sexual pleasure with a restaurant worker in Greece who fumbled "under my knickers" before being frightened away by her parents. Susan makes a list of all the sexual experiences she wants to share with Leo, including "I perform oral sex on you, and then you perform oral sex on me, and then 69 – if that is still what it is called." It is likely that Emma Thompson's film name (Mrs. Robinson) pays homage to Mike Nichols's *The Graduate* (1967).

"There are nuns out there more sexually experienced than me."

Emma Thompson (Susan Robinson) apologizes for her lack of sexual expertise, in *Good Luck to You, Leo Grande* (2022)

The Sessions (2012) stars John Hawkes as Mark, a man in an iron lung who has never experienced a mature sexual relationship. He discusses the situation with his priest, Father Brendan, played by William H. Macy, and decides to seek out the services of a sexual surrogate (played by Helen Hunt). The film, based on a true story involving a University of California student in Berkeley, delightfully explores nascent sexuality and makes the point that genuine and enduring love relationships can exist between people who are quite different.

"I have a feeling that God is going to give you a free pass on this one. Go for it."

Father Brendan encourages Mark to explore his sexuality, in *The Sessions* (2012)

(A)sexual (2011) is a documentary depicting people who do not experience sexual feelings (e.g., people who are not attracted to either men or women). **Asexuality** is not a disorder or diagnosis, because if you ask many of these

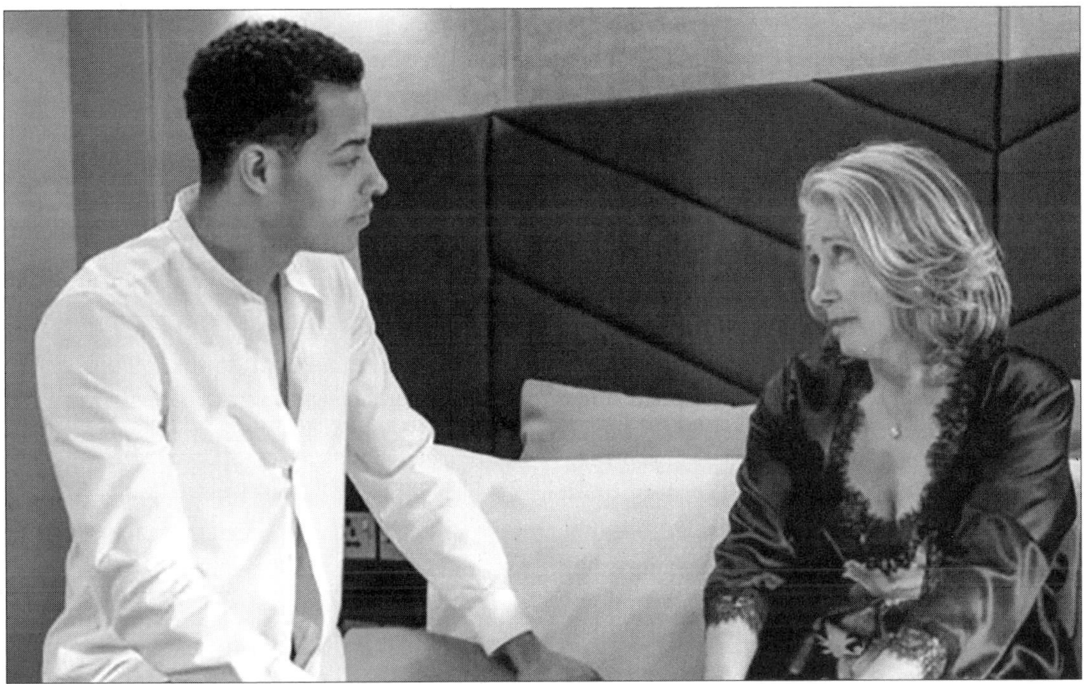

Figure 32. *Good Luck to You, Leo Grande* (2022, Genesius Pictures, Align, Cornerstone Films, Searchlight Pictures). Produced by Katy Brand, Sam Cornish, Kelly Duffell, Julian Gleek, et al. Directed by Sophie Hyde.

individuals, they will report that their lack of sexual desire is simply not a problem. Many of the female characters in *(A)sexual* would meet the main criteria for the DSM-5 condition, **female sexual interest/arousal disorder**: absent or minimal interest in sex, absent/minimal erotic thoughts/fantasies, reduced or no sexual initiation, etc. However, most of these females in the film are entirely comfortable with their asexuality and thus would not meet the key requirement that the symptoms causing significant distress. As a result, no diagnosis would be given. Asexual individuals do not seem to have a problem with sexual arousal. Some scientists have begun to study asexuality, a topic mostly neglected over the decades. One survey of the general population found that 1% of people report they are not attracted to men *or* women; this number suggests there are 3 million asexual people in the United States. Research reported in the film notes that these individuals do not have any higher rates of depression, anger, trauma, or any mental illness than the normal population.

International Films: Sexual Dysfunctions and Gender Dysphoria

Breakfast on Pluto (2005, Ireland/UK), Neal Jordan's adaptation of a novel by Patrick McCabe (1992), is an Irish film that presents the life of "Kitten," an orphan and a transvestite who enjoyed dressing up in women's clothes from an early age. This film is less a gender identity study than the story of societal abuse, ostracism, tragedy, and diagnostic misadventure. It is about an individual who cross-dresses and has gender issues and overcomes enormous stressful and tragic experiences, including serious life threats, prostitution, homelessness, job loss, and a fire that destroys his home. Kitten perseveres through all of this.

She Male Snails, originally released with its Swedish title *Pojktanten* (2011, Swedish), is a documentary about the life of a transgender artist named Eli Leven. The film's director, Ester

Martin Bergsmark, also identifies as transgender. *Tomboy* (2011, France) is a touching French film about a 10-year-old girl, Laure, who moves to a new neighborhood with her sister and mother. When Laure sets out to meet the other kids in her neighborhood, she meets Lisa who assumes Laure is a boy because of her pageboy haircut. Laure effortlessly slides into her new, masculine identity, and she introduces herself to Lisa as "Mikael."

Wild Tigers I Have Known (2006, UK), directed by Cam Archer, is a sensitive film that tells the story of Logan, a 13-year-old boy coming to terms with his sexuality. Logan keeps a wig and a tube of lipstick hidden in his dresser drawer, and it is never clear if he is gay or transsexual. He becomes romantically involved with another boy, Rodeo, because of a series of late-night phone calls in which Logan pretends to be a girl. Although this is a film worth seeing, we recommend you watch *Tomboy* first.

Rayan: "We hear you're a girl. We're gonna check that."
Lisa: "Stop it! What do you think you're doing?"
Rayan: "We're gonna check if she's really a girl."
Lisa: "Leave him alone."
Rayan: "You're right. It's YOU who'll check."
Lisa: "No, I won't."
Rayan: "If she's a girl, then you kissed her. It's disgusting. Right?"
Lisa: "Yes, it's disgusting."
Rayan: "Then, you're gonna do it."
[Lisa pulls down Laure's pants]

Children trying to make sense of the mystery of gender, in *Tomboy* (2011, France)

One of the boys in the film *That's the Way I Like It* (1998, Singapore) has gone through his life trying to please his parents. For example, he goes to medical school and works hard in school to get stellar grades. One day he announces that he has been hiding the fact that he is a woman. He then shares that he will be undergoing sex reassignment surgery involving genital surgery and hormone treatment. His father becomes quite angry in response to his son's disclosure. Later in the film, despite being disowned by his father, he shows up dressed fully as a woman. His father remains rigid in his disgust and exclaims that he will kill his son if he sees him again. Although this film is a comedy-musical, it depicts the significant impact of such interactions and decisions on the family. The young man then, distraught by the shame he believes he has brought upon his family, attempts suicide. However, he lives, and his brother provides the financial support he needs for the operation.

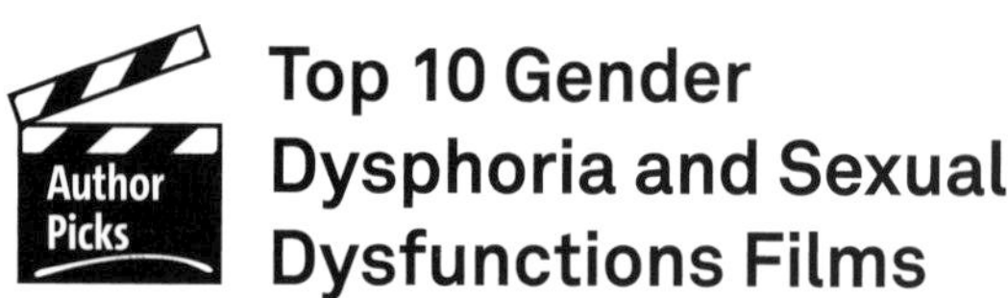

Top 10 Gender Dysphoria and Sexual Dysfunctions Films

Gender Dysphoria

The Crying Game (1992)
Boys Don't Cry (1999)
Normal (2003)
Soldier's Girl (2003)
Transamerica (2005)
Tomboy (2011)
Cowboys (2020)

Sexual Dysfunction

The Oh in Ohio (2006)
Love and Other Drugs (2010)
Good Luck to You, Leo Grande (2022)

Chapter 10

Disruptive, Impulse-Control, and Conduct Disorders

Eva: Why would you have something like that?
Kevin: I collect them.
Eva: Isn't that a weird thing to collect?
Kevin: I don't like stamps.
Eva: Well, what's the point?
Kevin: There is no point. That's the point.

Kevin tries to explain to his mother
why he collects computer viruses,
in *We Need to Talk About Kevin* (2012)

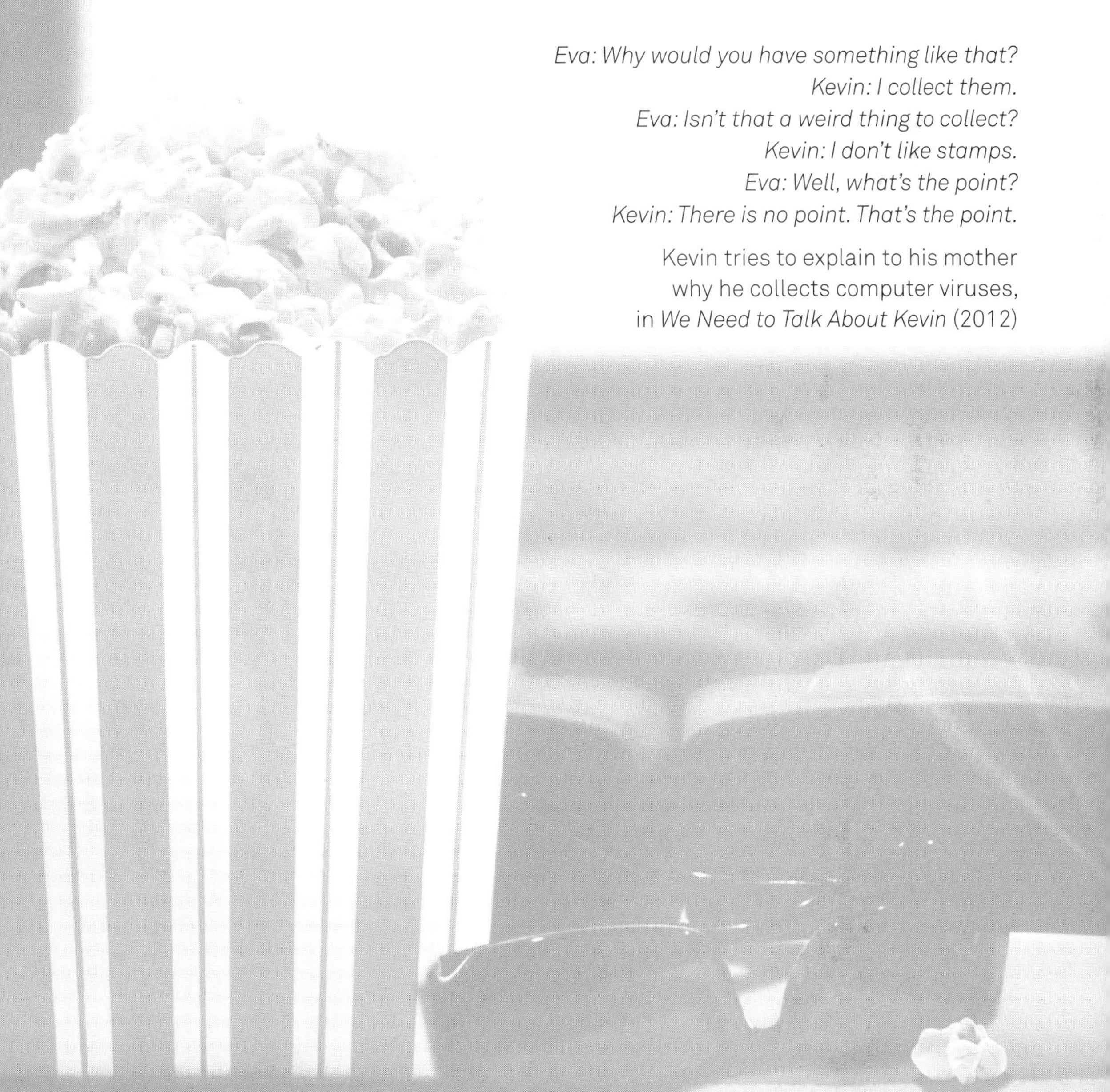

Child Mental Health

In most cases, the diagnoses discussed in this chapter originate in childhood. Psychiatric problems of children are not as easily diagnosed as those of adults, and the symptoms of mental illness in children are sometimes difficult to distinguish from those changes associated with normal growth and development. For example, it is normal for a 4-year-old to have an imaginary friend, but for an adolescent, an invisible friend that only he sees would be considered a psychotic hallucination.

Children who receive mental health treatment usually fall into one of the following categories:

- children whose behavior is a response to family disruptions, crisis, or dysfunction;
- children whose behavior does not conform to social norms and is troublesome to others (e.g., disruptive behaviors and conduct disorders);
- children who experience repeated and excessive depression, anxiety, or states of personal distress;
- children whose cognitive or neuromotor development is not proceeding normally (e.g., developmental disabilities).

Oppositional Defiant Disorder and Conduct Disorder

The diagnosis of **oppositional defiant disorder** (ODD) is typically given to children and adolescents who have a pattern of negativistic, hostile, and defiant behavior, such as losing their temper, being argumentative, and being easily annoyed and resentful. The DSM-5 requires the presence of four out of eight symptoms, and the aberrant behavior pattern must have existed for at least 6 months. People, most often children, who receive an ODD diagnosis lose their temper easily and often. They are quickly annoyed and are often angry and resentful. They refuse to comply with instructions or demands from authority figures. They annoy other people, and their peers typically dislike them. They blame other people for their mistakes and have a history of spiteful or vindictive behavior. These individuals have little insight into their own behavior and the reactions of other people. The DSM-5 suggests the prevalence of the disorder varies across studies, ranging from 1–11%; however, the average prevalence estimate is around 3.3% with males outnumbering females by about 40% until adolescence, when the number of males and females with the disorder becomes approximately equal.

A diagnosis of **conduct disorder** is given to children and adolescents who violate the basic rights of others or societal norms by engaging in aggression toward people or animals, destruction of property, theft, deceit, and/or truancy. The DSM-5 diagnosis requires the presence of three out of 15 criteria occurring in the past 12 months, with at least one criterion present in the past 6 months. (Note that five children could each receive this diagnosis without a single overlapping symptom among the five.) The criteria used in making this diagnosis include bullying, frequent fighting, use of a weapon, cruelty to people or animals, stealing, rape, fire setting, destruction of others' property, lying, stealing, truancy, and running away.

It should be clear that there is an overlap in these diagnoses (and with intermittent explosive disorder, discussed in the section Intermittent Explosive Disorder), and differential diagnosis is often challenging. In many countries, these diagnostic labels are not used. However, these behavioral problems are universal, as are the movies that depict them.

ODD in late teens is beautifully illustrated in the film *Don't Come Knocking* (2005), in which a young man displays outrage and defiance after his biological father, a washed-up actor, returns to town wanting to see him. In *Manic* (2003), the viewer gets an inside look at the adolescent unit of a psychiatric hospital. This well-acted independent film presents interesting questions about differential diagnosis, demonstrates friction between various adolescents with clashing behavioral problems (e.g., bipolar disorder, impulse-control disorder, conduct disorder, and depression), and offers a good portrayal of group psychotherapy.

My Flesh and Blood (2004) is a documentary about a woman who takes care of special needs children; one child, whose life is explored in detail, has a severe conduct disorder in addition to cystic fibrosis. His anger outbursts and sexual acting out are at times tempered by a needy softness and emotional vulnerability. His behavioral problems are related to the loss of his mother as a caretaker (she continues to visit him), the stress of his environment (one caretaker serves 11 special needs children), and the stress of his illness.

Holes (2002), an excellent Disney feature film, depicts various oppositional and rule-breaking youth who are sent to a working camp because of their disruptive and behavioral problems. One adolescent steals cars and has a tic disorder. *Beautiful Boy* (2012) is a film in many ways like *We Need to Talk About Kevin*; it deals with the way a couple is affected after learning that their son, who was away at college, has shot and killed 17 people and then killed himself.

We Need to Talk About Kevin

We Need to Talk About Kevin (2012) is a powerful and compelling drama directed by Lynne Ramsey that stars Tilda Swinton and John C. Reilly as Kevin's parents. The film is a horror story for any parent who sees the film, and every parent watching finds themselves wondering how they would have responded to the challenges presented by a child like Kevin. The film has frequent flashbacks that depict Kevin at various developmental stages, all of them difficult for his parents but especially for Eve, Kevin's mother. Kevin does not bond with his mother (or she with him); in contrast, he appears friendly and loving around his sister and father, presumably to underscore how very alienated he is from his mother.

Kevin is a skilled archer, and he eventually sets up a premeditated mass murder at his school, where he locks the gym doors and kills dozens of children before the police take him into custody. When his mother returns to the

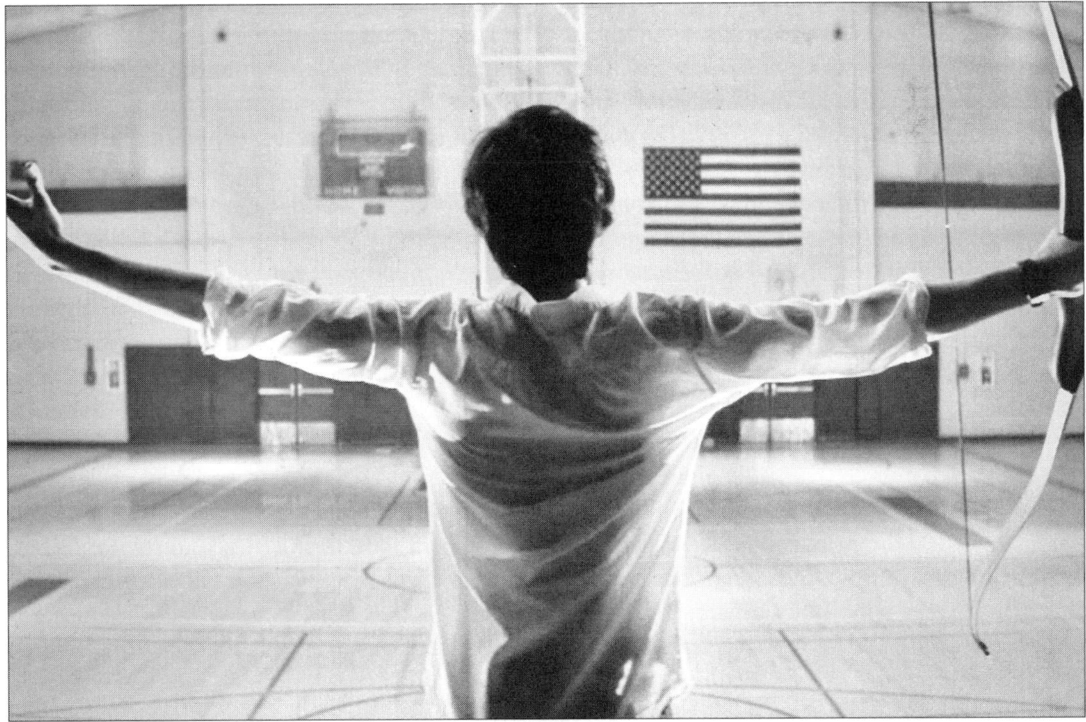

Figure 33. *We Need to Talk About Kevin* (2011, BBC Films, UK Film Council, Independent Entertainment). Produced by Suzanne Baron, Michael Corso, Molly Egan, Christopher Figg, et al. Directed by Lynne Ramsay.

family home, she discovers that her husband and daughter have also been killed. Kevin spared his mother's life because having her witness the full horror of the atrocity he committed was more hateful than anything he could have done, including murdering her. Figure 33 shows Kevin using his bow and arrow. The film's theme that some children are just "born bad" evokes memories of a 1956 film, *The Bad Seed*, in which an evil child turns out to be adopted and the daughter of a man who was a serial killer.

Life as a House and *My First Mister*

Two important films portray highly troubled, isolated, suicidal, and oppositional adolescents – *Life as a House* (2001) with the character of Sam (Hayden Christensen), and *My First Mister* (2001) with Jennifer (Leelee Sobieski) as the protagonist. Each film presents a highly troubled and alienated young person who is transformed through meaningful relationships. The major difference between the lead characters is their gender, and watching both films will help you appreciate the differences in psychosexual development between boys and girls.

In *Life as a House*, we are introduced to Sam, a character with a rebellious, gothic appearance as evidenced by his colored hair, lip ring, eye makeup, and tough exterior. In an early scene, he huffs paint while choking himself (**autoerotic asphyxiation**) in his closet. He resorts to this practice whenever he needs to escape from people and reality: He locks his door, plays loud music (e.g., Marilyn Manson), uses drugs (pills, pot, and huffing), and masturbates. With his extreme negativism and oppositional personality, it is easy to see how he believes that no one understands him and why he must come up with complicated ways to isolate himself. At one point in the film, he reveals he has been using drugs since the age of 12. He earns money to buy drugs through prostitution, finding this preferable to working hard to earn less money. Sam can articulate that he wants to become something he is not and does not know how; this leaves him to feel like "nothing." Beneath his rough exterior is a wounded and isolated adolescent longing for a meaningful connection. He finds the needed friendship and love when he establishes a relationship with his dying father; at that point, Sam's behaviors, attitude, and appearance are transformed.

My First Mister portrays a similarly troubled youth, 17-year-old Jennifer, who is also gothic in appearance. She wears mostly black and has multiple facial piercings. She is very isolated, with no real friends and no genuine interest in her needy mother or distant stepfather. She comments that she has never had a boyfriend or, for that matter, any friends. The closest Jennifer can get to people is when she views them through her binoculars. She fantasizes about living with the Partridge family. She has a blunted, sad affect and is highly negativistic and critical about life. She is preoccupied with death, and she writes melancholy poetry about dying, hopelessness, and "not existing." She likes to lie on gravesites, and exclaims, "I'm gonna go to hell anyway." More serious problems include self-injurious behaviors (cutting her arm) and visual hallucinations of her deceased grandmother. She finds meaning and purpose in a random, healthy relationship that blossoms with a man who she works with in a men's clothing store.

Both films include characters in search of their identity. These two teens work through oppositional and conduct problems to find themselves.

Thirteen

This film depicts a nightmarish reality for some parents; for others, it may serve as a wake-up call. *Thirteen* (2003), directed by Catherine Hardwicke, depicts a rapid transformation from childhood to adolescence and the pervasive influence of peer pressure during the teen years.

Tracy Freeland (Evan Rachel Wood), a 13-year-old seventh grader, is eager to be accepted by the "in group" in her school. She earns acceptance from this group when she rejects her current, less popular friends, and spontaneously steals money from a woman on the street. She takes her soon-to-be best friend Evie Zamora (Nikki Reed) on a shopping spree, buying clothing and shoes. A friendship soon develops, and an emotional roller coaster ride begins, characterized by rebellion, acting out, parental opposition, and misconduct. Tracy gets her tongue and belly button pierced, exhibits self-injurious behavior, abuses substances, tells numerous lies, and lets her grades plummet. She also becomes sexually promiscuous. An opening scene (a flash-forward) depicts Tracy and Evie getting high and amusing themselves by punching one another in the face.

> **"I'll die for you, but I won't leave you alone right now."**
>
> **Melanie Freeland (Holly Hunter) to her daughter, who has been used and betrayed, in *Thirteen* (2003)**

As these oppositional behaviors escalate, Tracy becomes more isolated from her mother (Holly Hunter). She becomes angry with her mother and resists any attempts to set parental limits on her behavior. The mother works hard to establish appropriate boundaries, yet frequently falls short because of her own struggles and limitations as a recovering drug addict. The mother and daughter eventually come to know each other better because of their frequent fights. Evie's mother, on the other hand, is a self-absorbed abuse victim who allows and even encourages the girls to drink and smoke. The plot culminates in a bitter betrayal by Evie, demonstrating that peer relationships can end as abruptly as they begin.

Elephant

The award-winning (Cannes Film Festival) 2003 independent film *Elephant,* directed by Gus Van Sant, is a realistic and artful portrayal of an American high school and the routine life of students just prior to a massive school shooting, reminding the viewer of Columbine, Sandy Hook, and subsequent tragedies. The film is eerie and foreboding in that it is much more about nonverbal behavior than about dialogue; this heightens the importance of the cinematic craft, a craft Van Sant has mastered, particularly in his unique camera work and use of **nondiegetic sound** (i.e., sounds whose source cannot be seen in the film). The viewer is taken along as the camera slowly follows several major characters going through their daily routines (e.g., walking down long hallways, greeting fellow students), and going in and out of buildings (into danger or safety zones, unbeknownst to them), often with nondiegetic music in the background. It is interesting to note the title outside the building reads simply "high school," letting this school represent every high school.

Two characters, Eric (Eric Deulen) and Alex (Alex Frost), are depicted playing a video shooting game and looking up information about guns on the Internet. They order guns without difficulty and receive them in the mail in a large package. Later, these two teens plot their shooting spree with a map of the school, planning to "pick off" as many classmates as possible in the school's high-traffic areas.

Although the film is realistic, the viewer is left with more questions than answers about causes, prevention, psychopathology, and etiology. At the same time, this is part of the director's craft, and he deliberately lets each member of the audience draw their own conclusions.

Kids and *Gummo*

These two movies are discussed together because both are extraordinarily disturbing films. Harmony Korine, who wrote the script for *Kids* (1995), was both writer and director for *Gummo* (1997). Both films provide a frightening perspective on the lives of adolescents, the former in an urban setting and the latter in a small town/rural setting.

Kids, directed by Larry Clark, is a fast-paced film that allows the viewer to experience the thoughts, words, and behaviors of young adolescents as they interact with each other. One unforgettable scene depicts 15 or so skateboarding teens who brutalize a man who made the mistake of criticizing one of the skateboarders. The plot revolves around the character of Telly (Leo

Fitzpatrick), a scrawny but confident adolescent who takes tremendous pride in his ability to seduce virgins. Unbeknownst to him, Telly is HIV positive, and he is rapidly spreading the virus to his vulnerable partners, most of whom have never had sex before. Telly is extremely narcissistic, and the viewer assumes he would not change his behavior even if he knew of his diagnosis. One of Telly's victims, a teenage girl, finds out she has been infected by Telly, and much of the film involves her frantic attempts to get him to stop spreading the disease. In this film, HIV is a metaphor for the spread of violence among inner-city youth.

Gummo is a realistic but disturbing film that portrays lower-class, antisocial children and adolescents. The film includes numerous disturbing scenes of animal torture, drug abuse, and bizarre behavior such as that exhibited by one man who has a fight with an inanimate object. The film's two main characters, Solomon (Jacob Reynolds) and Tummler (Nick Sutton), bicycle around shooting stray cats and collecting them in garbage bags to sell them to a storeowner so they can get high on glue or have sex with a girl with an intellectual disability. At times, these two characters are violent just for the sake of violence; they repeatedly whip a hanging dead cat and later take turns shooting a dead cat in the pouring rain. They break into the home of their competitor (another cat killer), masked with guns and a golf club, and unhook the life support of an infirm elderly woman. Each adolescent is reared by a single parent with limited parenting skills; Solomon's mother threatens to kill him with a toy gun for not smiling, and later washes him in filthy bathwater while serving him spaghetti and milk.

There are many other quirky and disturbed characters in the film, including a boy who dresses like a bunny, urinates on traffic from overpasses, drowns a cat, and fakes his own death, and a developmentally disabled girl who laughs while she shaves her eyebrows and compulsively treats her doll as if it were a real infant. The director, Harmony Korine, has a cameo appearance in the film as a drunken adolescent who randomly pours beer on his head while describing his history of sexual abuse and trying to seduce a gay, African American midget. Korine's character recollects throwing marbles on his mother's belly when he was a young child – if he hit her navel, he would get 5 dollars but whenever he missed, he was hit with a rolling pin.

These characters lack insight into their behavior, and they are not able to appreciate the consequences of their acts. Most lack empathy and have little regard for ethical or moral standards; it is reasonable to assume that many will become adults who qualify for a diagnosis of antisocial personality disorder.

Many viewers stay to the end of the credits of *Gummo* to confirm that the animal abuse scenes are simulated, that prosthetic animals are used, and that the characters and situations are fictitious; despite the assurance of the credits, viewers know that for some children, the scenes portrayed are all too real.

Dysfunctional Families in Contemporary Films

There are a myriad of dysfunctional families captured in films. We have included a handful of examples here. These films show the impact of familial problems on the children and provide a view of children with both healthy and unhealthy coping.

A child's behavior may appear to be symptomatic of a psychiatric disorder, but in fact be a response to parental marital discord or family dysfunction. Complex family relationships provide filmmakers opportunities to dramatically portray multiple plots and subplots with few characters. In Noah Baumbach's highly acclaimed film *The Squid and the Whale* (2005), two brothers, 16-year-old Walt (Jesse Eisenberg) and 10-year-old Frank (Owen Kline), are the center of their divorcing parents' feuds. The father, Bernard (Jeff Daniels), is an impossible character – jealous, self-absorbed, condescending, and narcissistic. He is a self-proclaimed novelist who feels victimized by being relegated to a college teaching position. The mother, Joan (Laura Linney), is emerging as a legitimate writer whose success only fuels her husband's animosity toward her. When the parents separate, Walt, who idolizes and imitates his father, chooses to live with Bernard. Frank, the more emotional of the two brothers, stays with his mother, Joan. Both boys develop abnormal behaviors. Frank drinks alcohol, masturbates, and smears his ejaculate on books and a locker at school. Walt plagiarizes a Pink Floyd song as his own, breaks up with his girlfriend, and refuses to see his mother because she had an affair while still married. Walt is referred to a therapist who helps him increase his self-awareness. In isolation, any of these abnormal behaviors could have been evaluated as symptoms of a mental disorder. Instead, these behaviors are all reactions to the chaotic family crisis.

Another interesting but disturbing film, one that explores a child's attempt to make sense out of chaotic and dysfunctional family interactions, is *Running With Scissors* (2006). This award-winning film is based on the real-life memoirs of Augusten Burroughs who was handed off to his mother's psychiatrist after his parents' divorce. Burroughs is the son of poet and writer Margaret Robison and the late John G. Robison, head of the philosophy department at the University of Massachusetts at Amherst. The Augusten Burroughs character, played by Joseph Cross, is a young gay child who is consumed with adoration for his mother Deirdre (Annette Bening), who is attempting to launch her career as a poet. Augusten spends his childhood skipping school and practicing becoming a performer. Augusten's father Norman (played by Alec Baldwin) teaches philosophy and abuses alcohol. The mother and father spend most of their time arguing. When the parents separate, Augusten, aged 12, is given to Deirdre's psychiatrist, Dr. Finch (Brian Cox), an eccentric physician. As Deirdre sinks into her mental illness, Augusten avoids school, keeps a diary, becomes sexually involved with one of Finch's patients, and develops a friendship with Finch's younger daughter. During this time, he has perfected his cosmetology skills. In real life, Burroughs dropped out of school after the sixth grade and obtained his high school diploma (GED) at age 17. He became a successful advertising executive, then left the field and became a successful writer.

> **"I want rules ... and boundaries ... because ... what I've learned is that ... without them ... all life is ... is a series of surprises ..."**
>
> **Augusten Burroughs**
> **in *Running With Scissors* (2006)**

The Academy Award–winning satiric comedy *Little Miss Sunshine* (2006) portrays a family in crisis. Olive Hoover (Abigail Breslin) has fantasized about winning a beauty pageant for her entire young life. Although she does not fit the stereotypic contestant profile, Olive does manage to become a finalist in the Little Miss Sunshine pageant. Her family takes off in an old Volkswagen bus to attend the pageant. The family characters are unforgettable – her father (Greg Kinnear) is an unsuccessful motivational speaker–author, her brother Dwayne (Paul Dana) is a lost soul who has not spoken for months but has dreams of being an air force pilot, and her uncle Steve (Frank Ginsberg), who has just been released from a psychiatric facility after a suicide attempt, requires close observation. One of the best performances is that of Olive's grandfather (Alan Arkin), who supports Olive's confidence and sense of self-worth. Olive, the healthiest member of the family, does not have a mental illness or emotional problem, but she is an example of a child much wiser than her years who helps an unhealthy family grow psychologically.

Intermittent Explosive Disorder

Intermittent explosive disorder is a diagnosis that requires recurrent behavioral outbursts characterized by verbal aggression or misbehavior such as destroying property or harming animals or other people. This behavior is grossly out of proportion to the provocation, and the outbursts are not premeditated and appear to be out of the individual's control. These outbursts are typically relatively short, but highly disruptive in family interactions or in the classroom. The diagnosis is more prevalent among young individuals (under age 35) than those older than 50 but can be applied to anyone with anger management problems over the age of 6. The DSM-5 estimated prevalence is 2.7%.

Anger is a normal emotion all humans experience. It can be a healthy indicator of internal stress, a sign that deep emotions are being tapped, or a cue that someone has offended us. In many instances, anger turns from thoughts and feelings into behaviors and is acted out in some form. Anger can be extraordinarily destructive, and this destructiveness comes across verbally or physically. Intermittent explosive disorder is diagnosed when there are several discrete episodes of aggressive impulses that result in serious assaults or property destruction. Several good films depict intermittent explosive disorder.

In *Boy A* (2007, Britain), a young boy, Eric, is frequently beaten up at school and becomes isolated. Desperate for social contact, Eric connects with another young boy who has a conduct disorder. The boys' behavior turns from "bad" (e.g., shoplifting, beating up kids) to despicable (e.g., killing a young girl). They are prosecuted and sent away, not as punishment but to protect others (and themselves). The prosecutor emphasizes that the two boys are evil and dangerous. Upon release, the newspaper announces that "evil comes of age" and shows a photo of Eric on the release day. Eric decides to change his name to Jack and create a new persona. He is shy, awkward, nice, and desperate to connect with others. He tries but struggles to overcome his past demons and previous instincts; in one instance he impulsively explodes and attacks a bully who is mistreating someone. He is supported by a social worker portrayed as caring, resourceful, and insightful.

Acclaimed director Ang Lee's *Hulk* (2003) is a commentary on anger and, more specifically, intermittent explosive disorder. The whole film is about raw anger: anger being unleashed, the dangers and detrimental effects of anger, the build-up and development of anger, and family of origin issues regarding anger. When Bruce Banner (Eric Bana) transforms into the Hulk, there is enormous destruction of property, and this occurs in intermittent episodes of rage as he shifts into the role of Hulk and then back to the scientist role after his anger subsides. If this film is viewed by someone eager to understand the psychological phenomenon of anger, the movie is educational as well as entertaining. A recent remake, *The Incredible Hulk* (2008), starring Edward Norton as Bruce Banner, also provides a useful perspective on this impulse control disorder.

"But you know what scares me the most? When I can't fight it anymore, when it takes over, when I totally lose control ... I like it."

Bruce Banner in *Hulk* (2003)

Two quintessential films about men who are angry with society (and people in general) and who impulsively decide to take matters into their own hands are *Falling Down* (1993) and *Noise* (2007). In the former film, Michael Douglas's character explosively attacks (sometimes with weapons) anyone who confronts or challenges him, as he can no longer tolerate anything or anyone that brings forth any degree of disagreement, tension, or offense. In *Noise*, the protagonist is portrayed by Tim Robbins who becomes fed up with the sounds and noises of New York City. He decides to act as "the rectifier," becomes a vigilante, and proceeds to smash in the windows of cars that have alarms going off. We highly recommend both films.

In *Punch Drunk Love* (2002), Barry Egan (Adam Sandler) is a quirky, serious character who alternates between extreme passiveness (often to his sisters' requests) and brief explosions of anger. Interestingly, when he is confronted with danger, he either runs away or explodes with rage (illustrating the fight-or-flight response).

In *Manic* (2001), an adolescent Lyle (Joseph Gordon-Levitt) is sent to an inpatient unit for intermittent explosive disorder: While angry, he smashed a peer's head with a baseball bat. Though Lyle does begin to relate and connect with others as well as understand himself in a deeper way, he continues to explode periodically with his rage directed toward others. Lyle is sporadic in his anger management attempts – sometimes he stops his anger, choosing not to fight, and at other times he provokes fights. Lyle reflects that the cause of his anger is that his father was physically abusive and his peers made fun of him. An authoritative psychologist (Don Cheadle) utilizes an intervention that involves telling Lyle he is "just like dad" regarding his anger outbursts.

Mateo (Djimon Hounsou), a man dying of AIDS, frequently screams, and destroys property in his apartment in the film *In America* (2003). Another man dying of AIDS, Roy (Keifer Sutherland) in *Behind the Red Door* (2001), has repressed rage resulting from his diagnosis and a family history of neglect and abuse. His outbursts emerge verbally and at random times (e.g., when his rice is not fully cooked).

The title character in *Antwone Fisher* (2002) exhibits explosive anger, attacking his fellow sailors in response to minor provocations. The viewer later learns that beneath the anger lies intense internal pain and unresolved abuse issues. The classic character of Bluto in *Popeye* (1980) could also be diagnosed with this disorder.

The female protagonist, portrayed by Julie Delpy, in *2 Days in Paris* (2007) has an intermittent explosive disorder. She has numerous anger outbursts and explosiveness in both private and public settings. Another woman with impulsive and explosive behavior can be seen in *Stuck* (2007), starring Mena Suvari.

Kleptomania

Kleptomania is the recurrent failure to resist impulses to steal objects that are not needed for personal use or for their monetary value. Feelings of tension precede the theft act, and pleasure or relief occurs at the time of the theft.

The independent film *Klepto* (2003) uses kleptomania as a major plotline. In an opening scene, a young woman, Emily (Meredith Bishop), steals some CDs; after spotting a camera, she runs out of the store and is chased by an employee. She does not steal because she needs the items or money, but because stealing is a way to manage her stress. It quickly becomes clear that Emily loves the rush she experiences whenever she steals something. Those with kleptomania feel a sense of increasing tension prior to stealing and pleasure or relief at the time of theft or immediately thereafter. After the pleasurable rush, Emily feels worse as she realizes how out of control she is; in turn, this leads her to steal more. She stores boxes of unopened and unused stolen items in her car trunk. Emily realizes she cannot stop herself from stealing, exclaiming, "I'm a pill freak with a bad habit," referring to an enormous collection of bottles of medications. Emily is an interesting contrast with her mother who is a compulsive shopper who accumulates a $100,000 debt but is unable to stop buying things (for an example of similar psychopathology, see the section Spending/Shopping Addiction in the next chapter). Emily later finds out that her father was a thief who died in prison. Emily eventually gets treatment for her impulse-control disorder – she takes medication and sees a therapist who comes across as supportive and inquisitive.

"I have a mental condition and I have to take things. I'm addicted to getting caught."

Emily explaining her kleptomania, in *Klepto* (2003)

It is uncertain whether the characters in the following films meet the full DSM-5 criteria for kleptomania, but they are at least interesting to consider: *Niagara, Niagara* (1997); *Female Perversions* (1996); and *Mortal Transfer* (2001). In *Mortal Transfer*, one of the psychiatrist's patients is undergoing psychoanalysis and cannot resist her impulses to steal, including stealing things from her psychiatrist's desk. Kleptomania symptoms can also be seen in *Virgin* (2003), although the protagonist would undoubtedly carry multiple psychological diagnoses.

> "I steal to stop me from killing myself."
>
> Maddie Stevens
> in *Female Perversions* (1996)

Pyromania

Pyromania is deliberate and purposeful fire setting on more than one occasion, in which there is tension prior to the act, pleasure or relief after it, and a fascination and curiosity with fire itself.

In *House of Fools* (2002), one of the patients at a psychiatric hospital, Mamud, is a veteran with pyromania. After burning the curtains in the hospital, he quickly exclaims, "It wasn't me!" Mamud is restricted from having any fire-setting materials, and the other patients are instructed not to give him matches. Francie in *The Butcher Boy* (1997) sets fires, but he would not qualify for this diagnosis as far as his aberrant behavior is better explained by other diagnoses. Figure 34 depicts Francie, an adolescent with multiple diagnoses and behavior problems, reading a letter from his mother and avoiding the task at hand while all those around him are hard at work. Francie would present a diagnostic challenge for any mental health professional.

International Films: Disruptive, Impulse-Control, and Conduct Disorders

The French film *The Chorus* (2004, France) is about life at a boarding school for troubled children. The school is headed by a dictatorial principal, M. Rachin (Francois Berléand). The movie depicts defiance, conduct problems, and running away, and children who draw obscene pictures of teachers and set traps for the teaching staff. Many of these children would qualify for a diagnosis of conduct disorder or ODD. Clément Mathieu (Gérard Jugnot) is hired to teach these rowdy children. With the superintendent's approval, he turns his 4 o'clock study hall into a chorus class. Pierre Morhange (Jean-Baptiste Maunier), the most problematic student, has a beautiful voice and after initial hesitation joins the choir. The choir and Mathieu are eventually able to expose Rachin's cruelty.

The 400 Blows (1959, France) is regarded as one of the best films ever made, and it is a classic among the **French New Wave** movement. It

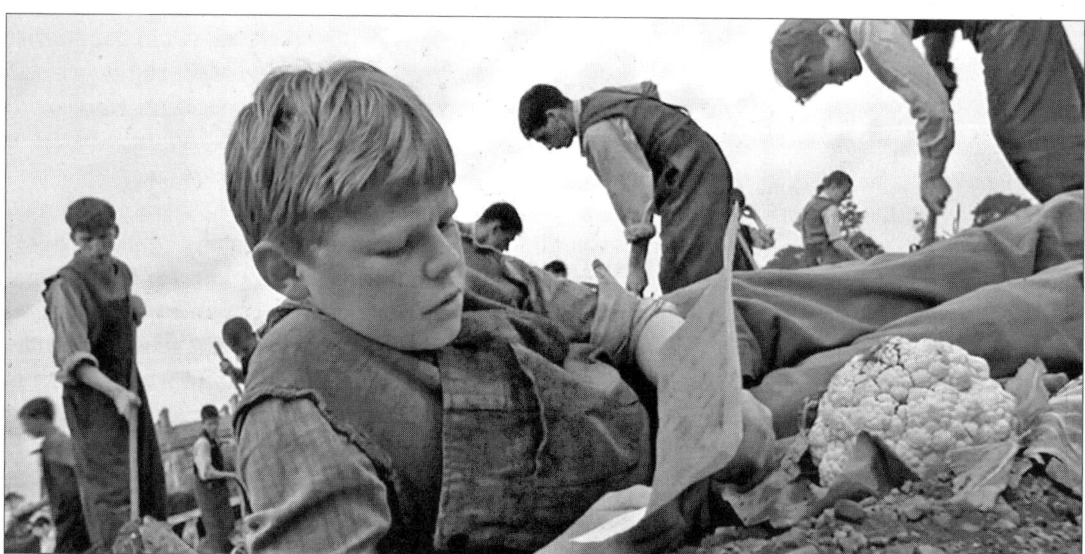

Figure 34. *The Butcher Boy* (1997, Geffen Pictures, Butcher Boy Film Productions). Produced by Neil Jordan, Redmond Morris, and Stephen Wolley. Directed by Neil Jordan.

was directed by François Truffaut. In the United States, the title is thought to reference corporal punishment; in French, it means "raising hell." The protagonist, Antoine, is a young boy with conduct disorder who is mischievous and gets into trouble frequently. His mother is harsh, unemotional, and does not appear to love her son; his father is playful and emphasizes humor in his interactions with his son. As the film progresses, Antoine's parents' behavior is inconsistent and unstable as well as immoral (e.g., he witnesses his mother's infidelity). He also receives strong negative and verbal-emotional abuse from a teacher. There are some pleasant times and positive interactions with his parents, and he makes some effort at school but is oppressed by the teacher. He runs away from home on more than one occasion, steals a typewriter, steals money from his family, frequently lies, sets fires, plagiarizes, and cheats, frequently misses school, and smokes.

Antoine is not a horrible child, and his behavior is a result of a combination of poor parenting and childhood rebellion. After running away from home, he is caught and sent away to a reform school. It is clear he has been outright rejected and abandoned by both of his parents. He then runs away from this strict facility, and the film concludes with his simply running; he is shown running through the woods, streets, and alongside the ocean. This can be viewed as a poignant symbol of autonomy and individuality, of self-reliance, and of rebellion (i.e., a refusal to be controlled, a rejection of authority). Viewers might want to compare the core themes of this film, and the boy's personality, with Paul Newman's classic depiction of rebellion in *Cool Hand Luke* (1967).

The short film *The Antichrist* (2002, Poland) depicts four boys exploring a field in which explosions are occurring because of excavations. One boy, who has a few ODD and conduct disorder symptoms, calls himself the Antichrist and challenges the other boys to engage in dangerous behavior. He catches a fish with his bare hands and then gleefully stabs it. He also buries himself alive, runs barefoot in thistles, and rides down a treacherous rocky hillside on his bicycle. It is highly likely that anyone like the child portrayed in this film would develop an antisocial personality.

The 2003 Brazilian film *City of God* looks at children and adolescents growing up in a poor, gang-infested area of Rio de Janeiro (called the "City of God") who must choose between a life filled with drug dealing, guns, and violence, and a life based on the hope that they will be able to escape their circumstances. These young children quickly learn to show no fear, and they do not seem to care if they live or die. The film depicts young children (referred to as "runts") running around with guns and talking about getting revenge by murdering their enemies. The film is especially disturbing because it is based on a true story (it is estimated that at least 100,000 people [about the seating capacity of the Los Angeles Memorial Coliseum] are involved in drug dealing in Rio), and conduct disorders are the norm for children and adolescents living in the City of God. The film contrasts two of the younger boys brought up in this culture: One, the protagonist, finds passion and meaning in photography and rejects gang life; the other, named Li'l Zé, achieves his life goal of rising to power to take over as drug boss in the City of God by killing his competition. The Rio police walk around in fear and ignore the drug dealers; before the dealers established their own power base, the police would come into homes and pillage them.

An interesting and provocative dilemma emerges for the children of *City of God*: A child can either choose an honest occupation and live in poverty or become rich by dealing drugs. If these children choose to deal drugs, there is a well-established career trajectory: First, they act as a drug delivery boy, then as a lookout, then dealer, soldier, and eventually manager. For many of these children, the life of a drug dealer is the more appealing option.

One of the most powerful cinematic portrayals of childhood psychopathology is found in the 1994 New Zealand film *Heavenly Creatures*, directed by Peter Jackson, and starring Kate Winslet. The film is based on the true story of two teenage girls, aged 15 and 17, who conspire to murder the mother of one of the girls. The older girl went on to develop a significant reputation as an author of murder mysteries, writing under the name of Anne Perry. The girl's confusion and mental illness in *Heavenly Creatures* is artistically captured in film through her interactions with life-size clay figures that inhabit a medieval fantasy land.

> **"The American dream never happened. The American nightmare is already here. I mean, look at the Washington Monument. It is 555 feet above the ground and 111 feet below the ground. 555 plus 111 is 666. 6-6-6, Poppy. 6-6-6"**
>
> **Scott, the explosive driving instructor, during one of his rants in *Happy-Go-Lucky* (2008)**

Happy-Go-Lucky (2008, UK) is an outstanding film by renowned British director Mike Leigh about a young woman, Poppy (Sally Hawkins), who faces life's stressors with a refreshing yet realistic optimism and humor. A supporting character in the film is Poppy's driving instructor, Scott (Eddie Marsan), who has an intermittent explosive disorder. On the surface, Scott is a fascinating contrast to Poppy's character, as he always has a frown on his face and comes across as very tightly wound, controlling, edgy, and angry. His anger emerges in each driving lesson he gives Poppy, usually taking the form of yelling and threatening. His mental illness becomes apparent when the viewer observes Scott's inability to control his impulses when he learns Poppy has a boyfriend. He speeds up the car, endangers himself and Poppy, becomes abnormally demanding, and at one point, grabs Poppy's hair and shakes her repeatedly. He screams at her on a public street, unable to control his anger, which is palpable. However, Scott is not merely a one-dimensional character; the viewer sees glimpses of his desperation and profound loneliness.

In a remarkable Norwegian film, *Elling* (2002, Norway), the character Kjell, upon being released from a psychiatric hospital, has explosive bouts of anger whenever he is frustrated. His condition would be diagnosed as intermittent explosive disorder.

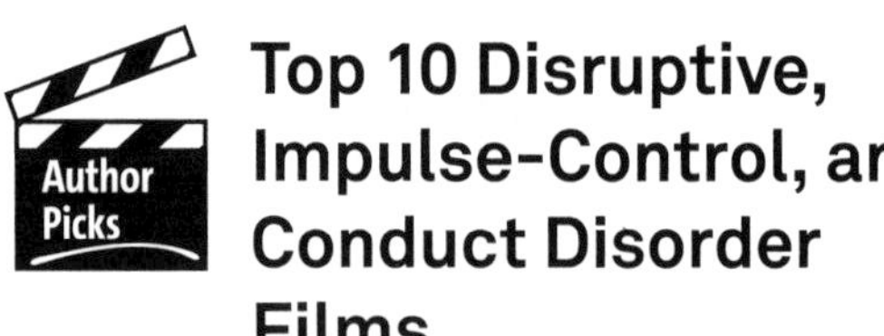

Top 10 Disruptive, Impulse-Control, and Conduct Disorder Films

Oppositional Defiant Disorder and Conduct Disorders

The 400 Blows (1959)
Kids (1995)
We Need to Talk About Kevin (2011)
Life as a House (2001)
My First Mister (2001)
The Chorus (2004)
Thirteen (2003)

Impulse-Control Disorders

Klepto (2003)
Punch Drunk Love (2002)
Happy-Go-Lucky (2008)

Chapter 11

Substance-Related and Addictive Disorders

Whip: I choose to drink! And I blame myself! I am happy to! And you know why? Because I choose to drink! I got an ex-wife and a son I never talk to! And you know why? Because I choose to drink!

Denzel Washington in the role of pilot Whip Whitaker, acknowledging the role of choice in his addiction, in *Flight* (2012)

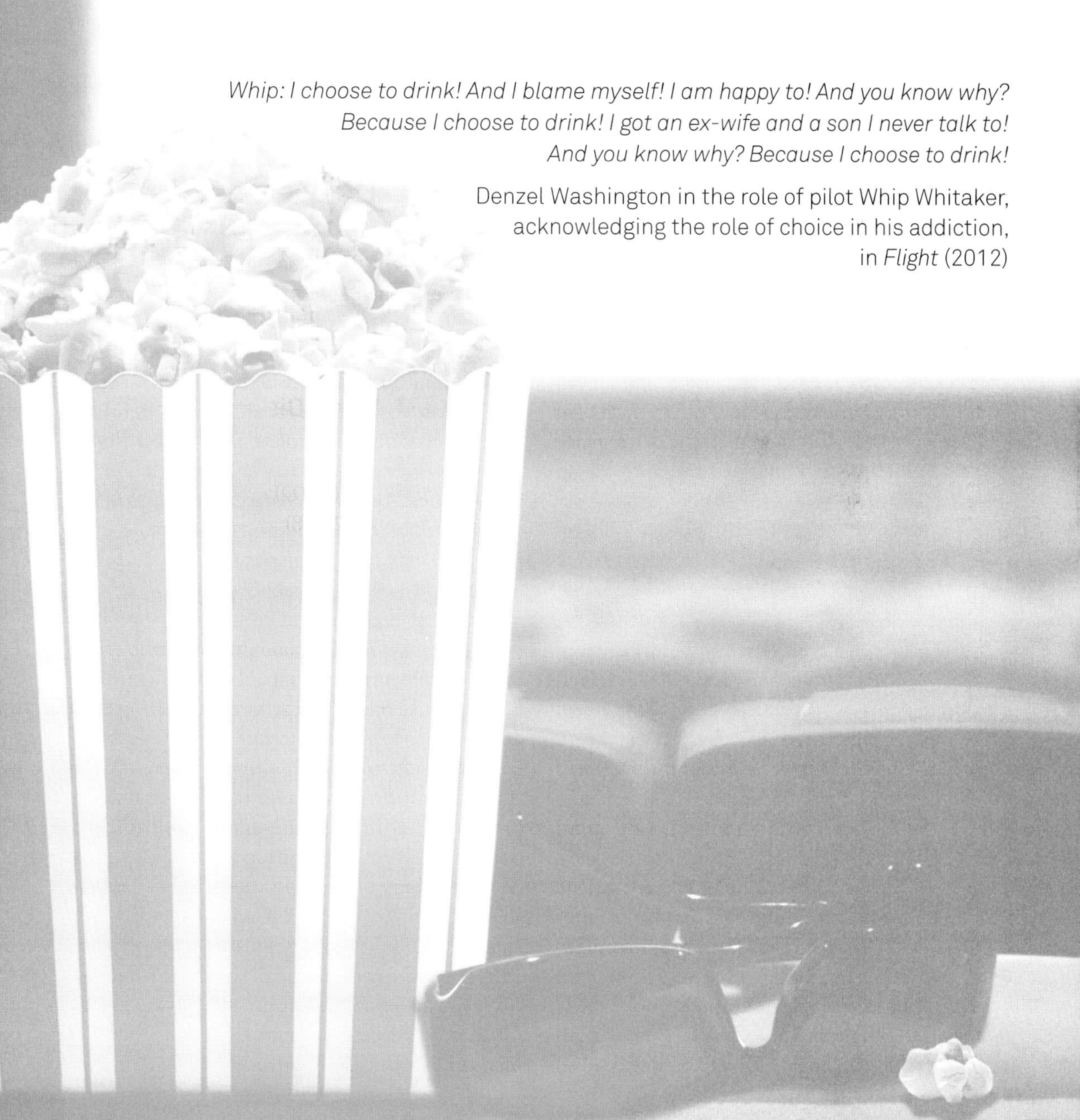

Alcohol Use Disorder

The use of alcohol can be traced back at least 5,000 years, and the relationship among alcohol, drugs, and mysticism has been explored in books such as William James's *Varieties of Religious Experience* (1902) and Aldous Huxley's *Doors of Perception* (1954). Oliver Wendell Holmes Jr. once remarked, "There is in all men a demand for the superlative, so much so that the poor devil who has no other way of reaching it attains it by getting drunk" (https://quotepark.com/quotes/1920942-oliver-wendell-holmes-jr-there-is-in-all-men-a-demand-for-the-superlative/).

In DSM-5, the diagnosis of alcohol use disorder requires at least two of 11 symptoms occurring within a 12-month period. These symptoms include using alcohol in larger amounts than intended or for longer periods than intended; the presence of a persistent desire to cut back on alcohol use; excessive time spent obtaining alcohol, drinking, or recovering from intoxication; craving; failure to fulfill major life obligations; and tolerance and withdrawal. Tolerance refers to the need to use increasingly copious amounts of a substance to obtain a desired effect (a buzz or the feeling of being high), or else to the fact that a given amount of a substance after continued use fails to produce the same effect it once did.

Alcohol and the Brain

Alcohol is quickly absorbed into the bloodstream and transported to the liver, which can metabolize about 1 oz of 100-proof alcohol in an hour. If a person consumes only one drink per hour, the liver can keep up, and alcohol has less of an impact on the brain. However, at consumption rates greater than one drink per hour, the brain is quickly affected, with obvious consequences. There is rapid uptake of alcohol in the cerebellum, and this results in staggering, diminished coordination, and slower reaction times. Judgment is impaired, and alcohol can trigger aggression in some individuals. Although alcohol may initially facilitate sexual interactions by reducing inhibitions, at higher levels there is clear impairment of functioning. In the words of Shakespeare: "Lechery, sir, ... [alcohol] provokes, and unprovokes; it provokes the desire, but it takes away the performance" (*Macbeth*, Act II, Scene 3).

Flight

Flight (2012) is a powerful film that portrays the life of Whip Whitaker (Denzel Washington), a pilot for a major airline who is also a functional alcoholic. He is high on vodka and cocaine when a plane he is flying crashes due to mechanical malfunction. Quick thinking on his part allows

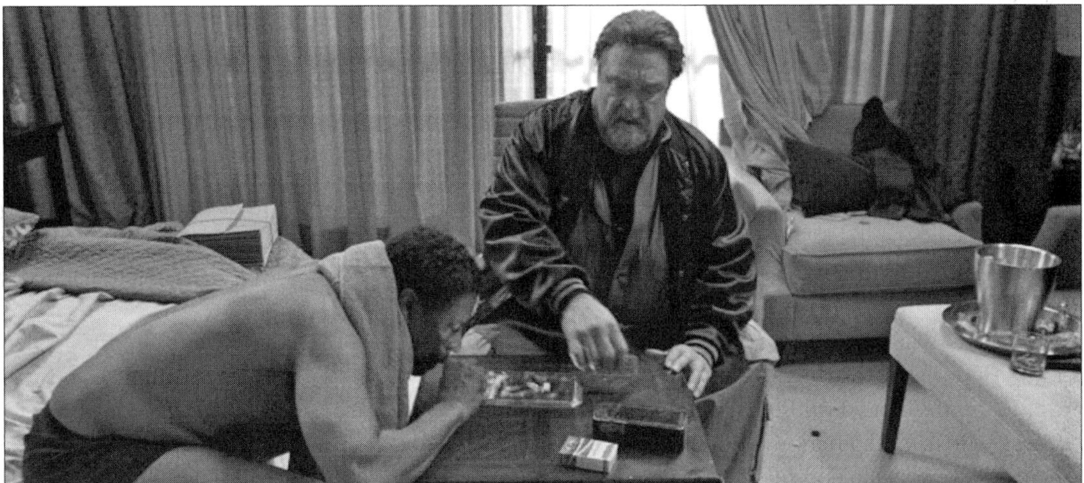

Figure 35. *Flight* (2012, Paramount Pictures, ImageMovers, Parkes-MacDonald Productions, Imagenation Abu Dhabi FZ, The Georgia Film Office). Produced by Heather Kelton, Laurie MacDonald, Cherylanne Martin, Walter F. Parkes, et al. Directed by Robert Zemeckis.

him to flip the plane and fly it upside down to avoid a crash that would have resulted in the death of everyone onboard. Although he could have been exonerated and walked away a free man, Whip confesses to his extensive history of alcohol and drug abuse and is imprisoned for manslaughter. Figure 35 depicts one of Whitaker's many relapses; in this instance, he is enabled by his "supplier," played by John Goodman.

Whitaker has a poor relationship with his ex-wife and no relationship with his son. He makes attempts to reconnect with his son, but the boy – upset after years of disappointments and neglect – angrily refuses his father's overtures. While Whitaker is in prison, his son finally decides to reach out to him and offers to interview his father for a class project. In a poignant, concluding scene, his son tells him that the title of the project is "the most fascinating person I *never* met." The first question makes the now-sober Whitaker pause: "Who are you?" his son inquires.

"It was as if I had reached my life-long limit of lies. I could not tell one more lie."

A sober Whip Whitaker commenting on his rock-bottom turning point, in *Flight* (2012)

The Lost Weekend

Billy Wilder's classic film *The Lost Weekend* (1945) is a powerful portrayal of alcoholism. The protagonist, Don Birnam (Ray Milland), is ready to sacrifice his brother's trust, his career as a writer, and the love of his girlfriend Helen (played by Jane Wyman) for one more drink. Early in the film, we see clear examples of denial, believed by many to be the characteristic defense mechanism of the alcoholic. Don Birnam minimizes the significance of his drinking if he can, but eventually he realizes that it is ruining his life. A scene in which Birnam watches an imaginary bat kill and eat a mouse is an effective illustration of the type of hallucinations characteristic of **delirium tremens**. Birnam eventually hocks his girlfriend's coat to get a gun and writes a suicide note. However, Helen arrives before he pulls the trigger, and the film ends with Birnam planning the novel he is going to write and, in a heavily symbolic gesture, dropping a cigarette in a glass of rye. Some of the symptoms that apply to Don Birnam's alcoholism are presented in Table 8. The symptoms of dependence are the same for all psychoactive substances (alcohol or drugs).

"One's too many and a hundred's not enough."

A bartender chides Don Birnam, in Billy Wilder's *The Lost Weekend* (1945)

Despite an ending that is too pat for contemporary viewers, the film is still a dramatic illustration of the destructive effects of alcohol. Ray Milland won an Academy Award for Best Actor for his portrayal of Birnam, and the film earned additional Academy Awards for best picture, best director, and best screenplay. Billy Wilder, the film's director, consulted with Alcoholics Anonymous before beginning work on the film.

Epidemiology of Alcoholism

Most American adults (about 65%) drink at least occasionally, and many adults consume alcohol daily. Men tend to tolerate alcohol more easily than women, in part because they typically weigh more, and the definition of a heavy drinker needs to be adjusted for males and females. However, it is generally accepted that individuals who average more than three drinks per day are heavy drinkers. Many individuals will consume far more than this average: 10% of all drinkers consume more than 50% of all alcohol consumed.

The DSM-5 estimates the prevalence of alcohol use disorder is 8.5% among adults in the United States (i.e., approximately one in 12 people). The disorder occurs far more frequently among men than women, and there are marked differences across ethnic groups, with Native

Table 8. Criteria for alcohol use disorder, with examples from *The Lost Weekend* (1945)

Selected criteria for alcohol use disorder from the DSM-5	Examples from *The Lost Weekend*
Alcohol is consumed in a larger amount or over a longer period than the individual intended.	Birnam is drinking when the film begins, and he drinks throughout the film.
People know that their use of alcohol is excessive but fail in their attempts to control their drinking.	Birnam tries repeatedly to go on the wagon and has "taken the cure" at least once without success.
A great deal of time is devoted to acquiring alcohol, drinking it, or recovering from its effects. In severe cases, almost all of the individual's waking hours are devoted to the substance.	Birnam is preoccupied with rye and has hidden it throughout his apartment. He thinks about little else, and he steals a purse and robs a liquor store to support his addiction.
Intoxication or withdrawal symptoms occur at work or in other inappropriate situations (e.g., while driving a car).	Birnam has quit writing altogether and has pawned his typewriter to buy whiskey.
Important social, occupational, or recreational activities are replaced by alcohol.	Birnam's relationship with his brother is seriously damaged by his drinking, and he avoids spending a weekend in the country with his family. He also comes close to destroying his relationship with his girlfriend.
Alcohol use persists, despite increasing awareness of the problems it causes.	Birnam describes himself as a "drunk," and he is acutely aware of his declining prowess as a writer.
Tolerance develops, and an increased amount of alcohol is required to produce the same effect. (Tolerance is less marked for alcohol than for some other drugs.)	The film shows Birnam drinking approximately 2 quarts of whiskey per day, far more than most people would be able to tolerate.
Withdrawal symptoms develop when the individual cuts back on their use of alcohol.	Birnam develops delirium tremens and hallucinates in the film.
After experiencing withdrawal symptoms, the individual begins to drink to avoid these unpleasant experiences rather than to produce the pleasant feelings initially associated with alcohol use.	When questioned by a bartender about drinking so early in the morning, Birnam remarks, "At night it's a drink; in the morning it's medicine."

Note. DSM-5 = *Diagnostic and Statistical Manual of Mental Disorders*, 5th edition.

Americans and Alaska Natives having the highest risk. The prevalence is lowest for Asian Americans and Pacific Islanders.

Alcoholism is one of the most serious public health problems in the United States, costing billions annually in lost productivity, increased health care costs, and accidents. Alcohol abuse contributes to about 30% of all motor vehicle accidents, and it is responsible for about half of all traffic fatalities.

About 10% of adults seeking treatment by physicians are dependent on alcohol, and about a third of admissions to general hospitals are for alcohol-related problems. The mortality rate for alcoholics is 2–3 times greater than that of the general population, and the life span of alcoholics is 10–12 years shorter. In addition, the children of alcoholic parents are at increased risk for hyperactivity, low IQ, emotional problems, child abuse, and fetal alcohol syndrome (National Institute on Alcohol Abuse and Alcoholism [NIAAA], 2000). Despite the severity of these problems, less than 10% of those addicted to alcohol will receive treatment for their problems.

Several states have proposed zero-tolerance policies for impaired drivers, dropping the blood alcohol concentration (BAC) permitted for drivers from 0.08% to 0.05%. Stringer (2022) has argued that these policies "reflect a net widening effect that will criminalize unimpaired drivers, divert criminal justice resources away from the most problematic impaired drivers, and will have little impact on impaired driving crashes." In contrast, Garrisson et al. (2022) assessed the effects of BAC levels between 0.05% and 0.08% and found that driving performance became significantly impaired at these levels, but drivers were unaware of their impairment.

Portrayal of Alcoholism in Films

Images of alcohol and drinking are ubiquitous in contemporary films, and one is hard-pressed to name adult films in which alcohol use is not portrayed. This may reflect the fact that alcohol affects everyone directly or indirectly.

The early success of *The Lost Weekend* (1945) led to other films with alcoholism as a central theme, including *Key Largo* (1948), *Harvey* (1950), *Come Back Little Sheba* (1952), *A Star Is Born* (1954), *Cat on a Hot Tin Roof* (1958), *Days of Wine and Roses* (1962), and the vicious alcoholism portrayed by Bette Davis as Baby Jane Hutson in *What Ever Happened to Baby Jane?* (1962). Other relevant older films include *Who's Afraid of Virginia Woolf?* (1966), *Arthur* (1981), *Barfly* (1981), *Tender Mercies* (1983), *Paris, Texas* (1984), *Under the Volcano* (1984), *Hoosiers* (1986), *Ironweed* (1987), *The Verdict* (1987), and *Clean and Sober* (1988).

"You can never lose your talent ... you can lose everything else but can never lose your talent."

Jane's father referring to her talent for musical performance. In fact, Jane's alcoholism contributes to the deterioration and squandering of her talent in *What Ever Happened to Baby Jane?* (1962)

In contrast to the sobering representations of alcoholism in films such as *Clean and Sober* (discussed later in this section), some films portray the alcoholic as happy and carefree. *Harvey* (1950) and *Arthur* (1981) are the two most obvious examples. Writing about *Arthur*, Vincent Canby (1981) noted,

> Not since Nick and Nora Charles virtually made the dry martini into the national drink ... has there been quite so much boozing in a movie without hidden consequences. Arthur drinks scotch the way people now drink Perrier.... When he goes giggling about town, sloshed to the eyeballs, he's not seen as a case history but as eccentric. (Canby, 1981, p. 10)

Unfortunately, the film presents Arthur as an appealing model driving around Long Island in his Rolls Royce. In the film, he has the good fortune to have a chauffeur; most of the teenage viewers emulating his example will not be so lucky.

Movies *reflect* social mores as interpreted by filmmakers, and this certainly applies to the use of alcohol. In the film *Revolutionary Road* (2008), alcohol plays an important role in anesthetizing the boredom and rigidity of gender roles of the 1950s. In turn, movies *affect* social mores in a cyclical manner. A film presentation of the ways in which families are affected by alcoholism is found in *When a Man Loves a Woman* (1994). Other powerful films about alcoholism and its treatment include *Leaving Las Vegas* (1995), in which Nicholas Cage willingly drinks through graphically depicted delirium tremens until his death; Steve Buscemi's *Trees Lounge* (1996); and *Drunks* (1997). This last film is an especially helpful introduction to Alcoholics Anonymous

(AA) and is highly recommended to anyone who has not had an opportunity to visit an open AA meeting. In addition, students interested in the way in which alcoholism is portrayed in films should read an excellent book by Norman Denzin, *Hollywood Shot by Shot: Alcoholism in American Cinema* (1991).

The functional impact of alcoholism is well-portrayed in the film *The Prize Winner of Defiance, Ohio* (2005), starring Julianne Moore and Woody Harrelson as the parents of 10 children growing up in the 1950s. Harrelson gives an impressive performance as Kelly Ryan, an alcoholic who spends his weekly paycheck on alcohol, to the point that the family cannot afford milk and risks foreclosure on their home. Kelly shows a childlike dependency, and he is unable to care for his children or take care of the house. He is enabled by a community that, true to the time and culture, had no diagnosis or solutions for alcoholism; a police officer arrives after a dramatic incident resulting from Kelly's alcohol abuse and simply talks about baseball; a priest takes it a step further in the wrong direction and places blame on Kelly's wife, Evelyn, saying she must try harder to give him a better home.

> **"This has been going on for a very long time. Every night he drinks a six-pack and a pint of whiskey and by the end of the week there's nothing left of his paycheck. It's all gone to the liquor store."**
>
> **Evelyn Ryan describing her husband's alcoholism, in *The Prize Winner of Defiance, Ohio* (2005)**

Everything Must Go (2011) stars Will Ferrell as Nick, a married man who is an executive vice-president for a corporation. At the film's onset, Nick is both fired from his job and separated from his wife who throws all his possessions on the front lawn. With frozen credit cards, no resources, and minimal support, he feels he has no choice but to live on his front lawn. He discovers that he can live on his front lawn for 5 days if he is having a yard sale, so he hastily identifies some things he can sell. He befriends a young African American boy, Kenny, who helps him sell his personal items. The viewer soon learns Nick is addicted to alcohol. This has frequently led to serious work problems, which often require treatment. His minimizing and denial are clear, and he notes, "I had had a couple slip-ups." His recent stressors lead to another relapse, and he begins to drink beer on his lawn chair in his front yard. He drinks first thing in the morning, while driving, and throughout the evening, despite having little or no money. The film has several redeeming qualities as it taps into the human condition, depicts the suffering and consequences of alcohol dependence, and portrays a unique, unlikely friendship between Nick and Kenny.

In *Crazy Heart* (2009), Jeff Bridges plays Bad Blake, a 57-year-old, four-time divorced, small-time musician. Blake is an alcoholic who travels around the southwest performing in bars and restaurants. He spends his days and nights drinking and womanizing, ending each night isolated and broke. He develops a meaningful relationship with a young woman (Maggie Gyllenhaal) and her son, but his alcohol dependence seriously affects his relationship with both. She continues to either enable him and give him second chances, but the last straw occurs when he loses her son at a busy mall after he becomes distracted due to his drinking. Some lyrics from one of his songs are particularly poignant and seem to describe Blake's alcoholism, suffering, and related behaviors: "Pick up your crazy heart and give it one more try; Falling feels like flying; Never see it coming till it's gone; Days and nights all feel the same."

When Blake does become sober and maintains his sobriety for an extended period, his transformation is evident: He returns to writing songs (which is his true passion), and he elevates his subjective well-being, increases his empathy levels, and becomes more generous. This film and the depiction of substance abuse/dependence can be compared with other excellent films portraying alcoholic musicians, such as *Ray* (2004), *Walk the Line* (2005), and *Tender Mercies* (1983), as well as other traveling-wandering figures with substance abuse problems who try to reclaim their life (e.g., *Don't Come Knocking* [2005]). Robert Duvall, the down-and-out musician in *Tender Mercies*, has a minor role as a bartender in *Crazy Heart*.

Following Meg Ryan's outstanding portrayal of an alcoholic woman in *When a Man Loves a Woman* (1994), several films have portrayed depressed women who are either dependent upon or abuse alcohol; powerful examples include *House of Sand and Fog* (2003), *Monster's Ball* (2001), *28 Days* (2000), and *Smashed* (2012). In *28 Days*, Sandra Bullock portrays Gwen Cummings, a writer who is remanded to a rehabilitation setting by a judge after a drunk driving accident. Bullock's character displays symptoms of intoxication and tolerance, including excessive drinking, blackouts, use of an "eye opener" in the morning, and drinking throughout the day. In addition to extreme denial, she is impulsive and enjoys taking risks. Her out-of-control behavior includes carrying a drink wherever she goes, creating a spectacle at her sister's wedding, and inadvertently starting a fire while drinking. Her withdrawal symptoms are depicted as shaky hands, cravings, agitation, and a powerful desire to immediately replace alcohol with pain medication, nicotine, or any other drug she can get her hands on. A complicating factor common for alcoholics is a partner who drinks heavily; in this film, her boyfriend is an alcoholic and significant enabler who is very rejecting and critical of treatment.

Helen Hunt plays an alcoholic working two jobs to pay her bills while secretly drinking in *Pay It Forward* (2000). Even a small amount of alcohol is associated with violence by Kim Bassinger's character in *Final Analysis* (1992). Tilda Swinton gives a dramatic and convincing portrayal of an alcoholic woman, in *Julia* (2009).

Alcohol abuse is evident in several lead characters, such as the title character (Robert Duvall) in *The Apostle* (1997), William Forrester (Sean Connery) in *Finding Forrester* (2000), Willie (Billy Bob Thornton) in *Bad Santa* (2003), and Matt Damon's character, Rannulph Junuh, in *The Legend of Bagger Vance* (2000), who drinks heavily upon returning from war. Alcohol only exacerbates his isolation and loneliness. Alex and his "droogs" use alcohol to "sharpen up" before committing violent acts in *A Clockwork Orange* (1971). *Love Streams* (1984) is a classic John Cassavetes film in which he plays a divorced man addicted to both alcohol and gambling. He finds meaning in his life after he reestablished his relationships with his son and sister.

Alcoholism is particularly common in Western films, and saloons, bar fights, whiskey bottles, drunken gunfighters, and town drunks are staples of the genre (Wedding, 2001). *High Noon* (1952), *Stagecoach* (1939), *Shane* (1953), *Rio Bravo* (1959), and *Unforgiven* (1992) are classic examples.

"Now it's thirty days later. I've been to a funeral, been on about nine million job interviews, I'm $52,000 in debt, and I've got this chip. Suddenly I've got this startling belief that I'm an alcoholic and a drug addict."

Daryl Poynter (Michael Keaton) referring to his 30-day sobriety chip from Alcoholics Anonymous, in *Clean and Sober* (1988)

Clean and Sober (1988) stars Michael Keaton as Daryl Poynter, an alcoholic and cocaine addict, and Morgan Freeman as an addiction counselor known simply as Craig. Some of the most interesting scenes in the film show Poynter at AA meetings and in group therapy. The film ends with Daryl getting his 30-day AA chip, acknowledging to the group that he is both an alcoholic and a drug addict, and realizing that each of us can be responsible only for their own behavior.

Some other films depicting alcohol use disorder include *My Name Was Bette: The Life and Death of an Alcoholic* (2011), a documentary about a nurse, wife, and mother whose life was destroyed by alcohol abuse; *There Will Be Blood* (2007), in which Daniel Day-Lewis's character pours whiskey into his adopted son's baby bottle; *Flight* (2012), in which Denzel Washington plays an alcoholic commercial pilot (see the section Flight, above); *California Solo* (2012); and *Smashed* (2013). Teenage alcoholism is portrayed in *The Spectacular Now* (2013), and alcoholism in a very wealthy playboy is found in the disappointing remake of *Arthur* (2011). *The Last Ride* (2011) tells the story of Hank Williams and documents the damage done to his life and his career by his heavy drinking, and *Country Strong* (2010) stars Gwyneth Paltrow as a country singer who tries to reestablish her career after leaving a rehabilitation facility early; she fails, resumes drinking heavily, and eventually commits suicide. *The Last Day of August* (2012) portrays a man who responds to his paralysis by retreating to the country and drinking heavily. *Bluebird* (2013) documents the ways many people use alcohol to cope with personal crises (in this case the death of a child due to a bus driver's negligence and a mother's alcoholism). *Suddenly* (2013) is a film about a small-town police officer who uses alcohol to cope with his PTSD; he is forced to turn in his badge because of his alcoholism, but he is given a shot at redemption when he is reassigned to duty to help the president of the United States who will be coming through town. *Family of Four* (2011) portrays an alcoholic mother who is generally able to keep her alcoholism hidden, and *Deep in the Heart* (2011) is a film based on the true story of Richard Wallrath, an alcoholic man who loses his family because of his drinking, but who later regains sobriety with the help of a 12-step program, establishes a successful business, and goes on to become a philanthropist, donating millions of dollars for 4-H and Future Farmers of America scholarships.

Numerous recent films have depicted alcoholism or drug abuse These films include cocaine, methamphetamine, alcohol, sex, and gambling addiction in *Dallas Buyers Club* (2013), alcohol dependence in *Nebraska* (2013), the horrifying effects of prescription drug abuse by Meryl Streep's character in *August: Osage County* (2013), and drug and alcohol abuse in *American Hustle* (2013) and *The Wolf of Wall Street* (2013). Excessive alcohol use leading to drunken, toxic homoerotic interactions between two isolated and suffering men is seen in *The Lighthouse* (2019). Regarding *The Lighthouse,* director Robert Eggers acknowledged that he was influenced by psychiatrist Carl Jung's work, and the phallic imagery of the lighthouse was deliberate. *Life Itself* (2018) includes a segment in which a grieving man copes with the loss of his wife with caffeine, alcohol, and Xanax – and eventually commits suicide on the couch of his therapist (played by Annette Bening) during a therapy session.

I strongly recommend that readers watch *Bill W.* (2012), a biopic about the lives of William Griffith Wilson (Bill W.) and Dr. Robert Holbrook Smith (Dr. Bob), the two men who founded Alcoholics Anonymous (AA). Reviewing this film in *PsycCRITIQUES*, Fred Frese wrote,

> AA members regularly identify each other among themselves as "friends of Bill"; and thousands of AA members converge on the city of Akron, Ohio, every June to celebrate Founders' Day. It was in Akron where Dr. Bob and Bill W. met and founded the AA organization in 1935. ... Bill W. died of emphysema in 1970 at the age of 76. The organization he cofounded has grown to having over two million members worldwide ... [and] spawned over 60 other recovery-oriented, anonymous self-help groups based on the twelve-step approach. (Frese, 2013)

I also recommend that you secure a copy of the limited release film *Bob and the Monster* (2011). This documentary portrays the life of Bob Forrest, a rock musician whose career was almost ruined by his alcoholism and drug addiction. After several failed attempts at rehabilitation, Forrest succeeded in overcoming his various addictions, and today he is both successful and sober, working as an addictions recovery counselor who specializes in helping musicians, actors, and other celebrities achieve sobriety. *Krisha* (2015) is another powerful film, which portrays a woman trying to reunite with her estranged family after a 10-year absence; sadly, her addiction to alcohol and drugs is too powerful, and she winds up drunk on Thanksgiving Day and ruins the holiday meal. This low-budget film by a new director offers a dramatic illustration of a dysfunctional family; in many ways it is like Jane Campion's 1989 film *Sweetie.*

In *Honey Boy* (2019), Shia LaBeouf plays his own abusive father. The film is clearly autobiographical, and the car wreck that landed LaBeouf in a mandatory rehabilitation facility is vividly portrayed in the film. LaBeouf is given a diagnosis of PTSD, but there is little unambiguous evidence justifying the diagnosis; the kind of parental verbal abuse LeBeouf the child experiences would lead to adult psychopathology, but not to the kind of symptoms that would justify a diagnosis of PTSD.

In *The Way Back* (2020), Ben Affleck plays Jack Cunningham, a former high school basketball star who works at a menial construction job. Jack spends every evening getting drunk at a local bar. When the high school basketball coach has a heart attack, Cunningham is offered the coach's job and a chance for redemption (Figure 36). He is clearly addicted to alcohol – he keeps each successive beer in the freezer to ensure it is cold before drinking, and he starts each day drinking beer while in the shower – and his wife has left him because of his drinking. The movie is partially autobiographical, and Affleck's divorce from Jennifer Garner, his personal struggles with substance abuse, and his repeated stints in rehabilitation hospitals have been well documented, as well as his strong family history of alcoholism and suicide (Barnes, 2020).

Drug Abuse

The use of mind-altering substances seems to have existed from when humans first became aware of the potent effects plants could have on human perception. Substance use disorders (alcohol or drugs) include substance abuse and substance dependence problems. **Substance abuse** is a *pattern* of use characterized by *recurrent adverse consequences* related to the substance's use. The DSM-5 diagnosis requires evidence of impairment according to one of the following four criteria: (1) failure to meet role obligations; (2) recurrent use in situations, such as driving, in which clear hazards are present; (3) recurrent legal problems; and (4) continued use, despite

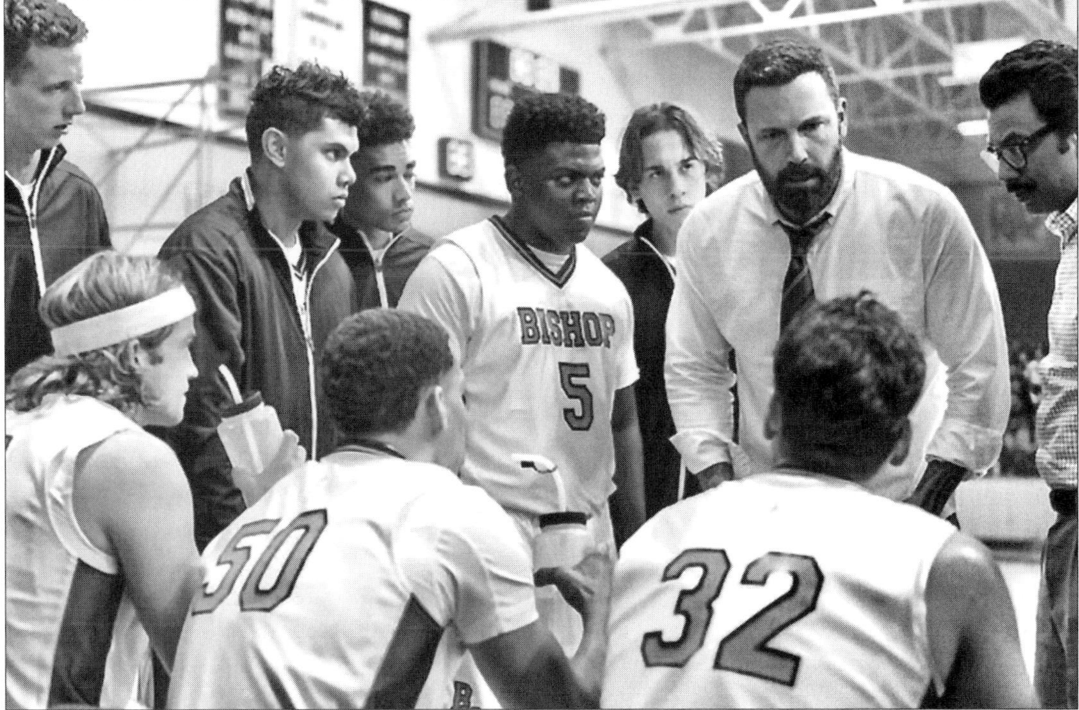

Figure 36. *The Way Back* (2020, Warner Brothers, BRON Studios, Jennifer Todd Pictures, Mayhem Pictures, Filmtribe). Produced by Madison Ainley, Mark Ciardi, Jason Cloth, Robert J. Dohrmann, et al. Directed by Gavin O'Connor.

social or interpersonal problems related to the substance. In addition, the symptoms must never have met the criteria associated with the diagnosis of substance dependence.

In addiction or **substance dependence,** tolerance, withdrawal, and compulsive drug-taking behavior are present. The symptoms associated with dependence on different drugs are similar (but not identical) across drug categories. Dependence is characterized by the presence of symptoms like those listed in Table 9.

Table 9. Symptoms of substance dependence, with examples from *Ray* (2004)

DSM-5 criteria	Examples from *Ray*
Tolerance, defined by (a) a need for ever increasing amounts of the substance to achieve intoxication or (b) diminished effect with use of a set level of the substance.	Throughout the film, Ray continues to use more and more heroin.
Withdrawal, defined by (a) specific effects associated with the substance being abused or (b) use of a substance to relieve or avoid the withdrawal symptoms.	Ray's withdrawal from heroin is life threatening. He refuses to use any medication to ease the physiological and psychological effects of his "cold turkey" withdrawal.
Using the substance in larger amounts or over a longer period than was intended.	He continues to use heroin more frequently throughout the movie, even when he intends to attend family functions.
A persistent desire to cut back or eliminate use of the substance.	Ray says he could quit whenever he wants, and he knows he should quit.
A great deal of time is devoted to acquiring the substance or recovering from its effects.	He is often intoxicated. He seems to have easy access to the drug.
Important social, occupational, or recreational activities are ignored because of the preoccupation with use of the substance.	He misses important family events when under the influence.
The substance use is continued despite recurrent physical or psychological problems resulting from its use.	He continues to use even though he is often scratching, unable to concentrate, and losing balance.

Opioids

The opioids are a class of drugs that includes opium, morphine, codeine, methadone, Percodan (a combination of aspirin and oxycodone), and heroin. They are highly addictive and lead to severe physical and psychological dependence.

Heroin is particularly dangerous and has taken the lives of countless people addicted to it, including stars such as Philip Seymour Hoffman, whom many consider one of the most talented actors of this generation. He overdosed and died alone in his Manhattan apartment at age 46 in February 2014. His films are described throughout this book, including several in this chapter.

These drugs are sometimes lumped together under the general rubric of narcotics. **Opium** is usually smoked; the other drugs are most often ingested or injected. In most countries, opioids are controlled substances. When used legally, these drugs are prescribed for pain or diarrhea, except for methadone, which is used to treat opioid addiction. **Fentanyl** and **meperidine** are opioid analogs (chemical compounds that are like other drugs in their effects but differ slightly in their chemical structure) that are legally prescribed for pain but are also illegally sold as recreational drugs. Fentanyl is especially dangerous because it is at least 50 times more potent than morphine.

Numerous films depict the use of opioids. Robert De Niro can be seen smoking opium in both the opening and the ending scenes of Sergio Leone's *Once Upon a Time in America* (1984), and opium plays a significant role in both *Indochine* (1992) and Bernardo Bertolucci's *The Last Emperor* (1987).

Katharine Hepburn plays a morphine addict with an alcoholic son (Jason Robards) in the film adaptation of Eugene O'Neill's *Long Day's Journey into Night* (1962). Morphine abuse is also portrayed in the science fiction thriller *Pitch Black* (2000).

An example of the ability to function despite being extremely high on drugs can be found in Quentin Tarantino's *Pulp Fiction* (1994). Vincent (John Travolta) shoots up before going out on a date with his boss's wife, Mia (Uma Thurman), who snorts cocaine before meeting him. The two wind up at Jack Rabbit Slims and maintain a coherent – if not stimulating – conversation. They even managed to win a dance contest. Later in the evening, Mia discovers the heroin in Vincent's coat pocket. Believing it to be cocaine, she proceeds to snort a line of the drug and goes into a coma. Vincent eventually saves Mia's life by plunging a syringe filled with epinephrine into her heart (see Figure 37).

One of the most compelling, yet still disturbing, portrayals of heroin addiction is in the classic film *Requiem for a Dream* (2000). Most of the main characters are substance dependent – prescription diet pills for Sara (Ellen Burstyn) and multiple other substances including heroin for the teenagers Harry (Jared Leto), Marion (Jennifer Connelly), and Tyrone (Marlon Wayans). In this film, Harry's arm is eventually amputated because of drug-related untreated infections that lead to gangrene.

A young Leonardo DiCaprio stars in *The Basketball Diaries* (1995), a film based on the life of writer Jim Carroll that chronicles his descent from a high school basketball star to a desperate heroin addict who loses everything he once held dear. Eventually Carroll overcomes his addiction with the help of an older friend.

Opioid withdrawal occurs when use of opioid drugs is discontinued or when an opioid antagonist (any drug that blocks the effects of an opioid) is administered. Complete withdrawal

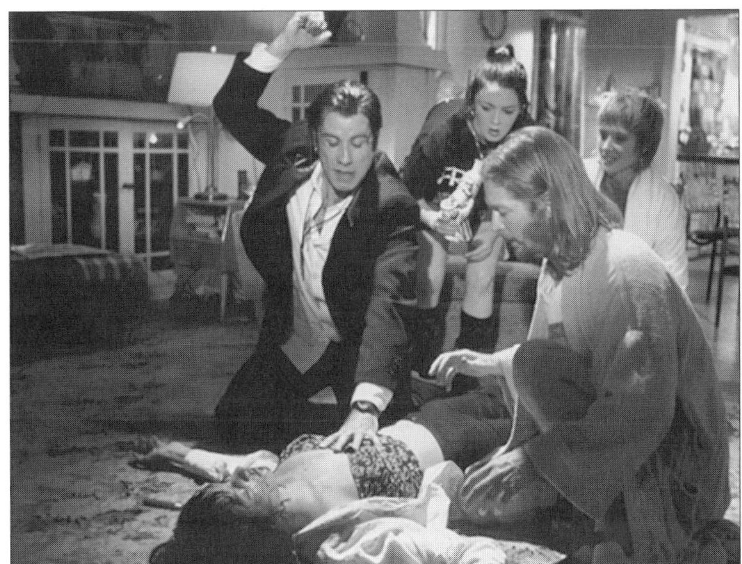

Figure 37.
Pulp Fiction (1994, Miramax, A Band Apart, Jersey Films). Produced by Lawrence Bender, Danny DeVito, Richard N. Gladstein, Michael Shamberg, et al. Directed by Quentin Tarantino.

usually takes 3–8 days. Opioid withdrawal can lead to the following symptoms: dysphoric mood, nausea or vomiting, muscle aches, lacrimation (crying) or rhinorrhea (runny nose), diarrhea, yawning, fever, or insomnia. Dramatic examples of opioid withdrawal can be seen in *Ray* (2004), *The Basketball Diaries* (1995), *Candy* (2006), and in the Frank Sinatra film *The Man with the Golden Arm* (1955).

The classic film about the heroin trade is William Friedkin's *The French Connection* (1971). Friedkin won an Academy Award for his directing, and Gene Hackman won the Academy Award for Best Actor for his role as police detective Jimmy (Popeye) Doyle. *The Connection* is a 1961 film about a group of junkies waiting for the arrival of a pusher. A more powerful and realistic presentation of teenage addiction and prostitution is *Christiane F.* (1981, Germany), which explores the drug culture of West Berlin. Other examples of films depicting heroin addiction include *High Art* (1998), *Who'll Stop the Rain* (1978), *Mona Lisa* (1986), *Chappaqua* (1966), and *Lady Sings the Blues* (1972).

One of the most powerful drug films ever made is Gus Van Sant's 1989 film *Drugstore Cowboy*, starring Matt Dillon as Bob, the leader of a group of four addicts who rob drugstores to maintain their habit. The film is especially memorable because of a very realistic cameo played by William Burroughs as an old, burned-out, addicted, and defrocked priest living in a seedy motel. Bob sees in the priest the image of the man he (Bob) will eventually become. His decision to go straight and the dilemmas he faces (including attempts by his friends to seduce him back to the world they formerly shared) are realistic and illustrative of the challenges ex-addicts face trying to go straight.

Pedro Almodóvar's *Pain and Glory* (*Delor y Gloria;* 2019, Spain) is an autobiographical film starring Antonio Banderas and Penélope Cruz. The film depicts a director (Banderas) coping with depression and chronic pain; he turns to smoking heroin to deal with his pain, and he soon becomes addicted. The film includes flashbacks to the director's childhood and his earliest sexual memories. It is interesting to contrast with other cinematic portrayals of older gay men including *Death in Venice* (1971), *Gods and Monsters* (1998) and *Love and Death on Long Island*.

Ray and Heroin Addiction

The Academy Award–winning film *Ray* (2004) is based on the first 35 years of the life of Ray Charles (Jamie Foxx), the legendary musical genius of rhythm and blues who lived until the age of 73. Charles's childhood years are marred with racial discrimination, extreme poverty, an absent father, the traumatic drowning of his younger brother, and the loss of his sight. A local café musician fosters Ray's early interest in music. At age 15, following the death of his mother, he leaves school and begins touring the South with several dance bands that play Black dance halls. Charles's second wife, Della Bea Robinson (Kerry Washington), struggles with his absence, addictions, and extramarital affairs. In the movie, she stays with him, but in life, Della Bea left the marriage. Throughout the movie, Ray's iconic success in music is contrasted with a struggle for a personal identity, multiple failed and conflicting relationships, a need for constant sexual gratification, and an overall fear of being alone. Figure 38 shows Ray Charles as a boy being nurtured by his mother as he struggles to cope with the realities of his blindness.

Ray Charles begins his 20-year heroin addiction in his teenage years with an injection from an older musician. Ray immediately experiences the surge of pleasure and the rush that occurs as heroin crosses the blood–brain barrier, is converted to morphine, and binds rapidly to the brain's opioid receptors. Ray also experiences other heroin effects. Clouded mental functioning is shown in the film, but nausea, vomiting, and suppression of pain (other short-term effects) are not. A user's response to heroin or other opioids will vary depending on dose level and experience with the drug. During a state of opioid intoxication, the user tends to be euphoric, drowsy, apathetic, and usually

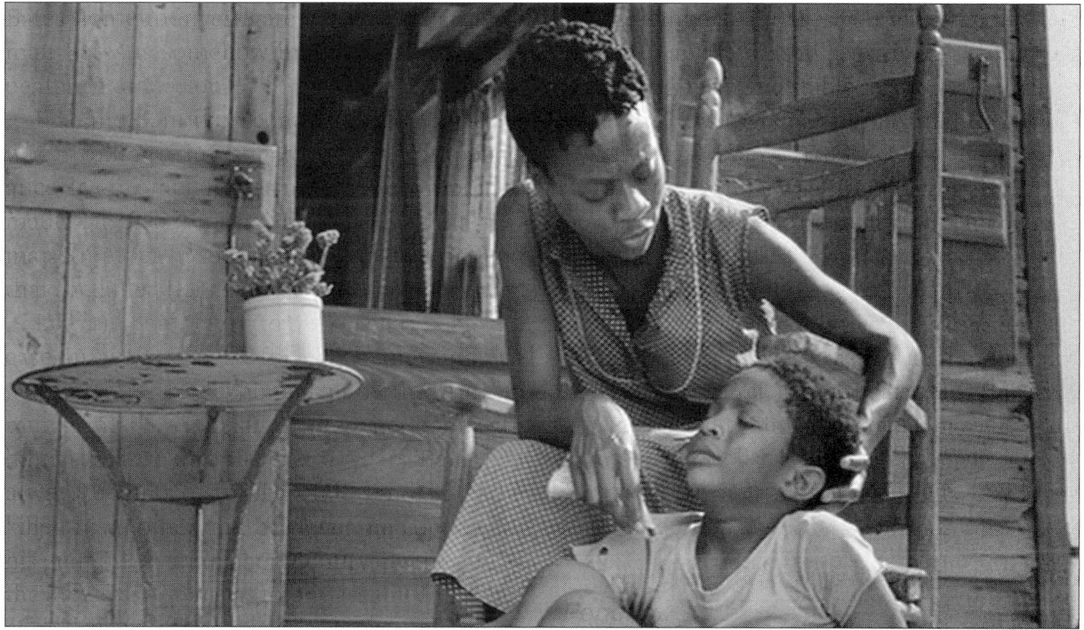

Figure 38. *Ray* (2004, Universal Pictures, Bristol Bay Productions, Anvil Films, Baldwin Entertainment Group, Walden Media). Produced by Howard Baldwin, Karen Elise Baldwin, Alise Benjamin, Stuart Benjamin, et al. Directed by Taylor Hackford.

indifferent to their surroundings. Constipation is common. The user's pupils become markedly constricted, and hallucinations may occur. Judgment is often impaired, although an experienced user may function in routine occupational and social roles.

The long-term effects of heroin are quite devastating and include addiction, infections (from dirty needles), collapsed veins, abscesses, infection of heart lining and valves, and arthritis. The primary long-term effect for Ray is addiction. All opioids produce significant tolerance, and withdrawal symptoms are common when drug use is discontinued. In *Ray*, withdrawal is graphically depicted. As tolerance develops, heroin users frequently require doses more than 100 times the amount that was originally necessary to produce a state of euphoria. In *Ray*, viewers can clearly see tolerance develop. Typical of addicts, Ray Charles becomes more impaired as he continues to use heroin. Unlike most people with heroin addictions, Ray has extensive financial resources and does not have to engage in typical drug-seeking behavior such as theft or prostitution. Eventually, the FBI arrests him for possession of heroin. Ray seeks treatment only because it is a better alternative than prison.

Sedative-Hypnotics

Sedative drugs produce a calm feeling of well-being in low doses and induce sleep in larger doses. These drugs include barbiturates such as Amytal, pentobarbital, and Seconal, as well as **anxiolytics** (anxiety-reducing drugs) such as the **benzodiazepines** (Valium, Librium, etc.). Xanax, a more recently developed anxiolytic with a short half-life, combines the anxiety-reducing properties of other benzodiazepines with a mild antidepressant effect. It has become one of the most widely prescribed drugs in the United States. Some of the problems associated with Valium addiction are portrayed in the autobiography of Barbara Gordon and film *I'm Dancing as Fast as I Can* (1982).

Barbiturates are muscle relaxants that induce feelings of well-being in small doses; with larger amounts, the user falls into a deep and profound sleep. Although tolerance develops extremely rapidly with barbiturates, the dose that is lethal remains constant. This puts the barbiturate abuser at elevated risk and is one of the reasons barbiturates are rarely prescribed for anxiety. However, they remain the medication of choice in some cases of epilepsy.

The effects of barbiturates mimic the effects of alcohol and include symptoms such as slurred speech and staggering gait. These effects may be especially pronounced when barbiturates are combined with alcohol, and this combination is likely to be lethal. Marilyn Monroe committed suicide using a combination of alcohol and sleeping pills. In addition, barbiturate withdrawal is more difficult and more painful than withdrawal from narcotics, and it is more likely to be life threatening.

Benzodiazepines have replaced barbiturates for the treatment of insomnia, because they are less addictive and not as likely to be successfully used in suicide attempts. Benzodiazepines are especially widely prescribed in the United States, and many people feel they are prescribed too often.

Stimulants

Stimulant drugs excite the central nervous system (CNS), fight fatigue, suppress one's appetite, and enhance mood. Cocaine, amphetamines, methamphetamines (meth), 3,4-methylenedioxy-*N*-methylamphetamine (MDMA; or ecstasy), nicotine, and caffeine are all stimulants with varying consequences of addiction. These substances activate the reward systems of the brain resulting in a pleasurable feeling. Cocaine and methamphetamine effects are highly addictive and can lead to grave consequences such as tremors, psychosis, and convulsions. Lethal overdose causes death from respiratory failure. Drug cravings and stress lead to drug seeking behavior. Methylphenidates (Ritalin, Concerta, etc.) are also classified as stimulants, but are legally prescribed for attention-deficit/hyperactivity disorder.

Cocaine

Cocaine is usually snorted or, more rarely, injected intravenously. Sigmund Freud's recreational and therapeutic use of cocaine has been documented and is described in the film *The Seven Percent Solution* (1976), a historical fantasy in which Freud and Sherlock Holmes share their love of cocaine and pool their deductive talents to solve the puzzle of a missing patient.

The film *Blow* (2001), named for the street name of cocaine and based on the life of a cocaine smuggler, George Jung (Johnny Depp), chronicles the rise and fall of one of America's most powerful drug traffickers. This movie portrays the influence of the seductive forces of money and power on a typical adolescent of the 1960s who would rather smoke marijuana on a California beach than work. He discovers that it is easy to make money selling marijuana. While imprisoned for his marijuana dealing, he was introduced to the world of cocaine trafficking. This film shows the social realities of the illegal, but highly profitable, drug culture. George also displays the physiological and psychological symptoms of addiction and withdrawal.

> **"The official toxicity limit for humans is between one and one and a half grams of cocaine depending on body weight. I was averaging five grams a day, maybe more. I snorted ten grams in ten minutes once. I guess I had a high tolerance."**
>
> **George Jung in *Blow* (2001)**

Other compelling films dealing with cocaine addiction include *The Bad Lieutenant* (1992), starring Harvey Keitel; Martin Scorsese's *Goodfellas* (1990), Brian De Palma's *Scarface* (1983), Alejandro Gonzalez Inarritu's *21 Grams* (2003), featuring a tormented woman played by Naomi Watts; and *The Wolf of Wall Street* (2013).

In Casey Affleck's mockumentary film, *I'm Still Here* (2010), Joaquin Phoenix announces his retirement from making films and instead turns to drugs and hip-hop music. The viewer sees a dramatic change in Phoenix who snorts cocaine any chance he gets, pays for prostitutes, slurs his words, and explodes angrily around his friends. Many viewers will assume this must be a hoax; however, several indicators show it to be real, as well as a major identity crisis, because these behaviors were maintained for about 18 months during the film's inception, production, and promotion. Just as the media rumors that this was a hoax began to subside, it was revealed that it actually was a hoax, and Phoenix admitted to this on the David Letterman Show, after having embarrassed Letterman 18 months earlier with his disheveled appearance, mumbling, and refusal to talk in the interview.

Crack cocaine, named after the sound made as the drug is consumed, takes the form of small rocks and is smoked. The effects of smoking crack cocaine occur almost immediately, but the high that is produced is brief. Although crack is inexpensive, crack addicts can quickly develop addictions that require hundreds of dollars each day to support. For many people, cocaine addiction leads to prostitution, theft, or violence. The day-to-day life of a crack dealer is portrayed by Djay (Terrence Howard) in *Hustle and Flow* (2005), a film about a man who tries to make money to support his family but begins to question what kind of life he wants to be leading. *Half Nelson* (2006) is a well-directed film in which Ryan Gosling portrays a drug-addicted teacher–coach of inner-city students in a racially diverse neighborhood. He uses cocaine regularly – alone and with strange women – and smokes crack in the girls' locker room after a game. While he is a creative and engaging teacher, his drug addiction leads him to be distant, avoidant, angry, tired in class, and disengaged from his family.

MacArthur Park

The independent film *MacArthur Park* (2001), depicts Cody, a man addicted to crack and struggling to leave both his addiction and the park where he lives with other homeless crack addicts. He has a good reason to leave: His son recently tracked him down, and his son has a home where Cody could recover. This film depicts the obstacles of crack addiction Cody must overcome in order to leave.

> **"I'm not homeless; I just don't wanna go home."**
>
> **Cody in *MacArthur Park* (2001)**

The film explores a world of crack addiction where extensive drug abuse and dependence – as well as drug selling and producing – are depicted. The film's characters use large amounts of crack to cope with their pain and to avoid withdrawal effects. A variety of characters are depicted, and each has a different relationship with the park's drug world: Some are leaving the lifestyle; others are trying to leave, entering the world, deteriorating in it, or have no interest in leaving; still others are simply lost causes.

The screenplay was written by Tyrone Atkins, a man who was homeless in Los Angeles' MacArthur Park and addicted to crack cocaine. Atkins wrote most of the story while in jail; after leaving jail, he returned to the park before entering a rehabilitation program.

Sweet Nothing

Another film illustrating the degradation associated with crack addiction is *Sweet Nothing* (1996), a true story based on a set of diaries discovered in an abandoned apartment in the Bronx. The film demonstrates the corrosive effects of the protagonist's addiction on his marriage, his relationship with his children, his friends, and his job. At one point, Angelo, the lead character, misses his father's funeral because he has an opportunity to get high, and this need supersedes all others. Angelo loses the ability to become sexually aroused by his wife, and we watch him become increasingly paranoid as the film progresses.

Cocaine has affected the lives and careers of numerous actors and directors. For example, Tommy Rettig (best known as Jeff, Lassie's master in the TV series) was sentenced to 5 years in federal prison for smuggling cocaine; Richard Pryor became severely burned because of an explosion related to smoking crack cocaine; and when Rainer Werner Fassbinder, considered by many to be Germany's finest director, died at the age of 37, his death was attributed to heart failure resulting from a combination of barbiturates and cocaine.

Amphetamines

Common amphetamines include **amphetamine** (Benzedrine), **dextroamphetamine** (Dexedrine), and **methamphetamine** (Methedrine). Amphetamines or their derivatives are commonly found in nasal decongestants and appetite suppressants. These agents are taken orally. Methamphetamine crystals (ice), a highly concentrated form of amphetamine, can also be smoked, injected or taken orally, producing a high that can last up to 14 hours. **Khat**, a shrub grown in Africa and the Middle East, produces leaves that can be chewed to produce an amphetamine-like effect. The use of khat is referred to in *Black Hawk Down* (2001). In *Walk the Line* (2005), a drama based on the life of Johnny Cash, Joaquin Phoenix is masterful in the role of the musician. The film tells the story of Cash's rise in the music business, his history of amphetamine abuse, and his love for singer June Carter (Reese Witherspoon). Cash chronically abused prescription drugs, among other substances, often using them to manage tension and stress. Tolerance and withdrawal (both physiological and psychological) are well-portrayed, as is intoxication as Cash falls over on stage in the middle of his performance. The film parallels *Ray* (2004) in that both depict renowned musicians who overcome trauma, rise to the top of the music business, fall dangerously into drugs, are unfaithful in their marriages, lead a double life, recover from drug dependence, make a comeback in their music, and inspire millions.

Winter's Bone (2010) is a compelling film that dramatically but indirectly portrays the ways in which methamphetamine abuse affects a family and a community. Ree (played by Jennifer Lawrence, in her breakthrough performance) is a 17-year-old girl who is highly resilient and takes on the dangerous role of trying to discover what has happened to her father. The viewer never actually sees the father (alive) in the film, but we learn he is an addict who cooks and sells crystal meth for a living, The viewer also comes to understand how this drug can affect (and ruin) entire rural communities. Amphetamines are highly addictive, and tolerance for drugs like methamphetamine develops rapidly. There is a characteristic withdrawal syndrome that includes depression, fatigue, nightmares, insomnia or sometimes hypersomnia, increased appetite, and either psychomotor retardation or agitation. This "crashing" effect is the price the user must pay for the euphoria that accompanies the initial drug use. Amphetamine-induced psychoses often produce symptoms that closely resemble those found with serious mental disorders such as schizophrenia.

The film *Dopamine* (2003) features a lead character who engages in heavy use of stimulants. He gets amphetamine pills from a drug dealer and stays up all night working; in one scene, he has lined up seven cups of coffee next to his computer. Two better films that offer more compelling portrayals of stimulant abuse are *Requiem for a Dream* (2000) and *Spun* (2002). *Beautiful Boy* (2018; not to be confused with an earlier film with the same name about a school shooter), is based on a true story and shows how a family can be torn apart by methamphetamine addiction.

Requiem for a Dream

The unforgettable film *Requiem for a Dream* (2000) tells the stories of four lonely, desperate characters, each on the wrong track and each destroying their life with drugs. Uppers are not the only drug portrayed in the film, which notably contains one of the most vivid and disturbing portrayals of heroin addiction; these characters will take any drug available. Drugs take the place of food, sex, life goals, and everything else. The effect of drugs on the body and mind is unrelenting. Sara (Ellen Burstyn) takes drugs to lose weight so that she can appear in a live broadcast of a television show. Her son, Harry (Jared Leto), repeatedly steals Sara's television set (even though it is chained to the wall) and pawns it for drugs.

Director Darren Aronofsky uses extreme close-ups to demonstrate the effects of drugs. He shows characters swallowing pills, injecting substances, and snorting drugs followed by predictable physiological effects (e.g., pupil dilation), all with exaggerated sound effects. Vigorous camera work, editing, and split-screen techniques allow the viewer to experience the confusion and fast-paced world of addicts abusing "uppers."

In the end, each character is alive but destroyed, well past the point of no return, living in a hospital, prison, psychiatric institution, or on the streets as a prostitute. In his review, Roger Ebert appropriately labels this film as "a travelogue of hell."

Spun

Spun (2002) is a devastatingly realistic portrayal of several methamphetamine addicts. Virtually every character is a meth addict – Mickey Rourke plays the cook, who sets up meth labs in various shady apartments until they blow up, and John Leguizamo plays Spider Mike, the addicted dealer. Another character dependent on methamphetamine is the cook's girlfriend, Nikki (Brittany Murphy), whose dog has turned green due to drug exposure in the meth lab. The lead character, Ross (Jason Schwartzman), is so preoccupied with always using and having meth available that he forgets he has chained a woman to his bed during sex. Ross wants to have another chance at a relationship with a different woman, Amy, who left Ross because of his methamphetamine abuse and moved on in her life; she can see through Ross's denial so patently evident in one of his comments, "You know what the best part is, Amy? I'm not hooked. I can stop anytime."

These characters are depicted doing meth around the clock – off a girl's body, off a urinal, and "doing a round" while driving. Symptoms of intoxication are present in each character: Inappropriate laughter, jerky, quick body language and movement, and completely trashed living quarters; this is a world in which no one sleeps, everyone talks fast, and no one has meaningful relationships. The postintoxication impairment following the repeated pattern of getting high on meth and crashing to sleep after several days of being awake is called being "spun." All of these characters surround themselves with meth – they all get spun. The consequences are clear: The meth addict will eventually be jailed, hospitalized, blown up, or (if lucky) they will find a way to escape the lifestyle.

"Spoof, dope, crank, creep, bomb, spank, shit, bang, zip, tweak, chard. Call it what you will, it's all methamphetamine. That's what I'm here for."

An opening quote from an addict in *Spun* (2002)

As in *Requiem for a Dream* (2000), the camera speeds everything up to let the viewer experience in some small way what it is like to take methamphetamines. A character inhales meth, and a close-up shows his eyes bloodshot and wide open; cartoon images accentuate thoughts and drug effects; other close-ups display spinning movements with pupils dilating and contracting.

Hallucinogens

Hallucinogens, sometimes referred to as **psychedelics**, are drugs that distort the perception of reality. Users report hallucinations involving all senses, **synesthesia** ("crossed" sensations, such as hearing sights and seeing sounds), and depersonalization. These drugs can also have profound effects on mood.

Hallucinogens can occur in the natural environment but are more often produced synthetically. Naturally occurring hallucinogens include **mescaline**, derived from the peyote cactus, and **psilocybin**, which is present in *Psilocybe* mushrooms. Some Native Americans use *Psilocybe* mushrooms in religious ceremonies.

Mescaline can also be produced in a laboratory. However, the best-known and most widely used of all synthetic hallucinogens is **lysergic acid diethylamide** (LSD). It is most often swallowed as a pill, but it can also be mixed with a fluid, licked off blotter paper, or swallowed in sugar cubes or gelatin sheets. LSD is colorless, tasteless, and extremely potent. It produces varied symptoms and can result in affective changes that range from euphoria to absolute terror. The most dramatic effects are often sensory in nature: When the drug experience is positive, it allows the user "to see a world in a grain of sand / And a heaven in a wild flower, / Hold infinity in the palm of your hand / And eternity in an hour" (William Blake, *Auguries of Innocence*). Unfortunately, the experience is not always this benign, and injury or death can result from bad decisions made while under the influence of the drug. Some users have also reported flashbacks in which they re-experience the sensory phenomenon associated with previous trips weeks or years after last using the drug. The drug is not addictive, but tolerance develops rapidly.

In a 1968 *Playboy* interview, the renowned director Stanley Kubrick made the following constructive observation about LSD:

> One of the things that's turned me against LSD is that all the people I know who use it have a peculiar inability to distinguish between things that are interesting and stimulating and things that appear to be so in the state of universal bliss that the drug induces on a good trip. They seem to completely lose their critical faculties and disengage themselves from some of the most stimulating areas of life. Perhaps when everything is beautiful, nothing is beautiful. (Agel, 1970, p. 346)

In the film *In the Name of the Father* (1993), prisoners cope with the monotony of prison life by licking LSD off the back of a jigsaw puzzle. The puzzle is a large world map, and the prisoners get high "one country at a time." The LSD experience is also portrayed in any number of films from the 1960s that document the youth culture of that period. In *Awakening the Beast* (1970), a psychiatrist tests his theory that drugs are the conduit for evil. He conducts research on four subjects who will take LSD as an experiment while he monitors their behavior for a book he is writing about addicts. He injects distilled water to deliver the drug. In the film he observes: "Drugs are but an excuse to release the instinct in all of us."

Phencyclidine (PCP), also known as angel dust, is another powerful hallucinogen that has been used since the early 1960s. It can be taken in pill form or dusted onto marijuana and smoked. The drug produces symptoms even more marked than those associated with LSD and may result in analgesia, depersonalization, paranoia, rage reactions, or schizophrenia-like psychoses. Hallucinogen use is depicted in *Easy Rider* (1969) and *Fear and Loathing in Las Vegas* (1998).

The stylized, partly computerized characters of *A Scanner Darkly* (2006) portray a science fiction–fantasy world characterized by paranoia, drug abuse, and government control. Richard Linklater directs Keanu Reeves, Robert Downey Jr., Winona Ryder, and Woody Harrelson in this story about a family man who is unhappy, so he leaves his life to become a narcotics agent. During his training, he learns that good agents do drugs in moderation. The made-up drug in the film is Substance D (D stands for despair, desolation, and death) to which 40% of the population is addicted. Many intoxication and withdrawal symptoms are dramatized including tactile hallucinations (e.g., bugs crawling all over the body), shakiness, bloodshot eyes, extreme paranoia, dramatic anger, and a suicide attempt. One character develops an extensive hallucination in which a foreign creature spends eternity reading out his life sins without ever pausing.

Inhalants

Common substances that inhalant addicts abuse include glue, gasoline, paint thinners, spray paints, cleaners, and spray-can propellants. Methods used to inhale the vapors include soaking a rag with the substance, placing the substance in a paper or plastic bag, inhaling directly from the container, or spraying the substance into the nose or mouth. The chemicals inhaled reach the lungs and bloodstream very rapidly.

Love Liza

In *Love Liza* (2002), Wilson (masterfully portrayed by Philip Seymour Hoffman) is a computer technician who becomes addicted to inhaling gasoline following his wife's suicide. This is a bizarre and atypical bereavement reaction. Wilson is an emotional wreck and puts all his energy and concerns into "huffing" gasoline. The method he uses is to soak a rag with gasoline and hold the rag over his face while he inhales. He is frequently shown bending over to smell gasoline at gas station pumps and the opening in his car's gas tank.

When intoxicated, Wilson's speech becomes slurred, distorted, inappropriate, and at times nonsensical. His interpersonal relationship skills dramatically diminish to a level that he appears confusing, rude, and distant to the person speaking with him. Cinematic elements enhance the effects of his blurred vision, and in one scene he experiences hallucinations. Wilson vacillates from complete euphoria from the gasoline highs, which lead to grossly inappropriate behavior such as swimming in a lake where remote-controlled boats are racing, and cheerfully attempting to converse with other drivers on a highway, to severe agitation and anger outbursts evident when he is not huffing or is awakening from a blackout. Wilson becomes more isolated as the film progresses and would probably be completely isolated if it were not for a few dedicated and long-suffering friends. His judgment is impaired in other ways, like when he supplies two young huffing adolescents banned from gas stations with the intoxicant.

The consequences of his huffing include the loss of a new job, damage to important relationships, and his house burning down. Wilson is experiencing so much pain that he cannot bring himself to read his wife's suicide note; instead, he carries it around with him as a constant reminder of her death. Upon eventually reading it, he knows exactly what to do. Overall, this portrayal of a serious and severe addiction is realistic, honest, and not unduly melodramatic.

Cannabis

Marijuana is obtained from the hemp plant *Cannabis sativa*. The active ingredient in marijuana is the drug **tetrahydrocannabinol** (THC). The greater the THC content, the more potent the drug. The THC content of marijuana purchased illegally varies widely, but in general, THC levels have been increasing over the past 3 decades, and the marijuana used today is approximately five times stronger than that widely available on street corners and on college campuses in the 1960s. The resin of the *Cannabis sativa* plant can be used to produce **hashish**, a stronger form of the drug.

Marijuana has medicinal value, and it can be obtained legally for the treatment of some disorders. The drug enhances appetite and is often helpful in controlling the nausea associated with chemotherapy. Other physical effects include tachycardia, sedation, and psychomotor impairment. Like hallucinogens, marijuana can produce markedly varied psychological effects, depending on the mood and situation of the user. Most often, the drug produces mild euphoria, giddiness, and a general sense of well-being. However, at a different time and in a different setting, the same drug can produce marked apprehension or paranoia.

Examples of marijuana use can be found in countless films. One especially memorable scene involves a group of characters (played by Dennis Hopper, Peter Fonda, and Jack Nicholson) sitting around a campfire and smoking marijuana in *Easy Rider* (1969).

The low-budget, antidrug exploitation film *Reefer Madness* (1936), formerly titled *Tell Your Children*, became a cult classic among young people who smoked marijuana in the 1960s. Many people believed the film was tongue-in-cheek; however, it was meant to be a serious film. It begins by dramatizing marijuana with introductory text referring to it as "ghastly," a menace to society, a "deadly narcotic," and "public enemy #1," followed by various mock newspaper headlines on the dangers and societal consequences of marijuana use. The film turns to a parent meeting in which an expert speaks of the dangers to concerned parents and the need for a united front against marijuana; the bulk of the film (which runs like a satirical story) revolves around a group of normal-looking drug dealers who get adolescents addicted to marijuana by throwing wild jazz parties. Everyone who uses marijuana has serious deleterious effects – laughing foolishly and uncontrollable, extreme shakiness, intense anger and edginess, pacing, terror and panic, and paranoia; the eventual effects include sexual abuse, suicide, and murder. Marijuana is clearly portrayed as a drug that directly changes one's character for the worse. The film ends with the same parent meeting noting that these are the dangers and consequences of addiction and concludes with a finger pointing at the camera and an admonition that the viewer's children could be next. Clearly this film does little to educate the viewer about marijuana, its side effects, or consequences; if it were ever taken at face value, it would mislead and confuse viewers. The film does document the misconceptions that people have had in the past and the power of group contagion and its ability to produce paranoia and hysteria.

Several Cheech and Chong movies celebrate marijuana use and ridicule its classification as a narcotic. Other movies emphasizing marijuana include the Coen Brothers' noir *The Big Lebowski* (1998) and the outlandish comedy *Half Baked* (1998). Kevin Spacey portrays a psychologist who is addicted to marijuana in *Shrink* (2009). He uses the drug in the opening scene and throughout the film – while driving, when he first wakes up after hearing the alarm clock, while showering, and while shaving. He uses it at good times and bad – for example, as a celebration after hearing about the success of his self-help book and to cope with stress. He has regular interactions with his drug dealers and enjoys hanging out with them. In one scene, he smokes "laced" weed which ends up putting him in the hospital. He eventually decides to give up smoking and dumps all his drugs down the toilet.

Polysubstance Dependence

Polysubstance refers to the use of three or more groups of addictive substances (excluding nicotine and caffeine) with no substance predominating.

Naked Lunch (1991), the David Cronenberg film adaptation of William Burroughs' book, is fascinating albeit not always tightly linked to the novel. William Lee, the protagonist, is a polydrug addict trying to go straight. Unfortunately, both he and his wife are addicted to bug spray, and Bill's job as an exterminator makes it almost impossible for him to avoid this drug. The cinematic representation of visual hallucinations in *Naked Lunch* is especially fascinating.

In the B movie, *Shadow Hours* (2000), a young man working as a gas station attendant is lured back into drug addiction by a wealthy, mysterious writer who advises the young man he must go into the abyss before he can get back to sobriety. The two men visit dance clubs, drug fests, strip clubs, fight clubs, sadomasochism clubs, and torture events.

Leonardo DiCaprio plays a wall street investor in Martin Scorsese's *The Wolf of Wall Street* (2013), a film based on the true-life story of Jordan Belfort. Belfort uses dozens of different drugs, at every opportunity, and some critics have complained that the film glamorizes drug use.

> **"On a daily basis I consume enough drugs to sedate Manhattan, Long Island, and Queens for a month. I take Quaaludes 10–15 times a day for my 'back pain,' Adderall to stay focused, Xanax to take the edge off, pot to mellow me out, cocaine to wake me back up again, and morphine ... Well, because it's awesome."**
>
> **Jordan Belfort (Leonardo DiCaprio) brags about his drug use, in *The Wolf of Wall Street* (2013)**

Tobacco

The drug most often portrayed on television and in films is tobacco. Epidemiological studies suggest it is also our most lethal drug. The US Centers for Disease Control and Prevention (CDC) estimates that tobacco accounts for 480,000 deaths annually in the United States, approximately one out of every five deaths (CDC, 2022). Although fatality rates are only one index of the severity of a drug problem, none of the drugs typically regarded as our most *serious* are as dangerous as cigarettes.

In part because of the pain of withdrawal, less than 5% of smokers are successful in their attempts to stop smoking, although about 35% try to stop each year (and 80% express the desire to stop). Some of the symptoms associated with nicotine withdrawal include dysphoric or depressed mood, insomnia, irritability/anger, anxiety, difficulty concentrating, restlessness, decreased heart rate, and increased appetite or weight gain.

The morbidity and mortality associated with tobacco use have been underscored by a series of reports issued since 1964 by the Office of the Surgeon General. Partially in response to the massive public education efforts spearheaded by the surgeon general, numerous Americans have stopped smoking. In addition, the American Medical Association and the American Public Health Association have been very vocal in their opposition to tobacco use.

Various films depict people smoking cigarettes, and it is difficult to find a standard drama or comedy where smokers are absent. *Coffee and Cigarettes* (2003), directed and written by Jim Jarmusch, explores the use of nicotine and another addictive substance, caffeine. Several separate vignettes about different characters are connected only by conversation and the use of coffee and cigarettes, with some characters using the substances more compulsively than others. There are comical interactions between musicians Iggy Pop and Tom Waits, between actors Alfred Molina and Steve Coogan, between Bill Murray and two members of the Wu-Tang Clan (where Murray drinks coffee straight from the pot), and between Cate Blanchett and herself. Gwyneth Paltrow's character, Margo, is addicted to nicotine and finds creative ways to hide her smoking habits in *The Royal Tenenbaums* (2001). Ironically, the satirical comedy *Thank You for Smoking* (2005), while being about a lobbyist who works for a marketing organization supported by major tobacco companies, does not portray a single character smoking in the film. Aaron Eckhart plays Nick Naylor, a master of spin, who can argue that cigarettes should be made available for patients with cancer. In one scene, he is abducted and covered with nicotine patches; however, what keeps him alive is the fact that he has a high tolerance from heavy smoking (though he is never shown smoking).

Substances Depicted in Films

Countless films depict characters abusing substances, and at times it is unclear what substance is being abused. Rather than labeling the character as a "drug addict," it is more important to decipher the substance being abused, as each substance has different characteristics (e.g., tolerance, withdrawal, and intoxication levels). Table 10 helps make this clarification with some of the best portrayals of substance abuse in films. The number of psi's (Ψ) provides a rating scale, further emphasizing the pedagogical importance of each film – see Appendix 6 for details on this scale.

Table 10. Substances abused, with film examples

Abused substance	Film example(s)	Comments	Rating
Alcohol	*Leaving Las Vegas* (1995)	Nicholas Cage as an alcoholic giving up	ΨΨΨΨ
	Born on the Fourth of July (1989)	Tom Cruise as a bitter veteran	ΨΨΨΨ
	House of Sand and Fog (2003)	Jennifer Connelly relapsing	ΨΨΨΨΨ
	Smashed (2012)	Kate (Mary Elizabeth Winstead) and Charlie (Aaron Paul) have a relationship built around a mutual love of alcohol	ΨΨΨΨ
Heroin	*Pulp Fiction* (1994)	Uma Thurman mistakes heroin for cocaine in a classic Tarantino scene	ΨΨΨΨΨ
	Quitting (2001)	Deterioration and withdrawals	ΨΨΨΨ
Sedatives and hypnotics	*I'm Dancing as Fast as I Can* (1982)	Valium addiction	ΨΨ
Cocaine	*Traffic* (2000)	Dynamic, integrated drug film	ΨΨΨΨΨ
	Blow (2001)	Johnny Depp as a famous cocaine importer	ΨΨΨ
Crack cocaine	*MacArthur Park* (2001)	Gripping realism in LA	ΨΨΨ
Amphetamine	*Walk the Line* (2005)	Johnny Cash mixing uppers & song	ΨΨΨΨΨ
	Requiem for a Dream (2000)	Ellen Burstyn's role is unforgettable	ΨΨΨΨ
	Spun (2002)	Methamphetamine addiction and lifestyle	ΨΨΨ
Hallucinogens	*Fear and Loathing in Las Vegas* (1998)	Normalizes drug use	ΨΨ
Inhalants	*Love Liza* (2002)	Philip Seymour Hoffman depicts gasoline huffing	ΨΨΨ
Steroids	*The Wrestler* (2008)	Mickey Rourke pumping for a fight	ΨΨΨΨ
Cannabis (Marijuana)	*The Big Lebowski* (1998) *Shrink* (2009)	Jeff Bridges as "The Dude"; Kevin Spacey as an addicted psychologist	ΨΨ ΨΨΨ
Nicotine (Tobacco)	*The Royal Tenenbaums* (2001)	Gwyneth Paltrow's character tries to hide her smoking habits	ΨΨΨΨΨ
Caffeine	*Coffee and Cigarettes* (2003)	Vignettes with both substances	ΨΨΨ
Polysubstance	*Naked Lunch* (1991) *Dallas Buyers Club* (2013)	Bug spray and other substances Addiction to cocaine, methamphetamine, alcohol, gambling, and sex	ΨΨ ΨΨΨΨ

Note. The psi ratings are based on the author's subjective impression of the pedagogical and artistic value of each film.

Substance Abuse Recovery

Many films depict characters who are former substance abusers in full recovery (i.e., sustained full remission) and are not depicted as abusing or relapsing in the film. Support groups are a key component for many individuals' recovery from alcohol and drug abuse. The founding of AA, by Bill Wilson and Dr. Bob Smith, which has paved the way for countless support groups over the decades, is portrayed in *My Name Is Bill W.* (1986). An early Louis Malle film, *The Fire Within* (1963) is about a depressed, alcoholic, and suicidal writer searching for intimate connections. He has been recovering from alcohol dependence for a few months following a treatment called "the cure," which involved having him drink until he "bursts." He decides to continue to stay at the treatment center because he feels safer there – he is simply too frightened to face the world. Malle discloses that the film was transformative for him to make and that it helped him to "clear away the clouds" in his mind.

Rachel Getting Married

Rachel Getting Married (2008) is a Jonathan Demme film that realistically portrays substance abuse recovery, emphasizing some of the family dynamics that can erupt when an addict returns home from rehabilitation. Kym (Anne Hathaway) leaves rehab for a few days to spend time with her family as they prepare for the wedding of her sister, Rachel. The family tries to accept her, although they cannot help but be hypervigilant, cautious, and tense at times. Kym has an explosive temper, and many issues emerge from the past (e.g., Kym's tragic incident years ago when she was supposed to be looking after her baby brother – instead, she drove off a bridge while high on drugs, and he died in the accident) and from the present (e.g., tension with her sister's best friend competing for Rachel's attention). At times, Kym's sickness emerges, such as when she gives a rehearsal dinner speech that is tangential and self-involved (and embarrassing for her family) before taking time to comment on the wedding couple. Remarkably, Kym maintains her sobriety throughout the party-filled weekend and the tensions and issues that come up. However, after a physical and emotional fight with her mother, she drives her car off the road, perhaps as a suicide attempt (symbolically atoning for the egregious behavior years ago that killed her brother). It is never clear what drug(s) Kym is addicted to, but the film alludes to alcohol and other substances. Despite the dreary topic, the film illustrates the importance of humor and hope, two important character strengths for an addict or a family dealing with an addict. The film is also strong in its portrayal of support group meetings, which are accurately portrayed as real, supportive, and helpful for those who participate. Individuals share their personal stories, recite the 12 steps, and common 12-step adages (e.g., "keep coming back; it works if you work it"), prayers (e.g., the serenity prayer), and themes (e.g., life can feel boring without substances) are shared. Kym is persistent in her life with her family, which is critical for substance abuse recovery, and puts forth good effort; she is difficult yet endearing for both her family and the viewer.

The film *28 Days* (2000), discussed earlier in this chapter (see the section The Portrayal of Alcoholism in Films), also depicts 12-step support groups; in this case, it is AA. In addition to the serenity prayer, inspiring AA adages include: "It works, if you work it, you're worth it"; "God never gives us more than we can handle"; and "We are better, together." An alcohol–drug counselor (Steve Buscemi) is a recovering addict (also common for alcohol–drug counselors) and shares his story as a source of inspiration.

Another film depicting a character trying to make it outside of an institution (although in this case it is a release from prison) is Sherry Swanson (Maggie Gyllenhaal) in *Sherrybaby* (2006). Sherry has been clean for 2 and a half years following a 6-year heroin addiction; however, she has strong urges within 4 days of her release. She tries to do what is right, but she has few coping resources, and she still craves heroin. She functions out of a survivor mentality – she is manipulative, lacks empathy, and displays poor social judgment; she has significant inner rage and aggression and frequently slams doors and curses. In one scene, her emotionally aloof father takes advantage of her and fondles her breasts during a vulnerable moment; the stress associated with her father's sexual abuse triggers an immediate relapse. The opening song of the film repeats the line "There's an angel on my left but the devil's on my right," which describes the inner struggles of the addict, particularly those who are trying hard to maintain sobriety.

Benicio Del Toro plays a recovery alcoholic and ex-con who becomes a born-again Christian in *21 Grams* (2003). In *A Mighty Wind* (2003), Eugene Levy's folk singing character, Mitch, has flat affect, slowed speech and thought, and presents with wide-eyed expressions, each assumed to relate to significant drug abuse in his past.

The 12 steps are a set of guidelines that have become a tradition for numerous support groups. These important beliefs have revolutionized the conceptualization and treatment of substance abusers and have contributed to saving the lives of countless addicts. Table 11 lists the 12-step approach used by AA; however, the word "alcohol" can be easily replaced by "drugs"

Table 11. The 12 steps of alcoholics anonymous

Number	Step
1	We admitted that we were powerless over alcohol – that our lives had become unmanageable.
2	Came to believe that a Power greater than ourselves could restore us to sanity.
3	Made a decision to turn our will and our lives over to the care of God *as we understood Him*.
4	Made a searching and fearless moral inventory of ourselves.
5	Admitted to God, to ourselves, and to another human being the exact nature of our wrongs.
6	Were entirely ready to have God remove all these defects of character.
7	Humbly asked Him to remove our shortcomings.
8	Made a list of all persons we had harmed, and became willing to make amends to them all.
9	Made direct amends to such people whenever possible, except when to do so would injure them or others.
10	Continued to take personal inventory and when we were wrong promptly admitted it.
11	Sought through prayer and meditation to improve our conscious contact with God *as we understood Him,* praying only for knowledge of His will for us and the power to carry that out.
12	Having had a spiritual awakening as the result of these steps, we tried to carry this message to alcoholics, and to practice these principles in all our affairs.

Note. The Twelve Steps are reprinted with permission of Alcoholics Anonymous World Services, Inc. ("A.A.W.S."). Permission to reprint the Twelve Steps does not mean that A.A.W.S. has reviewed or approved the contents of this publication, or that A.A. necessarily agrees with the views expressed herein. A.A. is a program of recovery from alcoholism only – use of the Twelve Steps in connection with programs and activities which are patterned after A.A., but which address other problems, or in any other non-A.A. context, does not imply otherwise.

(Narcotics Anonymous), "sex," "gambling," "money," or "food," depending on the person's addiction.

Nonsubstance-Related Disorders

Gambling Disorder

Gambling disorder is the only nonsubstance-related disorder included in the DSM-5, and its inclusion is controversial. Many authorities believe we can only become addicted to substances; others argue that we can just as surely become addicted to gambling or other behaviors such as sex, shopping, exercise, and Internet gaming. The DSM-5 panel did not believe there was sufficient peer-reviewed evidence to set diagnostic criteria and classify these addictive areas as mental disorders. Nevertheless, as in the last edition of *Movies and Mental Illness*, we continue to provide examples of some of these addictive behaviors in this edition as well, following the discussion of gambling disorder.

Gambling disorder is diagnosed when four or more of nine criteria are met over a 12-month period. Criteria include the need to gamble with increasing amounts of money; restlessness or irritability when attempting to cut back or stop gambling; repeated unsuccessful efforts to stop gambling; preoccupation with gambling; gambling to relieve guilt, depression, or anxiety; lying to conceal the full extent of one's involvement with gambling; and jeopardizing or losing a significant job, relationship, or opportunity because of gambling. The prototypical gambler with this diagnosis has made several unsuccessful attempts to stop gambling, gambles with increased amounts of money, "chases" losses, lies to cover up the problem, and escapes from personal problems or internal pain by gambling.

Gambling is frequent in movies. Although not all these films depict characters who would meet the criteria for a gambling disorder, one film is a particularly compelling example – *Owning Mahowny* (2002).

Owning Mahowny

The film *Owning Mahowny* is based on true events that occurred in Toronto between 1980 and 1982; the movie tells the story of a man who stole millions of dollars from his employer to support his gambling addiction. He eventually served a 6-year prison term for fraud.

Philip Seymour Hoffman stars as Dan Mahowny, a man described at the onset as having three lives: (1) a public life, (2) a private life, and (3) a secret life. Mahowny has a loving, dedicated girlfriend, and at work he is the youngest in his position as a loan officer, someone described as having an "impeccable record" and "excellent judgment." His secret life involves his serious, self-destructive gambling problem.

Psychologist: "How would you rate the thrill you got from gambling, on a scale of one to 100?"
Dan Mahowny: "Um ... a hundred."
Psychologist: "And what about the biggest thrill you've ever had outside of gambling?"
Dan Mahowny: "Twenty."

***Owning Mahowny* (2002)**

Mahowny accumulates a debt of US $10,300 by placing bets with shady bookies. He decides to write fake loans to pay off his debt. He then begins to gamble with this money at casinos to pay off the debt more quickly. He flies to Atlantic City numerous times to gamble. Along the way, he tells various lies to his girlfriend Belinda (Minnie Driver) and his boss to keep his secret life hidden. While gambling, Mahowny appears to be in a trance – he is extremely focused and absorbed in the experience, and he loses track of time. His losses progressively increase; he loses US $15,000 one night and then US $100,000 another night, unsuccessfully attempting to chase losses by doubling up on his bets. His denial is obvious to the viewer, such as when he frequently convinces himself that he is "in the zone." Mahowny deteriorates psychologically and behaviorally, and his behavior becomes erratic, his appearance disheveled and unkempt, and his self-care is poor. At one point, he gives a friend money to hold, making him promise not to give it back to him no matter what; soon Mahowny is screaming at his friend to "give me my money and stay away from me." Scenes like this dramatically display the intensity and power of this addiction. Mahowny is alone and depressed, he does not get enough sleep, and in one scene he falls asleep while driving. The film is a dramatic depiction of the despair of someone caught in the throes of a gambling addiction.

The casino realizes its potential profit and goes to great lengths to keep Mahowny gambling, following him; watching him; trying to entice him; offering him food, drinks, a free hotel stay, and women; and even sending him a friend to shadow him and keep him there. Mahowny rejects the women and alcohol; he is referred to as a purist in his gambling addiction because he does not mix sex, alcohol, or drugs with his gambling.

The addiction worsens when Mahowny takes his girlfriend on a special vacation and then neglects her; when she confronts him about this while he is gambling, he simply begs for a "few more minutes," choosing gambling over love and sex. This scene illustrates the huge disparity that has developed in their relationship; she continues to be focused on the relationship, while his addiction leaves him too engrossed in gambling to even care what happens to her.

In another movie based on a true story, *Two for the Money* (2005), a young, savvy football expert, Brandon Lang (Matthew McConaughy) is hired by Walter Abrams (Al Pacino) to work in a fast-paced business as a gamblers' advisor (helping gamblers make good bets on football games). Walter is a recovering pathological gambler of 18 years – though he is clearly experiencing similar highs from devoting his life to helping gamblers. Much of his life relates to gambling – he bets on his salesmen, he watches each football game closely, and his income is based on how successful his clients are. He sees the successes of Brandon, who beats the odds and predicts game outcomes at an 80% success rate, becomes attached to his new protégé, and obsesses about building an empire around Brandon. Walter is unable to quit, focused on riding the excitement he experiences when working with Brandon. Walter displays typical gambler self-sabotaging behavior, taking increasingly high-risk bets. He continues despite unmistakable evidence of a serious heart condition that he treats with medication. The film depicts a Gamblers Anonymous meeting in which one member speaks honestly of his struggles; however, Walter attempts to take advantage of the man by giving him his business card, tempting the man to reclaim his addiction. The deep sense of inherent defectiveness and shame common to this addictive behavior is portrayed convincingly in the film.

Oscar and Lucinda (1997), based on the 1988 Booker Prize–winning novel by Peter Carey, portrays two outcasts who connect through pathological gambling. Oscar Hopkins (Ralph Fiennes) copes with his anxiety disorder by gambling. He won his first bet on horse racing (this is common for those with the disorder) and is unable to stop gambling. He is quite distressed by his behavior, even breaking his own strict adherence to keeping the Sabbath holy and free of gambling. He rationalizes his gambling, arguing that belief in God is a gamble, so how could gambling not be accepted by God? Another rationalization is that he is not gambling for personal gain, because he gives away his winnings. When he has periods of sobriety during which he can stay away from gambling, he lives in constant fear that he will revert to his old habits and ways. Lucinda Lepastrier (Cate Blanchett) stays up all night gambling, tries to hide her behavior from others, and uses gambling to cope with loneliness. Oscar and Lucinda make a pact to not gamble or lead one another in that direction, and they attempt to put their energy productively into a floor-washing competition. Soon they break the pact and make the ultimate gamble – their inheritance.

In *Dinner Rush* (2001), a cook at an upscale New York City restaurant is unable to control betting on sports teams. This significantly affects his work performance, interpersonal relationships, and his ability to focus. He exhibits the common gambler's behavior of attempting to chase his losses. The impact on his life and functioning is clear: He continues to upset more people around him, and eventually he puts his life in danger.

In *21* (2008), an MIT student is accepted into Harvard Medical School but is unable to pay the steep tuition, so he reluctantly takes part in an illegal card counting operation, led by his teacher (Kevin Spacey). The teacher crosses many boundaries as he promotes this illegal activity, manipulates his students, fixes grades in his course, and orchestrates some nasty university politics. While the film is not particularly strong in portraying elements of pathological gambling, it does illustrate a common dynamic gamblers and other addicts experience – a double life. In addition to his normal life as a student, the protagonist creates a gambler's (or card counter's) life in which he spends time in exciting cities, takes on a variety of high-roller personas, and becomes invested in a new peer group. As is the case in many of these instances, all is well until the two lives converge. This film is based on a true story about six smart MIT students who took on the Las Vegas casinos and walked away with millions.

Sex Addiction

Sexual addiction is increasingly recognized as a growing problem in contemporary society. Patrick Carnes, one of the world's leading authorities on sexual addiction, has written extensively on the topic, addressing sexual compulsivity (*Don't Call It Love* and *Out of the Shadows*), Internet sex addiction (*In the Shadows of the Net*), and each of the paraphilias discussed in Chapter 14. There are movies that illustrate each of these clinical problems. Holt (2023) addresses the dividing line between enthusiastic sexual expression and addiction, challenges the medical framework used to treat sexual addiction, and offers a sex-positive approach to treat hypersexual behaviors.

I Am a Sex Addict (2005) is an autobiographical documentary film that emphasizes the role of compulsivity in sexual addictions – for the director–actor, the acting out was compulsive sex with prostitutes and compulsive masturbation. The importance of 12-step recovery groups (e.g., Sex Addicts Anonymous) is highlighted, as are several unhealthy and healthy coping strategies. A better movie, *De-Lovely* (2004), documents the numerous compulsive homosexual affairs of Cole Porter and the conflict he felt about reconciling these affairs with his very genuine love for his wife.

Good films on sex addicts will not only reveal the behaviors of the addict but also the consequences and realities of the decisions they make. Characters who are presented as male sex addicts include Joe Taylor (Ewan McGregor) in *Young Adam* (2003), the title characters in *Alfie* (2004) and *Don Juan DeMarco* (1995) (played by Jude Law and Johnny Depp, respectively), and Sammy Horn (Michael Des Barres) in *The Diary of a Sex Addict* (2001, Spain). *Don Jon* (2013) depicts the life of a man addicted to masturbation; he initially views this as a harmless habit, but eventually sees that it interferes with his ability to form a mature, adult loving relationship. The belief that there were deleterious health effects from compulsive masturbation lasted well into the middle of the 20th century (Hodges, 2005).

The classic Luis Buñuel film *Belle de Jour* (1967) portrays a married woman who takes a job as a prostitute. The film illustrates female sexual addiction and depicts the creation of a double life. As the protagonist sinks deeper into her new lifestyle and becomes more comfortable with her lies, she becomes unable to extricate herself. Other female sex addicts are depicted in *Swimming Pool* (2003), *Leap Year* (2011), and in one segment of *Personal Velocity* (2002); and Juliette Marquis plays the role of a confident, self-assured, and enthusiastic porn star in *This Girl's Life* (2003). A memorable female sexual addict can also be found in *Diary of a Nymphomaniac* (2008). This serious film reveals the loneliness, suffering, and emotional turmoil common to sexual addicts.

> **"I need sex. I see a man and I need him."**
>
> **An insatiable sexual appetite described in *Diary of a Nymphomaniac* (2008)**

On Line (2002) examines the serious problem of Internet addiction. In the film, a man is abandoned by his fiancée; consequently, he spends countless hours on the Internet, partly to help his roommate with a popular pornographic website designed to link people together with their fantasy. At the end of the film, the viewer learns that the fiancée had been a person online with a webcam whom he had watched all day and had never personally met. His compulsive fantasy had become so ingrained that it shaped his personal reality. The film accurately portrays the intense loneliness, isolation, and lack of intimacy or connection that Internet addicts and Internet sex addicts experience.

An important feature of sex addiction is the secrecy of the behavior. The link between secrecy and sexuality is explored in *Far from Heaven* (2002), *Unfaithful* (2002), and *The Secret Lives of Dentists* (2002). Film directors Pedro Almodóvar, Peter Greenaway, and John Waters are especially known for their creative depiction of sexuality, sexual addiction, and paraphilias (the last of which are a group of disorders discussed in Chapter 14).

Shame

Shame (2011) offers a memorable portrayal of sexual addiction. The film depicts Brandon (Michael Fassbender), the male protagonist, as someone whose suffering and sexual addiction are clear. The viewer can see all the signs and symptoms associated with alcohol or drug abuse, such as intoxication, dependence, and withdrawal, but in this case, sex is the substance. Brandon becomes high on sex, dependent in that he needs more frequency to meet his needs, and experiences withdrawal symptoms when he does not have access to sexual partners (e.g., negative isolation, irritability, explosiveness, loneliness, risk taking, and self-defeating behavior). He attempts to connect with others in a more meaningful way; however, when these attempts fail, he returns to the pursuit of meaningless, anonymous sex with women, multiple partners, and men, to cope with his failures.

Brandon's longest relationship lasts 4 months. After going on a second date with a woman and beginning to connect with her, this connection becomes too substantive and real for him, and he becomes impotent. He then curls up in a fetal position, cannot look the woman in the eye, and refuses to speak to her. His pathology worsens when he is faced with the stressor of his younger sister dropping in to temporarily live with him in his apartment. He treats her badly, is constantly irritable toward her, and he becomes physically abusive, explosive, and dismissive. The ending scene might be viewed as ambiguous to someone unfamiliar with sexual addiction as it shows Brandon making eye contact with an attractive woman on the subway whom he had seen before; she is married yet their protracted eye contact is clearly flirtation.

The final shot shows a serious looking close-up on Brandon's face that leaves the viewer wondering whether he has made a substantive change and whether he will resist temptation or if he will continue to pursue his addictive behavior. Yet, this also reveals one of the danger points of sexual addiction – Brandon is breaking a boundary by visually lingering and prolonging his eye contact. This is one step too far for the sexual addict. He does not display a coping strategy or quickly turn away, but instead he does what sex addicts call rubbernecking. This suggests he has made no progress and his sexual addiction is still a problem. Frank Lachmann (2016) wrote a detailed review of *Shame* published in *Psychoanalytic Psychology*; it examines the struggles of the two protagonists using the theories of Joseph Lichtenberg, Otto Kernberg, and Heinz Kohut.

Spending/Shopping Addiction

Maxed Out (2006) is a documentary that looks at the impulse control problem of compulsive spending. The film focuses on the problem of credit card debt, the cyclical patterns therein, and the factors that contribute to the development of this disorder. The film notes that a family living in today's world has less money for the essentials than a family living in the 1970s, that US $9,200 is the average American credit card debt, and that 10 million people filed for bankruptcy over a recent 10-year period. Some of the consequences of excessive credit card debt include depression and suicide. Problems with impulse control often play a significant role in the development of compulsive spending and the accumulation of massive debt.

International Film: Substance-Related and Addictive Disorders

The film *Quitting* (2001, China), by Chinese director Zhang Yang, depicts heroin abuse and withdrawal, intermixing both through flashbacks. A young man, Hongsheng, at one time a famous actor, is living with his parents to help him deal with his heroin addiction. He is bitter and verbally abusive toward his parents. Through flashbacks, the viewer learns of his deterioration due to heroin dependence and the ramifications of its abuse; his career is in shambles, he loses several friends, develops a delusional obsession with John Lennon, hallucinates, and has several anger outbursts.

Vodka Lemon (2003, France/Italy/Switzerland/Armenia) is a slow but engaging comedy-drama with an interesting and subtle vibrancy, from exiled Iraqi Kurd director, Hiner Saleem. The film takes place in Armenia, post-USSR, and depicts the romance of a widowed man and woman after they meet during their daily, separate trips to visit the graves of their former spouses. The background of this minimalist film is alcohol. It seems that all of the townspeople drink alcohol as a coping strategy that is accepted as an established part of daily life. Everybody drinks all the time, hence the need for the only store in town – a "vodka lemon" shop where people purchase vodka by the bottle. No unruly behaviors or symptoms result from the extensive alcohol use, barring one exception, and it is unclear if this incident is alcohol related.

No Such Thing (2001, Iceland/US), a film by independent auteur Hal Hartley, tells the story of a young woman (Sarah Polley) who goes to investigate the story of a "monster" who has killed a film crew (including her cameraman-fiancé) in a remote Icelandic village. She tracks down the monster, who is an isolated, grotesque alcoholic, and befriends it, bringing it home to America even though the monster breathes fire, kills people at will, and is described as indestructible, beyond science and unable to even commit suicide. It is interesting to reflect on what the monster (and alcohol) represents, as well as the dichotomies that arise – hope/fear, good/evil, comedy/tragedy, denial/reality, and humanity/inhumanity.

The film *16 Years of Alcohol* (2003, UK) portrays Frankie, an alcoholic, who as a child of an alcoholic observed his father's infidelity, alcoholism, and violence, and grew up to repeat the same patterns. The film pays homage to another film that involves violence and substance abuse, *A Clockwork Orange* (1971, US/UK); *16 Years of Alcohol* includes a scene in which an intoxicated gang of hoodlums severely beats up a bartender in a tunnel, similar to what Alex and his droogs do in an early scene in the classic Kubrick film. Women with alcoholism are portrayed in *Rain* (2001, New Zealand) and *Walking on Water* (2002, Australia).

Gervaise (1956, France) is a depressing film based on an Emile Zola novel about the deterioration of individuals and families because of alcohol addiction. Gervaise is a young, beautiful, and lame laundress who is left by her lover, Lantier, with their two boys. She then marries Coupeau, a roofer. Shortly thereafter, Coupeau falls off a roof, and although he recovers, he is too fearful and lazy to return to work, so he avoids work and turns to drinking full-time. His alcohol dependence threatens Gervaise, potentially ruining both their relationship and the new laundering business she has opened. He drinks day and night, prioritizes drinking over all other activities, becomes angry at any attempts to get him to slow down, makes poor decisions, displays a disregard for his children and the impact of his behavior on them, and he begins to treat Gervaise badly. He invites her former husband, Lantier, to join them at a special event party and then to live in their already-crowded home. Coupeau, in a fit of alcohol rage, ends up physically destroying the home and Gervaise's business. He later dies from alcoholism, but not before he has destroyed the family. In the final scene, the kind and gentle Gervaise is shown sitting haggard in the middle of the day at a pub, unkempt, unresponsive, and drunk for the first time in her life, paying no attention to her nearby daughter who is filthy and starving.

Mads Mikkelsen stars in *Another Round* (2020), a Danish film that depicts the lives of four middle-aged men who agree to try to maintain a blood alcohol level of 0.05%. They use alcohol to dull the pain and tedium of their quotidian lives. Initially, they find drinking during the day is adaptive; for example, a high school teacher discovers his classes are more interesting and he is more engaged when he is a little drunk. However, the film's acting is better than the film's premise, and viewers are not well served by any film that promotes daily drinking.

Gambling disorder is depicted in several international films. For example, the protagonist, Fugui, in *To Live* (1994, Hong Kong/China) is addicted to gambling and, chasing his losses, he loses everything. His family goes through major difficulties and many of their hardships are due to his gambling disorder.

The movie *2046* (2004, China) is Kar Wai Wong's portrayal of pathological, or at least excessive, gambling in which the protagonist loses most of his money playing cards. As is typical with many addicts, the gambler in this film is addicted to both card playing and sex.

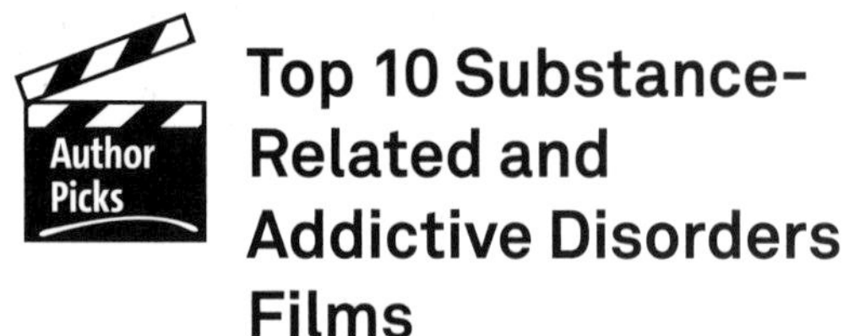

Top 10 Substance-Related and Addictive Disorders Films

Substance Use Disorders

Days of Wine and Roses (1962)
Clean and Sober (1988)
Leaving Las Vegas (1995)
Requiem for a Dream (2000)
Spun (2002)
Ray (2004)
Crazy Heart (2008)
Flight (2012)

Nonsubstance-Related Disorders

Owning Mahowny (2002)
Shame (2011)

Chapter 12

Neurocognitive Disorders

If we talk for too long, I'll forget how we started and the next time I see you I'm not gonna remember this conversation. I don't even know if I've met you before. So, if I seem strange or rude or something ... I've told you this before, haven't I?

Leonard Shelby in *Memento* (2000)

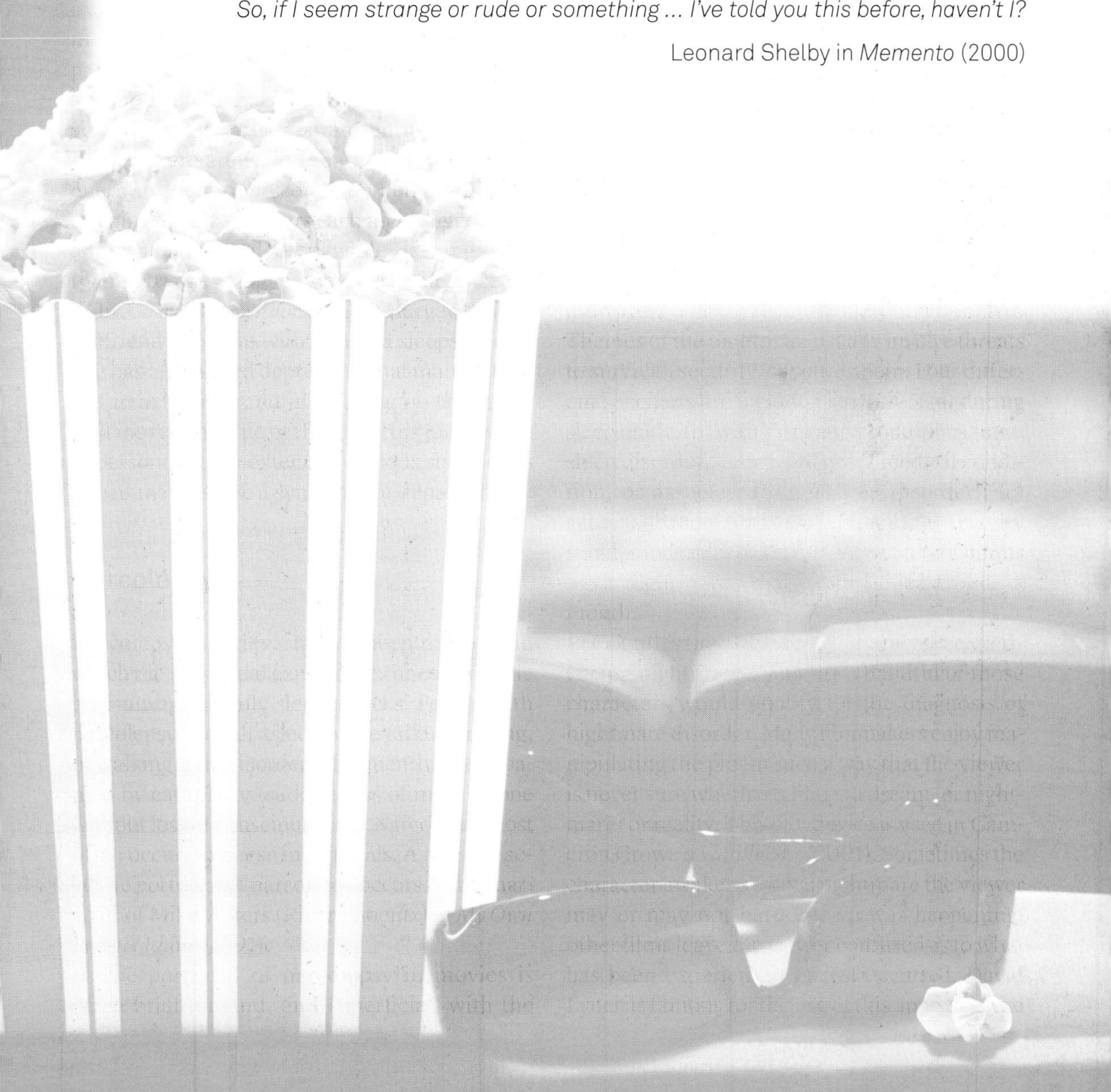

Neurocognitive Disorders

This chapter describes conditions that result in a significant deficit in cognition or memory and impact the individual's ability to function normally. **Neurocognitive disorders** are unique in the DSM-5 because the underlying pathology is almost always known, and the etiology of the disorder can usually be established (e.g., stroke, trauma, Alzheimer's disease). These disorders are always acquired rather than developmental, and they represent a decline from a previous level of functioning.

Neurocognitive disorders result in impairment in one or more of six cognitive domains: complex attention, executive functioning, learning and memory, language, perceptual-motor abilities, or social cognition. A deficit in **complex attention** might result in an individual who experiences significant distress in situations in which there are competing stimuli (e.g., multiple conversations occurring at the same time a television is playing). A person with deficits in **executive functioning** might need help in planning the day's activities or focusing on more than one task at a time. Deficits in **learning and memory** are clearly apparent in the film *Memento*; other examples might include repeating oneself often and or having trouble recalling three or four items after a brief delay on a mental status examination. Deficits in the **language** domain can be either expressive or receptive; patients with difficulties in this domain may use vague language and be unable to remember the names of celebrities, casual friends, or common household objects. Problems in the **perceptual-motor** domain result in difficulties navigating in unfamiliar territory, and difficulty using tools or driving a car. Perceptual-motor defects may worsen at sunset ("sundowning"). Finally, examples of problems in the **social cognition** domain include inappropriate social behavior (e.g., sexually touching the breast or leg of a nurse) or wandering in a cold, winter environment without proper clothing.

Neurocognitive disorders are first classified as major or mild; after that, specific codes are provided to indicate the presumed or known etiology of the disorder (e.g., major neurocognitive disorder due to Alzheimer's disease). The DSM-5 recommends that deficits be documented by standardized neuropsychological testing whenever possible.

The overall prevalence for major cognitive disturbance is estimated to be 1–2% at age 65 and as high as 30% by age 85. The overall prevalence for mild cognitive disturbance is 2–10% at age 65 and 5–25% by age 85 (American Psychiatric Association, 2013). The DSM-5 categorization of mild cognitive disturbance has been widely criticized because it pathologizes what many consider to be normal cognitive changes that accompany aging. Writing about the medicalization of ordinary life, Alan Frances notes,

> In the early 1980s, about a third of Americans qualified for a lifetime diagnosis of mental disorder. Now about half do. ... Some people think these are underestimates – more carefully done prospective studies double the lifetime prevalence. If you believe the results, our population is almost totally saturated with mental disorders. (Frances, 2013, p. 104)

Dementia

The term **dementia** refers to a collection of brain disorders characterized by memory disturbance, impaired judgment, and personality change. Insidious onset and gradual deterioration of cognitive abilities characterize dementia. Although some authorities believe the term should be applied only to those conditions that are nonreversible, the more customary practice is to use the term descriptively, without any implications for prognosis. Hence, brain dysfunctions from causes as diverse as nutritional deficiencies and Cushing's syndrome can be diagnosed as dementia.

In 2021, there were 55 million people (about twice the population of Texas) worldwide living with dementia, and this number is expected to double in the next 20 years (Shin, 2022). The *World Alzheimer Report 2021* notes, "Dementia is now the 7th leading cause of mortality globally and ... one of those with the highest cost to society. There is a perfect storm gathering on the horizon, and governments all over the world should get to grips with it" (Gauthier et al., 2021).

Dementia can be caused by any number of medical conditions, or they can be substance induced. Some of the more commonly known medical causes are cerebrovascular disease, head trauma, Parkinson's disease, HIV infection, Huntington's disease, frontotemporal lobar degeneration, and Creutzfeldt-Jakob disease. *Awakenings* (1990) offers excellent demonstrations of dementia and catatonia due to Parkinson's disease. The film is based on the experience of neurologist Oliver Sacks, best known as the author of *The Man Who Mistook His Wife for a Hat*.

The single leading cause of dementia is **Alzheimer's disease**, responsible for at least 60% of all cases of dementia. Alzheimer's is a public health problem of enormous dimensions, and one that is becoming an increasing problem as the average life span steadily increases. Advances in medical science and public health have resulted in dramatically longer lifespans around the world; unfortunately, for many of us our bodies will outlive our minds.

The brains of patients with Alzheimer's disease are demonstrably different from those of age-matched controls, and they contain **senile plaques** and **neurofibrillary tangles.** Although some neuronal loss is universal with aging, the brain of the Alzheimer's patient shrinks at a more rapid rate. Psychological tests are often the best indicators of the presence of Alzheimer's disease, especially in the early stages, as these patients will often maintain excellent social skills and use these skills to disguise the marked problems they develop with their memory. Other early signs of the insidious onset of Alzheimer's disease include diffuse generalized anxiety and inappropriate social behavior. An official diagnosis of Alzheimer's cannot be made until after the individual has died and an autopsy has been performed.

Other forms of dementia include **vascular dementia, dementia with Lewy bodies** (diagnosed at autopsy in Robin Williams), and **frontotemporal dementia**. The boundaries between different forms of dementia are indistinct and mixed forms often coexist (WHO, 2022). Dementia clearly increases the risk for exposure and contracting COVID-19 (Tahira et al., 2021), especially for elderly people in nursing homes, and preliminary data suggests that COVID-19 may enhance the likelihood of developing dementia (Hariyanto et al., 2021).

Gerritsen et al. (2014) used the IMDb to identify 23 movies released between 2000 and 2014 that dealt seriously with dementia. They concluded that "the clinical picture of dementia portrayed in fictional movies is mild and may be misleading" (p. 276).

The Alzheimer's Project (The Memory Loss Tapes) (2009) is a poignant and important documentary that integrates education with seven vignettes of individuals at various stages of Alzheimer's disease, along with their families. The vignettes help the viewer appreciate the variability in presentation and the extent of the degeneration caused by the disease. The film addresses both the suffering caused by Alzheimer's and challenges for the caregiver, including adult–child role reversal, wandering, loss of independence, and the grieving process.

Sunset Blvd. (1950) offers a classic portrayal of the lack of insight, the confusion, and the delusions that accompanied the dementia of an aging movie star. *The Iron Lady* (2011) is a biopic about the life of Margaret Thatcher; the sections of the film most relevant to this book show her as an elderly and demented woman having imaginary conversations with her deceased husband, Denis, played by Jim Broadbent. Jeffrey Tambor plays a demented client cheated by his attorney (Paul Giamatti) in *Win Win* (2011). Frank Langella plays Frank, a retired jewel thief with early dementia, in *Robot & Frank* (2012); Frank's son buys a robot to take care of his father, but this purchase has unforeseen consequences. *Quartet* (2012), directed by Dustin Hoffman, is a charming film about life in a home for retired musicians.

Some of the residents appear to have mild dementia.

> **"She was the greatest of them all. You wouldn't know, you're too young. In one week, she received 17,000 fan letters. Men bribed her hairdresser to get a lock of her hair. There was a maharajah who came all the way from India to beg one of her silk stockings. Later he strangled himself with it!"**
>
> **Max Von Mayerling commenting on the life of Norma Desmond, a washed-out movie star in *Sunset Blvd.* (1950)**

Paul Giamatti portrays Barney Panofsky, a small-time television producer in *Barney's Version* (2010). Barney would likely be diagnosed with substance-induced neurocognitive disorder. There seems to be a clear relationship between Barney's alcohol dependence and not only his languishing life and poor relationship skills, but also his failing memory. At first, he displays subtle forgetfulness for something he should have remembered, but he soon begins to deteriorate into what is clearly progressive dementia.

Iris

Iris Murdoch was one of the greatest writers and thinkers of the 20th century. She wrote 26 novels, six philosophical works, and several plays. The content and purpose of her intricate works can be simplified in one phrase: She wanted to teach humans how to be free and how to be good. Murdoch was a deep, complex, and gifted thinker. It is bitterly ironic to see such a brilliant and well-used brain deteriorate with dementia, as we observe in the film *Iris* (2001).

Some of the early signs of Iris's major cognitive disorder (i.e., dementia) are indicated in her experiences of memory loss – she would forget what she had just said and frequently repeat herself. She then began to talk to herself, exhibit blank stares and flat affect, display further language disturbance (i.e., babbling), and lose her ability to care for herself. Her writing, which had always flowed easily and extensively, came to be constricted and limited, and she would frequently sit at a table with blank pages in front of her. She stopped cleaning her house or caring about her appearance. The film depicts the development of increasingly serious symptoms and shows Iris (Judi Dench) in danger on several occasions – for example, jumping out of a moving car, trying to control the steering wheel when on the passenger side, and leaving her house to wander in the middle of traffic. The viewer sees Iris slowly retreat into a world of her own; at first, it is for brief periods, and she comes back to reality, but she experiences increasingly longer periods of isolation and quiet. She does emerge from her world at times to say, "I love you," to her husband in powerful cinematic moments.

The film *Iris* also speaks deeply to the challenges and responses of the caretaker of someone with Alzheimer's. John Bayley (Jim Broadbent), Iris's loving husband, joins Iris in denying her disease at first, saying, "she disappears into a mystery world ... [but] she always comes back." As he continues to watch his wife display more serious symptoms, his emotions catch up with him, and he screams out in anger. Several scenes show John Bayley deep in despair as he sits alone, helpless to do anything to stop the disease. He sadly repeats the phrase: "Love will soon be over." It is fascinating to watch him experience predictable stages of grief: denial, anger, questioning/challenging, sadness, and finally acceptance when he takes Iris to a nursing home. The movie asks a fundamental philosophical question, "What makes us human?" (Liao, 2011).

> **"She's in her own world now, perhaps that's what she always wanted."**
>
> **John Bayley on his wife's illness, in *Iris* (2001)**

Love and Dementia

Two other memorable films have portrayed husbands coping with their wives' dementia: Sarah Polley's *Away from Her* (2006) and Nick Cassavetes' *The Notebook* (2004). The first film portrays an Ontario couple who have been married for 44 years; the wife, Fiona (Julie Christie), is becoming increasingly forgetful, and she and her husband Grant (Gordon Pinsent) are acutely aware that whatever is happening, it is something far more serious than benign senescent forgetfulness. In addition to her forgetfulness, Fiona finds herself engaging in irrational behavior (e.g., putting a frying pan into the freezer after it is washed, being unable to retrieve the word "wine"). She realizes that she needs nursing home care, and she does not want to be a burden on her husband. The husband, a college English professor guilty about his history of infidelity during the marriage, eventually capitulates to this plan, agreeing that his wife needs to be in a setting in which she can confront her illness "with a little bit of grace." When Grant takes Fiona to the nursing home, he accompanies her to her room and they have sex ("I would like to make love," she says, "and then I'd like you to go. Because I need to stay here and if you make it hard for me, I may cry so hard I'll never stop"). No visitors are allowed for the first 30 days of residency in the nursing home, allegedly to facilitate the new resident's adjustment. (Visitor restriction is very unlikely in any nursing home.) During this time Fiona becomes romantically, albeit not sexually, involved with another resident in the facility. Part of the cinematic tension in the film involves the fact that it is never entirely clear whether Fiona's interest in Aubrey, the other resident, is simply due to her lost memories of her marriage and husband or a willful way to get back at Grant because of his history of extramarital affairs with his students. The film is also remarkable for the persistence and unconditional love of Grant – not dissimilar to John Bayley's – in visiting Fiona regularly despite her obvious intimate involvement with another man.

The Notebook (2004) stars Gena Rowlands and James Garner as a married couple coping with the wife's dementia. Allie Calhoun (Gena Rowlands) is in a nursing home; her husband, Duke, has moved in with her and spends each day reading to her out of a notebook. We later learn that she has written the story of their romance and life together so that she can continue to relive it even as her illness progresses. A series of flashbacks is used to tell the story of their initial love affair, separation, and eventual reunion. The film is sentimental and unduly romanticizes Alzheimer's, but it illustrates the dramatic loss of memory that is one of the disease's defining features.

The Savages

Laura Linney and Philip Seymour Hoffman play siblings confronting the dilemma of caring for an aging, demented father in *The Savages* (2007). The two siblings have never been close to their father, but when his girlfriend dies, decisions about his care are foisted upon them. They are initially notified of their father's condition when he begins writing on the wall with his own excrement; for many demented individuals, loss of bowel and bladder control become powerful metaphors for the "loss of self" associated with diseases like Alzheimer's. The movie illustrates how depressing some nursing homes can be – even expensive ones – and it provides a compelling example of the stress associated with the decisions children often must make when a parent develops dementia.

"People are dying, Wendy! Right inside that beautiful building right now, it's a fucking horror show! And all this wellness propaganda and the landscaping, it's just there to obscure the miserable fact that people die! And death is gaseous and gruesome, and it's filled with shit and piss and rotten stink!"

Jon Savage confronting his sister in *The Savages* (2007)

The tempo of life in a nursing home is captured in *Assisted Living* (2003), a pseudo-documentary filmed with real residents of a real nursing home in Kentucky. In one scene, Todd, an underequipped, pot-smoking orderly amuses himself by pretending to be God on phone calls with a resident. Despite Todd's antics, it is also clear that he cares about many of the residents, and he goes out of his way to help one of the residents who is quickly deteriorating with Alzheimer's.

Still Alice

In the 2014 film, *Still Alice,* Julianne Moore plays the role of Dr. Alice Howland, a brilliant 50-year-old linguist and a beloved professor. She has a cheerful home life with her husband and her three children; however, she realizes something is wrong when she begins to experience word-finding difficulty. It is a time in her life when she is at the height of her career, but after a visit with a neurologist she realizes that she – and her family – are going to have to cope with a diagnosis and the reality of early onset dementia. Because she is highly intelligent, she can hide her worsening symptoms, but only for a while. Alice's husband, played by Alec Baldwin, is minimally supportive, refusing to take a year off from his academic life to spend with Alice. She plans her own suicide, leaving instructions for how to do it and where to find the pills on a video on her laptop computer; however, when the time comes, she fails because the task is simply too difficult. She is especially concerned about her children's future because she realizes the condition is hereditary. (There are three specific gene mutations associated with early-onset Alzheimer's; if you inherit one of these mutated genes, you are at elevated risk for the disorder.) The movie ends with Dr. Howland giving one last speech at an Alzheimer's society conference. There is a special poignancy in the film because the codirectors, husband and wife team Richard Glalzer and Wash Westmoreland, know firsthand how devastating a neurodegenerative disease can be, because Glalzer was coping with amyotrophic lateral sclerosis (ALS) while making the film. Julianne Moore won an Academy Award for Best Actress for her role in the film, and she dedicated the award to Glalzer who died in 2015.

"All my life I've accumulated memories – they've become, in a way, my most precious possessions. The night I met my husband, the first time I held my textbook in my hands. Having children, making friends, traveling the world. Everything I accumulated in life, everything I've worked so hard for – now all that is being ripped away. ... But this is not who we are, this is our disease. And like any disease it has a cause, it has a progression, and it could have a cure. My greatest wish is that my children, our children – the next generation – do not have to face what I am facing. But for the time being, I'm still alive. I know I'm alive. I have people I love dearly. I have things I want to do with my life. I rail against myself for not being able to remember things – but I still have moments in the day of pure happiness and joy. And please do not think that I am suffering. I am not suffering. I am struggling. Struggling to be part of things, to stay connected to whom I was once. So, 'live in the moment' I tell myself. It's really all I can do, live in the moment. And not beat myself up too much... One thing I will try to hold onto though is the memory of speaking here today. It will go, I know it will. It may be gone by tomorrow. But it means so much to be talking here, today, like my old ambitious self who was so fascinated by communication. Thank you for this opportunity. It means the world to me."

Julianne Moore as Dr. Alice Howland giving a goodbye speech at an Alzheimer's Society event, in *Still Alice* (2014)

The Father

Anthony Hopkins and Olivia Colman star as father and daughter in *The Father* (2020), one of the most remarkable films released in 2020, and one of the most realistic and heart-wrenching depictions of the paranoia, confusion, and memory loss associated with dementia (see Figure 39). Hopkins is an octogenarian who forgets his own daughter's name, can't recognize her husband (who has lived in the same flat with him for 10 years), and becomes convinced that someone is plotting to take away his home. He wonders why his younger daughter doesn't come to visit him, not realizing that she died many years earlier. However, his social skills and sense of humor remain relatively intact, allowing him to partially hide his rapidly declining mental prowess. This seeming disconnect between intact social skills and profound memory loss is a common feature of dementia.

> **Anthony: "I feel as if I'm losing all my leaves."**
> **The Woman: "Your leaves?"**
> **Anthony: "Yeah."**
> **The Woman: "What do you mean?"**
> **Anthony: "The branches and the wind and the rain. I don't know what's happening anymore."**
>
> **Anthony Hopkins attempting to make sense of his all too rapidly changing reality, in *The Father* (2020)**

Hopkins won a Best Actor Oscar for his role in this film. It was his second award; the first was for *The Silence of the Lambs* (1991). The second award made Hopkins the oldest living recipient of an acting Oscar (Christopher Plummer had won the Best Supporting Actor Oscar at the age of 82 for *Beginners* [2010)] a decade earlier). Director Florian Zeller insisted on Hopkins for the role; the character's name in the film is Anthony, and his birthday is December 31, 1937, Sir Anthony's actual date of birth.

Dementia Versus Depression

One of the most important tasks confronting clinicians working with older patients is the difficult discrimination between dementia and **clinical depression**. Appropriate diagnosis is critical in these cases so that a depressed patient will not go untreated because they are inappropriately believed to be suffering from Alzheimer's disease (Drag & Bieliauskas, 2019). In most cases, the two disorders will present in ways that are different enough for the alert clinician to distinguish between them. For example, Alzheimer's has a more insidious onset, whereas depression

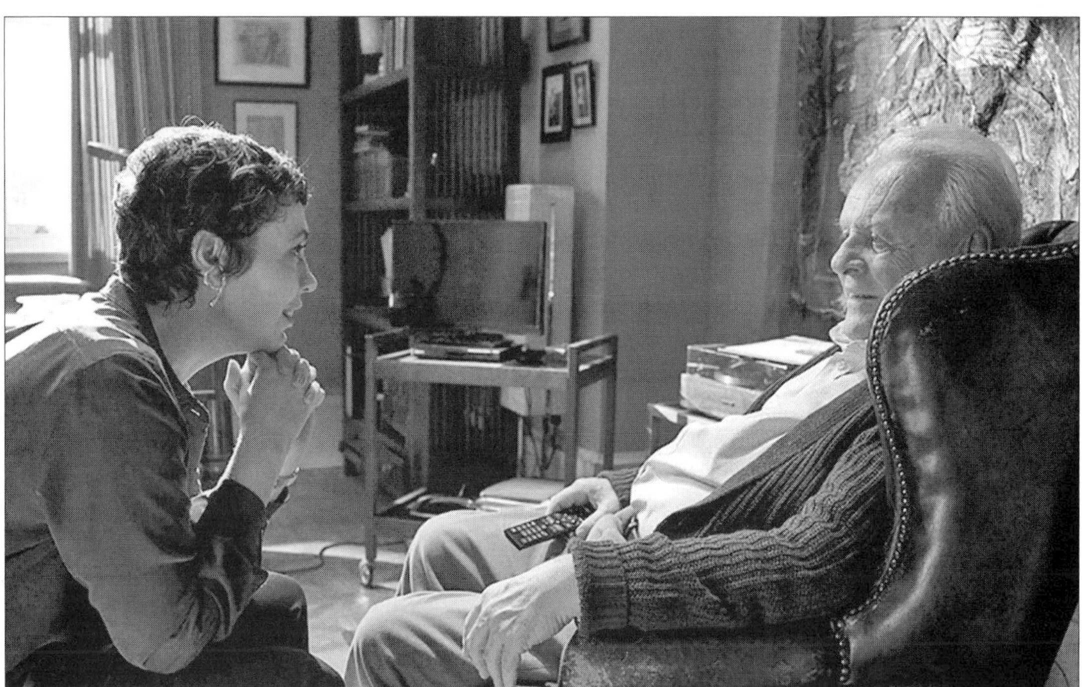

Figure 39. *The Father* (2020, Les Films du Cru, Film4, F Comme Film, Trademark Films, Cine@, Simon Friend Entertainment, Viewfinder). Produced by Daniel Battsek, Phillippe Carcassonne, Cleone Clarke, Lauren Dawson, et al. Directed by Florian Zeller.

may come on more rapidly. The patient with Alzheimer's will always have genuine cognitive deficits and have trouble learning new tasks. The depressed patient will lack motivation and may have trouble concentrating but should be able to learn, although slowly. The depressed patient is also more likely to experience loss of appetite and a fluctuating course, and they are far more likely to have a history of affective illness. In addition, depressed patients tend to acknowledge and sometimes even exaggerate their problems. In contrast, patients with Alzheimer's are far more likely to cover up their difficulties, deny that they are having problems, and may be euphoric. Finally, in the later stages of the illness, patients with true dementia will often have abnormal brain images and EEGs.

Another important film portraying Alzheimer's disease is a made-for-TV movie, *Do You Remember Love?* (1985), in which Joanne Woodward plays a college professor who develops Alzheimer's disease. Woodward's portrayal is sensitive and moving. There is also a memorable scene between Jane Fonda's character and her mother in *Agnes of God* (1985). Fonda plays Dr. Martha Livingston, a psychiatrist who goes to visit her mother in a nursing home. The scene opens with the mother watching a children's cartoon program. The disoriented mother gets Martha confused with her younger sister, who had died years earlier in a convent.

Jessica Tandy very convincingly portrays an old woman who eventually develops Alzheimer's disease and is placed in a nursing home in *Driving Miss Daisy* (1989). Tandy won an Academy Award for her performance in this film. A television series titled *The Last Days of Ptolemy Grey* (2022) stars Samuel L. Jackson as a man who undergoes a controversial and dangerous treatment to regain enough memory to avenge the killing of his nephew.

Treatment for Dementia

It is discouraging for patients, loved ones, and providers to realize that most dementias – and especially dementias of the Alzheimer's type – are progressive and irreversible, and their clinical course inevitably runs downhill. However, although cure is not possible, there are some interventions that hold promise for enriching the lives of patients with these disorders. Hallam and Shaw (2020) found that both movies and music benefit patients with dementia, and their Cinema, Memory and Wellbeing project used "a combination of archive film footage of Liverpool and clips from Carmen Miranda's spectacular Hollywood musicals to trigger memories and spark reminiscences among older, care home audiences (p. 37). These authors have provided a tool kit for occupational therapists and others working in nursing homes or memory care units.

Agency is one of the key elements in effective care for patients with dementia. In what has become recognized as classic studies, Ellen Langer and Judith Rodin examined the role of choice and responsibility in older adults in residential care facilities. As described by Mallers et al. (2014):

> In their early research, residents at a nursing home were randomly assigned to 2 groups: 1 group was told they could arrange their furniture as they wanted, go where they wanted, spend time with whom they wanted, and so forth and were given a plant to care for; the other group was told that the staff was there to take care of and help them, including watering a plant given to each of them. During this study, and 18 months later, residents who were given control and personal responsibility had improved health; among those for whom control had not changed, a greater proportion had died. Since these original studies, research has continued to support the need for personal control as we age. (Mallers et al., 2014, p. 67)

There are challenging legal, ethical, and due process issues that arise in the treatment of patients with dementia. For example, these patients are often not capable of giving informed consent for medication, medical procedures, or sexual intimacy, and they are at heightened risk for financial or sexual exploitation. These problems are compounded with patients who have limited English-language proficiency. In 2017,

Luis Gomez was sentenced to 23 years in prison for sexually violating two women, one of whom he had helped transfer from her bed to the bathroom (CNN, 2017). There were numerous other reports of sexual misconduct in numerous other nursing homes. CNN noted,

> Claims like theirs are often dismissed as drug-induced hallucinations, signs of dementia or attempts by lonely residents to get attention. And even when the cases of nursing home residents get to court, they can fall apart when victims' memories prove unreliable – or they are no longer alive to testify. (CNN, 2017)

Delirium

Delirium refers to the rapid onset of confusion and disorganized thinking (a "clouding" of cognition) and is often characterized by rambling, incoherent, or inappropriate speech. Emotions are often out of line with expectations; for example, the delirious individual may be anxious or euphoric in situations where these reactions would be inappropriate. Delirium can also cause illusions, hallucinations, or misinterpretations of sensory stimuli; for example, a doctor's look of concern may be perceived as extreme anger by the delirious patient. Most films depicting dementia will show some examples of delirium as well (e.g., *Iris*).

Marcontonio (2017), writing in the *New England Journal of Medicine*, noted,

> One third of general medical patients who are 70 years of age or older have delirium; the condition is present in half of these patients on admission and develops during hospitalization in the other half. Delirium is the most common surgical complication among older adults, with an incidence of 15 to 25% after major elective surgery and 50% after high-risk procedures such as hip-fracture repair and cardiac surgery. (Marcontonio, 2017, p. 1456)

Delirium most often (but not always) results from a disturbance of the metabolism of the brain, and causes can include infections, insufficient oxygen levels, ionic imbalances, vitamin deficiencies, and kidney disease. One common cause of delirium is either acute intoxication with – or withdrawal from – drugs. **Delirium tremens** is a frequent problem for alcoholics with a history of problem drinking. Patients experiencing delirium tremens ("the DTs") become disoriented, hallucinate, and display marked tremors. Other symptoms may include intense fear, fevers, and sweating. The intensity of delirium tremens is vividly portrayed in Billy Wilder's film, *The Lost Weekend* (1945), and in Nicholas Cage's character in *Leaving Las Vegas* (1995).

Amnesia

Patients with **amnesia** display marked impairment of short-term memory with intact long-term memory and preserved intellectual functioning. In its extreme form, the disorder results in the total inability to learn new information. A patient with an amnestic syndrome will be unable to recall a doctor's name, no matter how many times it is presented; simple learning tasks such as recalling the names of four objects become virtually impossible. The patient will be able to *repeat* the four items, suggesting intact understanding of the task and good receptive and expressive language skills; however, after dozens of trials the patient will still be unable to recall the four items from memory.

Patients with amnestic syndromes will sometimes **confabulate** and present detailed and plausible explanations for their obvious inability to acquire new information. The patient who cannot remember four numbers for more than a few seconds will explain that they were never any good at math, and the patient in a psychiatric hospital may say they are there because of problems with his kidneys. One of my patients with amnestic syndrome was asked four times during a 1-hr, taped interview what he had had for breakfast that morning. The patient responded by supplying four different menus during the interview, each equally plausible. On each occasion, he had absolutely no recollection of being asked this question earlier in the interview.

One of the most often encountered amnestic syndromes is **Wernicke-Korsakoff syndrome**. Patients with this disorder have great difficulty with new learning, fail to recall recent experiences, exhibit gait disturbances secondary to cerebellar dysfunction, and display a variety of ocular disturbances, including impaired conjugate gaze. This condition is found in older alcoholics after many years of substituting the nutritionally empty calories of alcohol for the protein, carbohydrates, vitamins, and fat found in a normal diet. The disorder is particularly related to deficiencies in thiamine (vitamin B_1), and some public health experts have recommended enriching spirits with vitamins in the same way we enrich bread. Although this could be done with minimal cost, the distillers have not been enthusiastic about this procedure, despite its potential benefit to alcoholics.

Other films have portrayed characters with amnesia, including *Spellbound* (1945), *Mirage* (1955), *Anastasia* (1956), and *Desperately Seeking Susan* (1985). *Eternal Sunshine of the Spotless Mind* (2004) is about a man who attempts to have memories of his girlfriend, Clementine, erased (after discovering that she has done the same with *his* memories). As his memories begin to fade, he realizes he still loves Clementine, and he attempts to subvert the process. The 1983 film *The Return of Martin Guerre* creatively explores the limits of memory and the extent to which it can be influenced by motivation and need. Dissociative amnesia (see Chapter 7) needs to be differentiated from amnesia caused by a substance or general medical condition (including head injuries).

Memento, Memory, and Viewer Empathy

Memento (2000) is a psychological thriller that centers on the life of Leonard Shelby (Guy Pearce), a man with **anterograde amnesia** that makes it impossible for him to transfer new experiences into long-term memory. The movie chronicles the psychological and social complications associated with this memory disorder and this man's efforts to get revenge for past offences against himself and his wife. This is the second film of director Christopher Nolan (see also *Following* (1998) and *Insomnia* (2002), discussed in Chapters 8 and 14, respectively), who amazingly created this incredibly complex film in 25.5 days. Nolan's most recent film, *Oppenheimer* (2023), portrays the mental health challenges associated with the life of a brilliant physicist known as the father of the automic bomb.

Memento is a cleverly edited film that begins at the end of the story and works backward: The color portions of the film progress backward in 10-minute segments, and these clips are juxtaposed with black-and-white clips that move forward in time.

Leonard has lost his wife and is struggling to avenge her loss by finding the killer. He does not remember that he is the person who killed her when she tested his amnesia by having him administer repeated doses of insulin until she went into shock and coma, and subsequently died. Leonard believes that Sammy Jenkins injected the insulin. Leonard also believes that Sammy Jenkins was malingering (with anterograde amnesia) when Leonard was a claims investigator. Leonard fuses his story with Sammy's and distorts reality. The film cleverly gives the viewer clues to the truth that Leonard is both denying and forgetting. For example, in one scene, one frame of Leonard is superimposed on the character of Sammy Jenkins, and it is unclear who is in the hospital. Another example involves a flashback at the end of the film (the beginning of the story) of Leonard and his wife lying in bed together; the camera focuses briefly on the words "I've Done It" tattooed on his chest, as if to give the viewer one final piece of direct evidence.

The film does a brilliant job of depicting the suffering of someone with a memory disorder and illustrates the painstaking discipline and detail-oriented approach necessary for someone to cope with such a disorder using compensatory strategies (e.g., tattoos and Polaroid photographs of people and places). Leonard's use of tattoos to record key facts in his life is illustrated in Figure 40.

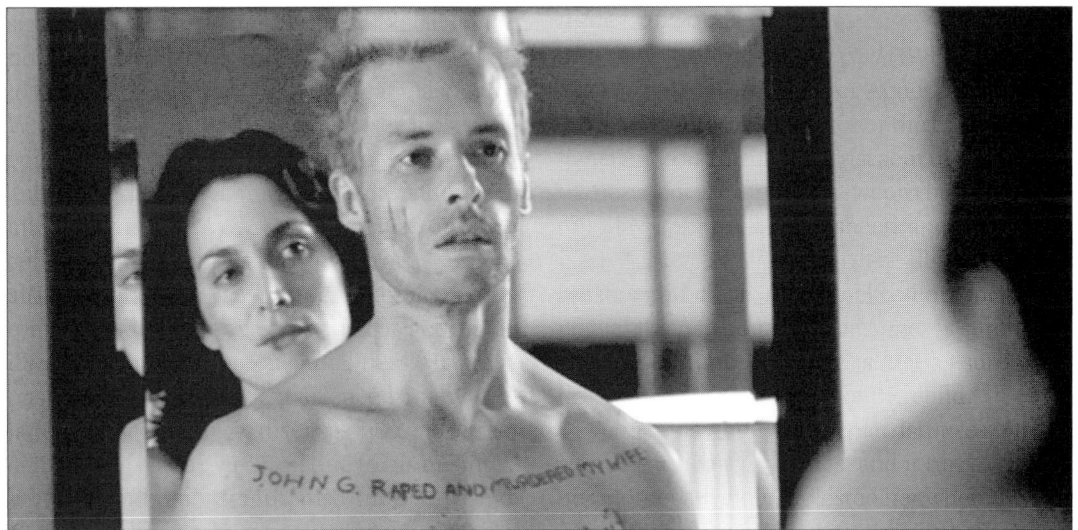

Figure 40. *Memento* (2000, Newmarket Capital Group, Team Todd, I Remember Productions, Summit Entertainment). Produced by Christopher Ball, Elaine Dysinger, Aaron Ryder, Emma Thomas, et al. Directed by Christopher Nolan.

As if Leonard is not facing enough as a man who has lost the ability to consolidate memories, he must also cope with others determined to take advantage of his illness, manipulating, and lying to him. He has no one he can rely on or trust, including himself, as those who help only "use" him (e.g., for drug deals, for murderous revenge, or to make some extra money, all at his expense). Eventually, he is confronted with a harrowing truth. A corrupt police officer, Teddy, tells him: "You don't want the truth ... you create your own truth." The viewer eventually comes to realize that Leonard has not known the truth from the beginning, and he is preparing to kill an innocent man.

The most remarkable aspect of this film is its ability to force the viewer to experience the world as someone with anterograde amnesia experiences it. The viewer experiences the protagonist's struggles, distortions, lapses, questions, and emotions as they try to put together the scenes going backward, while making sense of the juxtaposed black-and-white scenes that are going forward. The viewer is constantly reevaluating and rethinking what has just been seen. The film demands both strong concentration and memory from the viewer, who almost immediately begins to appreciate the majesty of something most of us take for granted: the ability to convert new information into long-term memory. Viewers experience the protagonist's confusion, in trying to decide who is manipulating whom, and they feel what the amnestic patient feels when trying to sort through conflicting distortions of time, place, person, and situation. Viewers question their own memory and must also adopt some cognitive strategy to keep all of the confusing aspects of the film straight. They also begin to lose trust in the film's characters, particularly the "unreliable narrator" (Leonard) who comes by the role honestly due to his anterograde amnesia.

This film's complexity extends further to address existential themes about our search for meaning, the loss of identity, the role of truth and lies (both to oneself and to others), the problem of coping with a cognitive disorder, and the ubiquitous power of denial.

Head Trauma

The link between head injuries, amnesia, and movies is strong, and numerous films have been produced in which someone experiences head trauma and becomes amnestic to their past – they can start over from scratch, they can try to rediscover life with a deeper appreciation, other people can manipulate them, etc.

Although not given a separate rubric in the DSM-5 nomenclature, it is common to see references to **dementia pugilistica** (punch-drunk syndrome) in the professional literature and in the medical charts of aging boxers. These patients, after a lifetime of repeated blows to the head (with concomitant brain injuries), often develop difficulty with movement and a tremor like that found in **Parkinson's disease**. They develop slurred speech and diminished mental agility, and they become especially sensitive to the effects of alcohol. Dramatic mood swings (referred to as **emotional lability**) are common, and these individuals are quick to become angry, engage in fights, and become paranoid. Many of these symptoms can be seen in Robert De Niro's portrayal of Jake LaMotta in *Raging Bull* (1980).

The repetitive head blows associated with boxing have been shown to cause brain injuries that may not be detected by magnetic resonance imaging (often referred to simply as MRI). There is evidence that microstructural damage exists in professional boxers when compared with an age- and sex-matched control group (Zhang et al., 2003).

> **"You don't understand! I could've had class. I could've been a contender. I could've been somebody, instead of a bum, which is what I am."**
>
> **Terry Malloy (Marlon Brando) in *On the Waterfront* (1954)**

This problem is so serious that the American Medical Association and other professional organizations have called for the elimination of professional boxing as an organized sport. Indeed, it is hard to find redeeming social value in a sport in which the express purpose is to damage the brain of an opponent. However, boxing remains a popular American pastime, and this popularity is reflected in films such as *The Great White Hope* (1970), *The Harder They Fall* (1996), *The Joe Louis Story* (1953), *Kid Galahad* (1937/1962), *On the Waterfront* (1954), *Requiem for a Heavyweight* (1962), the ever-popular *Rocky* films (1976, 1979, 1982, 1985, 1990, 2006), and many others.

When visualizing brain injuries, it is useful to remember that the cranium is a closed, solid container, and the brain is soft and consists of a jelly-like substance that moves inside the skull when the head is struck. The brain is fragile, albeit well protected by the skull and meninges (the three layers of protective covering found between the skull and brain).

Head injuries are usually classified as **concussions**, **contusions**, or **open-head injuries**. Concussions occur when the brain is jarred, and amnesia and loss of consciousness are common consequences. Impaired memory and concentration, headaches, fatigue, anxiety, dizziness, and irritability characterize the postconcussion syndrome. Contusions occur when the brain is bruised, most often because of an impact between the brain and the skull. Contusions produce more serious neurological consequences than concussions and can result in death. Contusions are characterized as **coup injuries** if the damage is at the site of impact (e.g., at the point where a baseball bat hits the skull). **Contrecoup injuries** occur opposite the point of impact. They most often result from acceleration injuries (such as occur when a moving head hits a stationary steering wheel). Open-head injuries occur when the skull is hit with sufficient force to open it and expose the underlying neural tissue. Open-head injuries from missile wounds are common in wartime, and much of what we know about the organization of the brain is the result of examination of soldiers injured in battle.

The effects of head injuries often become apparent only hours or days after the initial injury. This occurred in the case of actress Natasha Richardson, daughter of Vanessa Redgrave and wife of Liam Neeson. Richardson died 2 days after suffering a head injury because of a skiing accident during a Quebec holiday. Paramedics at the scene were turned away because the actress reported that she felt fine and was in no distress.

The Vow (2012) depicts amnesia following a head injury from a car accident that had left the protagonist, Paige (Rachel McAdams), in a coma. Paige is unable to remember anything after a certain point in her past (i.e., around the time she moved to New York City and later met her future husband) up to the day of her injury. She can recall everything prior to that point (e.g., high school friends and sweethearts, family interactions), and she can create new memories. This is based on a true story in which the woman was never able to regain the memories she lost. The film emphasizes the strengths of love and perseverance as her husband, Leo, works hard to support her and help her remember him. *The Business of Amateurs* (2016) is a documentary film examining the National Collegiate Athletic Association (NCAA) and the organization's exploitation of student athletes. Numerous players are interviewed and, as described by Reiss (2017):

> A good part of the movie addresses the devastating, permanent effects of multiple sports concussions. Not infrequently, serious and at times malignant depression and suicidal impulses emerge. While the film stands by itself as an important documentary regarding issues confronting student-athletes, the film can help prevent important formative psychosocial experiences of many youth from becoming "hidden histories" during clinical mental health evaluation and treatment later in life. (Reiss, 2017)

Raging Bull

Raging Bull (1980) is a Martin Scorsese film starring Robert De Niro (who won an Academy Award for Best Actor for his role in this film), Cathy Moriarty, and Joe Pesci. This engrossing drama portrays the life of Jake LaMotta (De Niro), a prize fighter confronted with the need to find purpose and meaning in life once he leaves the ring. LaMotta's marriage fails, his wife takes their children with her, sexual jealousy drives a wedge between him and his brother, and he is forced to mutilate and then hock the jewels in the belt he received for winning the world middleweight championship. The viewer is never certain whether LaMotta is a pathetic or a heroic figure, but the film ends with reconciliation between the two brothers and with the protagonist successfully performing a Broadway reading of the works of several notable authors. The recitation of one of Marlon Brando's monologues from *On the Waterfront* (a 1954 Elia Kazan film about the life of a down-and-out prizefighter) is Scorsese's way of paying homage to another great filmmaker and provides a dramatic conclusion for the film.

Raging Bull is replete with examples of LaMotta's poor judgment. Two especially vivid examples are his failure to defend himself in the final round of a fight with Sugar Ray Robinson (Johnny Barnes) and his decision to let two 14-year-old girls into his nightclub after each girl kisses him. Impaired judgment is common in aging prizefighters. It is also likely that LaMotta's history of repeated blows to the head (concussions) contributed to his sexual jealousy and paranoia and was responsible for the slurred speech he exhibits in the film as he ages.

Other Films Dealing With Head Trauma

In addition to *Memento* (2000), many films show characters who display serious neurological symptoms, such as the amnesia, that can result from a head injury. One of the best is David Lynch's challenging film *Mulholland Drive* (2001), which begins with an automobile accident. The amnestic female survivor, Rita (a name she takes from a movie poster) finds refuge in the condominium of an aspiring Hollywood actress, Betty (Naomi Watts). The two women befriend each other, and Betty takes a particular interest in helping Rita (Laura Harring) find answers to the questions regarding her identity. The already unique film takes a major surrealistic twist, and the viewer is left to either accept the events as they are portrayed or challenge them as illusions. Like director Christopher Nolan in *Memento*, Lynch creates a rich atmosphere that allows the viewer to experience the confusion and discomfort of amnesia as the person affected increasingly becomes disoriented to person, time, place, and situation. Lynch does not attempt to give answers or insights into amnesia but to depict the experience for a character and to give a particular experience to the viewer. It is the viewer who is challenged, like the amnestic character, to accept the film as an experience; this is more important than a pat explanation for what is happening in the film. This is reinforced at the film's conclusion (and final word) when a character on stage looks at the viewer and, with a finger to her lips, says, "Silencio."

In contrast to the unforgettable depiction of anterograde amnesia in *Memento*, *The Majestic* (2001) depicts **retrograde amnesia.** Jim Carrey plays disenfranchised screenwriter Peter Appleton, who, upon being accused of communist ties, goes for a drive away from his Hollywood home. His car topples over a bridge into a river, and he subsequently develops retrograde amnesia after he hits his head on a rock in the river and is washed up on the shore of a small town. The townspeople mistake Peter for a former townsperson, Luke Trimble, who had gone to war many years ago, and the town proclaims Peter (now Luke) a hero, someone who had been lost for almost a decade after going to war. Not remembering his past, Luke identifies with many of the townspeople and rebuilds the local theater. He does not go through the pain, confusion, mental torture, and frustration that one would expect with retrograde amnesia. Instead, Luke readily accepts his new role and does not seriously challenge himself to figure out where he was over the previous 10 years. A theory of "double amnesia" is hypothesized, whereby he could have gone to war, experienced PTSD, and memory loss, reestablished his life for years as a writer, and then, upon getting involved in an accident, experienced amnesia a second time.

Two 1991 films address the complexity of amnestic symptoms that result from head injuries: *Regarding Henry* and *Shattered*. *Regarding Henry* is a Mike Nichols film starring Harrison Ford as a high-powered attorney who suffers a major traumatic head injury. After coming out of a coma, he discovers that his life can never be the same. There are interesting scenes in a rehabilitation hospital, and the viewer gets some sense for the sequelae of a head injury. However, the film is flawed by an unrealistic presentation of the deficits following head injury and by the simplistic assumption that someone's personality could be *improved* by a head injury. In *Shattered*, an architect undergoes extensive reconstructive surgery of his face following an automobile accident. Amnesia symptoms mix with his memories (that may or may not be distorted) and the inconsistent stories relayed by various people in his life.

The Lookout (2007) presents the story of Chris Pratt (Joseph Gordon-Levitt), a talented and handsome high school hockey player who sustains a serious closed head injury after a car wreck that resulted from a school prank (drunk driving with the lights off on the night of the high school prom). The result of the injury is like that seen in *Memento,* in that Chris is unable to remember things for any extended period. As a result, he winds up as a bank janitor, the only job he can handle. He displays classic signs of head injury, coping with these problems by repeating a kind of mantra for people with head injuries: **Ritual. Pattern. Repetition**. One of the characteristics of head injuries is poor judgment, and the head-injured Chris Pratt displays extremely poor judgment as he gets caught up in plans to rob the bank at which he works. We also see his constant reliance on a notebook in which he frequently writes notes to himself, and he has put labels on almost everything in his apartment; these are valuable **compensatory strategies** (coping strategies) for people with head injuries. He also has problems with impulse control; for example, when meeting with his case worker, Chris blurts out "I want to fuck you." However, he is clearly acutely aware of his deficits, and at one point he notes, "I call tomatoes lemons, [but] I know it's not right."

Tell Me Who I Am (2019) is a compelling documentary about twin brothers, one of whom, Alex, loses all his memories after a near fatal motorcycle accident at age 18 that resulted in a significant traumatic head injury. Alex, the twin who sustained the injury, recognizes his twin brother Marcus after his injury, but he cannot recognize either of his parents and he has no other memories; this is an example of profound retrograde amnesia. However, while autobiographical memory has been totally erased, procedural memory is intact (e.g., Alex retains the ability to ride a bicycle and tie his shoes). Marcus looks after his brother and helps him reconstruct his past but leaves out significant – and harrowing – details about their shared past. At age 32, Marcus reveals that both boys had been victims of sexual abuse by their mother and her friends up until around age 14; however, the details of the abuse are not fully shared until age 54. The story will help viewers understand retrograde amnesia and learn more about pedophilia.

Brain Tumors

Aberrant behavior and abnormal sensations and perceptions can result from brain tumors **(neoplasms)**. The specific behaviors that result will vary across individuals as a function of lesion site, size, type, and rate of growth. Brain tumors often, but not always, result in headaches and seizures. However, fewer than one out of a thousand people who have headaches will be found to also have a brain tumor.

An individual's premorbid personality will determine how they react to a brain tumor. About half of all patients with brain tumors first complain of psychiatric or behavioral symptoms, especially when the tumor involves the frontal or temporal lobes. Hallucinations, depression, apathy, euphoria, social impropriety, and personality change can all result from brain lesions.

Patients who have **frontal lobe lesions** are likely to display personality changes. They may be passive, apathetic, depressed, and slow to respond. Paradoxically, frontal lobe lesions also may result in irritability and problems with anger control. **Temporal lobe tumors** are often misdiagnosed as psychiatric disorders, and this is especially likely to occur in those cases that result in **psychomotor seizures**. These tumors can produce hallucinations, stereotyped movements, feelings of unreality, and intense fear. Reports of **déjà vu** (feeling you are re-experiencing a former experience) and **jamais vu** (feeling that familiar settings and situations are now very strange) are common with temporal lobe tumors. Patients with **parietal lobe lesions** often report abnormal sensory experiences (e.g., smelling burning rubber), may have difficulty with simple copying tasks, and may exhibit **anosognosia** (denial of illness). **Occipital lobe tumors** produce few psychological symptoms, but these lesions may result in visual field defects.

"Brain cells. Why do healthy normal cells go berserk and grow wild? ... Nobody knows. But we call them cysts and gliomas and tumors and cancers. And we operate and hope to cure with a knife and half the time we don't even know the cause. Our patients have faith in us because we're doctors ... Someday, somebody will discover a serum that will be to these growths what insulin is to diabetes and anti-toxins to diphtheria, and maybe earn his title of Doctor of Medicine."

Dr. Frederick Steele describing his sense of professional impotence, in *Dark Victory* (1939)

Dark Victory (1939) stars Bette Davis as a 23-year-old socialite whose headaches and double vision are eventually diagnosed as symptoms of a glioma by her physician, Dr. Frederick Stelle. Other symptoms include loss of feeling in her right hand, inability to distinguish objects by touch alone, and eventual blindness. The physician and patient fall in love, but he hides her diagnosis. Eventually she discovers she only has 6 months to live. *Dark Victory* was reported to be Bette Davis's favorite film; it was nominated in 1940 for an Academy Award for Best Picture (then called "Outstanding Production"); however, it had formidable competition that year, including *Mr. Smith Goes to Washington*; *Wuthering Heights*; *Stagecoach; Goodbye, Mr. Chips*; *The Wizard of Oz*; *Ninotchka*; *Of Mice and Men*; and *Gone With the Wind* (the winner).

In *The Bucket List* (2007), Morgan Freeman plays the role of Carter, a blue-collar mechanic with cancer that eventually becomes metastatic, spreads to his brain, and kills him. Before he dies, he develops a friendship with Edward, played by Jack Nicholson, and the two men share a series of adventures in which they collaboratively attempt to do everything on their bucket lists (things to do before they "kick the bucket"). Edward survives his cancer, lives to be 81, and has his ashes buried alongside Carter's at the top of the Himalayas.

Rhapsody in Blue (1945) is a biopic about the life of George Gershwin who died at the age of 38 from a glioblastoma multiforme. Gershwin's first symptom was passing out while playing the piano; other symptoms included blinding headaches and olfactory hallucinations (he complained about the acrid smell of burning rubber). In *The Green Mile* (1999), a film based on a novel by Stephen King, John Coffee (Michael Duncan) plays a death row prisoner who heals the prison warden's wife by transferring her brain tumor to the body of a sadistic guard.

Stroke

A **cerebrovascular accident** (CVA), more commonly known as a **stroke**, occurs when there is an inadequate supply of blood and oxygen to the brain. Strokes are characterized by sudden onset and are often fatal. Cerebrovascular disease is currently the third leading cause of death in the United States, following heart disease and cancer. Twenty individuals will experience CVAs for everyone who develops a brain tumor.

Infarctions occur when arterial blood flow is blocked. This can occur when a piece of fat or cholesterol becomes lodged in a vessel. This sudden blockage of blood flow is called an **embolus.** Blood flow can also be impeded by the gradual buildup of **atherosclerotic plaque** along the inside of a vessel, resulting in a **thrombus.** Vessels sometimes burst, and the resulting cerebral hemorrhage can be life-threatening. Only about 20% of patients survive a cerebral hemorrhage. An **aneurysm** occurs when part of a vessel balloons and threatens to burst. Signs of a ruptured aneurysm include painful headaches, nausea, and vomiting.

Transient ischemic attacks (TIAs) are mini strokes that last for less than 24 hours. Many patients who experience TIAs will go on to have actual strokes. Other risk factors for CVAs include diabetes, heart disease, and the use of oral contraceptives in women who also smoke. The patient experiencing a TIA will become disoriented, confused, and sometimes amnestic.

In John Steinbeck's novel *The Grapes of Wrath,* Grandpa Joad dies from a stroke. We do not actually see the old man die in John Ford's film adaptation, *The Grapes of Wrath* (1940), but there is a memorable scene in which his relatives bury him alongside the road because they are too poor to do anything else. Tom Joad (Henry Fonda) writes a short, poignant note to leave at the grave: "This here is William James Joad, died of a stroke, old, old man. His folks buried him because they got no money to pay for funeral. Nobody kilt him. Just a stroke and he died."

David Lynch's *Blue Velvet* (1986) opens with a man watering his yard. As we watch, he has a stroke and falls to the ground. His dog comes over and proceeds to drink out of the hose, and at this point the viewer becomes aware that this will not be an ordinary movie.

Amour (2012) depicts the challanges associated with caregiving after one member of a loving couple experiences a stroke.

Epilepsy

People with **epilepsy** experience uncontrollable attacks of abnormal neuronal activity. These brainstorms can result from a variety of causes, and it is critical to remember that epilepsy is a *symptom* of a variety of brain disorders, not a disease.

Head trauma is the most common cause of epilepsy, and about half of all penetrating head wounds will result in seizures. Prodromal symptoms and auras often precede seizures. **Prodromal symptoms** are "feelings" that a seizure is about to occur and usually appear several days before the seizure itself. In contrast, an **aura** signals the imminent arrival of a seizure and occurs only minutes before the seizure itself. Auras are often auditory or gustatory sensations.

Jacksonian seizures occur when there is a motoric response, such as twitching or jerking that is confined to one side of the body. A "Jacksonian march" results when minor motor movements in a finger or toe become more exaggerated and spread to other parts of the body on the affected side. If the initially isolated abnormal brain activity spreads to the other hemisphere, the entire body may stiffen or jerk; this attack is referred to as a **grand mal seizure**. Grand mal seizures typically last from 2 to 5 minutes and are sometimes referred to as **tonic-clonic** seizures because of their alternating periods of rigidity and jerking. In contrast, **petit mal seizures** (absence seizures), which are common in young children, do not result in falling, jerking, or loss of muscle tone. The child experiencing a petit mal seizure will be, for a very brief period (usually 2–10 seconds), very unresponsive to the external environment.

Complex partial seizures (also referred to by the older terms "psychomotor" or "temporal lobe seizures") are of considerable interest to anyone working in the field of mental health, because these disorders often mimic psychiatric diseases. The patient with complex partial seizures may hallucinate, engage in stereotyped motor behavior, experience feelings of unreality, or become extremely anxious. The sensations of **déjà vu** and **jamais vu** are often reported. The EEG is typically found to be normal in these patients, and about one in five will experience auditory or visual hallucinations. Unlike the hallucinations of the patient with schizophrenia, however, auditory hallucinations in the patient with a complex partial seizure will be localized within the head (rather than from an external source), and they will rarely contain bizarre, threatening, or accusatory material.

Fritz Dreifuss, one of the world's leading experts on epilepsy was fond of relating a story about a patient who had a genuine seizure disorder that could be documented on an EEG. However, she only seized when she heard Mahalia Jackson singing "My Heart Has a Life of Its Own." The song could be sung by anyone else, and the patient would not seize. Likewise, she could listen to Mahalia Jackson sing anything else, and she would not experience seizures. After several weeks in the hospital, someone asked the patient what was so special about Mahalia Jackson singing "My Heart Has a Life of Its Own." "Didn't you know?" she replied. "That was the song they played at my mother's funeral as her casket was being lowered into her grave."

A character in independent auteur Hal Hartley's *Simple Men* (1992) suffers from epilepsy, and a diagnosis of temporal lobe epilepsy is made in *Happy Accidents* (2001) due to a character's petit mal seizures and heightened sense of emotion. Interestingly, the diagnosis in *Happy Accidents* is made by a psychologist who, in addition to practicing outside of her competence, loses additional credibility by stating that the man is delusional. The made-for-TV movie *First Do No Harm* (1997) stars Meryl Streep and depicts a young boy with a type of epilepsy where there is no known cause. The film explores types of diet in the treatment of epilepsy. The depiction of seizures in movies is common and is portrayed for a variety of reasons: as a response to insulin-shock treatment in *A Beautiful Mind* (2001); to ECT in *One Flew Over the Cuckoo's Nest* (1975); and after brain surgery in *Molly* (1999).

International Films Depicting Neurocognitive Disorders

The inspirational Argentinean film *Son of the Bride* (2002), which was nominated for an Academy Award for Best Foreign Language Film, follows a man too busy for his family until he suffers a heart attack. This brings him to reevaluate his life and his relationships, one of which is with his mother, who is suffering from Alzheimer's disease. He had always found his mother to be cynical, controlling, and demanding, and he managed this situation by distancing himself from her. He is inspired by his father who ritualistically and lovingly visits his wife every day, showing nothing but faithful love and devotion to her despite her rambling speech, distant stares, and frequent inability to recognize her family. This is a touching, realistic, and emotional portrayal of Alzheimer's disease and the family members' reactions and coping.

In the Finnish film *The Man Without a Past* (2002), a man is robbed and brutally beaten while sleeping outside. He suffers a severe head injury, and physicians pronounce him medically dead and walk out of the room; suddenly, the man wakes up, rises, and simply walks out of the hospital beyond the sight of staff. He has had **retrograde amnesia** since the time of the injury and is forced to recreate his life. Although he is an outcast in society, he manages to cope with a greedy landlord, works at the Salvation Army, dates a woman, and finds a trusted companion in a dog and eventually a community. Pieces of memory return to him as he begins to find, reject, and come to terms with his past.

A Separation (2011, Iran) centers around marital tension. The film opens with a woman telling her husband that she has finally received her green card and wishes for the family to head to the United States to attain a much better life. Her husband insists he must stay in Iran to take care of his ailing father who suffers from Alzheimer's; he also insists on raising their daughter in Iran. The film has several subplots, one of which involves the rigors and challenges of caretaking for a parent with dementia – the challenges of finding and maintaining a good caretaker, managing practical issues such as going to the bathroom, handling the organization of busy work schedules within everyday life, attempting to block escapist behaviors of the person with Alzheimer's, and managing problems such as encopresis.

The sequelae of head injury secondary to a motor vehicle accident are portrayed in the French film *The Accidental Hero* (2002).

A Spanish film, *The City of No Limits* (2002), depicts a family patriarch, Max, who is dying of a brain tumor. Max displays paranoia and quirky behavior. Medical doctors describe his psychological state as "verging on derangement." He stares at objects, carefully touches walls, speaks of video cameras watching him, calls a phone number that does not appear to exist, and tries to escape the hospital. He has a concerned and paranoid expression on his face, does not trust others, is constantly fearful, and is dishonest. Some of his comments appear random: "I'll never tell you where they are," and "Don't speak in front of them." He becomes preoccupied with escaping from the hospital to meet with someone named Rancel, wanting to warn him "before it is too late." He is not compliant with his medications. Though the viewer does not know his psychological condition prior to the brain tumor's onset, it is to be assumed most of these symptoms have emerged because of his tumor. Overall, Max's condition waxes and wanes: At times, Max is coherent and oriented; on other occasions, he confuses novels with reality. Important family secrets are uncovered due to Max's seemingly random and ridiculous comments.

The Belgian film *The Memory of a Killer* (2003, Belgium) portrays a hit man in the early stages of Alzheimer's. He is repelled by his last assignment – he has been told to kill a 12-year-old girl forced into prostitution by her father – and he knows that his increasing forgetfulness puts him at great risk. The protagonist is all too familiar with the progression of Alzheimer's because he regularly visits his older brother who has the same disease.

Another Belgian film, *No Home Movie* (2015, France/Belgium), was directed by feminist filmmaker Chantal Akerman. The film portrays Akerman's mother's slow decline into dementia at age 86. Her mother, "Maman," was a Polish survivor of Auschwitz. The film portrays mundane activities and conversations between mother and daughter, and much of the film was captured using a smartphone and Skype video. Akerman committed suicide in 2015, and *No Home Movie* was her last film.

Bille August, the Danish director of the heart-wrenching *Pelle the Conqueror* (1987), turned to the tragedy of Alzheimer's disease with the film *A Song for Martin* (2002). The film depicts the life story of a composer, Martin, who falls in love with his first violinist. The two divorce their spouses to be together, and the relationship is idyllic until Martin begins to show early signs of forgetfulness, and eventually it becomes clear that he is the victim of a dementing illness. The film provides an excellent illustration of the demands Alzheimer's disease can place on a caregiver. Film critic Shelley Cameron called this film one of the most moving portraits of human relationships ever chronicled.

A powerful, haunting Japanese film, *The Ballad of Narayama* (1983, Japan), deals with the village practice of taking old people to the top of a mountain on their 70th birthday where they are left to die. As the US population ages, nursing homes are increasingly serving as our own mountain top.

Amour

Amour (2012, France) is a remarkable film directed by Michael Haneke, and it presents one of the most compelling illustrations of dementia in film history. This movie is about the life and love of Georges and Anne, two retired music teachers sharing a good life in Paris. They are both in their 80s, and they have an adult daughter who occasionally visits. Their life begins to change dramatically after Anne experiences a minor stroke one morning during breakfast; this event marks the beginning of the end of their long and happy life together. The film documents mature love between a man and his wife, but it also illustrates the stress and tension associated with caregiving (see Figure 41). *Amour* stars Jean-Louis Trintignant and Emmanuelle Riva. Trintignant is best known for his role in *A Man and a Woman* (1966), and Riva is celebrated for her role in *Hiroshima Mon Amour* (1959). *Amour* will stay with you long after the viewing, and it will leave you thinking about – and talking with your friends about – both dementia and euthanasia.

Anne: "There's no point in going on living. That's how it is. I know it can only get worse. Why should I inflict this on us, on you and me?"
Georges: "You're not inflicting anything on me."
Anne: "You don't have to lie, Georges."

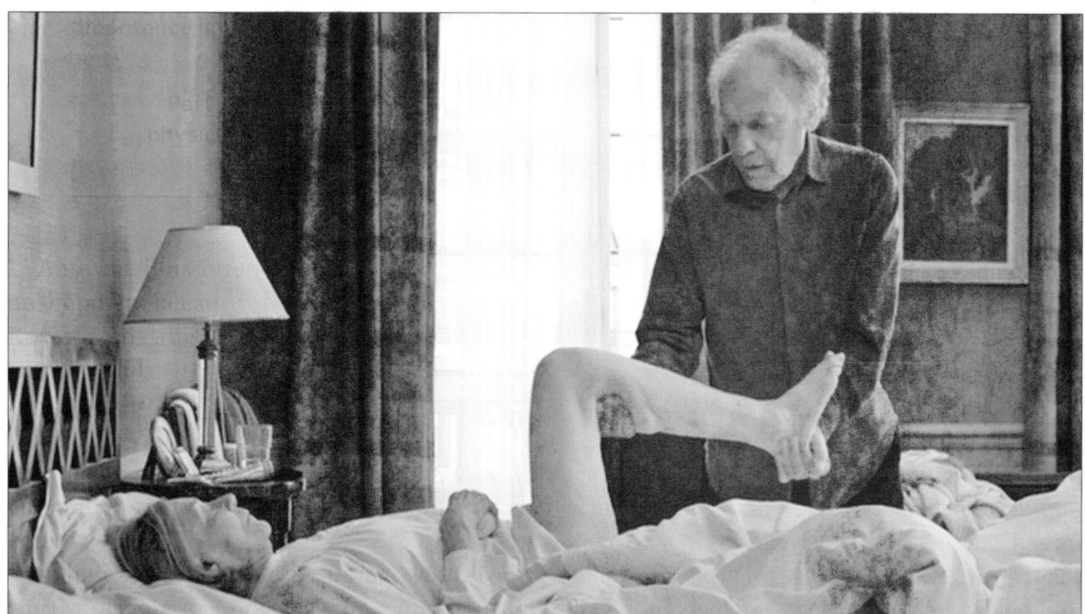

Figure 41. *Amour* (2012, Les Films du Losange, X-Filme Creative Pool, Wega Films, France 3 Cinema, ARD Degeto Film, Bayerischer Rundfunk, Westdeutscher Rundfunk). Produced by Michael Andre, Stefan Arndt, Rodin Bingol, Alice Girard, et al. Directed by Michael Heneke.

> **Georges: [looks down at the floor contemplatively] "Put yourself in my place. Didn't you ever think that it could happen to me, too?"**
> **Anne: "Of course I did. But imagination and reality have little in common."**
> **Georges: "But things are getting better every day."**
> **Anne: "I don't want to carry on. You're making such sweet efforts to make everything easier for me. But I don't want to go on. For my own sake, not yours."**
> **Georges: "I don't believe you. I know you. You think you are a burden to me. But what would you do in my place?"**
> **Anne: "I don't want to rack my brain over this. I'm tired, I want to go to bed."**
>
> A husband and wife share their anxiety over her symptoms, in *Amour* (2012)

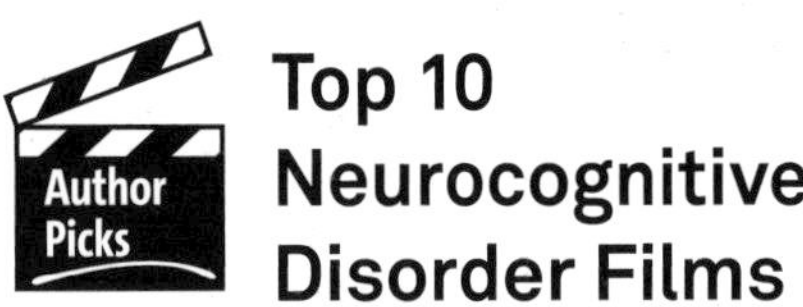

Top 10 Neurocognitive Disorder Films

Head Trauma and Stroke

On the Waterfront (1954)
Raging Bull (1980)
Memento (2000)
The Lookout (2007)
Amour (2012)

Dementia

Iris (2001)
The Notebook (2004)
Away From Her (2006)
Still Alice (2014)
The Father (2020)

Chapter 13

Personality Disorders

No, no, no. You don't understand. You can't make a deal with him. Even if you gave him the money, he'd still kill you. He's a peculiar man. You could even say that he has principles. Principles that transcend money or drugs or anything like that. He's not like you. He's not even like me.

The psychopath Anton Chigurh is described in *No Country for Old Men* (2007)

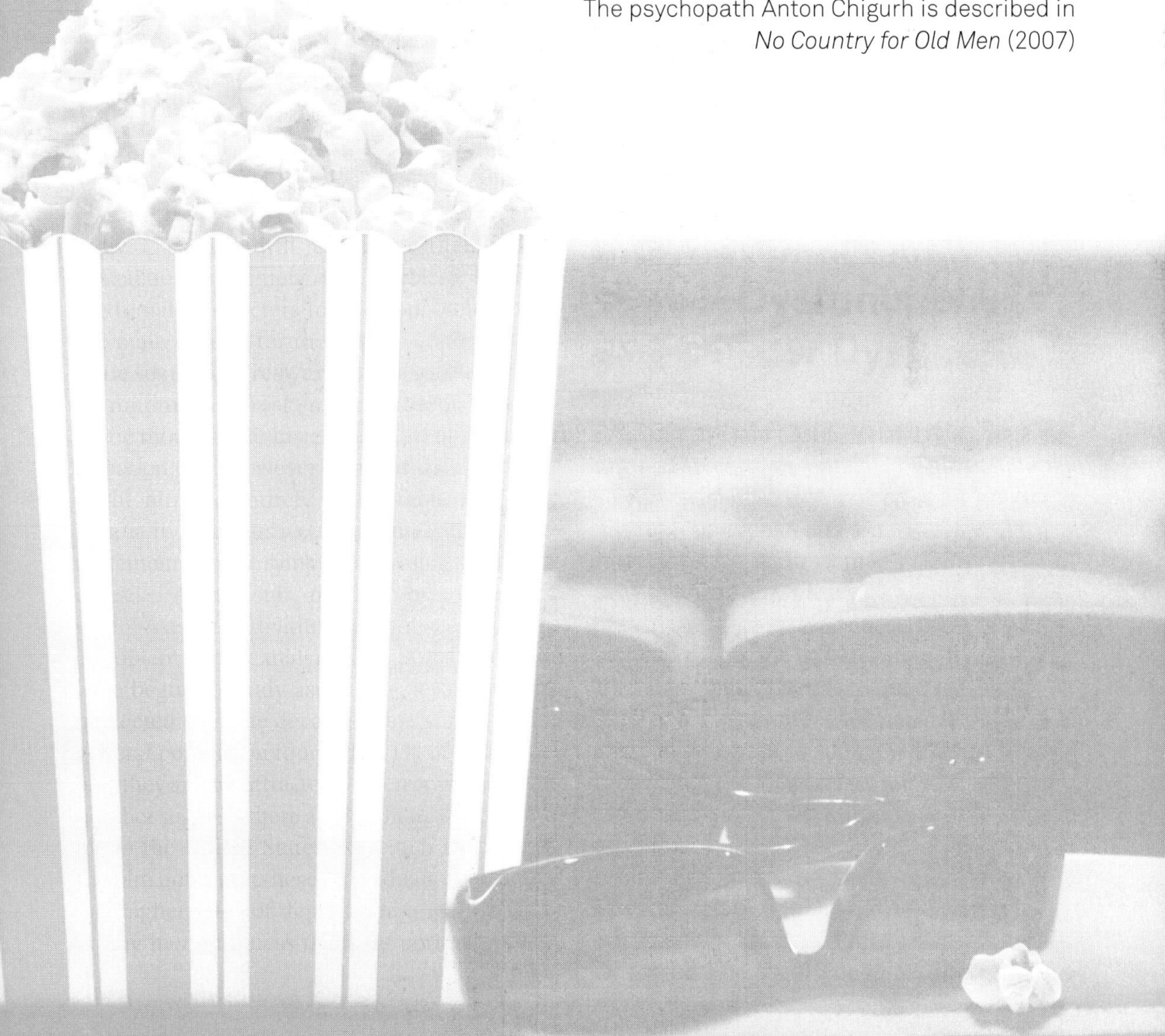

Types of Personality Disorders

All of us have unique personalities and our own individual personality traits. On occasion, these personality traits get us in trouble. For some individuals, their personalities result in a persistent pattern of recurring interpersonal difficulties. When there is a persistent pattern of inflexible and maladaptive behavior that *continually* gets an individual in trouble or that causes them considerable subjective distress, a diagnosis of personality disorder may be appropriate.

People with personality disorders exhibit enduring, pervasive, and inflexible patterns of behavior that deviate markedly from societal expectations. Their behavior seems odd, unusual, or peculiar to most other people. However, to the individual, the experience is so ingrained that it is **ego-syntonic**; it does not bother them – that is, they have learned to be comfortable with their own pathology.

The list of 10 personality disorders in Table 12 is not arbitrary but is based on a conceptual model that groups all personality disorders into one of three distinct clusters. **Cluster A** (for *odd or eccentric behavior*) includes the paranoid, schizoid, and schizotypal personality disorders. **Cluster B** (for *dramatic, emotional, or erratic behavior*) includes the antisocial, borderline, histrionic, and narcissistic personality disorders. **Cluster C** (for *anxious or fearful behavior*) includes the remaining personality disorders: avoidant, dependent, and obsessive-compulsive. Students sometimes find it instructive to remember these three clusters using the helpful (but potentially offensive) mnemonic "*weird, wild and wimpy*" for clusters A, B, and C, respectively.

DSM-5 also presents a dimensional model of personality disorders to accompany the standard taxonomy presented in the core manual. This represents an attempt to have it both ways. The core taxonomy preserves continuity with current practice (and is identical to the categorical classification of personality disorders found in

Table 12. Characteristics of personality disorders, with examples from both classic and contemporary cinema

Disorder cluster	Personality disorder	Characteristics	Classic film examples	More recent film examples
A	**Paranoid**	Distrust and suspiciousness about the motives of others	Lt. Cmd. Philip Francis Queeg (Humphrey Bogart) in *The Caine Mutiny* (1954); Fred C. Dobbs (Humphrey Bogart) in *The Treasure of the Sierra Madre* (1948)	Paul (John Diehl) in *Land of Plenty* (2004); Dell Spooner (Will Smith) in *I, Robot* (2004)
	Schizoid	Detachment from social relationships and a restricted range of emotional expression	Will Penny (Charlton Heston) in *Will Penny* (1968)	Bartleby (Crispin Glover) in *Bartleby* (2001); Ed Crane (Billy Bob Thornton) in *The Man Who Wasn't There* (2001)
	Schizotypal	Acute discomfort in close relationships, cognitive or perceptual distortions, and behavioral eccentricities	Jack Arnold Alexander Tancred Gurney (Peter O'Toole) in *The Ruling Class* (1972)	Willy Wonka (Johnny Depp) in *Charlie and the Chocolate Factory* (2005); Charlie Fineman (Adam Sandler) in *Reign Over Me* (2007)

Table 12. Continued

Disorder cluster	Personality disorder	Characteristics	Classic film examples	More recent film examples
B	**Antisocial**	Disregard for, and violation of, the rights of others	Alex (Malcolm McDowell) in *A Clockwork Orange* (1971); Bruno Anthony (Robert Walker) in *Strangers on a Train* (1951)	Patrick Bateman (Christian Bale) in *American Psycho* (2000); Chris Wilton (Jonathan Rhys Meyers) in *Match Point* (2005); Andy Hanson (Philip Seymour Hoffman) in *Before the Devil Knows You're Dead* (2007); Richard Kuklinski (Michael Shannon) in *The Iceman* (2013)
	Borderline	Instability in emotions and interpersonal relationships, inadequate self-image, fear of abandonment, and marked impulsiveness	Alex Forrest (Glenn Close) in *Fatal Attraction* (1987)	Barbara Covett (Judi Dench) in *Notes on a Scandal* (2006); Margot (Nicole Kidman) in *Margot at the Wedding* (2007)
	Histrionic	Excessive emotionality and attention seeking	Blanche DuBois (Vivien Leigh) in *A Streetcar Named Desire* (1951)	Carolyn Burnham (Annette Bening) in *American Beauty* (1999); Countess Sofya Tolstoy (Helen Mirren) in *The Last Station* (2009); Jasmine (Cate Blanchett) in *Blue Jasmine* (2013)
	Narcissistic	Grandiosity, a need for admiration, and lack of empathy for the problems and needs of others	Norma Desmond (Gloria Swanson) in *Sunset Blvd.* (1950)	Bud Fox (Charlie Sheen) in *Wall Street* (1987); Troy Duffy as himself in *Overnight* (2003); Ron Burgundy (Will Ferrell) in *Anchorman: The Legend of Ron Burgundy* (2004)

Table 12. Characteristics of personality disorders (continued from previous pages)

Disorder cluster	Personality disorder	Characteristics	Classic film examples	More recent film examples
C	**Avoidant**	Social inhibition, feelings of inadequacy, and hypersensitivity to criticism or negative evaluation	Laura Wingfield (Jane Wyman) in *The Glass Menagerie* (1950)	Amélie Poulain (Audrey Tautou) in *Amélie* (2001); William Forrester (Sean Connery) in *Finding Forrester* (2000)
	Dependent	Submissive and clinging behavior and fears of separation	Bob "Bobby" Wiley (Bill Murray) in *What About Bob?* (1991)	Claire Richards (Renée Zellweger) in *White Oleander* (2002)
	Obsessive-compulsive	Preoccupation with orderliness, perfectionism, and control	Felix Ungar (Jack Lemmon) in *The Odd Couple* (1968)	Al Fountain (John Turturro) in *Box of Moonlight* (1996)

DSM-IV); the newer, dimensional model aims to address numerous shortcomings of the current approach to personality disorders (APA, 2013, p. 761). One of these shortcomings is that *patients who meet diagnostic criteria for one diagnosis often meet criteria for other personality disorders.* This can be seen in Cate Blanchett's title character in Woody Allen's film *Blue Jasmine* (2013); Jasmine clearly meets the criteria for histrionic personality disorder; she just as clearly meets the criteria for narcissistic personality disorder.

The general criteria for the diagnosis of personality disorder, of any type, include the presence of "an enduring pattern of inner experience and behavior that deviates markedly from the expectations of the individual's culture" (APA, 2013, p. 646). The pattern must be present in at least two of four areas: cognition, affectivity, interpersonal functioning, and impulse control. In addition, the pattern must be inflexible and pervasive.

Just as it is a challenge for clinicians to diagnose a personality disorder in a single meeting with a client, it is challenging to diagnose cinematic characters with personality disorders in films that take place over a brief period of time. Films that show the developmental course of a character from childhood to adulthood and that depict the character in a variety of settings leave the viewer in a better position to make the diagnosis – for example, *Red Dragon* (2002), *The Silence of the Lambs* (1991), *Hannibal* (2001), and *Hannibal Rising* (2007) – the four films documenting the life of Hannibal Lecter.

Morten Hesse and two colleagues reported an interesting study in which they found that psychology students with little formal training in psychopathology could achieve reasonable levels of agreement when using rating scales to diagnose personality disorders in film characters (Hesse et al., 2005). The characters and films evaluated were Sarah Morton in *Swimming Pool* (2003), Aileen Wuornos in *Monster* (2003), Suzanne Stone in *To Die For* (1995), and Coleman Silk in *The Human Stain* (2003). These authors suggest that Morton's character would be diagnosed as "personality disorder, not other specified" (a DSM-IV diagnosis); the character of Aileen Wuornos would be diagnosed as having comorbid borderline and antisocial personality disorder; Stone's character would be diagnosed as someone with a narcissistic personality disorder (with histrionic features); while Silk's character was not believed to meet the criteria for any of the personality disorders.

A personality disorder diagnosis is inappropriate in any situation in which aberrant behavior results from transient situational factors (e.g., an individual who repeatedly gets their tax returns audited may become understandably paranoid about the government). Finally, it is critical that cultural variables be considered when a diagnosis of personality disorder is being considered. For example, the Italian film *Down and Dirty* (1976) includes a protagonist who has an antisocial personality. However, his behavior must be understood in terms of the culture of southern Italy and the debilitating and corrosive effects of poverty.

Some personality disorders are more common in men (e.g., antisocial, and narcissistic personality disorders), while others are found more often in women (e.g., borderline, histrionic, and dependent personality disorders). This is quite consistent with cinematic portrayals, as we will soon show.

Cluster A Disorders

These **odd and eccentric** disorders are rare and hence their depiction in cinema is uncommon (unlike other disorders such as DID, which, though rare, are often shown in movies).

Paranoid Personality Disorder

People with a paranoid personality are isolated and suspicious. They are convinced that others are talking about them behind their backs or plotting against them. The behaviors of others are scrutinized for evidence of intent to harm, and overtures of friendship or good will by other people are rejected as manipulative gestures or parts of a plot. Ironically, because paranoid individuals behave in peculiar ways, a self-fulfilling prophecy occurs, and people *do* begin to discuss the paranoid individual behind their back. Paranoid people tend to have few or no friends. They personalize everything and misinterpret casual remarks to make them fit into their belief structure.

Land of Plenty (2004, US/Germany) is a Wim Wenders film about misguided post-9/11 patriotism and paranoia in the United States. A young woman, Lana (Michelle Williams), returns to the United States from Tel Aviv with a mission to meet her Uncle Paul and deliver a letter to him on behalf of her mother. Paul is a highly suspicious and paranoid man whose life is preoccupied with searching for individuals with bombs or who may be attacking the city of Los Angeles. He has an irritable disposition, often characteristic of those with this personality disorder. When he communicates with others, his verbiage is intense and convincing. Paul lives in a dilapidated van, uses a makeshift camera with a joystick and monitor, and covers the walls of his van with newspaper clippings. Some of these come from the garbage cans he digs into looking for evidence. He racially profiles Arabic men, and when he encounters a homeless man wearing a turban, he immediately concludes the man is a terrorist. He later watches a drive-by killing of the man – and since he was taping the man's every move, he can keep the tape to rewatch for his own amusement. Paul notes he had been exposed to Agent Orange in Vietnam; therefore, a physical disorder would need to be ruled out before any psychological diagnostic conclusions could be made.

"They're trying to infect our country. They're trying to destroy us. I won't let them do that."

Paul revealing his paranoia, in *Land of Plenty* (2004)

Lakeview Terrace (2009) stars Samuel L. Jackson as Able, a paranoid LAPD officer in this Neil LaBute film. LaBute offers good character development of this multifaceted man, allowing the viewer to build some stereotypes and negative impressions of Able who then reveals his honest, genuine concern for his children, his inner pain, and his rationale for his frustration with interracial couples. Tension mounts between Able and an interracial couple who move in next door as Able begins to terrorize them. Able displays a high degree of rigidity and irritability and insists on all rules being followed. He is oversensitive in interpersonal communications and is hypervigilant and skeptical everyone's motives. Subsequently, he is quick to react negatively to any conversation. LaBute is known for using subtlety and metaphor in his films to parallel key themes. In this film, forest fires get closer and closer to Able's neighborhood as the film progresses; this adds to a sense unpredictable danger.

The dangers associated with having a leader with a paranoid or antisocial personality disorder become clear in *The Last King of Scotland* (2006), in which Academy Award winner Forest Whitaker portrays the leader of Uganda, Idi Amin. On the one hand, Amin is quite charismatic as he tries to convince the people that he is their rightful leader and the "father" of Uganda. He is also often fun-loving, friendly, jovial, and teasing. On the other hand, he is shown to be a ruthless dictator, explosive, and unpredictable, who murdered over 300,000 Ugandans during his reign. Paranoia was a significant part of this man's personality, and he used his paranoia to justify his horrendous actions.

"But a man who shows fear. He is weak ... and a slave"

Idi Amin's ironic observation, in *The Last King of Scotland* (2006)

A convincing portrayal of paranoid personality disorder is found in Detective Del Spooner (Will Smith) in *I, Robot* (2004). Spooner is a highly suspicious, judgmental, and angry person, particularly around robots, which are a mainstay in this world of 2046. Spooner's frustrated mistrust of robots leads him to push away a friendly robot delivering a package. His misperceptions bring him to randomly chase down and tackle a robot running with a purse, which he has assumed is a robbery even though no robots had ever committed a crime at this point in history. Much of the plot unfolds around Spooner's paranoia, which other characters recognize. One man, Dr. Alfred Lanning (played by James Cromwell), counts on Spooner's paranoia to save humans from robots. As with many films depicting paranoia (e.g., Jerry Fletcher, played by Mel Gibson, in *Conspiracy Theory* [1997]), the psychopathology is often distorted by the entertainment value of the plot, which results in a character's paranoia proving to be accurate and justified in the end.

Ben Stiller's character Chas Tenenbaum in *The Royal Tenenbaums* (2001) displays numerous paranoid characteristics that seem stable over time. He feels an underlying anger and rage toward his father, unrealistic fears, and displays excessive concern and hypervigilance.

Humphrey Bogart's role as Captain Queeg in *The Caine Mutiny* (1954) is a wonderful illustration of the paranoid personality. Queeg becomes preoccupied with trivial misdemeanors by sailors while he ignores the important parts of his job – such as maintaining the morale of his men. He eventually falls apart under pressure when he is called to the witness stand to testify in a court martial hearing for an insubordinate junior officer. There is a famous scene in which Queeg takes two ball bearings out of his pocket and begins to move them around nervously in his palm, and everyone in the court senses that this man is not well adjusted. Bogart plays another paranoid personality in *The Treasure of the Sierra Madre* (1948) in which he becomes obsessed with the idea that his partners are out to steal the gold all three men have agreed to split between them.

Pawn Sacrifice (2015) stars Tobey Maguire as chess prodigy Bobby Fischer, grandmaster, world champion and arguably the best player of all time. Despite his success and acclaim, Fischer led an unhappy life characterized by paranoia, explosive outbursts, anti-Semitism (even though he was Jewish), and "progressive psychosocial decline to the point of self-neglect and vagrancy" (Anand, 2017). He was odd and eccentric, estranged from his mother, and he alienated the few friends he had. Fischer was suspicious of everyone, and especially the Soviets he competed against. He found hidden meaning in the most trivial events and held lifelong grudges. He clearly meets DSM-5 diagnostic criteria for **paranoid personality disorder**. Students wanting to learn more about Bobby Fischer's life and mental problems are referred to psychologist Joseph Ponterotto's compelling psychobiography (Ponterotto, 2012). It is also interesting to compare Fischer's life to that of another mentally ill chess genius, Paul Morphy (Abbott, 2011).

"By the time Paul Morphy was felled by a stroke on July 10, 1884, he had become an odd and familiar presence on Canal Street in New Orleans: a trim little man in sack suit and monocle, muttering to himself, smiling at his own conceits, swinging his cane at most who dared approach. Sometimes he would take a fancy to a passing woman and following her for hours at a distance. He lived in fear of being poisoned, eating only food prepared by his mother or sister, and he believed that neighborhood barbers were conspiring to slit his throat."

A description of chess champion Paul Morphy (Abbott, 2011)

Schizoid Personality Disorder

The individual with a schizoid personality has little interest in and avoids close interpersonal relations. They are likely to be described as a loner who lacks meaningful ties to a family, community, or value system. These individuals are unlikely to display strong emotions or tenderness to others; they appear apathetic, diffident, and indifferent. They most often have little or no interest in sexual encounters, and few marry.

There are some excellent portrayals of schizoid personality in the cinema. Two examples come from two films both titled *Bartleby* (1970, 2001); both are remakes of a Herman Melville short story, "Bartleby the Scrivener." The 2001 version is a fascinating, cult film about a quiet, passive man named Bartleby (Crispin Glover) hired for a mundane office job. He thoroughly does his job at first but soon begins to refuse doing extra work, simply repeating the phrase, "I would prefer not to." This quirky behavior continues as he stares for hours at an air conditioning vent and displays no interest in socializing with his work peers. Schizoid individuals are often isolated from society, and an opening scene symbolizes Bartleby's isolation as he is depicted enclosed and caged on an overpass bridge above a busy, productive society represented by an expressway below. His speech is slow, eye contact is limited, and affect is flat and emotionless throughout the film. At times, he displays an incongruent, distant, random smile or two, but he does not engage others interpersonally with smiles or laughter. Often, there is no understandable reason for a person behaving in a schizoid manner, and the film parallels this idea, as no explanation is overtly given for Bartleby's behaviors, lack of emotions, or social apathy. The earlier, 1970 version portrays similar schizoid traits for the lead character, and the plot is like that of the later version. The older film is black and white, dark, slow, and gloomy.

Another classic example of someone with a schizoid personality is found in the Coen brothers' film noir *The Man Who Wasn't There* (2001), where even the title of the film suggests a schizoid quality. Billy Bob Thornton plays Ed Crane, an aloof, taciturn barber who appears disinterested in life and claims he dislikes most things and that his life has been one of "no excitement." He is unemotional with flat affect and a monotone voice. He moves slowly and stiffly, and even the way he smokes cigarettes is a slow, unconscious, steady ritual. His responses to others are dull with heavy sighs, and he is passive when criticized. He does not seem very bothered by the fact that his wife is cheating on him with his best friend. He allows himself to be exploited by a traveling salesman. The only relationship he seems to invest emotional energy in is with a young girl; he appears committed to helping her pursue her dream of becoming a musician. Also consistent with schizoid characteristics is the fact that no one "really knows him"; this is reinforced by his inability to share anything of himself with others.

Eraserhead (1976) is a cult classic created by innovative director David Lynch. The film is surreal, not only in direction but also in characterization, lighting, sound, imagery, and story.

The plot involves a young man, Henry, who visits his girlfriend's family, and discovers a premature, alien-like fetus in the home. Henry has a schizoid personality disorder – he is a loner and socially awkward, with no idea how to interact with people (including his girlfriend), and he displays flat and inappropriate affect throughout the film. There are multiple themes of birth and fetuses, as well as umbilical cords, blood, and womb images in various scenes.

Crispin Glover plays another socially awkward, schizoid character in *Willard* (2003). Willard is isolated from others, and his only companions are the rats that congregate in his basement. After one rat, whom he names Socrates, saves him from a suicide attempt, he distances himself further from people and rallies the rats to help him get revenge.

In the film *Heavy* (1995), the lead character displays a schizoid reaction to his mother's death. He becomes frozen, emotionless, sexually disinterested, and isolated with flattened affect. To qualify for a diagnosis of schizoid personality disorder, his bereavement would need to be evaluated and his personality assessed prior to his mother's death. The film offers another interesting schizoid description about the lead character's isolation, through his belief that you can be as "big as an ox and no one sees you."

The figure of the loner is a staple in Western films, and many of these characters would meet the criteria for schizoid personality disorder. These individuals avoid close relationships, prefer solitary activities, lack close friends and confidants, and appear indifferent to the praise or criticism of others; the title character (Charlton Heston) in *Will Penny* (1968) is one example; the eponymous lead (Robert Redford) in *Jeremiah Johnson* (1972) is another.

Schizotypal Personality Disorder

People with **schizotypal personality** have schizophrenia-like characteristics but do not typically meet the diagnostic criteria for schizophrenia. They hold odd or peculiar beliefs, thoughts, and/or behaviors. They are often very superstitious, have unusual perceptual experiences, and are suspicious and paranoid.

In the DSM-5, schizotypal personality disorder is included *both* in the chapter on schizophrenia and in the chapter on personality disorders (where it is fully described). Its inclusion in the chapter on schizophrenia results from its clear presence on the lower end of the schizophrenia spectrum. In his *PsycCRITIQUES* review of the new DSM-5, Greg Neimeyer (2013) noted,

> The scope and scale of the challenges faced within (and between) the 13 different work groups that revised the DSM-5 are scarcely imaginable. Numerous disorders were brought into this game of diagnostic musical chairs; when the music stopped, participants must surely have looked around to see who had found a seat and where they were located. At least one disorder seems to have found itself in two chairs: Schizotypal personality disorder is now listed twice, once under the Personality Disorders and again under the category Schizophrenia Spectrum and Related Disorders. The irony of this latter designation is not lost on those who have cut their eyeteeth on earlier versions of the DSM, where schizotypal personality disorder was fashioned from the long-defunct diagnosis of borderline schizophrenia. Quizzically, it now returns again to its homeland, though its tandem location obligates it to live out its current dissociative life in a *Tale of Two Identities*. (Neimeyer, 2013)

Adam Sandler's portrayal of Charlie Fineman in *Reign Over Me* (2007) is an impressive portrayal of someone with a schizotypal personality disorder. Charlie has lost his whole family – three daughters and his wife – in the 9/11 tragedy, but the viewer sees the character's deterioration and not his immediate reaction to the tragedy. Instead, the story picks up years later, and the viewer observes a man who would qualify for the diagnosis of schizotypal personality. Charlie exhibits eccentric and bizarre behavior, is odd in his appearance (e.g., he is unkempt and constantly wears headphones while riding around on a motor scooter) and seems childlike. He is clueless socially and interpersonally – brutally cold and inappropriate at times (e.g., he eats with his new friend's family but sits at the counter while singing to himself with his headphones on). When he speaks with others, it is only to ask random trivia questions. He repeatedly remodels his kitchen and spends his time in one of two activities: death metal drumming or playing solitary video games. The features of personality disorders in each cluster may merge and overlap at times. For example, Charlie has no desire to connect with others (schizoid) and is highly suspicious of others (paranoid). Before making a diagnosis of schizotypal personality disorder, the clinician would need to discern how much of Charlie's personality features result from prolonged bereavement, or the extent to which they might be related to severe depression or PTSD, and the therapist would need to know what Charlie's personality was like prior to the tragedy.

An outstanding illustration of a schizotypal personality can be found in Johnny Depp's unique portrayal of Willy Wonka in Tim Burton's *Charlie and the Chocolate Factory* (2005), a portrayal that is much clearer in terms of this diagnosis than the portrayal by Gene Wilder in *Willy Wonka and the Chocolate Factory* (1971). Depp's Wonka has a quality of desperate aloofness in which his isolation, unusual perceptual experiences, and odd thinking are much more apparent. He lives alone, and his only friends are a culture of dwarfs (Oompa-Loompas). He is quirky when he does communicate – for example, he exhibits disorganized speech, uses note cards to compensate for his poor social skills, talks to himself in public, and is unable to say the word "parents." His appearance is colorful and eccentric. The film depicts a familial root for Wonka's personality in that he lived alone with his father who was distant and authoritarian. His father showed no concern when he decided to run away from home.

In *The Royal Tenenbaums* (2001), Owen Wilson plays Eli, a man who wears flamboyant outfits and uses unusual words. He has a quirky tone of voice, exhibits odd and eccentric behavior, and often does not have a firm grasp on reality. His apartment has numerous odd paintings covering the walls. It is uncertain to what extent these qualities result from his drug abuse; regardless, his behavior and interactions are quite schizotypal.

Denis Leary plays a truly fascinating man who has paranoid schizophrenia in *Final* (2001). He displays some interesting schizotypal traits as well, but to qualify for a diagnosis of schizotypal personality, these traits could not occur exclusively in schizophrenia episodes.

The character Ernest (Maury Chaykin) in *Bartleby* (2001) displays many schizotypal traits. He has a poor use of logic and when he gets upset, he speaks in a verbal salad, mixes words, and is somewhat nonsensical. His appearance is disheveled. He is easily overwhelmed by stress. His behavior is often inappropriate for the situation, as he never is working when he is at the office, he displays no reaction after spilling water and copier ink, and he is later repeatedly and genuinely scared by a pop-up spin toy. He presents himself with a constant paranoid, concerned look on his face and has blunted affect throughout the film.

A schizotypal personality is demonstrated in Flannery O'Conner's novel *Wise Blood* (1952) and in the 1979 John Huston film adaptation also titled *Wise Blood*. A Southern preacher works hard to convince people to join his "Church Without Christ." He has numerous peculiar beliefs, odd speech, constricted affect, strange behavior, and few close friends. These five characteristics would be sufficient to justify the diagnosis of schizotypal personality. Hyler (1988) uses DeNiro's portrayal of Travis Brickle in *Taxi Driver* (1976) to illustrate the schizotypal personality. He feels this film is such a useful tool for teaching medical students about psychopathology that he has incorporated it into a computer program that can be used to teach students to perform and record a complete mental status exam (Hyler & Bujold, 1994).

Cluster B Disorders

Each of the personalities in this cluster is often lively and colorful, fitting the description "dramatic, emotional, and erratic." Consequently, individuals with Cluster B disorders are common in movies, as they tend to make fascinating, stimulating cinematic characters. They are often attention grabbing, conflicted, manipulative, charming, and charismatic – many of the qualities the moviegoer typically loves or hates. In addition, they often have troubled pasts, and the viewer gets to observe them escape from present pain or make impressive changes, either way making for good drama.

Veterans have an age- and sex-adjusted suicide rate that is 50% greater than for nonveteran US adults (VA Office of Mental Health & Suicide Prevention, 2020), and suicide prevention is a high priority for the Veterans Health Administration. Nelson et al. (2022) found that veterans with a diagnosis of personality disorder had over a 3 times greater risk than those veterans without a personality disorder, and veterans with Cluster B diagnoses, which includes borderline and antisocial personality disorders, were at the greatest risk. In a similar study, Edwards et al. (2021) documented that veterans with both a personality disorder *and* a substance use disorder had dramatically higher rates of suicide attempts, incarceration, and homelessness relative to other veteran groups. Ansell et al. (2015) studied personality disorders as a risk factor for suicide attempts over a 10-year period and found both borderline and narcissistic personality pathology uniquely contributed to suicide-related outcomes.

The Talented Mr. Ripley (1999) is a wonderful example of a film's character (Tom Ripley, played by Matt Damon) who displays characteristics of each of the disorders in this cluster. Even the opening credits get at the complexity of this disorder, listing the following adjectives to replace "talented" in the title: mysterious, yearning, secretive, lonely, troubled, confused, loving, musical, gifted, intelligent, beautiful, tender, secretive, haunted, and passionate.

Antisocial Personality Disorder

People with antisocial personalities break the law, can be physically aggressive, manipulate others, lie, take senseless risks, and have little or no sense of remorse or guilt about the consequences of their behavior. These individuals violate the rights of others and appear to experience distress only when their behavior results in punishment or incarceration. They are impulsive, thrive on the "pleasure principle," and have a great deal of trouble planning their future behavior or anticipating its consequences. Individuals with antisocial personality disorder find it difficult to learn from their mistakes and find themselves dealing with similar legal and interpersonal problems throughout their lives. To examine the drivers of deviant behavior and the influence of social factors in the context of the Ben Affleck film, *The Town* (2010), read the *PsycCRITIQUES* review of the film by Swenson and Schwartz-Mette (2011).

Daniel Day-Lewis is the only actor in history to win three Academy Awards for Best Actor (*Lincoln* [2012]; *There Will Be Blood* [2007]; and *My Left Foot* [1990]). In addition to being one of the world's most versatile actors, he has been exemplary in the role of characters with antisocial personalities, such as *Gangs of New York* (2002; a film for which he was nominated for Best Actor) and *There Will Be Blood*. In the latter film, he portrays Daniel Plainview, an ambitious prospector who calls himself "an oil man" and gets rich after purchasing a family's oil rich ranch. As the film progresses, Plainview becomes increasingly greedy, violent, and selfish. He abandons his son at an early age and eventually rejects every significant person in his life. His approach is to kill or eliminate or abandon anyone who gets in his way. He becomes a despicable character who, like the Joker and Anton Chigurh, represents a beastly, immoral, wretched human being.

"I have a competition in me.
I want no one else to succeed. I hate most people"
"There are times when I look at people and I see nothing worth liking."
"I want to earn enough money to get away from everyone."

Plainview's description of himself, in *There Will Be Blood* (2007)

The Assassination of Jesse James by the Coward Robert Ford (2007) portrays the obvious antisocial characteristics of a well-known train robber, Jesse James (Brad Pitt), and it also illustrates James's calm manipulation and defiant recklessness, as well as an elevated level of paranoia. He becomes suspicious that his followers and fellow criminals are out to get him. His paranoia leads him to become more controlling, impulsive, and unpredictable, especially as the price on his head increases. James would be diagnosed with an unspecified personality disorder with antisocial and paranoid traits.

Before the Devil Knows You're Dead (2007) is an intense Sidney Lumet melodrama in which the story defines the characters (in a drama, the characters define the story). Two brothers struggling financially and craving a better life scheme to rob a mom-and-pop jewelry store; however, the owners are their own mom and pop. After things go wrong with the robbery, the antisocial tendencies of each brother strongly emerge, and their deceit, impulsivity, and recklessness run rampant. Lumet reveals how each character is a flawed human being, and each becomes terrible in their revenge, decompensation, or inaction.

People with antisocial personality disorder often have multiple sexual partners and tend to use others for sexual gratification, with little concern for the needs or feelings of their sexual partners. They can be superficially warm and charming but become distant and aloof after their sexual conquest. This is evident in Johnny, the intellectual, philosophical, and antisocial character portrayed by David Thewlis in *Naked* (1993). Robert Duvall plays a complicated, antisocial minister who philanders, abuses, and projects his problems onto other characters and God in *The Apostle* (1997). Duvall's character, Sonny, is driven but flawed. He is a "spiritual antisocial" in that he passionately preaches, and his manipulation and charm often take the form of genuinely wanting to help others have more meaningful lives; however, he externalizes his problems by blaming Satan and not taking responsibility for his life. He abuses alcohol, is unfaithful to his wife, threatens her with a gun, throws an object through a window, and, most seriously, grabs his wife roughly by the hair and attempts to drag her away from a baseball game and then hospitalizes his wife's boyfriend by hitting him on the head with a baseball bat. He lies to others about his past, despite their trust in him as their spiritual leader. Sonny certainly embodies the qualities of narcissism as well, with his grandiose speech, and in his preaching, and he feeds off others' admiration and his ability to stake out a position on center stage. This film will remind some of the role of the much more psychopathic preacher played by Robert Mitchum in the classic film *The Night of the Hunter* (1955).

The fascinating film *Tape* (2001) takes place in one setting (a motel room) with only three characters (played by Ethan Hawke, Robert Sean Leonard, and Uma Thurman). Despite this simplicity, the film is a complex look at a devious, antisocial personality, Vince (Hawke), and his manipulation of two high school friends. Vince is a 28-year-old without a job who volunteers as a firefighter. He presents as unstable, using drugs, jumping and running around the small motel room, chugging beers, and throwing the cans around. He has a history of drug dealing and reports that he has anger tendencies and unresolved issues. At times, he is sweet and soft spoken, but the viewer soon realizes he is purposefully acting this way to manipulate his friends. With extreme craftiness, he secretly tape records his friend John (Leonard) revealing some vulnerable information (about a date rape in high school) after Vince interrogates him in cross-examination style; displaying a total lack of empathy, he blackmails John and calls another old friend (Vince's ex-girlfriend and John's date rape victim), Amy (Thurman), with the hopes of continuing his plotted manipulation.

Jonestown: The Life and Death of Peoples Temple (2006) utilizes old footage, tapes, writings, and interviews with several survivors and family members of those involved in what has been called the largest mass suicide in modern history. On November 18, 1978, in Jonestown, Guyana, 909 members of Peoples' Temple killed themselves, as did their evangelical leader, Jim Jones. Members of the church adored Jones for his charisma and his messages of integration, hope, equality, and justice. Many embraced him as godlike and considered him a savior. What was missed by those who died, and many others, was that Jim Jones was a vicious antisocial personality. He abused power and used the congregation to meet his own sexual needs (in one case explaining to a woman shivering while he had sex with her, "I'm doing this for you"). He frequently humiliated, shamed, and manipulated the congregants, finding pleasure in spanking or beating people in front of the congregation as punishment for petty transgressions. Jones once staged a blind woman in a wheelchair and performed a fake healing. He convinced people to sell their homes for the church, and in return he promised that the church would take care of elderly family members. He encouraged people to not think for themselves so that he could think for them; he reflected that he was happy to play whatever role the congregant needed – friend, brother, savior, or God. Jones exhibited significant pathological traits as a child; for example, he killed cats so that he could officiate at their funerals.

The true story of Danny Burrows (played by Ryan Gosling) in *The Believer* (2001) speaks to the serious love–hate relationship a young man has with himself as he adopts a dramatically contradictory role as a Jewish Nazi. In the opening sequence, the viewer sees Burrows, who presents as a stereotypic skinhead displaying Nazi symbols, seek out and beat a young Jewish man in the middle of the street. He embraces repugnant Nazi beliefs, ranking races by worthiness in the following order: Whites, Asians, Blacks, and Jews. At the same time, Burrows is highly intelligent and articulate, speaking charismatically to adults many years older than he is about Nazi order, discipline, and values, articulating "kill your enemy" and "Judaism is a sickness" messages. His aggressiveness and impulsivity lead him to instigate numerous fights. Burrows displays little remorse for any of his antisocial behaviors until, while ransacking a synagogue with a Fascist group, he begins to show concern for how people treat a scroll containing sacred Jewish writings. He brings the scroll home, takes painstaking care of it, and begins to teach his girlfriend Hebrew. From here, he must face his internal contradiction and deal with the consequences of the lifestyle he has created for himself.

Another film illustrating an antisocial personality, which is based on a true story, is the film *Shattered Glass* (2003) about Stephen Glass (Hayden Christensen), the *New Republic* magazine writer who went to extensive lengths to fabricate and embellish stories. Both the film and Christensen do a remarkable job of depicting not only the elaborate deceit, fantasy, and double life associated with this personality disorder, but also the neurotic quality of the "antisocial in trouble." The latter phrase refers to anxiety mixed with a façade of change that comes about when a person with an antisocial personality disorder is caught or about to be caught. Glass's response is to become emotional, obsequious, and/or apologetic. His manipulations take many forms, from trying to emphasize his need for the editors' support and how important it is (when he is lying), to trying to play others against one another to the incessant repetition of the question "Are you mad at me?" Glass does not see the consequences of his actions as he continues to tell various lies and stories to cover up earlier lies, digging himself deeper into deception with each interaction; we later see the tremendous impact of his behavior on the *New Republic*.

Another "caught" antisocial is Edward Norton's character in *25th Hour* (2002), who has 24 hours before he must begin a prison term for trafficking marijuana. Since he has been caught, he is forced to face some of his shame, guilt, and anger. In one unforgettable scene, he externalizes intense anger, blaring out "fuck you" to every race, group, district, and borough in New York City, as well as his father and girlfriend. We can infer he is saying this to himself as well, especially since he is looking at himself in the mirror while talking, but the acceptance of personal responsibility is missing – as it often is in the antisocial personality. This Spike Lee film brings up critical issues of regret and choice, and brilliantly leaves many questions unanswered.

Catch Me If You Can (2002) is another film about a character with an antisocial personality disorder. The film is based on the true story of Frank Abagnale Jr., a con man who used his charm and good looks to defraud banks of millions of dollars in the 1960s. The role of Abagnale is played by Leonardo DiCaprio, who successfully impersonates a Pan Am copilot, a physician, and an attorney. Abagnale is pursued for 6 years by FBI agent Carl Hanratty (Tom Hanks) before he is eventually captured, and he winds up consulting with the FBI on fraud crimes.

In the remarkable film *Dogville* (2003), Lars von Trier directs the depiction of a woman (Nicole Kidman) trying to escape the destiny her mob boss father has planned for her. She is clearly *not* antisocial, and she works hard to be accepted into the little community that she hides in after fleeing her father's control. However, she is exploited and abused by the community she works so hard to serve, and she eventually turns on them, murdering everyone in the village with little apparent remorse.

An interesting contrast of antisocial personalities occurs in *Levity* (2003), a film in which Billy Bob Thornton plays a person with an antisocial personality trying to make amends for his actions (a murder many years ago), and Morgan Freeman plays an antisocial preacher who uses a fake identity to hide from the police. Likewise, Tom Hanks is a charming person with an antisocial personality who cleverly uses sophisticated speech and extensive rationalizations to manipulate an old woman for his own purposes in *The Ladykillers* (2004).

A less dramatic illustration is found in the callous manipulation of naïve home buyers vividly portrayed by Jack Lemmon, who plays a desperate and unhappy real estate salesman in *Glengarry Glen Ross* (1992). The manipulation of others for personal gain without concern for the consequences of one's behavior is a characteristic feature of antisocial personality disorder. Natasha Richardson and Mia Farrow play two consummate con artists in *Widow's Peak* (1994).

Many films depict antisocial behavior, but it is often unclear as to whether these characters would meet all the criteria for the disorder. *Compulsion* (1959) depicts two antisocial fraternity men, Artie and Judd, who are intent on showing that the perfect crime is "the true test of the superior intellect." They believe they should be able to manipulate the system to get away with murder simply because "we can." Each has an antisocial personality disorder, although Artie's case is more severe. He is cool, smooth, and calculating under pressure, and enjoys listening to the police discuss the murder of which he is the perpetrator, taking pleasure in their confusion and the chaos.

Some actors like Kevin Spacey have made a career out of playing antisocial characters. Though Spacey can play a variety of characters with vastly different personalities, he has played an impressive range of roles that illustrate some dimension of the antisocial personality; for example, he portrayed an arrogant writer in *The United States of Leland* (2004), an unhappy man who becomes obsessed with "the pleasure principle" in *American Beauty* (1999), a devious serial killer in *Se7en* (1995), a con man in *The Usual Suspects* (1995), a brutal executive in *Swimming With Sharks* (1994) , and an ineffectual, unethical, and depressed therapist in *Shrink* (2009). Spacey's remarkable career as an actor has been marred by allegations of sexual misconduct, many of them involving minors. Anthony Rapp (lead actor in the movie *Rent*) sued Spacey for sexual assault in 2020. On the same day, Spacey came out as gay, stating, "I have had relationships with both men and women. I have loved and had romantic encounters with men throughout my life, and I choose now to live as a gay man" (Convery, 2017). Following the accusations of sexual assault, Spacey's role in filming was suspended on the sixth and final season of *House of Cards*.

While the film *Enron: The Smartest Guys in the Room* (2005) describes the antisocial behavior of various executives in a corrupt organization, the film *The Corporation* (2004) demonstrates that the typical corporation meets the criteria for psychopathy (e.g., callous unconcern for others, failure to conform to social norms).

> **"The fatal flaw at Enron, if there was one, you'd say it was pride, but then it was arrogance, intolerance, greed."**
>
> **The underlying issues for the executives in *Enron: The Smartest Guys in the Room* (2005)**

Psychopathy, Antisocial Personality, and *No Country for Old Men*

Javier Bardem's 2007 Academy Award-winning performance as Anton Chigurh is one of the most chilling portrayals of psychopathology and evil in cinema history. It is hard to imagine Chigurh not being named as one of the top five villains on the next list by the American Film Institute of the top 50 heroes and 50 villains in cinema history (see Appendix 1). His portrayal is as engaging as it is frightening. On one level, he is a man after money, simply doing a job; on another level, he is a cold-blooded, psychopathic serial killer; on still another, he symbolizes evil itself. It is fair to call him amoral – he is someone devoid of a moral code; on the other hand, some might say he is a man of principle, following his belief in one thing – fate. At times, Chigurh uses a coin toss to determine whom he will kill; at other times he simply kills anyone who gets in his way. He does not show a hint of goodness, morality, or care for anyone with whom he comes into contact; meaning and purpose are the furthest thing from his mind. He employs a unique weapon – a penetrating captive bolt pistol that is normally used to stun or kill cattle. A confrontation with a gas station proprietor, played by Gene Jones, is unforgettable (Figure 42); this scene underscores how difficult it is for most people to understand the motives and behavior of someone with an antisocial personality disorder.

The character of Chigurh is a fascinating film portrayal – he has a deep, harsh voice, penetrating eyes, and a steady, self-assured gait. He is usually taciturn; when he does speak, he chooses his words carefully. His nationality and ethnicity are intentionally left unclear so he could potentially be from anywhere. His behavior is incredibly resourceful with an important level of "negative ingenuity" (creativity in the moment and for malicious purposes). He appears unstoppable, and he adeptly uses everyone he encounters. There are no walls or locked doors that can slow him down or block him; his bolt gun blows through every lock he encounters. It makes no difference where a person goes if Chigurh is

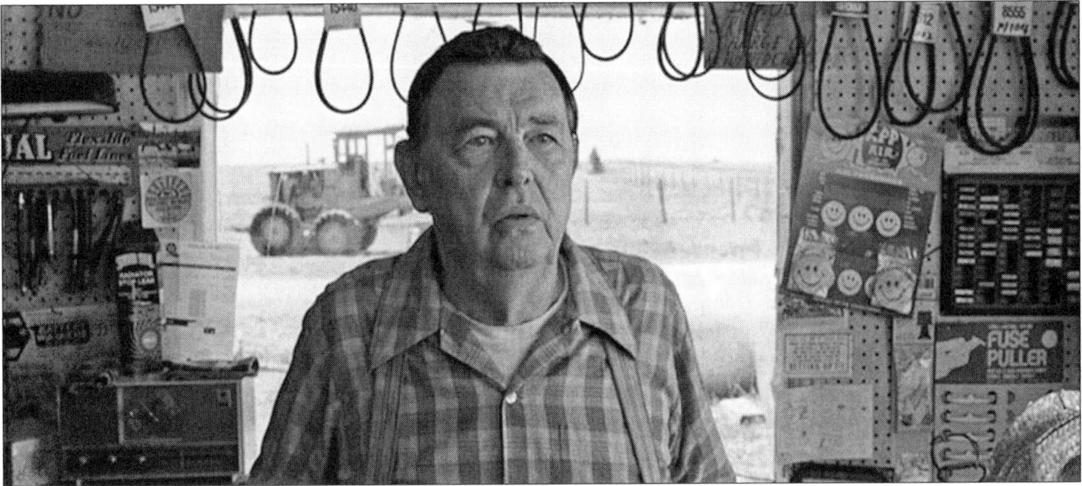

Figure 42. *No Country for Old Men* (2007, Paramount Vantage, Miramax, Scott Rudin Productions, Mike Zoss Productions). Produced by Ethan Coen, Joel Coen, David Diliberto, Robert Graf, et al. Directed by Ethan Coen and Joel Coen.

waiting there to deliver their fate. In one scene he is put on the defensive, yet he finds a way to disappear. This is another critical aspect of his character. Just as one does not necessarily see *pure evil*, but forms of evil, we do not see Chigurh, and he does not want to be seen. One character refers to him as a ghost. Indeed, the first shot of him in the film (and several other shots) is a shadow as he sits in the back seat of a police officer's car, just before an escape and a brutal killing. He follows his subjects silently and then suddenly is present; just as quickly as he appears, he disappears. When asked if he was going to kill a man, Chigurh responds "That depends, can you see me?"

When reading these descriptions, one can see that Chigurh is not a typical antisocial personality. He not only displays a pervasive pattern of breaking rules, irresponsibility, impulsiveness, and aggressiveness, but he is also a serial killer devoid of any hint of humanity. The diagnosis of psychopathic personality (not a formal DSM-5 diagnosis, but something discussed later in this chapter, in the section Antisocial Versus Psychopathic Personality) provides a more accurate and apt description.

No Country for Old Men (2007) won several awards, including Academy Awards for Best Director, Best Picture, and Best Adaptive Screenplay. Directed by the Coen Brothers, the film merges several genre elements – thriller-suspense, crime drama, and western.

Anton Chigurh's character can be compared with the late Heath Ledger's Academy Award-winning performance as the Joker in *The Dark Knight* (2008). The Joker is an incredibly engaging – and more charismatic – villain who clearly fits the dimensions of the psychopathic personality. He displays no remorse or hint of human goodness and kills at will. Both characters would be on the severe end of this personality disorder dimension. Viewers are very curious about each of these characters and eagerly anticipate each scene in which they appear. There are several explanations for viewers' fascination with these two characters and those of other psychopaths such as Hannibal Lecter in *The Silence of the Lambs* (1991) and Alex in *A Clockwork Orange* (1971). Curiosity researcher Todd Kashdan (2009) offers three explanations:

> **Exposure:** Movies are a safe place for the viewer to experience one's greatest fears and this opportunity is often relished since the viewer always knows at some level that what they are seeing is not real. These films combine curiosity and fear, producing a blended emotional state that can be a very pleasurable and positive experience. The viewer's anxiety amplifies the pleasure of the intrigue, and the resulting positive experience is more intense and long-lasting.
>
> **Thrill seeking:** Some viewers enjoy taking personal and emotional risks for the sake of the experience. Since much of life falls into the neutral category and there are typically few instances in which we can experience intense emotions (e.g., hatred), these movies let us fill out the full spectrum of experiences allowing the viewer to experience intense sensations.
>
> **Social scripts:** We know that courage and overcoming fear can lead to positive outcomes. Some viewers get to tap into this positive social script, while for others who don't necessarily enjoy the experience, it is nothing more than a test of courage. There are few occasions in which we get to do this, so the viewer will often seek them out, even if he or she doesn't particularly enjoy the experience. This occurs when a viewer has an emotional profile of high curiosity and low pleasure. (Kashdan, 2009)

Antisocial Versus Psychopathic Personality

Although **psychopathic personality disorder** is not an actual diagnosis, it is a commonly used term, and there is often confusion when the labels antisocial personality, sociopath, and psychopath are all lumped together. Robert D. Hare, the world's leading authority on psychopathy, has been doing research on psychopaths for over 50 years. Hare explains that most psychopaths fit the criteria for antisocial personality; however, the reverse is not necessarily true. Hare adds that cross-cultural studies have noted that psychopathy is generalizable. He cites several criteria for psychopathic personality including shallow emotions, glibness, manipulativeness, a parasitic lifestyle, episodic relationships, persistent violation of social norms, egocentricity, lack of remorse or empathy, low frustration tolerance, and lying (Hare, 2006).

Kavanagh and Cavanna (2020) have defined psychopathy as "a construct used to describe individuals with a conscience, who knowingly harm others via manipulation, intimidation, and violence, but feel no remorse" (p. 273). They analyzed psychopathy in James Bond novels and conclude that psychopathic traits are essential to Fleming's narrative scheme because they highlight the Bond/Evil dichotomy. However, they note that Bond himself has several psychopathic traits. Of course, this same dichotomy is found in the James Bond films.

In movies, psychopaths and sociopaths are often described as people who have "no conscience." Consider *Pirates of the Caribbean* (2003, 2006, 2007, 2011, 2016) and contrast Johnny Depp's character as the antisocial pirate with many of the pirate zombies led by Geoffrey Rush's character. The latter are clearly psychopathic. Table 13 uses contemporary films to illustrate the difference between antisocial personality disorder and psychopathy.

People have been fascinated with the topic of serial killers since Jack the Ripper strangled and cut the throats of five London prostitutes in 1888. More recent serial killers include Albert De Salvo (the Boston Strangler), David Berkowitz (the Son of Sam killer), Henry Lee Lucas, John Wayne Gacy, Ted Bundy ("the Preppie killer"), Wayne Williams, Charles Manson, and Jeffrey Dahmer, a harmless-looking young man who killed dozens of other young men, ate their body parts, and kept other parts in his refrigerator. The FBI defines a serial killer as anyone who has committed three or more separate murders. It seems that if a serial killer is well known, a movie will eventually follow: for example, *Dahmer* (2002), *Ted Bundy* (2002), *Gacy* (2003), *Monster* (Aileen Wuornos; 2003), *The Night Stalker* (Richard Ramirez; 1987), *Summer of Sam* (David Berkowitz; 1999), and *Zodiac* (2007).

"I believe what doesn't kill you makes you stranger."
"Do I really look like a guy with a plan? You know what I am? I'm a dog chasing cars. I wouldn't know what to do with it if I caught it. I just do things."
"Madness is like gravity; all it takes is a little push."

Comments made by the Joker revealing his psychopathology, in *The Dark Knight* (2008)

James Iaccino has written several *PsycCRITIQUES* film reviews examining the portrayal of serial killers according to different classification systems and serial killer typologies. Examples include an analysis of the *female serial killer* in *Scream 4* (2011; Iaccino & Dondero, 2013a) and the *mission-oriented and hedonistic serial killer* who matches wits with Edgar Allan Poe in *The Raven* (2012; Iaccino & Dondero, 2013b).

Anthony Hopkins plays one of the most terrifying serial killers ever filmed, in *The Silence of the Lambs* (1991), *Hannibal* (2001), and *Red Dragon* (2002). *American Psycho* (2000) is a quality film depicting a serial killer if the film is taken literally by the viewer. Another possibility in that film is that all of the murders committed by the fictional character Patrick Bateman are simply fantasies rather than reality; there are numerous cinematic elements to support this hypothesis, although few viewers leave the theater with this impression.

Contrary to media presentations and popular opinion, few if any serial killers are psychotic. (David Berkowitz was a salient exception.) In contrast, many are sexual sadists who derive sexual excitement from the murders they commit, and most are sociopaths who experience little remorse or regret after their crimes. Both John Wayne Gacy and Jeffrey Dahmer were homosexual pedophiles as well as serial killers.

Some serial killers commit multiple murders for utilitarian reasons – that is, they are "hit men" who kill for money. This is the kind of serial killer portrayed by Jack Nicholson in *Prizzi's Honor* (1985) and in *The Iceman* (2013), a film

Table 13. Differentiation of antisocial personality from psychopathic personality through movies

Personality type film		Personality characteristics
Antisocial	Jack Sparrow (Johnny Depp) in *Pirates of the Caribbean* (2003, 2006, 2007)	Manipulative and devious, though Jack Sparrow does show qualities of trust, care, allegiance, and teamwork
	Monty Brogan (Edward Norton) in *25th Hour* (2002)	History of not conforming to laws/rules, impulsive, irritable, and reckless disregard but shows remorse and care for others
	Johnny (David Thewlis) in *Naked* (1993)	Deceitful, impulsive, self-centered, lacks empathy, irresponsible; also shows fleeting concerns and care for others and for the betterment of society
	Euliss "Sonny" Dewey – The Apostle E.F. (Robert Duvall) in *The Apostle* (1997)	Heavily deceitful, impulsive, and dangerous in words and behaviors; also shows genuine care for others, love for God, and exhibits remorse
Psycho-pathic/ Sociopathic	The Joker (Heath Ledger) in *The Dark Knight* (2008); Barbossa (Geoffrey Rush) in *Pirates of the Caribbean* (2003, 2007)	Kills, tortures, manipulates, and creates mass confusion and terror, for his entertainment and pleasure. Kills at will for own gain, embodies the seven deadly sins, particularly greed
	Vann (Owen Wilson) in *The Minus Man* (1999)	Serial killer with no conscience and no reason or purpose, kills randomly
	Mickey Knox (Woody Harrelson) and Mallory Knox (Juliette Lewis) in *Natural Born Killers* (1994)	Torture and kill anyone who gets in their way or bothers them, without hesitation or regret
	Elijah Price (Samuel L. Jackson) in *Unbreakable* (2000)	Complete disregard for human life as he commits mass murder out of a self-serving need to find his "better half"
	Richard Kuklinski (Michael Shannon) in *The Iceman* (2013)	Based on a true story; Kuklinski murdered more than 100 people when working for the Gambino family

biography of the life of Mafia contract killer Richard Kuklinski.

Quality documentaries addressing the lives of sociopathic serial killers include *In Cold Blood* (1967) and *Henry: Portrait of a Serial Killer* (1986). The latter is loosely based on the life and confessions (since called into question) of Henry Lee Lucas. Henry (Michael Rooker) shares a cheap room with Otis (Tom Towles), a man he had met in prison in Vandalia. The film is controversial because it presents graphic details of several murders, including one in which Henry and his roommate, Otis, pretend their car is not running and then kill a man who stops to help. In a subsequent scene, Henry and Otis videotape the murder of an entire family. The film portrays the triangular sexual tension that existed between Henry, Otis, and Becky (Tracy Arnold), Otis's sister, a woman down on her luck who has come to live with her brother. In the final scene of the movie, Henry decapitates Otis. The movie is especially powerful as far as it trivializes murder, as in the scene in which Henry and Otis murder two prostitutes, then go out and casually share an order of French fries.

A family of serial killers can be seen in Rob Zombie's horror films, *House of 1000 Corpses* (2003) and *The Devil's Rejects* (2005). Serial killers also are depicted in numerous other popular films, such as *Se7en* (1995) and the *Scream* films (1996, 1997, 2000, 2011).

Two particularly powerful films pose interesting questions relevant to this distinction: *Monster* (2003) and *American Psycho* (1999). *Monster*'s Aileen (Charlize Theron) might be a rare example of a serial killer who seems more antisocial than psychopathic. She can express and share love for another (her lover, played by Christina Ricci), and in the film she claims that her killings were in self-defense (as did serial killer Aileen Wuornos in real life). In *American Psycho*, Patrick Bateman (played by Christian Bale) is shown killing many people throughout the film. If we are to take this literally, then he is clearly a psychopathic personality. Interestingly, the film also suggests that all of the murders depicted in the film are Bateman's fantasies, which is supported by plot elements, by his extensive fantasy doodles, and cinematically at the end through close-up shots of Bateman's head. The viewer is left to believe that Bateman is very narcissistic and has heavy antisocial traits but is not a psychopath.

The cinema is replete with examples of characters who illustrate the psychopathic personality. Some salient examples include Kurt Dussander (Ian McKellen) in *Apt Pupil* (1998), a film that depicts the rekindling of a suppressed psychopathic personality; *In Cold Blood* (1967); *The Boston Strangler* (1968); *Henry: Portrait of a Serial Killer* (1990); Fritz Lang's child serial killer in *M* (1931); Dennis Hopper as a sociopath in both *Blue Velvet* (1986) and *Speed* (1994); and Michael Shannon playing hit man Richard Kuklinski in *The Iceman* (2013). Charles Manson, as portrayed by Steve Railsback in the film *Helter Skelter* (1976), is another example of the indifferent disregard for social values and moral behavior found in people with psychopathic personalities. (Manson, responsible for the death of nine people in 1969, has never shown any remorse for his behavior or the deaths of his victims.)

"A door had been opened that couldn't be shut."

Kurt Dussander (Ian McKellen), a reclusive former Nazi henchman in hiding, in *Apt Pupil* (1998)

The legendary director Stanley Kubrick frequently depicted psychopathic personalities in his films. Perhaps his most famous is the street hoodlum, Alex, in *A Clockwork Orange* (1971); other characters in his films with strong psychopathic tendencies include the senior drill instructor, Gunnery Sergeant Hartman, in *Full Metal Jacket* (1987); the deteriorating character of Jack Torrance (Jack Nicholson) in *The Shining* (1980); the deceptive computer, Hal, in *2001: A Space Odyssey* (1968); the obsessed pedophile in *Lolita* (1962); and the generals who confront Kurt Douglas's character in the antiwar masterpiece *Paths of Glory* (1957).

A classic example of a psychopathic personality is found in Alfred Hitchcock's *Strangers on a Train* (1951). Bruno Anthony (Robert Walker), who repeatedly engages in unlawful behavior (including murder), is deceitful and glib and shows impulsivity, and there is never any reason to suspect he feels any remorse for the murder he commits or his plan to have his father murdered.

A recent Netflix film, *The Good Nurse* (2022), is based on a true story about one of history's most prolific serial killers, a nurse who practiced for 16 years and who may have been responsible for as many as 400 patient deaths before he was arrested in 2003. One of the most chilling aspects of the film is that the Charlie Cullen, dubbed "The Angel of Death" by the media, worked at nine hospitals where an alarming number of "codes" resulted in his repeated dismissals, but none of the hospital administrators notified the authorities because of fear of litigation. In the film, a "good nurse," Amy Loughren (played by Jessica Chastain), helps two detectives prevail in identifying and arresting Cullen

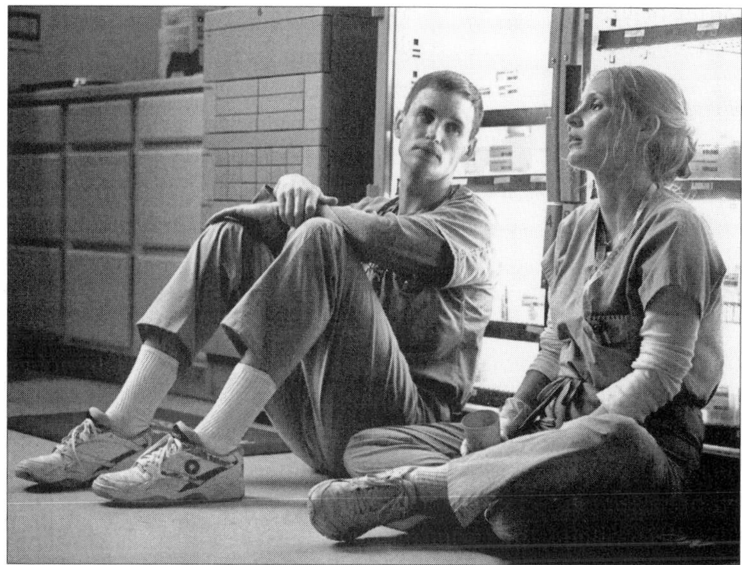

Figure 43.
The Good Nurse (2022, FilmNation Entertainment, Protozoa Pictures). Produced by Darren Aronofsky, Glen Basner, Ignacio de Medina, Jonathan Filley, et al. Directed by Tobias Lindholm.

(played by Eddie Redmayne; see Figure 43). The tension in the film is heightened by Loughren's serious cardiac problems; she badly needs medical care, but she is a single mom raising two daughters, and she must wait for a year before her health benefits kick in. Cullen becomes her friend and confident, helping her care for her children. When he was finally arrested, Cullen claimed he had engaged in "mercy killings," and he was only murdering people to help ease their pain. The film is based on a book by Charles Graeber titled *The Good Nurse: A True Story of Medicine, Madness, and Murder*.

Criminal proceedings have never been filed against any of the nine hospitals involved. Cullen agreed to plead guilty to 29 murders to avoid the death penalty; he was sentenced to 18 consecutive life sentences, and he won't be eligible for parole until 2403. Loughren received the cardiac surgery she needed and is currently living and working in Florida. She is still a good nurse, and she is interviewed along with the detectives involved in the case in a documentary film, *Capturing the Killer Nurse* (2022).

Borderline Personality Disorder

Borderline personality disorder is characterized by unstable but intense interpersonal relationships, labile mood, impulsive behavior, and erratic emotions. These individuals are easily angered, but their anger may pass as quickly as a summer storm, leaving no sign of its recent presence. Fear of abandonment is a pathognomonic characteristic of borderline personalities. These individuals become overly attached in almost all of their relationships: When they initially become romantically involved, their partners are apt to feel smothered by the intensity of the relationship and perplexed by the wild swings between affection and anger; when they enter therapy, therapists quickly become concerned about their excessive dependence and inappropriate adulation. These are the patients most likely to call in the middle of the night, insisting on an emergency consultation or late-night office visit. This is most apt to occur when the patient feels isolated or alone (e.g., when the therapist is about to take a vacation). They often vacillate between indiscriminate adulation and active hatred, sometimes within the space of a few hours.

Suicidal gestures and self-injury are common in people with borderline personality disorders. These gestures cannot be ignored, because completed suicide occurs in about 10% of borderline personality disorder cases. However, it is more common for the patient to behave in ways that are more attention seeking than life threatening, such as swallowing 20 Valium pills and then calling a crisis center, or making superficial cuts on their upper arm before calling a suicide hotline. Self-mutilation is also a common and serious problem with borderline personalities. The symptoms of borderline personality disorder overlap with those of both depression and bipolar disorders, and some borderline personality patients respond to treatment with either antidepressants or mood stabilizers. Women are diagnosed with borderline personality disorder much more often than men.

Glenn Close's character Alex Forrest in *Fatal Attraction* (1987) offers one of the best available depictions of borderline personality disorder. Michael Douglas plays Dan Gallagher, a happily married New York attorney who becomes sexually involved with Alex Forrest, a glamorous and sexually aggressive publishing executive. What starts out as a simple, one-night affair for Dan turns into a nightmare for him and his family, as Alex becomes increasingly possessive and manipulative. Dan tries to extricate himself from the affair, but Alex resorts to verbal threats, telephone calls to his wife, a suicide gesture (slashing her wrists after Dan tells her the affair is over), and intimidation of his wife and child. The performance by Close dramatically illustrates many characteristics of patients with a borderline personality disorder: anger, impulsivity, emotional lability, fear of rejection and abandonment, inappropriate behavior, vacillation between adulation and disgust, and self-mutilation. Although people with borderline personality disorder can be dangerous to others (as displayed dramatically in *Fatal Attraction*), this is not typically the case, and these individuals are more likely to be dangerous to themselves. If the individual has strong antisocial personality characteristics as well (which Alex Forrest does), the risk of danger to others rises.

Nicole Kidman portrays the title character in *Margot at the Wedding* (2007). Margot, a borderline personality, has separated from her husband, and she and her son are spending time at her sister's home for a wedding. As noted earlier in the chapter, it is difficult to diagnose a personality disorder with only a snapshot of the individual's life (e.g., a period of just a few days). Margot has very loose boundaries, labile affect, and is impulsive in her speech, and she shares the confidential news of her sister's pregnancy. Her mannerisms, speech, and behavior frequently reveal tension, anger, impulsivity, and reactivity. It is clear there has been significant tension over the years between the two sisters and a history of abuse which they discuss casually in front of their children. Margot roars with uncontrollable laughter when describing a rape. Margot also displays her fear of abandonment at the end of the film when she goes running uncontrollably after her son on a bus after just having sent him off, leaving her handbag and other items behind her on the ground. Most of her behavior and reactions are at least mildly inappropriate and have a significant impact on her life.

A more intense example of borderline personality disorder can be found in the character of Rae (Christina Ricci) in *Black Snake Moan* (2006), a film that exposes the protagonist's character flaws through a mixture of tragic scenes and beautiful interpersonal scenes. Rae is an unstable young woman whose fear of abandonment intensifies when her boyfriend Ronnie (Justin Timberlake) leaves for war. She covers over her fear with alcohol, drug abuse, and casual sex with multiple men. Sex is the only way she knows to relate to others. She has a history of abuse and allows others to take advantage of her. She displays a high level of explosive behavior and transient dissociative symptoms, both characteristic of people with borderline personality disorders. Also interesting is that over time she reverts to her same pervasive patterns of seductiveness and explosiveness.

Christina Ricci has also been successful elsewhere at portraying borderline personality, as demonstrated by two other films. In *Prozac Nation* (2001), her character, Elizabeth "Lizzie" Wurtzel, displays an intense fear of abandonment, is emotionally labile, possesses and then rejects her boyfriend, sabotages her friends, experiences multiple crises, has a deep underlying self-hatred, and reports a history of self-injurious behavior. She also suffers from comorbid depression. Likewise, her character Amanda Chase in Woody Allen's *Anything Else* (2003) displays borderline personality qualities in her interpersonal relationships and her affective instability. She has some attention-seeking qualities, is dishonest, manipulatively takes advantage of a dependent man, uses drugs, and is defensive and self-righteous in explaining her decisions and behaviors.

Another Woody Allen character – albeit deeper and darker – displaying a borderline personality disorder is Maria Elena, played by Academy Award winner Penélope Cruz in *Vicky Cristina Barcelona* (2008). She is unstable, intense in relationships, sexually impulsive, affectively labile, has rage-like temper and revengefulness, and is briefly suicidal with dissociative symptoms.

A more manipulative illustration of borderline personality can be found in Barbara Covett (Judi Dench), in *Notes on a Scandal* (2006). Barbara, a veteran teacher, discovers a younger teacher, Sheba Hart (Cate Blanchett), having an affair with a 15-year-old student, and the two women engage in a battle of manipulation and deceit. Barbara is a lonely woman with no friends or intimate contacts and seems to crave touch and emotional connection; she feels an intense attraction toward Sheba, sexualizes her, and engages her in a touching/stroking game. People with borderline personality disorders often misread and distort the realities of interpersonal situations, particularly those involving intimacy, and Barbara misreads their friendship as evidence of a deeper, more intimate connection. At the same time, she has no qualms about taking advantage of Sheba's trust and loyalty, and she betrays Sheba's trust, just as Shakespeare's Iago betrays Othello. Barbara also displays the pathognomonic symptom of fear of abandonment, even with respect to her cat. The viewer peers into Barbara's internal world through voice-over narration associated with her thinking and her journaling. In watching this film, the viewer is reminded that people with personality disorders exhibit repetitive behavioral patterns over time, and we learn that Barbara had often been obsessed with younger teachers and that in the past her behavior had led to a restraining order against her by another teacher; in a concluding scene, the viewer sees Barbara grooming her next victim.

The hospital staff in the film *Girl, Interrupted* (1999) apply the diagnosis of borderline personality disorder to the lead character, Susanna (Winona Ryder). It is difficult to justify this diagnosis, as Susanna only seems to display two behaviors fitting this diagnosis – a suicide attempt and sexual promiscuity. However, she is clearly depressed and has serious relationship problems. A rare depiction of male borderline personality can be found in Tom Ripley (Matt Damon) in *The Talented Mr. Ripley* (1999). Ripley has a tremendous fear of abandonment and even commits a murder to prevent himself from experiencing the pain of abandonment. Other potential examples of borderline personalities include Theresa Dunn (Diane Keaton) in *Looking for Mr. Goodbar* (1977), Marilyn Monroe in *My Week With Marilyn* (2011), and several of the female supporting characters in Martin Scorsese's *After Hours* (1985). Catherine Tramell (Sharon Stone) in *Basic Instinct* (1992) and *Basic Instinct 2* (2006) displays a number of borderline characteristics (not all of which meet explicit DSM-5 criteria) – for example, she is interpersonally manipulative, sexually exploitative and impulsive, seductive in therapy sessions (in the latter film), emotionally labile, angry, and vengeful.

Welcome To Me (2014) stars Kristen Wiig as a woman with a borderline personality disorder. Wiig's character, Alice Klieg, has not turned off her television set in a decade, and she loves Oprah. When she wins US $83 million dollars in a lottery, she stops taking her psychotropic medications, buys a talk show, and uses the show to broadcast her own odd ideas. The film is surprisingly engaging, and it puts many of the features of borderline personality disorder on full display.

Histrionic Personality Disorder

The defining feature of **histrionic personality** is dramatic attention-seeking behavior. These individuals are self-centered and preoccupied with their appearance. They feel uncomfortable in any situation in which they are not "center stage," and they can quickly turn their emotion on or off and with little provocation. They resent attention directed at others and will often engage in excessive behavior to have the focus of attention redirected to themselves. They initially are spontaneous and interesting people, not unlike Rosalind Russell's portrayal of the title character in the film *Auntie Mame* (1958). However, true histrionic personalities soon find that others quickly tire of their desperate attempts to remain at the center of attention and are angered by their inability to engage in equitable social interaction.

Carolyn Burnham (Annette Bening) in *American Beauty* (1999) is very melodramatic and clearly a character with a histrionic personality. She is unhappy and bored in her marriage, and she is having an affair with a man whom she admires for superficial reasons – he is rich, successful, charming, and highly narcissistic. She ruins a rare intimate moment with her husband Lester (Kevin Spacey) when she shows obsessive concern that he might spill beer on the couch. She is exact in her appearance, dressing in elegant clothes that make her stand out. At work as a real estate agent, Carolyn attempts to sell a house by exaggerating the house's appearance to unimpressed customers. She shows excessive emotionality and breaks down when faced with the reality that bright smiles and superficiality do not sell houses, and she goes into an emotional fit, crying, slapping herself in the face, stomping on the floor, and yelling, "Shut up! Stop it! You're weak! You baby! Shut up! Shut up! Shut up!" In social situations, Carolyn displays a very loud laugh that can be heard across a crowded room. She is socially inappropriate and overly critical of family members, such as when she greets her daughter after her daughter's dance routine, "I watched you closely. You didn't screw up once," with a big smile on her face as if she has just made an important, helpful observation. Her daughter looks at her in disgust.

In addition, rapid shifting from one extreme emotion to another is common in people with histrionic personality disorders. Carolyn quickly switches from hysterical laughter to blatant seriousness with a man she desires, and later from tearful crying to anger and slapping her daughter's face. Histrionic personalities are often very suggestible as well. Carolyn displays a ridiculous level of awe for another real estate agent's mantra, "You cannot count on anyone except yourself," and she follows and teaches this as the most important lesson to learn in life. In summary, appearance and style are far more important than substance for a person with a histrionic personality disorder.

Another precisely accurate example of histrionic personality is Katharine Hepburn's portrayal of a dying mother in *Long Day's Journey Into Night* (1962). Family life centers around the mother, and her two sons and her husband dote on her. She is extremely concerned with her appearance, openly fishes for compliments, and makes frequent references to her lost beauty. If she were being clinically evaluated, Hepburn's character Mary Tyrone would be diagnosed as someone with histrionic personality disorder and opioid addiction (morphine) with physiological dependence.

In *White Oleander* (2002), Robin Wright Penn plays Starr (an appropriate name for a histrionic character), the first mother figure for a young adolescent, Astrid (Alison Lohman), whose biological mother has been incarcerated. Starr is a former stripper, recovering alcoholic, and born-again Christian who encourages Astrid to read the Bible and accept Jesus as her savior. At first, Starr is kind and overly helpful in her care for Astrid; soon the viewer realizes these are superficial overtures that develop into a dangerous murder attempt when Starr becomes threatened as she realizes that Astrid's emerging sexuality excites her husband.

The classic example of histrionic personality disorder is found in Blanche DuBois's character (played by Vivien Leigh) in Elia Kazan's *A Streetcar Named Desire* (1951) based on Tennessee William's play by the same name. Blanche is clearly attention seeking, and she likes to be the center of attention. Her behavior is seductive and sexually provocative, and the sexual tension between her and Stanley, her brother-in-law, played by Marlon Brando, is present from the earliest moments in the film. Her emotions are shallow and shift often (such as when she screams when a glass of cola overflows onto her dress). There is a theatrical quality to every interaction, and she imbues even casual interactions with a significance that simply would not be there for most people. Woody Allen plays homage to *A Streetcar Named Desire* in *Blue Jasmine* (2013), a film in which Cate Blanchett plays the title role of Jasmine, a woman widowed and left broke after her husband's suicide, who still flies first class when she comes to San Francisco to stay with her sister. Jasmine – like Blanche DuBois – would also qualify for a diagnosis of narcissistic personality disorder. Her exhaustion and apprehension about an uncertain future are captured in Figure 44.

> **"Anxiety, nightmares and a nervous breakdown, there's only so many traumas a person can withstand until they take to the streets and start screaming""**
>
> **The histrionic Jasmine reflects on her troubles, in Woody Allen's *Blue Jasmine* (2013)**

Narcissistic Personality Disorder

People with a narcissistic personality have an intense need for admiration, are often self-centered, and have an exaggerated sense of their own importance. They may spend a great deal of time fantasizing about success or power. They feel entitled to special treatment and expect that others will automatically comply with their expectations; this often leads to their appearing conceited and pretentious. Their preoccupation with themselves leads them to overlook or devalue the contributions of others. The name of this disorder is taken from the Greek myth of Narcissus, who fell in love with his own reflection. Mirrors are often used in films portraying narcissists to symbolize self-reflection and infatuation with self and distorted or broken mirrors are used to represent a fractured sense of worth or esteem.

Although presenting as confident and secure, people with narcissistic personality disorder have low self-esteem and harbor unconscious feelings of insecurity, unworthiness, and self-doubt. Consider the film *Phone Booth* (2003), which is worthwhile for the ending in which a highly narcissistic New Yorker is stripped of his defenses and completely unravels, admitting to all his deceits, manipulations, and cover-ups, from the expensive clothes he wears, to his deep relationship fears, to keeping a young male sidekick around to feel better about himself. Suddenly, all his grandiosity, entitlement, and conceit are gone. He had never admitted these deeper issues even to himself in a conscious way,

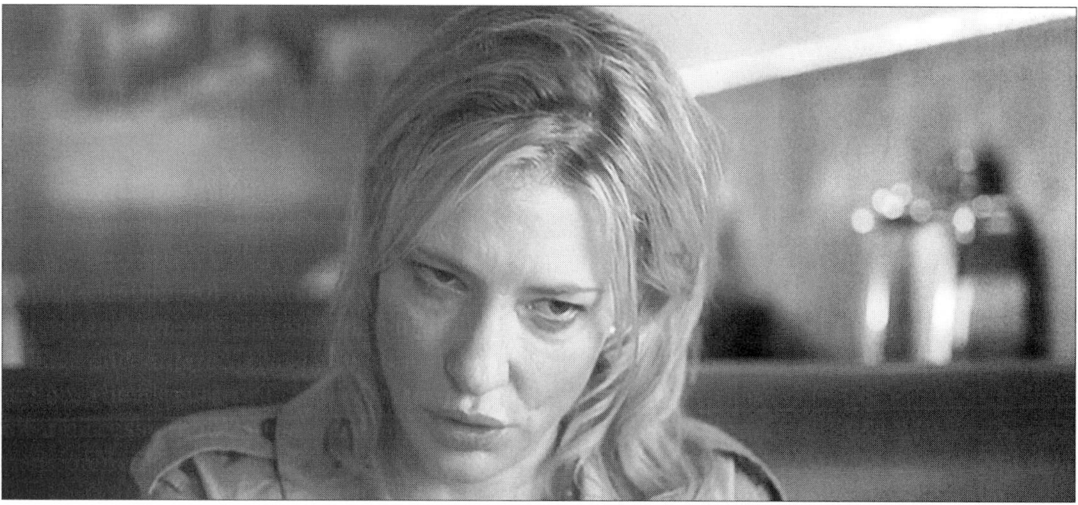

Figure 44. *Blue Jasmine* (2013, Gravier Productions, Perdido Productions). Produced by Letty Aronson, Helen Robin, Jack Rollins, Leroy Schecter, et al. Directed by Woody Allen.

and they remained present but deeply embedded. It took an extreme situation to trigger awareness and admission. Of course, most narcissists do not come to such insights about themselves, and when they do, it is not long before they return to their old patterns.

The narcissistic wound is also exhibited in *Overnight* (2003), a docudrama that tells the rags to riches to rags story of Troy Duffy, a bartender offered an attractive deal by Miramax for his screenplay. Nevertheless, it is Duffy's narcissism - his grandiose sense of self-importance, preoccupation with success, entitlement, and his willingness to exploit others to get his own way - that leads to his downfall and the likelihood he will never work in Hollywood again. The film does an excellent job depicting a deeply troubled and wounded man who is completely unaware of his shortcomings.

Contemporary cinema is replete with examples of narcissistic personality disorders: Andy Garcia's fascinating character, Byron, in *The Man from Elysian Fields* (2001), is a narcissistic, struggling writer who eventually realizes his narcissism and subsequent self-inflicted destruction and makes a change; Michael Douglas's portrayal of narcissistic personalities in *Solitary Man* (2009) and *Wall Street* (1987, 2010); Nicholas Cage's corporate character Jack Campbell in *The Family Man* (2000) states that his only concerns are "or money and power, nothing deeper"; Ben Stiller's ridiculous character Derek in *Zoolander* (2001), is too self-absorbed to realize he has been brainwashed; and John Turturro's character Dante Dominio is a narcissistic opera singer and performer in *The Man Who Cried* (2000). Robert Downey Jr.'s superhero character in the *Iron Man* (2008, 2010, 2013) films has a strong need for admiration, is grandiose, feels superior and special, and approaches relationships in an egotistical way. The consequences of his narcissism emerge when he insists that no one in the world can mimic or replicate his amazing technology; this is disproven, and it almost results in his death. In *Watch Out* (2008) we see an extreme example of narcissism in the film's protagonist, who masturbates while admiring polaroid photos of himself and who at one point has sex with an anatomically correct blowup doll with a pasted image of his own face pasted over the doll's face. In *American Psycho* (2000), Christian Bale's character would clearly qualify for a diagnosis of narcissistic personality disorder, as well as antisocial personality disorder - and several other diagnoses as well.

"Underneath all that bravado beats the heart of a guy who's not nearly as cocky as he wants everybody to believe."

Liz (Susan Sarandon) calling out the narcissism of Alfie (Jude Law), in *Alfie* (2004)

In *Roger Dodger* (2002), Roger Swanson (Campbell Scott) is a classic narcissistic personality - a womanizer who is teaching a 16-year-old adolescent boy about how men think and see the world. He teaches the boy to see, think, and perceive sex everywhere he looks. Roger creates various "opportunities" for the boy to seduce women - at the bar, at a party, and then with prostitutes. He has no qualms about encouraging the boy to take advantage of a drunken woman who has passed out. Roger displays little true empathy for the boy as he thrusts him to adulthood. Underneath Roger's inflated self-image and conceit is his rage at being rejected by his attractive boss (Isabella Rossellini) who has put an end to their love affair.

In *Lovelife* (1997), Alan (Jon Tenney) is a minor writer and professor who believes his work is especially important. He seems to care only for himself and his writing. He treats women badly and exploits them through seduction, deceit, and manipulation, and he eloquently explains his approach and craft to a barfly. In denying his own arrogance, Alan believes he is compassionate and sensitive because he must struggle to manage a relationship with two women (the real issue is that one of the women is not as fawning as the other). He believes women should be at his "beck and call" (one character describes him by saying, "he says what he wants, and everybody jumps").

> **"I want somebody to think I'm the greatest thing that ever happened to them and without me they couldn't go on."**
>
> **The narcissistic writer Alan in *Lovelife* (1997)**

The film accurately portrays the underlying sensitivity to criticism and inherent low self-esteem of the narcissist (which frequently results in narcissistic injuries). Alan gets terribly upset, stubborn, and passive-aggressive when his girlfriend does not come to his lecture; he expresses an intense fear of abandonment as he makes a big production about his girlfriend leaving a party without him, he then grovels on his knees with the girl standing over him, and later lies on a girl's lap to receive the motherly nurturance and attention he so deeply craves.

Director Neil LaBute created unforgettable and cruel narcissists in two of his bitterly satirical movies: *In the Company of Men* (1997) and *The Shape of Things* (2003). Though there are two male narcissists in the former movie, Chad (Aaron Eckhart) is more pathological as he convinces his friend that they should seduce a vulnerable, deaf woman and get her to fall in love with both, planning to subsequently dump her. Chad feels entitled to do this, blaming women for being rejecting, controlling, and manipulative, believing he and his partner can restore dignity to men through revenge and the pain of the innocent. In *The Shape of Things*, a character named Evelyn (Rachel Weisz) transforms Adam (Paul Rudd), an anxious, insecure, shy person, into a physically attractive, stylish, confident man. Without any qualms, she shocks Adam, the viewer, and the audience to whom she is giving a presentation when she reveals that her relationship with Adam has been a class "project" in which she used a human subject to prove that people are like clay and can easily be molded and manipulated. When talking with Adam afterward, Evelyn has a strongly stubborn, confident, and resentful expression on her face. She believes she has made him a better person and thus should be thanked for her behavior. The characters in each film have strong antisocial qualities evident in their complete disregard for others and social convention and in their pathological manipulation. They are predators who consciously seek out their prey - a vulnerable, neurotic individual with poor esteem. The endings of both movies reveal just how pathological both characters are as they reveal their manipulative "game," devoid of empathy. A similar plot line depicting extensive female manipulativeness can be found in *My Summer of Love* (2004).

Female narcissists are less common, but include Madonna portraying a grandiose, striking Eva Peron in *Evita* (1997). Eva emphasizes physical appearance, presentation to others, and her posture as critically important features. She manipulates people throughout the film for her own advantage - to help her rise in her career and look better in front of others. Annette Bening as Julia Lambert in *Being Julia* (2004) is another example of a female narcissist. Julia is a star of the theater who relishes her success and revels in her fame; however, feelings of self-loathing break through whenever she is rejected. She has been addicted to work most of her career but taking a break and having an affair revitalizes her, and her narcissism seems to shift. The character also has some histrionic qualities, as throughout the film it is often difficult for the viewer to discern when Julia is acting and when she is feeling and expressing real emotions. In addition, Mena Suvari's adolescent character, Angela Hayes, in *American Beauty* has narcissistic traits clearly seen in her preoccupation in becoming a model, her lack of empathy for a new student who has been hospitalized, and her strong beliefs that she is somehow special and important.

Other classic narcissistic characters include Norma Desmond (Gloria Swanson) in *Sunset Blvd* (1950) and (initially) arrogant and self-serving Whitey Marsh (Mickey Rooney) in *Boys Town* (1938). In *The Doctor* (1991), William Hurt plays Jack MacKee, a self-centered and narcissistic physician who cares little for anything except himself and his career until he develops a tumor in his throat and discovers what it feels like to be a patient. Warren Beatty plays Bugsy Siegel, a narcissistic and self-centered gangster in *Bugsy* (1991). Finally, Nicole Kidman plays the role of Suzanne Maretto, a narcissistic television personality who will stop at nothing to achieve her ambitions in *To Die For* (1995).

Cluster C Disorders

As is true in clinical settings, characters in films will have symptoms and personality characteristics that overlap with more than one disorder in each cluster. For example, Robin Williams' milquetoast character in *One Hour Photo* (2002) has a personality disorder; however, he has characteristics of several disorders, most of which are found in Cluster C. He lives alone, being too scared to take the risks that relationships require (avoidant); he is obsessed with a pseudo family (dependent); and he is orderly and rigid in handling photos at work and hoarding photos at home (obsessive-compulsive). Add in some depression with psychotic features, a probable history of past sexual abuse, and voyeuristic elements, and Williams' character becomes even more complex.

Avoidant Personality Disorder

People with **avoidant personality disorder** have a tremendous fear of being exposed as inadequate and inferior. They are hypersensitive to criticism and shape their lives around fear of rejection and disapproval. They avoid intimate relations, convinced that they would be ridiculed as inadequate lovers. They conceptualize the world (and especially interpersonal relationships and interactions) as unsafe and threatening. They have diminished self-esteem and describe themselves as inept, incompetent, and inferior. They are apt to spend much of their time at home and alone, in large part because of their concern that their personal deficiencies will be revealed if they venture out in public. These pervasive feelings of inferiority typically originate in childhood. In Adlerian terms, the person with an avoidant personality lacks the *courage to be imperfect*. However, it is important for clinicians to be sensitive to cultural differences that may affect a client's behavior. For example, in some Asian cultures, self-deprecation and extreme modesty about one's own achievements are normative behaviors and not indicative of a maladaptive personality trait.

This diagnosis overlaps with the diagnosis of **social phobia, generalized type**. The overlap is so substantial that many clinicians find the distinction between the two diagnoses to be meaningless, and the two diagnoses may be simply diverse ways of conceptualizing the same (or similar) conditions. Keep this in mind as you read about the characters in the following films.

Avoidant personality can be distinguished from schizoid personality in that although both avoid interpersonal contact, the avoidant person craves the intimacy lacking in life. *Finding Forrester* (2000) is about a high school student, Jamal, who befriends a reclusive, retired professor and writer, William Forrester (Sean Connery), who wants more intimate connections. This film is about people who are trying to get "unstuck" from their avoidance patterns. In *Finding Forrester*, Connery's character does not leave his apartment and can only be seen by others when he is cleaning his windows. He wrote an award-winning book 50 years ago but has not been published since then. He seems to have given up, perhaps because of fear of rejection. He avoids other people and denies being interested in any life other than his own. When he does eventually go out, he has a panic attack when in a crowd. He is socially inappropriate, such as when he closes the door in the face of Jamal without saying goodbye. There is a fundamental sadness in William's isolation in his apartment; he does look for connection as a voyeur, watching others outside with interest and keeping his windows clean so he can continue observing the outside world. The viewer begins to wonder how much of William's isolation is loneliness. The protagonist frequently drinks alcohol alone, often while working. He avoids discussing personal issues such as his family history or his work. He is reluctant to risk interpersonal sharing, and although this changes significantly as the friendship with Jamal develops, William keeps the secret of his cancer to himself.

Dependent Personality Disorder

Dependent personalities have extreme difficulty making decisions. They are submissive and look to others for structure, meaning, and direction in their lives. They tend to be passive and clinging. These people lack assertion skills and submit to the will of others. They sometimes submit to verbal, physical, or sexual abuse by their spouses and others. They lack self-confidence and feel they cannot manage on their own. They fear the loss of approval that may occur if they express their own opinions or beliefs. They invest tremendous time and energy in maintaining a relationship with the person upon whom they are dependent. When a close, dependent relationship ends, they almost immediately seek out another relationship that supports their chronic need for succor.

An amusing illustration of a dependent personality occurs in the 1991 film *What About Bob?* Bob, played by Bill Murray, is the patient of a psychologist played by Richard Dreyfuss. Bob pursues the beleaguered psychologist across the country when he tries to take a short family vacation. All therapists have had overly dependent patients, although they are unlikely to have encountered a case as extreme as that of Bob. The film is an interesting starting point for a discussion of transference and countertransference.

> **"I've been seeing myself through him for years."**
>
> **A dependent personality in *Lovelife* (1997)**

In *Lovelife* (1997), a female bartender, Molly, maintains an elevated level of obsequiousness toward her narcissistic boyfriend, Alan, doing everything she can for him and losing her own identity in the process. Molly believes Alan can do no wrong and that he has no flaws; in addition, she subjects herself to his unrelenting criticism. Like many other dependent personalities, she finds herself rejected by her boyfriend who takes up with another woman; when he loses that other woman, he shows up, and Molly takes him back.

In *White Oleander* (2002), Renée Zellweger plays Claire Richards, a foster mother with a dependent personality. Claire's submissiveness to her husband, her inability to confront or challenge his decisions, and her vulnerability to manipulation by others leads her to commit suicide. Jason Biggs' agreeable, people-pleasing character Jerry Falk in *Anything Else* (2003) is so dependent he must be "tricked" into being alone, into asserting his needs, and into challenging himself.

Obsessive-Compulsive Personality Disorder

A person with **obsessive-compulsive personality disorder** (OCPD) has enduring, inflexible, and maladaptive personality traits that involve perfectionism, orderliness, and an excessive need for control. They display exacting attention to detail and may devote a great deal of time to making lists and plans. Time is seen not as the fabric of life but rather as an enemy and something to be conquered. All this psychological energy is expended in a futile attempt to achieve a sense of control over the exigencies of life and the vicissitudes of fortune. Two films that are solid depictions of OCPD are *The Odd Couple* (1968) and *M*A*S*H* (1970). *The Odd Couple* presents a memorable performance by Jack Lemmon as Felix Unger, the neurotic roommate of Oscar Madison (Walter Matthau), who roams the house with a can of air freshener, determined to eliminate any unpleasant smells. In *M*A*S*H*, Major Frank Burns (Robert Duvall) spends the entire war fretting about the antics of "Hawkeye" Pierce (Donald Sutherland) and "Trapper" John McIntyre (Elliott Gould) and the inability of the system to set limits on their exuberant behavior. He is obsessed with rank and bitterly resents any undue familiarity by enlisted men or junior officers. He also works hard to ensure that the enlisted men do not fraternize with Korean women. He is self-righteous, moralistic, and rigid, even though he is having an ongoing affair with "Hot Lips" Hoolihan (Sally Kellerman). He becomes furious when he does not get his way, and he is ineffectual in responding to the cavalier attitudes of his tent mates.

Another classic film to portray OCPD is *Mommie Dearest* (1981), which stars Faye Dunaway as Joan Crawford. Joan pursues a life devoted to extrinsic values - appearance, fame, money, and possessions are what matter most to her. She senses she is missing one thing in her life - a child; following two divorces and many miscarriages, she finally adopts two children after using her power and lawyer boyfriend to pull some strings. Her attempts at being a good parent vanquish quickly, and her OCPD takes over. She is deeply perfectionistic of herself (e.g., her personal appearance, the cleanliness of her house, her relationships, and her children). She drives her daughter harder and harder, and her behavior becomes monstrous and abusive. She displays rigidity, perfectionism, and orderliness in every situation. In addition, there is an underlying anger that drives her behavior. Joan would be diagnosed with comorbid conditions of alcohol dependence and borderline personality disorder, the latter diagnosis supported by her deep fear of abandonment, emotional instability, sexual promiscuity, and push-pull messages in her relationships (e.g., in one scene with her boyfriend, she alternates between begging and threatening).

Ben Stiller portrays a character with OCPD in *Greenberg* (2010). Rastogi (2011), in her *PsycCRITIQUES* review of the film, finds that Greenberg shows that he meets the criteria for OCPD, as evidenced by those scenes in which his sensitivity to imperfections becomes pathological and affects his daily life. He copes with this by writing complaint letters to institutions: for example, he writes to American Airlines detailing a problem with the button on his reclining seat on an airplane, and he writes to government officials because too many Los Angeles drivers are honking their horns.

It is important to understand the difference between OCPD and OCD. The first reflects a maladaptive personality style; the second indicates the presence of a serious mental disorder characterized by recurrent and persistent thoughts, images, or impulses (obsessions) and repetitious behaviors or mental acts (compulsions) that the individual cannot avoid or suppress. For example, an obsessive-compulsive personality may need to be constantly cleaning the house and "picking up." This is maladaptive (when excessive) but may not significantly impair the person's life and may be mildly adaptive in some roles. However, the patient with an **OCD** - for example, Nicholas Cage's character Roy Waller in *Matchstick Men* (2003) - spends much of the day focused on their obsession or engaged in compulsive behavior. This individual is significantly distressed by their problem and realizes that the behavior or thoughts are abnormal and out of control. In contrast, people with OCPD are far less likely to be troubled by their condition.

John Turturro plays Al Fountain, a man with OCPD, in *Box of Moonlight* (1996). Turturro's character is rigid, overly conscientious, and rule-driven in both his work as a manager and in his family life with his wife and children. Al is rigid about the way his child learns using flashcards and obsessively asks about their use; he seems unable to handle joking and must rehearse a social situation before its occurrence. He is awkward and rigid at his job, bossing others around, seems robotic and machine-like, and is stiff in behavior (e.g., walking). The depiction of the effect of these OCPD traits on the family and coworkers is clear: Family members are avoidant, passive, or hesitant around him, and his coworkers make fun of him behind his back.

Al takes time off work and away from his family to loosen up as he goes on a journey to search out his past. Along the way, two Jehovah's Witnesses quickly and accurately get at his pain and sense of loss over the years (confronting the etiology of his OCPD), but they soon turn religious and begin proselytizing, which only alienates him. In a couple of scenes, Al sees things going backwards – for example, water being poured and a child riding a bike. Does this represent his life going backwards? It is a fascinating cinematic example of the lack of progress that occurs when one is so stuck in routine that it seems as if one is going backwards. Moreover, it is a metaphor for time, one of the biggest enemies to someone with OCPD.

Films Portraying Various Personality Disorders

Some readers may want to see films that depict several personality disorders in one viewing for educational and clinical purposes. These films present interesting dynamics in their portrayal of interactions between different pathologies. Some examples follow.

Bartleby (2001) displays a classic example of schizoid personality in the lead character, Bartleby, portrayed exquisitely by Crispin Glover. Surrounding Bartleby, in a colorful office, are co-workers who are narcissistic (Joe Piscopo as Rocky, a self-inflated womanizer), schizotypal (Ernie, a disheveled man who often speaks in word salad), and histrionic (Vivien, seductive and attention seeking, and dependent.

In *White Oleander* (2002), we see a young girl under the care of various mother figures, each with their own personality flaws. The child goes from her biological mother, Ingrid (an antisocial manipulator), to Starr (a dangerous histrionic), to Claire (a dependent personality with low self-esteem), and eventually to Rena (an antisocial personality who forces her foster children to sell clothes on the street to make money). The eyes of each mother seem to say it all, from the penetrating eyes of Ingrid to the downtrodden eyes of Claire.

The Royal Tenenbaums (2001) portrays the ultimate dysfunctional family, with pathologies that include narcissism, dependency, incest, suicidal behavior, paranoia, addiction, depression, and antisocial behavior, along with a schizotypal friend.

Woody Allen's *Anything Else* (2003) portrays an older man with a narcissistic personality disorder who befriends a young person with a dependent personality disorder in a relationship with someone with a borderline personality.

French director Jean Pierre-Jeunet purposefully creates films with very interesting and quirky personalities who play their roles on elaborate, often fantastical, set designs. For examples, see *Amelie* (2001), *The City of Lost Children* (1995), and *Delicatessen* (1992).

International Films: Personality Disorders

Cluster A

The character Joseph (Dominique Pinon) in *Amélie* (2001) meets the criteria for a paranoid personality, as he is so suspicious of his ex-girlfriend dating and meeting other men that he sits all day in the café where she works and watches her closely. He carries a small tape recorder in his pocket and records her various laughs, comments, and conversations with his own play-by-play and time-of-day voice-over. The viewer sees this is a pattern (thus providing additional weight for the diagnosis) as he continues similar suspicious behavior with the next woman he begins to go out with and then again with the first girlfriend when the new girlfriend dumps him. Anger and quick defensive reactions are common in the paranoid personality and are clearly part of Joseph's personality.

Cluster B

A classic in film history is *Breathless* (1960, France) by Jean-Luc Godard, one of the leading directors of the French New Wave cinema of the 1960s. This movement involved filmmakers who shifted toward being more abstract and experimental in writing style and narrative structure and emphasized psychological and social issues such as psychopathology and alienation rather than hard sciences and technology. In *Breathless*, the protagonist, Michel Poiccard (Jean-Paul Belmondo), is a young hoodlum and an antihero. He steals, gets in police chases in which he glibly kills one of the officers, and spends his time on the run from the authorities. He becomes truly fascinated by an American girl (Patricia Franchini, played by Jean Seberg) and tries to convince her to escape to Rome with him. This character is devoid of empathy and is characterized by selfishness, rudeness, blaming, and objectification of women.

Polish director Krzysztof Kieslowski created *The Decalogue* (1989), an extraordinary work composed of ten 1-hr films portraying a variety of tenants in an apartment complex. Each film relates loosely to one of the Ten Commandments. There are several antisocial characters scattered throughout the films, such as the mother who uses deceit and manipulation to keep her daughter's child from her, and the young vagabond who wanders the streets and randomly strangles a taxicab driver. *Perfume: The Story of a Murderer* (2006, Germany) is an interesting film from independent director Tom Tykwer, about a boy who grows up with a superior olfactory sense. He becomes obsessed with this ability, smelling anything in the environment, near or far. As the character, Jean-Baptiste Grenouille (Ben Whishaw), matures to adulthood, he develops a mission to "preserve scent" and to "keep smell" as he searches for the ultimate perfume. Along this journey, he directly and indirectly begins to cross boundaries (e.g., he inappropriately grabs the arm of a woman on the street without speaking to her and carefully smells her arm) and kill people – in one scene, he obsessively smells a woman after accidentally killing her by covering her mouth to prevent her from screaming; he then strips her naked and smells her whole body carefully. Recklessness, irresponsibility, and lack of remorse are key features of this character.

The Robber (2010, Germany) is based on a true story of a solo bank robber who is also an accomplished marathon runner. His one connection in life is his ex-girlfriend. His antisocial personality is dramatically portrayed in a scene in which he kills his parole officer and experiences no remorse. He displays flat affect and does not consider the consequences of his actions on others. *Animal Kingdom* (2010, Australia) is a well-directed story of a diabolical crime family; the family includes numerous psychopathic killers and drug addicts. The plot involves a 17-year-old boy whose mother has just died of a drug overdose; he is sent to live with this crime family consisting of his grandmother and uncles. Upon learning how deeply pathological, manipulative, and dangerous they are, the young man realizes he must either join them or escape.

Tsotsi (2005, South Africa/UK) is a movie about an African gangster who kills others when needed and brutally beats a fellow gang member to a pulp. One day Tsotsi (Presley Chweneyagae) robs a woman and steals her car but discovers there is an infant in the back seat. He reluctantly decides to care for the baby, and this experience slowly transforms his character. Through flashbacks the viewer learns of Tsotsi's painful past – his longing for a connection with his mother, his physically abusive father, his observation of his father abusing animals, and the neglect his father orchestrated in intentionally keeping Tsotsi separate from his mother despite living in the same household. The viewer begins to feel some sympathy for this brutal character, and this experience for the viewer intensifies when Tsotsi's caring and nurturing of an infant lead him to make a connection with a caretaking mother in his village, renew a friendship with the man he beat up, and sacrifice his livelihood by returning the infant to its mother.

Another young person with an antisocial personality disorder is portrayed in a film that won the Palm d'Or at Cannes, *The Child* (2005,

France). An endearing, petty street thief, Bruno (Jérémie Renier), becomes much less likeable when he sells his newborn for money. The film shows an interesting depiction of selling a baby: Bruno makes a phone call, goes into an abandoned house, walks up several flights of stairs, places his baby on his jacket in a room, walks into the next room and closes the door. He makes a call on his smartphone, saying "it's done," waits a brief time, and then goes back into the first room and picks up his jacket and money.

Luis Buñuel is regarded as one of the greatest directors in cinema history. In the filming of *That Obscure Object of Desire* (1977, France/Spain), the lead actress walked off the set and Buñuel jokingly remarked that her role should be played by two women. This comment became a reality and marked his signature style of surrealism. In the film, Mateo (Fernando Rey) pursues a young Spanish woman, Conchita (who is played by two actresses who do not look alike). The use of two actresses is helpful in depicting the character's borderline psychopathology. Conchita displays a mix of teasing, controlling, avoiding, manipulating, taunting, and erratic fighting. When she attempts to get the couple to agree they will never leave each other, it is clear fear of abandonment is the underlying issue. Conchita is seductive, reeling Mateo back to her – but then refusing to be intimate with him. Her push–pull behavior becomes so significant that the viewer begins to wonder when Mateo will leave the relationship.

Love Exposure (2008, Japan) is a little-known film that is surprisingly accurate in its depiction of borderline personality disorder. A dramatic woman, Kaori, falls in love with a priest and attempts to seduce him by wearing provocative clothing. She admits she goes to confession so she can be close to him in a tiny room. In the confessional, she puts his hand to her chest (so he can feel both her rapidly beating heart and her breast) and speaks of being in love with someone who cannot return her love. After the confession, she asks for his smartphone number and calls him immediately after she leaves the church. She invites him to a park where she jumps on him. He initially rejects her sexual overtures, but she persists. The two eventually move in together and hide out from the church-going community. Shortly thereafter, she becomes controlling, angry, and aggressive, and moves out of the home to be with a younger lover. Several scenes later, she reappears, admitting she has slept with many men in the interim. She is emotionally labile with him – expressing sadness, hopelessness, anger, and joy – cycling around and around. She desires immediate satisfaction of all her whims, and she insists that they be married immediately. She also has an intense fear of abandonment, as shown by her statement: "Don't leave me! I won't let you!" She once again gets her lover to abandon his role as a priest; predictably, once they are living together, she becomes labile and agitated and walks out of their relationship.

Kaori: "Father, listen to my confession! If you turn away from me, I'll kill myself. Please listen to me."
Priest: "What can I do?"
Kaori: "I'm in love with you. I know I really am a hopeless woman. What can I do about it? Please listen to my confession."

The manipulative verbiage of Kaori, a borderline personality, in *Love Exposure* (2008, Japan)

The intriguing movie *Swimming Pool* (2003, France/UK) portrays a young woman, Julie (Ludivine Sagnier), who is seductive, provocative, and has a desire for excitement. She presents as nonchalant and laid back, but she is also someone who can be easily hurt or angered. She is sexually impulsive and promiscuous, having sex with a different man each night. She throws herself at older men, even when they express disinterest. One night she appears with a bruise on her face around her eye, and the viewer is left to speculate as to what sort of danger she had been involved in while staying out the whole night. She is manipulative and jealous when her roommate begins to dance with a man. Julie acts out in anger when she is rejected. Her instability leads to a dissociative episode where she thinks she sees her mother (who is deceased) and expresses happiness at the prospect of her mother's return, screams when she is told that her mother is not there, and then faints. Julie also experiences a loss of memory, in which she is unable to remember killing her lover.

Zaza (Michel Serrault), the gay transvestite performer in *La Cage aux Folles* (released in US with the title *Birds of a Feather*; 1978, France/Italy), provides a wonderful example of a histrionic personality. She is dramatic and flamboyant, and everything she does is exaggerated. When her partner Renato (Ugo Tognazzi) tells her that he plans to invite his ex-wife to an important dinner with his son's future in-laws, Zaza is highly insulted and announces her intention to commit suicide. Neither Renato nor the viewer thinks for a minute that she is serious about her threat.

Cluster C

Sheila McCarthy plays Polly Vandersma, an insecure, socially awkward, temporary worker with avoidant traits in the popular Canadian film *I've Heard the Mermaids Singing* (1987). She is naïve, socially inhibited, and seems to have fragile self-esteem and self-concept. The voice-over narration done by McCarthy provides insights into her thinking and feeling when she is interacting with others.

Audrey Tautou's whimsical and endearing title character in *Amélie* (2001, France) has many avoidant personality characteristics. Amélie wants contact with others, especially intimate love, though she is unable to take the risk. The emphasis in the film is on her thoughts and the challenge involved in meeting a man; the key theme, which the movie cleverly portrays cinematically, is her constant avoidance of meeting a man who comes into her life. After doing a good deed, Amélie appears nervous and looks away, ignoring an opportunity for human interaction; she simply does not know how to interact socially. The film is rare in its sophisticated exploration of the causes of Amélie's anxiety and avoidant behavior. It notes that, from birth, she was trapped between a neurotic mother (who had "shaky nerves" and was anxious about everything) and an iceberg father, who avoided all feelings. In addition, she had no playmates or social life and therefore became used to isolation, fantasy, and imagination. Other contributing etiologies are presented when she is tricked by a neighbor into feeling guilty as the "cause" of natural disasters, when her mother is dramatically killed in front of her, and when she has ongoing problems in relating and communicating with her father.

A common pattern for people with avoidant personalities is the problem of self-sacrifice – devoting oneself to helping others and losing sight of one's own struggles and self-care. Amélie epitomizes self-sacrifice as she devotes herself to being a regular "do-gooder," helping others find joy and become "unstuck" from their life patterns. Amélie is personally stuck in her avoidant pattern and does not know it. Eventually, she learns to reach out to others for support and develops the courage necessary to face her fears.

Tautou also portrays a Cluster C character, Michèle, in another French film, *God Is Great and I Am Not* (2002), in which she has a quirky element of dependent personality (but not the disorder) as far as she repeatedly compromises her beliefs by conforming and converting to the religion of her partner at the time. She is shown trying to dedicate herself to Catholicism and Buddhism before finding a Jewish man and converting to Judaism. Her fear of being alone leads her to become suicidal after the end of an intimate relationship.

In the Spanish period film *Mad Love* (2002), a woman compulsively attaches herself to her husband despite continuous evidence of his philandering. She becomes preoccupied and worried about his whereabouts, yet she maintains an elevated level of excitement when he returns from a journey that has obviously involved infidelities. In one scene, he resists a warm embrace despite her clinging and affectionate behavior, and she asks him to lie to her about where he has been. Even when she is rejected by him, she obsessively continues to love him and believe they will be reunited upon her death.

> **"I want to love you, even if you loathe me."**
>
> **A classic dependent quote from "Joan the Mad" in *Mad Love* (2002)**

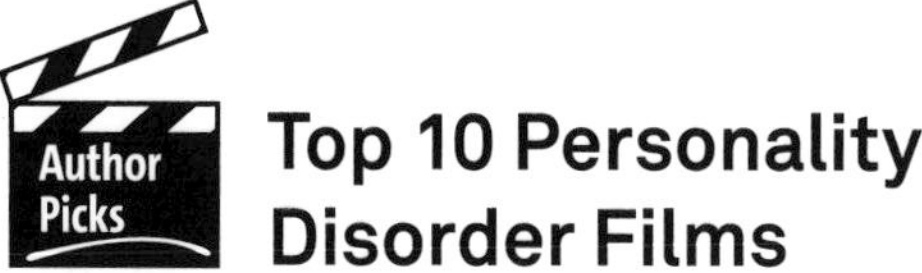

Top 10 Personality Disorder Films

Sunset Blvd. (1950)
A Streetcar Named Desire (1951)
The Odd Couple (1968)
A Clockwork Orange (1971)
That Obscure Object of Desire (1977)
The Talented Mr. Ripley (1999)
American Beauty (1999)
No Country for Old Men (2007)
Blue Jasmine (2013)
The Iceman (2013)

Chapter 14

Paraphilic Disorders

Why is that day marked in red?

Arturo asks Laura about the significance of February 29th, in *Leap Year* (*Año Bieiesto*; 2011)

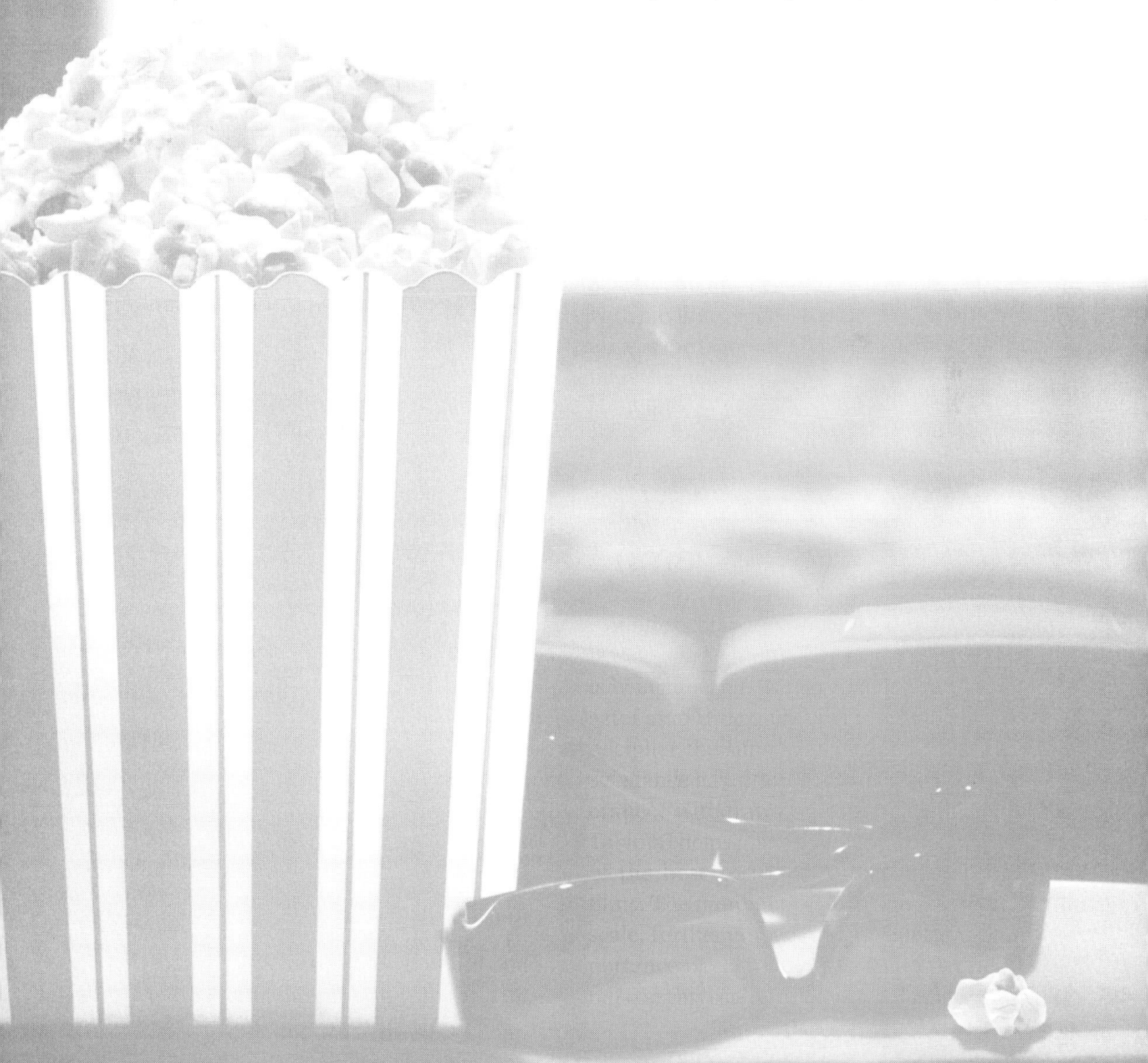

The Range of Normal Sexual Behavior

Few areas of human behavior are as complex, varied, and interesting as sexual behavior, and filmmakers, social scientists, and the public are all fascinated by the multitude of possibilities inherent in our sexuality. It is important to appreciate that the range of normal sexual behavior is exceptionally broad, and many behaviors that seem unusual or are disturbing to most people do not qualify for a DSM-5 label (e.g., rape, incest). As a rule, remember that complex or elaborate sexual fantasies are commonplace and do not suggest that any type of psychological disturbance is present. A psychological problem exists when a person acts on their fantasies with unwilling partners or behaves in ways that distress other people.

Filmmakers have been quick to exploit our fascination with sexual behavior, and contemporary cinema is replete with examples of sexual psychopathology. A serious student can learn a great deal about abnormal psychology from selective viewing.

Paraphilic Disorders

The term "paraphilia," according to the DSM-5, "denotes any intense and persistent sexual interest other than sexual interest in genital stimulation or preparatory fondling with phenotypically normal, physically mature, consenting human partners" (p. 685). The paraphilic disorders included in the DSM-5 are **voyeuristic disorder, exhibitionistic disorder, frotteuristic disorder, sexual masochism, sexual sadism disorder, pedophilic disorder, fetishistic disorder,** and **transvestic disorder**. Sexual desire has many faces, and there are numerous other ways it can manifest (e.g., necrophilia); however, these eight disorders are the most common paraphilias, and they are included in the DSM-5 because clinicians frequently encounter them in clinical practice, and because many of them are illegal and sometimes can result in prosecution and incarceration. Clients frequently present with two or more paraphilias; these sometimes are logically related (e.g., the person with a foot fetish may also have a shoe fetish), but often are quite disparate (e.g., a pedophile may also be a sadist).

It is important to note that at some time in their lives, most people have had fantasies or have engaged in a behavior that may fit one or more of the categories listed above. However, sexual fantasies per se are not a psychological problem – and do not warrant a diagnosis – unless a person has acted on their fantasies or is significantly distressed by them. The male who has fantasies about peeping through a window and watching his neighbor undress, for example, is not engaging in deviant behavior. In fact, fantasies of this type are common among males. The behavior would be deviant if the man could be aroused *only* by the fantasy, or if he acted out and spied on his neighbor.

Voyeuristic Disorder

A **voyeur** is a "peeping Tom" who experiences arousal and derives sexual satisfaction from spying on unsuspecting people, usually strangers, as they are getting undressed, using the toilet, or having sexual relations. Although it is normal to want to look at the bodies of others (e.g., at the beach), the voyeur goes to great lengths to find surreptitious hiding places from which they can watch others without being detected. Arousal is always associated with the clandestine aspects of the situation; voyeurs report little interest in watching pornographic films, visiting topless or nude beaches, or attending topless bars – all experiences where public voyeurism has been sanctioned. Voyeurism is the most common illegal sexual behavior, and the DSM-5 estimates that the highest possible lifetime prevalence is 12% in men and 4% in women. The diagnosis requires a minimum age of 18 years, because viewing associated with sexual curiosity in puberty is both age appropriate and developmentally normal.

As is the case with exhibitionism and obscene phone calls, it is rare for the voyeur to attempt to initiate sexual relationships with the victim. The voyeur will most often masturbate while viewing the arousing scene or sometimes later, when replaying the scene in memory. Although it is rare for voyeurs to progress to crimes of sexual violence, more than two thirds of males who commit sex-related murders report early experiences with voyeurism (Ressler et al., 1986).

Pulp Fiction (1994) depicts a sadist who derives sexual pleasure from watching Marsellus Wallace being raped, and *Psycho* (1960) includes a classic scene in which Norman Bates watches Marion Crane undress, spying through a peephole in the hotel office. In Gus Van Sant's 1998 remake of the film, Norman is obviously masturbating while spying on Marion. (It is interesting to note that Alfred Hitchcock used a 50-mm lens on a 35-mm camera to film every scene in which Norman spies on Marion; this method replicates human vision, and filming in this way draws in the viewer and makes them a fellow voyeur.)

In David Lynch's *Blue Velvet* (1986), Jeffrey watches from a closet while Frank (Dennis Hopper) inhales amyl nitrate and abuses Dorothy. The scene in which a confused and naked Dorothy is walking on a Wilmington Street was based on a childhood memory of the director who had been with his brother when they saw a naked woman walking toward them.

In *American Beauty* (1999), the character of Ricky Fitts is clearly a voyeur, and he films his neighbor Jane through her window (and eventually persuades her to undress while he films her). Finally, *The Truman Show* (1998) is a classic example of extreme voyeurism in which Ed Harris's character devotes his life to filming and viewing every moment in the life of Jim Carrey's character. Films like *Porky's* (1981) depict adolescent boys drilling holes in the wall to watch girls showering, while a more serious film, *Sex, Lies and Videotape* (1989), introduces Graham Dalton (James Spader), a character who is otherwise impotent and can only become aroused when listening to videotapes in which women he has interviewed talk about the personal details of their sex lives.

An interesting variation of voyeurism is **troilism**, or sexual gratification derived from watching other people have sex (or allowing others to watch oneself engage in sexual activity – behavior more logically linked to exhibitionism than voyeurism). This practice is sometimes referred to as **scoptophilia**. Variations on these themes include the **ménage à trois** ("family of three"), swinging, and couples that have monogamous sex in each other's presence. Swinging or mate swapping is widespread, although AIDS and other sexual diseases have presented serious obstacles to this form of sexual expression. A failed attempt at swinging is portrayed in Paul Mazursky's 1969 film *Bob and Carol and Ted and Alice*, starring Robert Culp, Eliot Gould, Dyan Cannon, and Natalie Wood. The film celebrates social permissiveness and the mores of the late 1960s more than sexual freedom; in the final scene, Bob, Carol, Ted, and Alice, all in bed together, reaffirm their commitment to monogamy.

The pain of voyeurism is evident in the film *Voyeur Confessions* (2001). Other films depicting voyeurism include *Lovelife* (1997) and the Canadian film *The Adjuster* (1991). Most films that have dealt explicitly with voyeurism have been misleading presentations that perpetuate common myths. For example, *Peeping Tom* (1960) presents the story of a voyeur, Tom (who was raised by a sadistic psychologist who constantly filmed Tom as he was growing up), who tortures his victims and then photographs them as they are dying. This is an example of sexual sadism, not voyeurism.

Some films depict a strong voyeuristic component without depicting explicit sexual fantasy or gratification. (If there is no sexual arousal, a diagnosis of voyeuristic disorder is *not* made.) Christopher Nolan's debut film, *Following* (1998), tells a creative story about a man who enjoys picking out one person in a crowd and then following this individual for a day. The voyeur is a lonely writer who convinces himself he follows people to get character ideas for his stories. His habit has qualities of an addiction as far as it becomes "irresistible" to him, he is unable to keep it under control, he obsesses about it, and he employs various cognitive justifications for maintaining this inappropriate and disturbing behavior.

Another nonsexual (possibly impotent) voyeur is displayed in Hitchcock's classic film *Rear Window* (1954). Voyeurism is clearly portrayed, James Stewart's character watches his neighbors incessantly, and he cannot pull away from his window (although it results in part from boredom and a broken leg). His whole life revolves around looking into others' lives, and he satisfies his psychological needs in this way. He also resists and rejects a beautiful, caring woman who is a society debutante who cannot join him as he travels to photograph international conflicts. If the viewer assumes Stewart's character is wrong about the murder he thinks he sees, and that all his behavior was pure voyeurism with no positive, beneficial outcome, it is hard to avoid the conclusion that this is a film about voyeurism. Brian De Palma's *Body Double* (1984) pays homage to Hitchcock and portrays an interesting connection between a male voyeur and a female exhibitionist.

Exhibitionistic Disorder

The exhibitionist's preferred form of sexual gratification is exposing his genitals to unsuspecting strangers. Masturbation often occurs during or after exposure. The exhibitionist will almost never attempt to have intercourse with the person intimidated and would be personally intimidated and frightened by an opportunity for an adult sexual encounter. Although reports of exhibitionism in a neighborhood usually result in increased concern about the possibility of rape, exhibitionism and rape are dramatically different behaviors and are almost never linked.

The DSM-5 requires that exposing one's genitals to unsuspecting persons occur for at least 6 months before the diagnosis of exhibitionistic disorder can be made, and specifiers are used to stipulate whether the behavior occurs with prepubescent children, physically mature individuals, or both. The prevalence of exhibitionistic disorder in males is estimated to be at most 2–4%, and the disorder in females is dramatically lower (DSM-5).

Exhibitionism can occur at any age, but typically develops in males in their mid-20s. Despite the popular image of a "dirty old man in a raincoat," the incidence of exhibitionism falls off rapidly after the age of 40 and is rare in older males who are cognitively intact. Many exhibitionists have never had meaningful or satisfying adult sexual relationships; others have normal psychosexual development histories.

Reports of true exhibitionism in females are quite rare, although exposing their breasts or legs in public may arouse some women. Exhibitionism in females can also be used as a way of establishing dominance in a nonsexual encounter with males. The potential for psychological manipulation through exposure is dramatically portrayed during Sharon Stone's interrogation scene in *Basic Instinct* (1992). Brief scenes of exhibitionistic behavior are depicted in *Natural Born Killers* (1994) and *Morvern Callar* (2002).

The Good Mother (1988) raises interesting questions about the boundaries between healthy sexuality and exhibitionism. Diane Keaton plays Anna Dunlap, the divorced mother of a 6-year-old daughter. Anna falls in love with an artist and starts to live a bohemian life that includes nudity in front of her daughter. Her new lover at one point innocently lets the daughter touch his penis when he is getting out of the tub, and she expresses natural childhood curiosity. When the ex-husband learns about this event, he sues for custody, and Anna is forced to renounce her lover to maintain visitation rights with her daughter.

Frotteuristic Disorder

The **frotteur** is someone who derives sexual pleasure from brushing or rubbing against others in an inadvertent but clearly sexual manner. This rubbing typically involves a man's pelvis or erect penis. Frotteurs frequent crowded stores, escalators, buses, and subways, where their behavior can be attributed to crowding. The DSM-5 lists frotteurism as an independent paraphilia, although many authors view it as a variation of exhibitionism. In *All Out!* clinical psychologist Albert Ellis describes being an enthusiastic teenage frotteur (Ellis & Ellis, 2010).

The film *Dummy* (2003) portrays an unemployed man who is a frotteur. The man is balding and wears thick glasses. He is included in the film purely for laughs. Though his behavior is not depicted cinematically, the character clearly meets the DSM-5 criteria for frotteurism.

Sexual Masochism Disorder

The **sexual masochist** becomes sexually excited when they are humiliated, beaten, bound, or made to suffer. It is important to appreciate that the diagnosis of sexual masochism is made only when patients engage in these behaviors. As is the case with other paraphilias, masochistic fantasies are both common and harmless, and moderate sadomasochistic behavior (e.g., scratching and biting) can be a rewarding part of normal sex play.

Masochists allow themselves to be abused in a variety of ways, including bondage, whipping, handcuffing, spanking, cutting, and burning. They are often verbally abused as well as physically mistreated. Humiliation may be necessary for arousal to occur – for example, a masochist may be forced to wear a diaper, or his partner may defecate or urinate on the masochist. Whips, chains, leather, and rubber accouterments often play a key role in the sexual activity of the masochist, who is happiest with a (mildly) sadistic partner. A woman who caters to the sexual preferences of masochistic men is referred to as a **dominatrix**. Masochists may be gay or straight, although most sadomasochistic encounters are heterosexual. Among homosexuals, masochists outnumber sadists (Innala & Ernulf, 1992). There are no good estimates of prevalence of the disorder; however, the DSM-5 cites data from Australia suggesting about 2% of males and 1% of females had been involved in bondage and discipline, sadomasochism, or dominance and submission during a 12-month period.

Secretary (2002) is an intriguing film about a young woman (Maggie Gyllenhaal) who is depressed and seriously self-injurious. She takes a job as a secretary working for a successful attorney, Mr. Grey (James Spader). She begins to enjoy his harsh criticism of her mistakes, and a sadomasochistic relationship develops. Grey enjoys spanking her, yelling at her, and engaging in other sadistic behavior, but he prohibits her from injuring herself (paradoxically using his sadism to control her masochism). The film opens with her nicely dressed at work, arms tied to a long bar behind her neck. She picks up items with her teeth or by turning her torso horizontally. Through a variety of sadomasochistic behaviors, she matures, stops her self-abuse, and develops a meaningful relationship with her boss, eventually marrying him. Hart and Cutler-Broyles (2021) have argued that films like *Secretary* can offer healing for members of the bondage, discipline, and sadomasochism (BDSM) community by reframing the discourse on pathology surrounding these practices and creating a space in which community members can explore their desires without stigma.

Quills (2000) depicts the last years of the Marquis de Sade (Geoffrey Rush), who spent years in an institution. The protagonist engages in a variety of paraphilias that give his life meaning and pleasure. In Lars von Trier's *Dogville* (2003), Nicole Kidman plays the role of Grace, a woman who becomes involved in a masochistic relationship with an entire community in her efforts to become accepted by the community and escape her mob pursuers. Peter O'Toole plays T. E. Lawrence in *Lawrence of Arabia* (1962), and the film hints at his masochism. Paul Schrader's biopic, *Mishima: A Life in Four Chapters* (1985), accurately presents Mishima as a bisexual masochist; the final scene in the film shows Mishima committing ritualistic suicide *(seppuku)* by disemboweling himself before having himself beheaded by one of his followers.

Extreme masochism is present in the documentary *Sick: The Life and Death of Bob Flanagan, Super masochist* (1977), a film about a Los

Angeles performance artist who used masochism to cope with his cystic fibrosis. Flanagan was involved in a love relationship with Shree Rose, a woman who collaborated in his need to embrace pain as a way of coping with his illness.

> **"I want a wealthy collector to finance an installation in which a video camera will be placed in the coffin with my body, connected to a screen on the wall, and whenever he wants to, the patron can see how I'm coming along."**
>
> **One of Bob Flanagan's last wishes in *Sick: The Life and Death of Bob Flanagan, Supermasochist* (1977)**

Replika, Robots, Sex Dolls, and Human Sexuality

The parallel development of artificial intelligence (AI) and advances in robotics technology has opened new arenas for sexual expression. This sometimes takes the form of chatbot companions who come to know their user, learning about his or her personality with increased use. Over time, the AI companion accrues considerable knowledge, and the recommendations made (movies, for example) can become increasingly sophisticated. Most of these AI companions are available on the internet at no cost for basic services; they are easily accessible on smart phones, making them virtually omnipresent. They are all programmed to be warm, empathic, and (seemingly) genuine – all characteristics of effective psychotherapists!

Replika is currently the most popular of these programs, and it has been available since 2017. However, competition is intense and new AI chatbots are constantly being developed. Although such bots initially target friendly companionship, flirting is commonplace, and your bot – for an additional fee – can undress, "talk dirty," and simulate orgasm (i.e., "Get romantic with Replika Pro"). The addition of voice messages significantly enhances the illusion that one is speaking to a caring, devoted human companion. The "friend" option is free; interacting with any other option (girlfriend, wife, sister, or mentor) requires an additional fee.

Chatbot interaction moves into new, provocative, and potentially promising arenas with the development of sex dolls and sex robots. Although cheap plastic sex dolls have been available for decades, newer models draw on advances in silicone and thermoplastic elastomer technology to produce robots that look and feel much more realistic than earlier models. In addition, eye movements can be made to track movement by the person being spoken to, and robotic genitals can be programed to be warm and moist. Such robots may have utility in sex therapy, and robots offer avenues for safe sexual expression for incels, isolated individuals (e.g., prisoners, explorers), and people with disabilities like cerebral palsy that are likely to limit sexual opportunities and options.

Eichenberg et al. (2019) surveyed sex therapists and physicians about the potential therapeutic benefits of sex robots. They found about half of their respondents could imagine themselves recommending purchase and use of sexual robots in the future; female therapists, older therapists and psychologists (as opposed to physicians) tended to be more critical about the use of sex robots in therapy. The authors highlight the ethical and moral issues associated with robotics and sex therapy.

Desbuleux and Fuss (2023) conducted one of the first empirical studies to examine the relationship between sex doll use and criminal behavior, responding to bans on the use of child-like sex dolls in some countries and calls from scholars to also ban adult-like sex dolls and robots. They found,

> Users reported an overall reduction in sexuality-related behaviors (e.g., porn consumption or visiting of sex workers) in response to doll ownership. Users in a relationship with a human were less affected by doll use, while those in a relationship with a doll reported greater effects. ... These self-reported data challenge the view that doll use is

> dangerously affecting human sexuality and instead suggest that dolls may be used as a sexual outlet for potentially dangerous and illegal (sexual) fantasies. (Desbuleux & Fuss, 2023)

Harper et al. (2022) examined the psychological characteristics of individuals who owned sex dolls, noting that this is a multi-million-dollar industry. They contrast prevailing models and note that doll owners frequently purchased their dolls following divorce or separation. Their data paint a picture rooted not in a hatred or contempt of women, but in a confusion or insecurity about them. In addition, "these data are indicative of a potentially attenuating effect of doll ownership on offending proclivity, with doll owners being less likely to express a behavioral willingness to engage in sexual aggression" (p. 201). They conclude their article by noting,

> We hope that our data can advance a more evidence-informed social conversation about sex doll ownership, shifting the focus away from blanket criminalization and stigmatization and toward a functional analysis of how, why, and under what conditions dolls are incorporated into healthy sexual expression. (Harper et al., 2022, p. 202)

Romantic relationships between dolls/robots and individuals are explored in numerous films including *Westworld* (1974), *Her* (2013), *Ex Machina* (2015), *Lars and the Real Girl* (2007), and *The Stepford Wives* (2004). It is likely that we will see more movies address similar themes as sexual robots become cheaper, more anatomically correct, widely available, and more socially acceptable.

Leap Year (Año Bisiesto) and Sadomasochism

Leap Year (Año Bisiesto) is a powerful film about a 25-year-old woman who lives in Mexico City. Laura is a journalist who spends every evening in bars where casual meetings with new men inevitably lead to one-night stands. She is deeply dissatisfied with her loneliness, and she frequently masturbates while watching a happily married couple kiss in a nearby apartment. She thinks there may be potential for a more substantive relationship when she meets Arturo, a sadist who introduces her to the world of sadomasochistic sex. She initially has reservations, but soon joins in with abandon, embracing the role of the masochist. This low-budget film was directed by Michael Rowe, an Australian expatriate living in Mexico City, and many reviewers

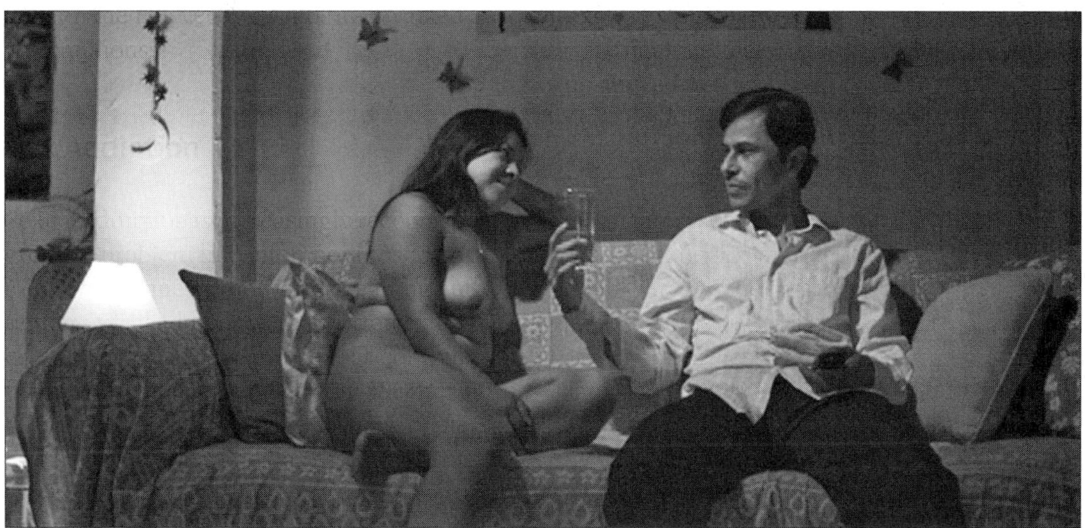

Figure 45. *Leap Year* (Año Bisiesto; 2011, Machete Producciones, Instituto Mexicano de Cinematografía [IMCINE], Bh5). Produced by Roger Bello, Edher Campos, Gustavo Campos, Olga González, et al. Directed by Michael Rowe.

have compared it to Bernardo Bertolucci's *Last Tango in Paris* (1972). The entire movie takes place in Laura's apartment. It is a difficult film to watch, but the viewer comes away with a deep appreciation for the depth of Laura's loneliness and a better understanding of how it might lead to a masochistic relationship. Figure 45 depicts the unequal, degrading but surprisingly symbiotic relationship between Arturo the sadist and Laura the masochist.

The Piano Teacher

In *The Piano Teacher* (2001), Erika Kohut (Isabelle Huppert) is a highbrow, successful pianist. She performs concerts for standing-room-only crowds and gives demanding lessons to her students. Erika clearly presents as a sexually repressed and conservative woman with a stern, controlling presence. The film takes its time in getting to important themes and core issues, allowing the viewer to be gradually introduced to her world and values. The viewer sees her go to a porn shop briefly in which she chastises a young male student before she leaves. In another scene, she goes into a booth in the shop to watch a video. These scenes progress to acting out sexually with a male student in a public restroom; in this scene, she is mildly sadistic and very controlling. A relationship begins, and it is only then that her deepest fantasies (and true diagnosis) are revealed. She is in fact masochistic. In one scene, she sets up a blockade so her nosey, controlling mother is unable to burst into her room. Erika gives her lover a letter revealing her fantasies about sadomasochistic behavior. As he reads the letter, he learns about her desires to be reminded of her powerlessness, to be gagged, and to be hit if she disobeys any of his commands or rules. Next, she reveals her stash of ropes and other sadomasochistic toys. He responds by telling her that he feels both love and repulsion, and that she is "sick" and needs treatment.

"The urge to be beaten has been in me for years."

***The Piano Teacher* (2001)**

The film makes inferences about etiology, mostly surrounding a forceful, controlling mother who needs to know every detail about her adult daughter. The mother is physically controlling, aggressive, and quick to criticize everything from Erika's attire and her piano playing (although Erika is an expert pianist), to a benign conversation she has with a young man. She instructs her daughter, "No one must surpass you, my dear." Erika's father had died from an unspecified mental illness in an asylum.

Autoerotic asphyxia, using self-strangulation to produce excitement or to intensify erections or ejaculation, is an unusual but not uncommon paraphilia, often related to masochism. It is estimated that autoerotic asphyxiation results in 250–1,000 deaths per year in the United States (Uva, 1995). Blanchard and Hucker (1991) were able to review the cases of 117 males who died during autoerotic asphyxia. Autoerotic asphyxia is especially significant because most of the deaths that result from this practice are assumed to be accidents. Chater (2021) has suggested that intentional asphyxiation by strangulation is addictive, and Baxendale et al. (2019) maintain that knowledge about the practice is usually acquired from the Internet, and the behavior is best conceptualized as a subtype of masochism.

Most of what we know about the practice of autoerotic asphyxia is derived from police reports following death investigations. The victims tend to be young White males. Bondage accouterments are often employed, along with mirrors and cameras. Transvestism is a widespread practice in these cases. There is often evidence that ejaculation occurred before death. **With asphyxiophilia** is included as a specifier for the diagnosis of sexual masochism disorder in DSM-5.

Robin Williams stars in *World's Greatest Dad* (2009), a black comedy in which a high school English teacher discovers his son has died from autoerotic asphyxiation. To avoid humiliation for his son, William's character hangs his son in a closet, writes a suicide note, and pretends his son has been writing in a journal. This leads to notoriety and fame for the father, but he eventually comes clean and confuses his duplicity.

Sexual Sadism

Sexual sadism presents the mirror image of sexual masochism. The sadist derives sexual pleasure from the suffering and humiliation of their victims. Partners may be consenting or nonconsenting. If the partner is consenting, the diagnosis requires that sexual sadism be "repeatedly preferred or exclusive" and that "bodily injury that is extensive, permanent, or possibly mortal is inflicted in order to achieve sexual excitement."

The terms **sadism** and **masochism** were first used by a German sexologist, Richard von Krafft-Ebing, in the 19th century. Krafft-Ebing, who wrote *Psychopathia Sexualis*, the first medical school textbook on sexuality (1886), took the term "sadism" from the name of the French author Marquis de Sade. De Sade's novels and short stories are replete with abuse, torture, and murder, all of which are linked with sexual gratification. One of his works, *The 120 Days of Sodom*, was made into the controversial and repugnant movie *Salò, or the 120 Days of Sodom* (1976), the final film of Italian director Pier Paolo Pasolini.

Sadomasochistic sex often involves elaborate sex toys such as chains, whips, rubber and leather garments, and spike heels. Flagellation and bondage are common practices.

Although some sadists are also rapists, it is important to understand that rapists do not derive sexual pleasure from the rape itself. Rape is an act of violence in which sexual arousal may play almost no role. In contrast, the sexual sadist derives intense sexual pleasure from the suffering of the victim.

It is important to distinguish between *minor* sadism and masochism (sex play involving bondage and discipline or dominance and submission) and *major* sadism and masochism involving torture and the risk of death and bodily injury (Arndt, 1991). There is some evidence that at a minor level, there are more women who dominate males; at an extreme level, men are more likely to abuse women.

The Girl with the Dragon Tattoo (2011) depicts rape scenes in which the rapist is clearly sadistic, and *Tesis* (1996, Spain), *Vacancy* (2007) and *8MM* (1999) all deal with **snuff films**, a particularly odious form of sadism in which people are filmed while being murdered, most often after or while being raped. Other films depicting sexual sadism include *Belle de Jour* (1967, France), *Venus in Furs* (1969), *Last Tango in Paris* (1962), *The Night Porter* (1974), *The Story of O* (1972), *In the Realm of the Senses* (1976, Japan), *Tie Me Up! Tie Me Down!* (1990), and *New Tokyo Decadence - The Slave* (2007, Japan).

The public's interest in sadomasochism is reflected in the popularity of the erotic romance novel *Fifty Shades of Grey* (2011) by E. L. James, the fastest selling paperback of all time. The novel is part of a trilogy that sold over 90 million copies worldwide and has been translated into 52 languages. A film based on the novel was released in 2015; *Fifty Shades Darker* followed 2 years later, and *Fifty Shades Freed* came out in 2018. Sprott and Berkey (2015) reviewed the movie *Fifty Shades of Grey* for the journal *Psychology of Sexual Orientation and Gender Diversity* and noted,

> There are two reasons why a review of this movie makes sense in the context of this journal. The first is recognition of the cultural history of intersectionality between sexual orientations/identities, and alternative sexuality practices/identities, including BDSM. The second is the impact on therapeutic contexts, as people come out increasingly around kink to their therapists or attempt to try kink for the first time, encouraged or inspired by the books and movie. (Sprott & Berkey, 2015, p. 506)

Writing in *Sexuality & Culture: An Interdisciplinary Quarterly*, Carey Noland (2020) describes the success of the *Fifty Shades* triology and argues that the sexual scripts in these books and films provide women with self-help tools that allow them to expand and enhance their sexuality.

Films depicting sexual sadism are common in the United States, and they play for large audiences in Europe and Asia as well. Many of these films are heavy-handed and crude and have little social value. A salient exception is David Lynch's *Blue Velvet* (1986; see the next section, Blue Velvet).

Willem Dafoe and Robert Pattinson portray two lighthouse keepers ("wikies") in *The Lighthouse* (2019); Pattinson's character frequently masturbates with a mermaid figurine, and he has fantasies about having sex with a mermaid who washes up on the shore – until he sees her enlarged vagina and runs away screaming. There is considerable sexual tension between the two men, which becomes most apparent when they are both drunk and fighting. Their attraction to one another can only be acknowledged and permitted when it is sadomasochistic. In the final scene, Pattinson's character has beaten Dafoe's character into submission, and Pattinson leads Dafoe around on a lease, requiring him to perform several demeaning and degrading tasks.

Blue Velvet

Blue Velvet opens with Bobby Vinton's song of the same name and scenes of a bucolic Midwest neighborhood. This idyllic scene is soon interrupted, and the viewer is never really allowed to relax again until the film concludes.

The plot of the story involves a student, Jeffrey Beaumont (Kyle MacLachlan), who is home from college to care for his father who has just had a stroke. While walking in a field near his house, Jeffrey discovers a severed ear. It turns out to be the ear of the husband of a cabaret singer, Dorothy Vallens (Isabella Rossellini). Dorothy's husband and son are being held hostage to force her to comply with the sexual demands of a local gangster, Frank Booth (Dennis Hopper). Dorothy, one of the most complex characters in the film, discovers Jeffrey in her apartment after he goes there in a foolish attempt to solve the crime. In a controversial scene, Dorothy discovers Jeffrey and uses a knife to force him to have sex with her. She displays many of the features of masochism previously discussed; these become more prominent later when Frank arrives and proceeds to savagely abuse her. Frank, both obsessed with Dorothy and fixated on the song "Blue Velvet," has cut off a piece of Dorothy's blue velvet bathrobe. It is a fetish that Frank carries with him and uses during other sexual encounters. Hopper is unforgettable as Frank Booth, who is addicted to inhalants as well as sadistic sex.

"I have a part of you with me. You put your disease in me. It helps me. It makes me strong."

A masochistic and troubled Dorothy, in *Blue Velvet* (1986)

One troubling aspect of the film is that both Dorothy and Jeffrey seem attracted to sadomasochistic sex after they have been exposed to it. A subplot involves Jeffrey's involvement with Sandy, the daughter of a corrupt local detective. The relationship with Sandy seems pale and insipid after the intensity of a sexual encounter with Dorothy.

The film won the National Society of Film Critics award for Best Film of 1986, and Lynch was selected as Best Director of the year by the same group. It is a brutally honest film, but not one that will appeal to all viewers. However, it is a film rich in psychopathology and one worth seeing by anyone interested in the complex world of the sexual psychopath.

Pedophilic Disorder

The **pedophile** is sexually aroused by children and has acted on these desires or is markedly distressed by them. The pedophile can be attracted to girls, boys, or both, although heterosexual pedophilia is more common than homosexual pedophilia. The DSM-5 stipulates that the child must be prepubescent (age 13 or younger) for a diagnosis of pedophilia to be appropriate. In addition, the diagnosis is not used unless the perpetrator is at least 16 years old and at least 5 years older than the child involved. Specifiers are used to indicate whether the sexual attraction to children is exclusive or nonexclusive, and whether the individual involved is sexually attracted to male children, female children, or both. The true prevalence is unknown, but this disorder is far more common among men than among women. Pedophilia is a difficult condition to treat, and in most clients, it will be a lifelong condition that can be controlled but not eliminated.

Although not a formal diagnostic label, the 19th-century term **ephebophilia** is sometimes used to describe a person attracted to postpubescent adolescents; the ephebophile's attraction is exclusive and specific to this age group (ages 15–19). The phrase **Lolita syndrome** is also used to describe men attracted exclusively to female adolescents. Though often illegal, ephebophilia is not seen as pathological and is even normative in some societies in which adolescent girls routinely marry older adult men. Ephebophilia illustrates the conflict that often exists between biological and societal norms. This conflict is convincingly portrayed in *One Flew Over the Cuckoo's Nest* (1975), in which Jack Nicholson is arrested and subsequently hospitalized for having sex with a child who was "15-years-old, going on 35 ... and very willing."

Norja et al. (2021) studied responses to facial photos of children aged 12–18 years and found that their subjects *overestimated* the age of the adolescents by an average of 3.5 years. The age of girls was more likely to be overestimated than boys, and smiling faces and those with makeup were most likely to be overestimated. These authors conclude that the ability of individuals to estimate the age of adolescents is low, and this has obvious important legal implications.

While typical adolescents achieve sexual maturation (puberty) at or before age 13, most mental health professionals believe adolescents are not prepared to deal with the demands of sexual intimacy at such an early age and recommend a slow transition to adult sexuality; however, there is wide variation in the ages at which diverse cultures define the age of consent for sexual intercourse, and the minimum age of consent varies across countries from age 12 to 21. A dozen countries (e.g., Iran, Yemen, Afghanistan) outlaw premarital sex entirely, but have no age restrictions on marital sex (World Population Review, 2022).

Van Roost et al. (2022) examined US laws that allow children to marry before they are old enough to have sex under state law, and argued, "The simultaneous legality of child marriage and marital exemptions to statutory rape laws provide legal loopholes for sexual acts with children that would otherwise be considered crimes. Marital exemptions to statutory rape laws may also incentivize a substantial portion of child marriages" (p. 72).

Chrysanthi Leon analyzed sex crime policies in the United States in her book *Sex Fiends, Perverts, and Pedophiles* (2011), and she divides them into three historical periods: the **sexual psychopath era**, featuring a plethora of approaches toward sexual offenses; the **rehabilitative era**, during which the belief that propensity to commit sex offenses was curable led to a focus on clinical approaches; and the modern **containment era**, in which mass incarceration and numerous restrictions are related to a belief in incurability (Aviram, 2012, p. 931, emphasis added).

Ephebophilia is portrayed in the coming-of-age film *Towelhead* (aka *Nothing Is Private*; 2007), the first film directed by Alan Ball (who also produced and cowrote *American Beauty*, a film that deals with the emerging sexuality of two young girls; see next paragraph). In *Towelhead*, several adults abuse Jasira, a 13-year-old girl, including her mother's boyfriend, who feigns paternal concern while he is shaving Jasira's pubic hair. "Towelhead" is a contemptuous term for someone of Arab descent; the protagonist's father is a strict Lebanese American who is ill prepared to deal with his daughter's sexual maturation or the challenges of menstruation.

Venus (2006) stars Peter O'Toole as a septuagenarian actor with prostate cancer who becomes romantically and erotically involved with a woman 53 years younger than he is; the movie makes this relationship seem entirely plausible. *American Beauty* (1999) has Kevin Spacey playing the role of a middle-aged suburban father who becomes infatuated with his teenage daughter's best friend, who is beautiful but sexually inexperienced.

Hard Candy (2005) illustrates the ways in which the Internet has opened new avenues for pedophiles to exploit their victims. The film involves an online relationship between a 14-year-old girl and a 32-year-old photographer who is a pedophile. The two eventually meet, and both understand from innuendo that they are meeting to have sex; however, in a curious twist, the precocious 14-year-old winds up in control of the situation and proceeds to castrate the older man (who may have been involved in the disappearance of a child whose photo is included in his files), and the man eventually commits suicide.

While most cases of ephebophilia (and most movies with this theme) involve older men who are attracted to young girls, two films have successfully explored relationships between older women and teenage boys. *Private Lessons* (1981) is a movie about a French maid who seduces a 15-year-old boy; the film depicts grooming, boundary violations, and sexual abuse of a minor. *The Reader* (2008) is a powerful, engaging, and compelling film in which Kate Winslet plays Hanna Schmitz, a 36-year-old woman who becomes involved with a 15-year-old boy. They have an affair one summer, and then she drops out of his life, only to reappear 8 years later when she is on trial for war crimes committed as a concentration camp guard. The film's title comes from the fact that Hanna and her adolescent lover begin each of their trysts with him reading to her. Kate Winslet won an Academy Award for her role in this film.

> **"She had favorites. Girls, mostly young. We all remarked on it, she gave them food and places to sleep. In the evening, she asked them to join her. We all thought – well, you can imagine what we thought. Then we found out – she was making these women read aloud to her. They were reading to her. At first, we thought this guard ... this guard is more sensitive ... she's more human ... she's kinder. Often, she chose the weak, the sick, she picked them out, she seemed to be protecting them almost. But then she dispatched them. Is that kinder?"**
>
> **A witness describes Hanna Schmitz's odd behavior, in *The Reader* (2008)**

Other films in which older women become romantically or sexually involved with younger men include *White Palace* (1990), in which a 43-year-old woman (Susan Sarandon) seduces a 27-year-old man (James Spader); *Don Jon* (2013), starring Scarlett Johansson and Julianne Moore; *Good Luck to You, Leo Grande* (2022) with Emma Thompson; *The Age of Adaline* (2015), with Michiel Huisman and Harrison Ford; *I Could Never Be Your Woman* (2007) starring Michelle Pfeiffer; *P.S.* (2004), starring Laura Linney; *The Rebound* (2009), with Catherine Zeta-Jones; *Film Stars Don't Die in Liverpool* (2017), with Annette Bening; *Judy* (2019) with Renée Zellweger; *Something's Gotta Give* (2003) with Diane Keaton, Jack Nicholson, and Keanu Reeves; *Adore* (2013) in which Robin Wright and Naomi Watts become sexually involved with each other's sons; *The Good Girl* (2002), with Jennifer Aniston and Jake Gyllenhaal; *The Mother* (2003), starring Anne Reid and Daniel Craig; and *Bull Durham* (1988), with Susan Sarandon, Kevin Costner, and Tim Robbins.

Another nondiagnostic variation of pedophilia is the rare condition called **infantophilia**; this term is applied to adults with a primary sexual attraction to children from birth to age 5. The movie *Bliss* (1997) includes a scene illustrating infantophilia.

Most pedophiles report being sexually and emotionally abused as children (Grady & Levenson, 2021). Pedophiles who have been attracted to children since adolescence are identified as **fixated pedophiles**. In contrast, if an individual has satisfying adult sexual experiences, but then reverts to a sexual preoccupation with children, the person is classified as a situational or **regressed pedophile**.

Hundreds of thousands of children are sexually abused in the United States each year, and it is likely that the actual number of cases of childhood sexual abuse (CSA) are 3 times greater than the number of cases investigated by Child Protective Services. Approximately 28% of 14- to 17-year-olds report lifetime sexual violence victimization (Latzman et al., 2017).

Most people consider the practice of pedophilia reprehensible, perhaps because children are among the most vulnerable members of the human family. However, the widespread availability of "kiddie porn," despite the social opprobrium associated with pedophilia, suggests that sexual interest in children is as common as most other paraphilias. Empirical data document the extent of sexual attraction to children by adults. For example, Briere (1989) surveyed undergraduate males and found that 21% acknowledged being sexually attracted to children, 9% had sexual fantasies involving children, and 7% would consider having sex with a child if certain they could avoid being detected or punished. More recently, Savoie et al. (2021) reviewed 30 studies and reported a mean prevalence rate of sexual interest in children of between 2% and 24%. Sexual interest in children was correlated with mental health problems and adverse childhood experiences.

Pedophiles and ephebophiles seduce their victims using play, food, or gifts, which are followed by appropriate touching eventually leading to inappropriate touching and assault. The seduction of an adolescent is powerfully and realistically portrayed in *Blue Car* (2003), in which a young, vulnerable girl is seduced by her teacher. Most viewers are not aware that the teacher is manipulating the adolescent from the very beginning of the film. The seduction of adolescents is also depicted in *American Beauty* (1999), *Lolita* (1962), *Lolita* (1997), *Y Tu Mamá También* (2001), and *Manic* (2003). In *The Magdalene Sisters* (2002), a priest has sex with a vulnerable, emotionally, and physically abused adolescent girl.

Child sexual abuse is portrayed in the powerful and riveting documentary *Capturing the Friedmans* (2003). In *Capturing the Friedmans*, a father, Arnold, and his son, Jesse, are accused of pedophilia. When their house is searched, child pornography is found hidden throughout the home. The movie does not fully indict or acquit either individual. In *Happiness*, Dylan Baker plays a married psychiatrist who is also a pedophile who masturbates to teen magazines and fantasizes about raping the friends of his 11-year-old son.

Mysterious Skin (2004) tells the story of two boys growing up in a small Kansas town. Both boys are molested by their Little League coach, but they respond in quite different ways. Brian repressed the experience and only remembered waking up with a nosebleed; he accounts for the missing 5 hours in his life by developing a deep conviction that he has been abducted by aliens. Neil responds by becoming a teenage prostitute, working at first in local parks before moving to New York where his clients are older White men. The film presents an evenhanded and unsensationalzed examination of the effects of CSA.

Two films offer especially sensitive portrayals of the problem of pedophilia: *Little Children* (2017) and *The Woodsman* (2004). Director Todd Field's *Little Children* is a powerful film that shows how difficult it is to find and maintain long-term love relationships. Kate Winslet plays Sarah Pierce, a disenchanted stay-at-home mother whose husband is addicted to online pornography. One of the characters in the film, Ronnie, lives with his mother after completing a prison term for exposing himself to a little girl. Ronnie's mother is convinced that he will become attracted to adult women if he only starts to date one; however, the date she arranges for him turns into a disaster when he asks his date to drive him by a playground so he can masturbate. Before his mother dies from cancer, she writes him a short note, simply asking him to "be a good boy." He responds to his grief by castrating himself, and his life is saved by Sarah, who can set aside her previous repugnance and aversion to relate to Ronnie as a genuinely suffering human being. One of the most memorable scenes in the film occurs when Ronnie visits a public swimming pool, frightening both the mothers and the children, almost all of whom know he has been identified as a pedophile (Figure 46).

The Woodsman stars Kevin Bacon as a pedophile who has just been released from prison after serving a 12-year sentence; the film shows him continuing to struggle with his demons, while at the same time he is trying to establish a mature sexual relationship with a woman with whom he works. The movie underscores the

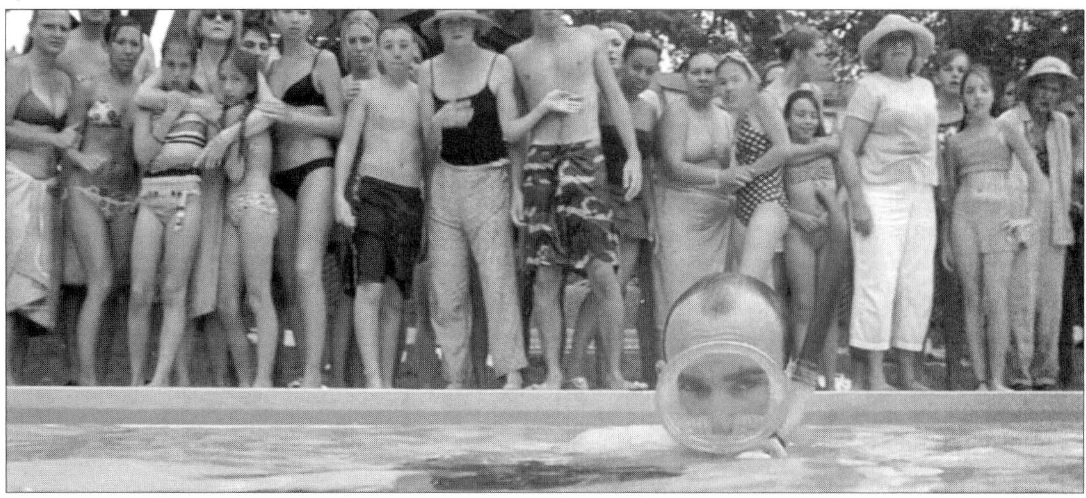

Figure 46. *Little Children* (2006, New Line Productions, Bona Fide Productions, Standard Film Company). Produced by Kent Alterman, Albert Berger, Toby Emmerich, Todd Field, et al. Directed by Todd Field.

complexity of the problem without providing pat solutions or a feel-good ending.

> **"Little Red Riding Hood! That's it! That's it. The Woodsman, he cuts open the wolf's stomach, the girl comes out without a scratch ... [But have you ever seen] a seven-year-old sodomized in half? She was so small, just broken. I saw 20-year vets on that job. Hard guys, they just broke down and cried. I was there, I cried ... There ain't no fucking woodsman in this world."**
>
> **A police sergeant describing the stress involved in working with children victimized by pedophiles, in *The Woodsman* (2004)**

Pervert Park (2014) is a documentary that interviews residents of a St. Petersburg, Florida, trailer park community, all of whom are all registered sex offenders. The community offers security and counseling, and it was originally set up by a mother for her sex offender son. According to the film, the recidivism rate for community members is less than 1%, which is significantly lower than that for the general population of sex offenders.

A 2019 British documentary, *Leaving Neverland*, caused considerable controversy when it was released. The film, released by HBO, depicts two men, now in their 30s, who make allegations of sexual abuse by Michael Jackson when they were children visiting Jackson's Neverland Ranch during the 1990s. The alleged abuse began when the boys were aged 7 and 10 and is reported to have been continued for many years. The Jackson estate condemned the film as tabloid character assassination.

Olver et al. (2011) completed a meta-analysis of predictors of offender treatment attrition and its relationship to recidivism. They found a history of prior offenses and a diagnosis of antisocial personality were significant positive predictors of recidivism, while older offenders who were more intelligent and more motivated were less likely to repeat offenses. They conclude, "The clients who stand to benefit the most from treatment (i.e., high-risk, high-needs) are the least likely to complete it" (Olver et al., 2011, p. 6).

Laura Dern plays an adult named Jennifer, in *The Tale* (2018), a film that includes numerous flashbacks to her childhood with her childhood role as Jenny played by Isabelle Nélisse (see Figure 47). Director Jennifer Fox based the story on her own vague memories of sexual abuse as a child, and the film is semiautobiographical. Jenny's childhood abuse only comes back to her after her mother (played by Ellen Burstyn) comes across letters Jenny wrote at age 13, a time when she visualized her involvement with two adults as romance rather than rape. This graphic film provides excellent illustrations of the way sexual abusers groom their victims, and Jennifer was abused by a both male and a female adult, both of whom she eventually confronts. The male abuser, her running coach, is confronted at a dinner party after he received a major award. The film is about the vagaries of memory as much as it is about sexual abuse, and it appears quite plausible that the adult Jennifer conveniently repressed her memories of molestation.

The concept of repression can be traced back to Sigmund Freud. His most noted case of repression was "Anna O," a woman paralyzed on her right side. Freud treated her with hypnosis, and she regained some use of the right side of her body. John Huston asked Marilyn Monroe to play the role of Anna O in a film about the life of Freud (*Freud: The Secret Passion,* 1962), but she turned down the role because she had heard Freud's family disapproved of the plan.

Repressed memories are hotly debated in clinical psychology and psychiatry, and the courts have become involved when parents have been accused of sexual abuse of their children, often years after the abuse is said to have occurred. Psychologist Elizabeth Loftus has become famous for her work on the misinformation effect, false memories, and criticism of recovered memory therapies, and she is frequently called on as an expert in cases involving recovered memories of incest or CSA. Her 2013 book *The Myth of Repressed Memory: False Memories and Allegations of Sexual Abuse* is a classic work documenting that there is little or no scientific support for the notion that memories of trauma are repressed and years later recovered in psychotherapy (Loftus & Ketcham, 1994; Loftus, 1996).

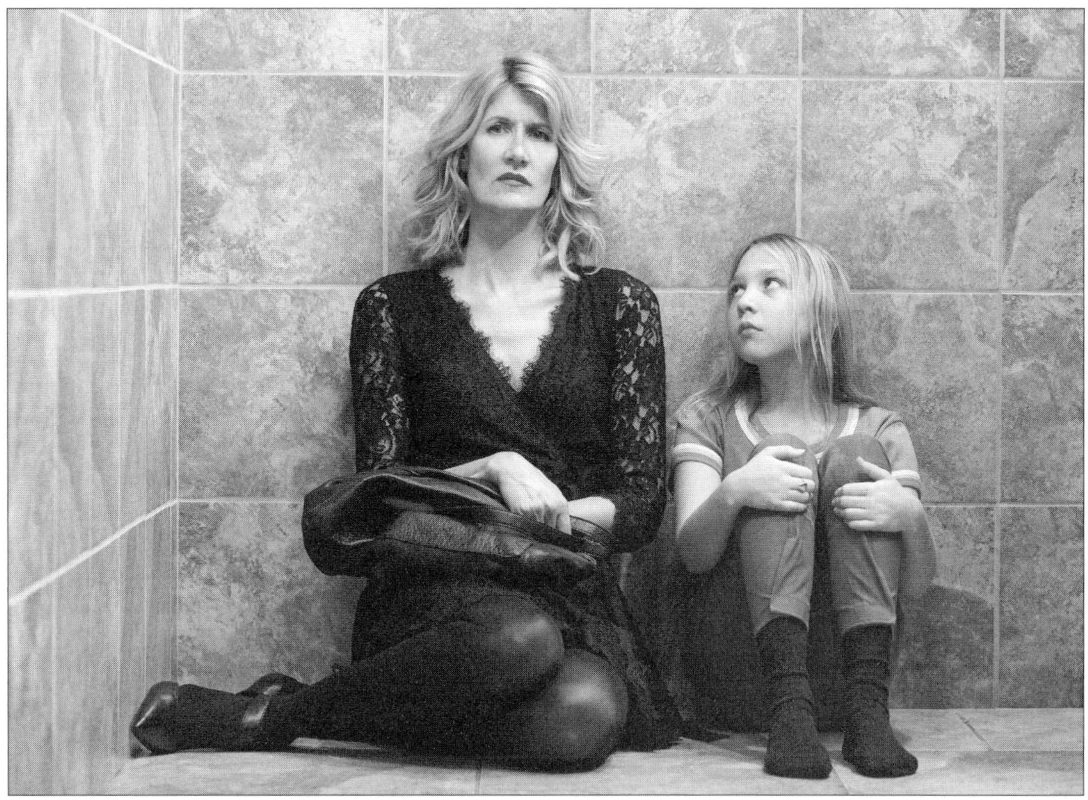

Figure 47. *The Tale* (2018, Gamechanger Films, A Luminous Mind production, Untitled Entertainment, Blackbird Films, ONE TWO Films, Fork Films, Artemis Rising Foundation, Blackbird, Chicago Media Project). Produced by René Besson, Dan Cogan, Ron Dempsey, Stefanie Diaz, et al. Directed by Jennifer Fox.

Katz (2022) argues that therapeutic relationships often promote and sustain pseudomemories. These therapeutic relationships tend to be "intense and dependent, with frequent contact and compromised professional boundaries" (p. 114). Therapists in these relationships use incest as a unitary explanation for the patient's problems, and Katz notes that "contrary to popular media depictions of trauma, total psychogenic amnesia is a rare occurrence after childhood sexual abuse, and memory distortion more often takes the form of intrusive memories, flashbacks, and symptoms of PTSD rather than amnesia" (Katz, 2022, p. 114).

An American Psychological Association Working Group on Memories of Childhood Abuse identified five points on which all members could agree:

1. Controversies regarding adult recollections should not be allowed to obscure the fact that CSA is a complex and pervasive problem in America that has historically gone unacknowledged.
2. Most people who were sexually abused as children remember all or part of what happened to them.
3. It is possible for memories of abuse that have been forgotten for a long time to be remembered.
4. It is also possible to construct convincing pseudomemories for events that never occurred.
5. There are gaps in our knowledge about the processes that lead to accurate and inaccurate recollections of childhood abuse (American Psychological Association, 1998).

Little has changed in the quarter century since this task force report was published, and the debate rages on (e.g., Otgaar et al., 2022; Ross, 2022). Movies like *The Tale* pay homage to this controversy.

Fetishistic Disorder

An individual has a **fetish** when an inanimate object habitually arouses them. A diagnosis is justified only if the sexual arousal associated with the object or fantasies about it is intense, recurrent, and lasts for at least 6 months. Sex often involves masturbation with the fetish, or the fetish may be incorporated into sexual activity with one's partner. The term "fetish" is used to refer to both the object itself and the inordinate attraction to it. However, the true fetish involves inanimate objects such as panties, silk stockings, garter belts, high heel shoes, or rubber items of clothing or body parts not normally associated with sexual activity (e.g., hair, feet, or the stumps of amputated limbs). Normally the link to sexuality can be surmised, but occasionally a patient will report sexual arousal to stimuli as obscure as file cabinets or baby buggies, and it is difficult to determine (a) how arousal initially could have been paired with the stimulus or (b) the potential symbolic value of the fetish. The fetish is often used for masturbation, but it may also be worn, worshipped, put in the rectum, hoarded, fondled, or sucked.

The DSM-5 requires at least a 6-month history of sexual arousal from nonliving objects or a specific focus on nongenital body parts, for the diagnosis. In addition, clinically significant distress must be present or impairment in important life tasks (e.g., keeping a job). Specifiers are used to indicate whether the fetish involves body parts (e.g., feet) or nonliving objects (e.g., bras and panties). As with most other paraphilias, fetishes occur far more often in men than in women.

Some authorities have speculated that fetishism is related to the same psychological impulses that trigger transvestism and kleptomania (an overwhelming desire to steal, usually insignificant or inexpensive objects). The differences among the three conditions seem trivial in comparison with the similarities that link the disorders. The person with a sexual fetish longs to relate to the object sexually, the transvestite longs to wear it, and the kleptomaniac longs to steal it.

Several films have included either leading or secondary characters with a fetish. One of my favorites is *Claire's Knee*, a French film directed by Eric Rohmer and released in 1971. This charming movie details the obsession of a soon-to-be-married writer for his friend's daughter – or, more exactly, the daughter's right knee. He becomes increasingly attracted to her because he cannot have her, and he has difficulty speaking when she is around. He focuses on her knee as the fulcrum for her beauty; in one scene, he massages her knee with considerable erotic glee, but does not move his hand anywhere else. The erotic elements in the film are handled with delicacy and good taste, and the writer's fixation on the girl's knee soon seems entirely plausible.

Peter Greenaway's *Pillow Book* (1997) portrays a woman with a fetish for calligraphy. She melds calligraphy with sex, and the calligraphic pen symbolizes the instrument of pleasure. She develops a passion for calligraphy and experiences withdrawal without it. She searches for the ideal mate to write on her; she rules out the old for not having enough energy, and the young for their distracted nature. She captures and tests out a graffiti writer and other random people to write on her in her search. "You're not a writer, you're a scribbler," she tells one candidate.

Another not-to-be-missed film demonstrating a sexual fetish is Steven Soderbergh's *Sex, Lies and Videotape* (1989). This intelligent film, which won the Best Picture and Best Actor awards at the 1989 Cannes Film Festival, was written, directed, and edited by Soderbergh. The film describes how the lives of three people (a man, his wife, and her sister, with whom he is having an affair) are changed forever by the arrival of the man's college roommate, Graham Dalton. Dalton is an impotent male who can achieve orgasm only by masturbating while he is watching the videotapes he makes of women discussing the intimate details of their sexual lives. Dalton has decided to live his life with absolute honesty, and he shares the details of his sexual life with Ann, the rejected wife. The two eventually become lovers, and there is a dramatic confrontation between Dalton and his old roommate (Ann's husband). Dalton is transformed through his relationship with Ann, and eventually he can move out of his isolation and into an emotionally satisfying and sexually mature relationship.

An equally powerful film is *Equus* (1977). This movie stars Richard Burton as Martin Dysart, a disillusioned psychiatrist who has lost all traces of passion in his life. The film revolves around Dysart's treatment of Alan Strang (Peter Firth), a young man arrested for blinding six horses. This cruel act is linked to Strang's fascination with horses; he finds them both threatening and sexually exciting. The film offers some insight into how an animal fetish might develop.

Some films utilize fetishes solely for comic purposes and offer little insight into the paraphilias, as in the depiction of a woman who claims to have a "Santa fetish," in *Bad Santa* (2003).

Crash (1996) is a controversial NC-17 (no children 17 and under) David Cronenberg film about people who have developed fetishes for cars and car wrecks. The film is based on a novel by J. G. Ballard, and the opening scene shows a woman rubbing her breasts against the wing of a plane and then licking metal while an anonymous lover enters her from behind. She later relates this experience to her husband, who in turn shares his day's sexual adventures. The husband later becomes involved in a serious car accident in which the driver of the other car is killed. This man's wife, Helen, survives the accident but is hospitalized and must walk on crutches while she recovers. Shortly after leaving the hospital, she becomes sexually involved with James, the man who had been driving the car that had killed her husband. Helen arouses James by telling him stories about all the men with whom she has had sex in cars. Both individuals find themselves sexually aroused by crashes and the accouterments of highway deaths (ambulances, flares, fire trucks, etc.). They are increasingly drawn into a deviant subculture that shares their sexual fascination with metal, cars, and crashing. This group is led by an unusual man who amuses himself and others by reenacting the 1955 death of James Dean in his sports car named "Little Bastard." In addition to its main theme of fetishism, the film involves exhibitionism, voyeurism, troilism (pleasure in having sex in front of others), and homosexuality. The film ends with a suggestion of necrophilia – James deliberately drives his wife's sports car off the road at high speed, and she is thrown from the car. He determines she is alive, and then embraces her unconscious and injured body while muttering, "Maybe the next one, darling, maybe the next one."

Feed (2005) portrays a man with a fat fetish who houses and feeds morbidly obese women who grow even fatter, eventually eating themselves to death. He films the women and puts videotapes of them on a pornographic website, and he takes bets on how long it will take the women to die.

Transvestic Disorder

Unlike transsexuals, **transvestites** are comfortable with their anatomic sex. However, transvestites derive pleasure and satisfaction from cross-dressing and being identified as a female, and cross-dressing and fantasies about cross-dressing play a prominent role in the sexual lives of transvestites. The transsexual male may cross-dress, but this is not done for purposes of sexual arousal but, rather, because female clothes are important in establishing a female identity. In contrast, the transvestite is likely to be a masculine, heterosexual male who becomes sexually excited when he dresses up in women's clothes. The transvestite does not desire to *be* a woman, but merely wants to be admired as one, or to experience the sexual excitement associated with wearing women's clothes. Brown (1994) maintains that most wives who discover their husband's cross-dressing after marriage come to accept the behavior and suggests there are no ill effects on children from these marriages. The children of transvestites engage in appropriate sex-role behavior as adults and are unlikely to cross-dress themselves.

As with transsexualism, transvestites may be heterosexual or homosexual, although most are clearly heterosexual. Transvestites can never be asexual since sexual arousal is part of the definition of the syndrome. The DSM-5 used specifiers to document **with fetishism**, when arousal is triggered by the feel of women's garments, and **with autogynephilia**, when arousal results from the thoughts and images associated with thinking of oneself as female.

The cross-dressing behavior of the transvestite almost always begins in childhood, although few little boys who dress up in the clothes of their mother or sister will grow up to be confused about their sexual identity. While transsexualism is found among both males and females, the diagnosis of transvestism is inevitably reserved for males, and there are very few case studies of women who become sexually aroused by wearing men's clothes.

Many transvestites cross-dress only on special occasions, and they may attempt to suppress the behavior, yielding to the impulse only when anxious, during periods of stress, or when separated from a sexual partner. The preferred objects of clothing include nightgowns, panties, bras, hose, and high heels. These garments are often the stimuli associated with fetishes, and in the DSM-5, transvestism is referred to as **transvestic fetishism.** It is like other forms of fetishism in that sexual arousal is associated not with an individual but, rather, with inanimate objects (women's clothing).

The topic of cross-dressing (but not necessarily transvestism) is surprisingly common in films, where it is treated with humor and never as a serious issue. One comedy that addresses cross-dressing is the popular film *Tootsie* (1982), in which an unemployed actor played by Dustin Hoffman pretends to be a woman to get an acting job. The counterpart to this film is Blake Edward's *Victor/Victoria* (1982) in which Julie Andrews portrays a starving cabaret singer who gets her big break when she manages to land a job singing as a male female impersonator. Both films are sensitive analyses of the complex relationships linking gender and role.

Other films that have explored cross-dressing include *Some Like It Hot* (1959) directed by Billy Wilder and starring Marilyn Monroe, Tony Curtis, Jack Lemmon, and George Raft. This is the classic example of this genre. More recently, *Mrs. Doubtfire* (1993) starred Robin Williams as a man who passes himself off as a "nanny" to spend more time with his children. The movie *Yentl* (1983) stars Barbra Streisand as a woman who must dress in male clothes and pretend to be a man to achieve an education. *To Wong Foo,*

Thanks for Everything, Julie Newmar (1995) is an entertaining film that examines the lives of three transvestites whose car breaks down in a small town filled with bigots. This film stars Wesley Snipes, Patrick Swayze, and John Leguizamo. In Jane Campion's *Holy Smoke* (1999), Harvey Keitel's authoritarian character falls into a sexual obsession and begins to cross-dress as he regresses and deteriorates.

> **"I'm the Latina Marilyn Monroe. I've got more legs than a bucket of chicken!"**
>
> **Miss Chi-Chi Rodriguez in *To Wong Foo, Thanks for Everything, Julie Newmar* (1995)**

Unfortunately, some otherwise good films, such as Brian De Palma's *Dressed to Kill* (1980), starring Michael Caine and Angie Dickinson, link transvestism with violence and sociopathy. There is no evidence that transvestites are more likely than the average individual to be homicidal, although, like others whose sexuality may be viewed as deviant by the majority culture, they are significantly more likely to be victims of crime.

Incest

Incest refers to sexual relations between persons too closely related to marry, and it is estimated that from 10% to 15% of the general populations has had at least one sexual contact with a family member, with less than 2% involving intercourse or attempted intercourse (Nemeroff & Craighead, 2001). Seto (2018) notes,

> Girls are more likely to have been sexually abused than boys, with an average rate of 18% versus 8%. Intrafamilial child sexual abuse accounts for a large proportion of total child sexual abuse cases, especially for younger children, where relatives have much more access to potential victims than for older children who go to school and participate in routine activities outside the home. Comparative studies find that intrafamilial child sexual abuse cases involve younger victims, proportionally more girls, more psychological harm, and more incidents over a longer time span, again reflecting relative access and opportunity. (Seto, 2018)

Incest is considered immoral in most faith traditions, and it is illegal in the United States and most countries. There is an increased risk of genetic disorders in children that result from incestuous relationships. Some societies, such as those in ancient Egypt, Samoa, and Hawaii, have accepted some degree of incest, most often to protect royal lineage.

A rough measure of interest in incest can be gauged by the number of pornographic websites that feature brother–sister, mother–son, or father–daughter themes, sometimes overlaid with themes of violence. Most often, perhaps for legal reasons, these sites focus on stepmothers, stepfathers, and stepsiblings.

Pornographic websites circumvent laws prohibiting sexual exploitation of children by including a "Barely Legal" category that often features incest. In many of these videos, teen performers experience degrading treatment and risky sex acts.

> Teen performers were more than twice as likely to be in anal penetration scenes and five times more likely to be in forceful anal penetration scenes. They were also approximately 40% more likely to be in scenes in which the male performer ejaculated in their mouth or on their face. (Rothman, 2021, p. 56)

Vera-Gray et al. (2021) conducted one of the few studies examining online pornography, and they found that "one in eight titles shown to first-time users on the first page of mainstream porn sites describe sexual activity that constitutes sexual violence" (p. 1243). Huntington et al. (2022) studied adolescents who viewed pornography with their romantic partners and found lifetime joint pornography viewing was associated with higher rates of dating violence, abusive behaviors from one's partner, and more verbal conflict in current dating relationships.

Mondragon et al. (2022) applied lexical analysis to over 20,000 French tweets with the hashtag **#MeTooIncest.** They concluded that incest victims found a safe space for disclosure in the #MeToo movement, and that "this wave of testimonies represents a turning point as it has broken the law of silence and allowed the victims to exist in the media space without being questioned." Middleton (2013) studied cases of parent–child incest that extended into adulthood and found that these cases are not rare. In addition, they frequently result in pregnancy, and often involve ongoing violence and death threats.

Stanley Kubrick's *Lolita* (1962) is a classic example of incest in a contemporary movie. The film takes liberties with Vladimir Nabokov's novel, but the changes were made with the permission of the great writer, who served as screenwriter for the movie. A psychoanalyst has argued that Nabokov himself was a pedophile because of CSA by an uncle (Centerwall, 1992). Considered quite daring when it was released more than 6 decades ago, the film portrays the love of Humbert (James Mason) for Lolita (Sue Lyon). Shelly Winters plays Lolita's mother, and Peter Sellers has two roles in the film. Like many actual incestuous stepfathers, Mason's downfall comes from the restrictions he places on his daughter's emerging sexuality and his paranoia about her sexual experience with anyone else. *Lolita* was remade in 1997 with Jeremy Irons playing the role of Humbert.

There are vivid scenes of bathroom seduction by a stepfather (Karl Malden) in Barbra Streisand's film *Nuts* (1987). The classic example of the combination of pedophilia and sociopathy is found in the 1931 Fritz Lang film *M*, in which Peter Lorre plays a child molester stalking the streets of Berlin. A riveting presentation of the fate of child molesters when they are caught and incarcerated is found in the 1977 prison drama *Short Eyes*.

AKA (2002) is a creative film that depicts a father who sexually abuses his son. In *Dolores Claiborne* (1995), a father sexually abuses his daughter in numerous ways; one scene occurs when the father makes his daughter masturbate him while riding on a ferry in chilly weather, claiming her hands are needed to keep him warm. In *Precious* (2009), a teenage girl gets pregnant twice, and her father is each baby's father. Incest also figures conspicuously in other excellent films including *Angels and Insects* (1995; brother–sister), *Murmur of the Heart* (1971, France; mother–son), *La Luna* (1979, Italy; mother–son), *The Dreamers* (2003, Italy; brother–sister), *Oldboy* (2003, Korea; father–daughter), *Antonia's Line* (1995, Netherlands; brother–sister), *The Royal Tenenbaums* (2001; brother–sister), *Aguirre, the Wrath of God* (1972, German; father–daughter), *Dogtooth* (2009, Greece; brother–sister), and *Chinatown* (1974; father–daughter). The potential for incest is treated humorously in *Back to the Future* (1985) when Marty McFly (Michael J. Fox) goes back in time and discovers his mother has a crush on him.

The drama in the controversial film *Priest* (1994) in part derives from the fact that a young girl tells her priest that she is being abused by her father (who attends mass every Sunday), and the priest is deeply troubled by his inability to break his vow of confidentiality to protect the child. The plot is complicated further by the fact that this same priest is involved in a sexual relationship with a gay friend, while his superior has broken his vows of celibacy and become sexually involved with his housekeeper.

The Falling (2014, UK) is a film about mass hysteria (fainting) that overtakes students in a Catholic Girls' school. There is an incestuous tryst between a brother and sister; after the agoraphobic mother discovers the siblings having sex, she makes her son leave home.

Other Paraphilias Not Specifically Classified in the DSM-5

Telephone Scatologia and Sexting

Most American women and a considerable number of men have experienced obscene phone calls (although it appears this will be replaced by offences committed on the Internet). The practice of making obscene calls for sexual gratification is referred to as **telephone scatologia**. Clinical assessment of 19 male adolescent sexual offenders who had committed exhibitionism or telephone scatologia showed that the majority were maladjusted, had committed numerous sexual offenses, and came from dysfunctional families. Several of them appeared to be sexually deviant. Antisocial traits, sexual deviance in the family, homosexual conflicts, repressed sexuality, and sexual deviance were contributing factors to their offending (Saunders & Awad, 1991).

People who engage in telephone scatologia tend to be males with low self-esteem. They often feel sexually inadequate, and the outrage of their victims gives them a feeling of power. These feelings of power are like those that accompany exhibitionism; however, the man making obscene phone calls is far less likely to be apprehended, and the practice provides similar thrills with far fewer risks. Obscene phone callers seldom seek out contact with the individuals they call, and the perpetrator typically masturbates when making the call.

Another variation of telephone scatologia-involves "dial-a-porn" services. These 900 numbers allow one to engage in paraphilic behavior without risk and with an enthusiastic partner. The lead character in Spike Lee's *Girl 6* (1996) and a woman supporting her family in Robert Altman's *Short Cuts* (1994) work as phone sex operators handling such calls. In the latter film, the woman moans, groans, and sighs at the same time she is changing the diapers on her baby and cooking her family's supper. Adam Sandler's character Barry Egan connects with a phone sex company in *Punch Drunk Love* (2002).

Philip Seymour Hoffman portrays a lonely man who is addicted to telephone scatologia in *Happiness* (1998). He initiates innocuous phone conversations, and then probes for more intimate details while he masturbates.

In the 21st century, telephone scatologia has been replaced by **sexting**, sometimes referred to as **technology-mediated sexual interactions** (TMSIs; Lefebvre et al., 2022), a practice in which explicit sexual images are transmitted electronically. The practice is especially troubling for parents because of the risk their children may be exposed to if sexually explicit photos are widely shared in a classroom or on social media. Bouchard et al. (2023) studied over a thousand adolescents and reported that one in four had produced or sent sexting, and approximately 3% of their sample had retransmitted sexting. Being female, impulsive, and having a sizable number of sexual partners increased the likelihood of sexting, while higher self-esteem, virginity, or having few casual sexual encounters decreased the likelihood. Mori et al. (2022) conducted a meta-analysis and reported youth sexting rates of 19.3% for sending, 34.8% for receiving, and 14.5% for forwarding without consent.

King and Rings (2022) have examined the legal and ethical implications of sexting. They note,

> Sexting has become a prominent part of adolescent culture. Under current laws, adolescents caught sexting are being arrested, facing child pornography charges, and having to register as sex offenders. State laws on child pornography and child abuse differ throughout the United States and conflict with federal laws, making the ethical obligations for psychologists unclear. (King & Rings, 2022, p. 469)

Gámez-Guadix and Incera (2021) studied a sample of 1,779 adolescents between 12 and 18 years old, including 146 adolescents who identified as a member of a sexual minority group (bisexual, homosexual, pansexual, asexual, or queer). They found that four out of 10 adolescents in the sexual minority group had experienced sexual orientation discrimination. Of those, 40% experienced discrimination. Of these, 9% were victims of **sextortion** (sexual exploitation by threatening to release sexual images or information), and over 5% had been targets of **revenge porn** (distribution of sexually explicit images or videos of individuals without their consent).

Widespread availability of cameras and miniature recording devices (e.g., smartphones) have made it easy to take covert recordings of body parts and sex acts, and dissemination of these images via social media platforms is both easy and fast. Regulating these reprehensible acts has proven extraordinarily difficult (Najdowski, 2017). A related issue occurs when someone willingly consents to having videos of private sex acts recorded, only to discover later that those videos have been distributed on the web (**nonconsensual pornography**). Gius (2022) describes the case of an Italian woman whose private videos were uploaded on the web without her consent. The woman went to court to have the videos removed, and she changed her name. However, she was unable to live a normal life because of the widespread notoriety generated by the videos, and she committed suicide in 2016.

Weiner (2016) is a documentary film about Anthony Weiner, who resigned from Congress in 2011 after evidence of sexting came to light. The film highlights Weiner's subsequent attempt to become mayor of New York City; this campaign was also derailed after new evidence of sexting. In 2017, Weiner pleaded guilty to a charge of transmitting obscene material to a minor, and he was sentenced to 21 months in prison. Weiner's misbehavior resulted in divorce from his wife, Huma Abedin, a consultant and a friend to Hillary Clinton and vice chair of Clinton's 2016 campaign for the US presidency.

Sexting in Suburbia (2012) is a made-for-TV movie about a young girl who commits suicide after her boyfriend shares nude photos she had made solely for him. When she comes to class the morning after sending her photos, all of her classmates clap. The film may have been inspired by the case of Megan Meier, a teenager from Missouri who committed suicide by hanging shortly before her 14th birthday. Megan was the victim of **cyberbullying** on social media. She "friended" a fellow MySpace account holder who claimed to be a 16-year-old boy named Josh Evans. The friend was fictitious, and in fact the account had been created by a female teenage rival who made hateful comments about Megan on the fake MySpace account. At the time, there were no laws prohibiting impersonating someone on the Internet or cyberbullying.

Deepfake Technology

It is possible to use technology to misrepresent people and events in very convincing ways, altering our perceptions of reality. For example, a rejected boyfriend can superimpose his former girlfriend's head on a pornographic film star's video, making it appear that the erstwhile girlfriend is engaging in the acts depicted on screen. Artificial intelligence and the use of neural networks make it possible for even unsophisticated users to make convincing reproductions. The altered videos can be easily distributed on the Internet or via smartphones. These practices use what is sometimes referred to as **deepfake technology.** Most often, deepfake technology has been used to put faces of female celebrities onto porn performers bodies, with the image of both being typically used without their consent (Dickson, 2019). Deepfake technology poses significant risks for victims of domestic violence because perpetrators can use deepfakes to threaten, blackmail, and abuse victims (Lucas, 2022). An especially pernicious application of deepfake technology occurs when pedophiles use artificial intelligence to make videos of children engaged in sexual acts without ever using an actual child, thereby circumventing laws aimed at curbing sexual exploitation of children (Ratner, 2021). Behun and Owens (2020) have written a book examining the ways in which sexually explicit Internet material affects adolescents, and the book explores the consequences of deepfake exposure. There is also a very real potential for using this technology to influence elections and determine political outcomes.

Miscellaneous Paraphilias

Other paraphilias include **coprophilia** (feces), **urophilia** (urine), **klismaphilia** (enemas), **partialism** (exclusive focus on part of the body), **necrophilia** (corpses), and **zoophilia** (animals). Alfred Kinsey investigated zoophilia (bestiality) and found that in some rural areas up to 65% of boys had experienced sexual contact with animals. One quirky character in *The Ballad of*

Narayama (1984, Japan) has sex with a neighbor's female dog.

Necrophilia is believed to be extremely rare, although estimating the prevalence of the disorder is difficult for obvious reasons. In *Kill Bill: Vol. 1* (2003) a hospital aide sells the right to have sex with patients in comas; this behavior would be a variant of necrophilia. Public interest in necrophilia was heightened by the arrest of Jeffrey Dahmer, someone who murdered his victims, had sex with their corpses, mutilated their bodies, and ate various body parts. Dahmer was tested with the **Minnesota Multiphasic Personality Inventory** (MMPI), a psychological test widely used to assess psychopathology. A computerized assessment of Dahmer's test results reported: "[This patient] is likely to have significant psychological problems ... He typically deals with frustration by acting out in an extra punitive way ... [He is] quite conflicted over sexual issues." *Dahmer* (2002), a film based on the life of Jeffrey Dahmer, has little value as either entertainment or pedagogy.

John Waters is a director whose films are often designed to shock viewers, and he has produced interesting cult films with sexual themes (e.g., *Pink Flamingos*, 1972). Another of his films, *A Dirty Shame* (2004), is about a woman who becomes a sex addict after a head injury; although the film portrays many fetishes, the viewer learns little about fetishism from watching this insipid movie. The film stands in marked contrast to Molly Parker's sensitive portrayal of necrophilia in *Kissed* (1966). Parker's character, Sandra Larson, first becomes fascinated with death observing dead sparrows and chipmunks; she buries the animals but later digs them up and rubs her body with them. Sandra eventually gets a job in a funeral home where she has sex with the corpses but treats the sex act as a quasireligious ritual. This film makes necrophilia seem more plausible than most of us believe it to be.

Necrophilia is sometimes portrayed or alluded to in vampire movies. One of the best of these is *Bram Stoker's Dracula* (1992), directed by Francis Ford Coppola. There are several case studies of people who are aroused by the sight of blood; this phenomenon is sometimes referred to as **vampirism** or **Renfield's syndrome**. Kazğan et al. (2021) have reported a case of autovampirism in which a patient with a borderline personality disorder engaged in pleasurable self blood sucking that eventually had to be treated as self-mutilation.

International Films and Paraphilic Disorders

Edouard Molinaro's *La Cage aux Folles* (*The Birdcage*; 1978, France/Italy) is a comedy that portrays the relationship between two middle-aged homosexual lovers, Renato and Albin. Renato owns and manages La Cage aux Folles, a nightclub in the south of France in which all of the performers are male transvestites who perform as women. Albin, whose stage name is Zaza, is the star performer at La Cage aux Folles, as well as Renato's lover and longtime companion. Albin cross-dresses both on and off stage and has adopted an exclusively feminine identity.

It is important to understand that this film is a farce and not an accurate presentation of either homosexual relationships or transvestites. Albin's role as a drag queen is as exaggerated as his feminine mannerisms and served to perpetuate many of the stereotypes about homosexuality that existed when the film was released in 1978. However, despite reliance on stereotypes, the film can be credited for its presentation of an enduring, loving relationship between its two lead characters. Both men are secure in their sexual identity, even though it does not conform to conventional norms, and they know the life they have made for themselves is the right one for them. At one point Renato remarks, "Yes, I use make-up. Yes, I live with a man. Yes, I'm an old fag. But I know who I am. It's taken twenty years and that deputy isn't going to destroy it."

The film also highlights the sanctimonious hypocrisy of many of those people who are so quick to limit sexual expression in others and illustrates the perils inherent in denial of one's true sexual identity. The film is best viewed as the hilarious farce it is, and one does the film a disservice by insisting that it portray too strong a social message.

Breakfast on Pluto (2005, Ireland/UK), Neal Jordan's adaptation of a novel by Patrick McCabe, is an Irish film that presents the life of "Kitten," an orphan and a transvestite who enjoys dressing up in women's clothes from an early age. This film is less a gender identity study than the story of societal abuse, ostracization, tragedy, and/or diagnostic pathology. It is about an individual who happens to cross-dress and have gender issues and overcomes enormous stressful and tragic experiences, including serious life threats, prostitution, homelessness, job loss, and his house being burned down. Kitten perseveres through all of this. Transvestites also are portrayed in the award-winning film *All About My Mother* (1999, Spain) and in *House of Fools* (2002, Russia).

Breaking the Waves (1996) is a powerful Danish film that examines troilism in a situation in which a formerly virile man paralyzed from an industrial accident insists that his wife have intercourse with other men so he can derive vicarious satisfaction from her stories. The wife, a devout Catholic, goes along with her husband's demands because she is convinced that these voyeuristic pleasures are the only thing keeping her husband alive.

Korean director Chan-wook Park's unforgettable film *Oldboy* (2003) presents a man caught up in a terrible situation in which he unwittingly and unavoidably becomes involved in an incestuous relationship with his daughter, someone he has not seen for 15 years. Another film from Korea is the comedy *Sex Is Zero* (2002), a cult film about the sexual energies and promiscuity of adolescents and college students. The film depicts several normal and abnormal sexual behaviors, including rubbing against others on a subway (frotteurism), sex with a blow-up doll, men gawking at women doing aerobics and sunbathing, compulsive masturbation, priapism, and young males' obsession with female breasts. The film's director claims that 80% of what happens in the film is based on real experiences.

Pedro Almodóvar's *Tie Me Up! Tie Me Down!* (1990) is a provocative investigation of the relationship between a mildly masochistic woman and the man who kidnaps her and holds her hostage, hoping she will eventually come to love him. The theme is ancient, present in other movies, such as William Wyler's 1965 film *The Collector*. However, few directors have developed the concept with as much skill as Almodóvar, who previously directed another complex psychological investigation of the relationships between men and women, *Women on the Verge of a Nervous Breakdown* (1988). *Tie Me Up! Tie Me Down!* tells the story of Ricky, a young man released from a mental institution, whose only ambition is to find a woman, Marina, he had slept with once when he had escaped from the institution. Marina, an actress and a former drug addict, now stars in pornographic movies and has no memory of her tryst with Ricky. Their interactions after the kidnapping present the viewer with an odd mix of sexual violence and comedy, and the film constantly jumps between the themes of love and control. Love eventually wins out, and Ricky and Marina develop a healthy, satisfying relationship. The movie's description sounds misogynistic, but Almodóvar very skillfully demonstrates the power Marina maintains throughout her captivity.

"All the way in. I take him in like a slave. I play my part faithfully, so I, too, can get to his heart. Every time he hurts me till I bleed and scream. Then he is satisfied. Then he feels alive."

A sexual masochist describes her relationship with a sexual sadist in *Lust, Caution* (2007)

Sexual sadism is depicted in Ang Lee's *Lust, Caution* (2007, China/Taiwan/Hong Kong), which is set at a time immediately prior to the Chinese revolution (i.e., during the Chinese resistance to the Japanese). A group of mainland Chinese attempt to take down Mr. Yee, a spy from Hong Kong. Yee is very cautious and careful, looking out for anything suspicious; he accounts for his unusual behavior by explaining that he is afraid of the dark. He is sexually sadistic, and at the end of each sexual act he becomes further aroused when he hurts his sexual partner.

Sadomasochistic behavior is also portrayed in Lars von Trier's film, *Antichrist* (2009, Denmark), a movie about a couple whose toddler falls out of a window to his death while the couple is having sex. Their sexual behavior and treatment of one another deteriorates and becomes deviant and dangerous, including sadomasochistic sex that is mostly related to grief and punishment rather than sexual pleasure. Roger Ebert described the film as a movie built around "torture porn."

The David Cronenberg film, *A Dangerous Method* (2011, UK/Germany) addresses the split in the relationship between Freud and Jung as well as Jung's alleged affair with a patient, Sabina Sprielrein, who suffered from a severe mental illness. During her treatment, Sabina spoke of the abuse and humiliation she endured from her father. She seemed to have internalized her father's criticism, and her self-deprecating behavior is clearly apparent throughout the film (e.g., her sexual masochism).

Warm Water Under a Red Bridge (2001), a Japanese film directed by Shohei Imamura, tells the story of a woman who retains water in her body that she can only release by "doing something wicked" like stealing things or having sexual intercourse. The woman's water is a symbolic life force; fish flourish and plants grow larger when exposed to it. This fictional character's diagnosis, if any, is unclear. Despite its unusual plot, this is a film well worth seeing.

There is a fascinating portrayal of autoerotic asphyxia in another Japanese film, Nagisa Oshima's *In the Realm of the Senses* (1976). This movie documents the sexual obsessions of two Japanese lovers who are preoccupied with sexual pleasure. The woman increasingly resorts to strangulation to prolong the erections of her lover, and he dies during one of these episodes. In one graphic scene, the woman severs off the man's penis. The film is based on the true story of a woman who accidentally strangled her lover and then wandered around in a daze, carrying her lover's severed penis with her. Oshima was tried for obscenity in Japan when the film was released, but he was eventually acquitted. His stature as a filmmaker was vindicated by the critical and commercial success of the film in Europe and the United States.

A Short Film About Love (1988), a Polish movie directed by Krzysztof Kieslowski, is about Tomik, a shy and withdrawn 19-year-old voyeur who uses a telescope to spy on an older woman who lives in a nearby apartment. He becomes increasingly obsessed with the woman and eventually confesses that he has been watching her have sex with her numerous lovers. She is at first outraged, then intrigued. She later repositions her bed so he can observe her more easily when she is having sex with her lovers. Eventually the teenager has brief physical contact with her, but it is an unsatisfying, humiliating experience, and he flees from her apartment and attempts suicide by slitting his wrists. He survives, and while he is in the hospital recovering, the woman, Magda, becomes increasingly obsessed with him, using binoculars to watch his apartment to see when he will return. The first part of the film is presented from his perspective; the second from hers. The film is reminiscent of Hitchcock's masterpiece *Rear Window* (1954).

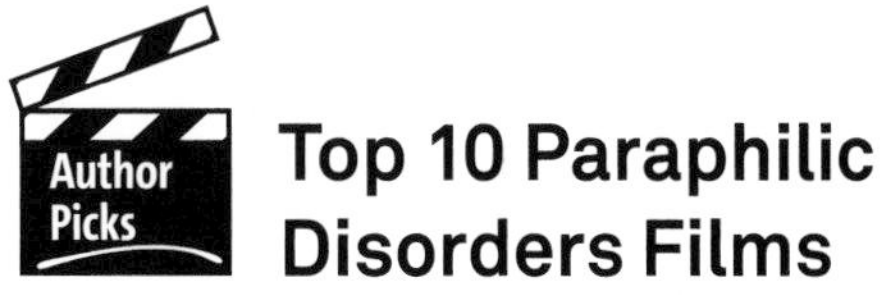

Top 10 Paraphilic Disorders Films

Lolita (1962)
Blue Velvet (1986)
Breaking the Waves (1996)
The Piano Teacher (2001)
Secretary (2002)
The Woodsman (2004)
Hard Candy (2005)
Towelhead (2007)
The Reader (2008)
Leap Year (2011)

Chapter 15

Violence and Physical and Sexual Abuse

When I woke up, I went on what the movie advertisements refer to as a roaring rampage of revenge. I roared and I rampaged, and I got bloody satisfaction. I've killed a hell of a lot of people to get to this point. But I've only one more ... the last one ... the one I'm driving to right now. The only one left. And when I arrive at my destination, I am gonna kill Bill ...

Beatrix Kiddo, the bride, in *Kill Bill: Vol. 1* (2003)

Violence

Violence is present in thousands of movies and documenting the presence of violence in films seems unnecessary and gratuitous. However, recent studies have shown there has been an increase in violent content in films over the past 2 decades. Riddle and Martins (2022) updated the National Television Violence Study by coding 765 television programs and movies airing on 21 different networks. They found a slight increase in the overall prevalence of violence, but many more programs "saturated" with violence. They relate these increases to the influx of highly violent movies on cable channels. This is hardly surprising because violence sells. Barranco et al. (2020) found that violent content in movies significantly correlated with ticket sales. A September 2023 search of the Internet Movie Database (IMDb) identified over 12,000 feature films tagged with the keyword "violence."

Violence and Racism

Kanye West (who changed his name to Ye) is an example of a celebrity who has used his social prominence as a platform to spew hateful rhetoric. He has made numerous anti-Semitic comments, wears "White Lives Matter" T-shirts, and in 2022 he dined at Mar-a-Lago with former President Trump Donald Trump and the noted White supremacist Nick Fuentes. Ye has repeatedly denied the Holocaust, and he publicly praises Adolf Hitler. He has been treated for bipolar disorder, and this condition may be sufficient to explain his impulsiveness during manic episodes – but it does not explain his racism and hatred. Most people with bipolar disorder do not spew hatred when they are interviewed. Hate and violence are often gendered and racialized, and sometimes politicized (witness the behavior of the Proud Boys and Oath Keepers and their attempts at insurrection on January 6, 2021). These problems are exacerbated when politicians make statements supporting xenophobia and violence toward minority groups; for example, hate crimes against Asian Americans surged after former President Donald Trump referred to COVID-19 as the "China Virus" and "Kung Flu."

In 2021, eight massage parlor workers were murdered by a 21-year-old White male and self-described sex addict who blamed the murders on the "temptation" the women had caused. The perpetrator was described as a devout Christian driven to commit murder because of his religion, his guilt, and his contrition. Inexplicably, the local sheriff's office denied that this was a racially motivated crime.

To understand events like this, Hwang and Parreñas (2021) analyzed the ways in which the theme of the "villainous temptress" has played out in cinema history, and they identified three cinematic archetypes of Asian femininity: the Lotus Blossom, the Dragon Lady, and the Little Brown Fucking Machine (LBFM). They illustrate the Lotus Blossom with *The Toll of the Sea* (1922), a silent film but one of the earliest color movies. In the film, a demure Chinese woman has a son with an American she has rescued from the sea. They fall in love and marry in an unofficial Chinese ceremony. He later returns to the United States, meets an American woman, and marries her. When he returns to China with his new wife, they persuade Lotus Blossom to give up her son so the boy can have a better life in America. Lotus Blossom commits suicide at the end of the film. In marked contrast, the Dragon Lady is characterized by excessive sexuality, as illustrated in *The Thief of Bagdad* (1924), a film starring Douglas Fairbanks and Anna May Wong (who had starred in *The Toll of the Sea* two years earlier). Wong "portrayed the scantily clad Mongol slave" whose "captivating sexuality is also threatening as she projects a treacherous foreign femininity that imperils an unguarded white man" (Hwang & Parreñas, 2021, p. 568). Hwang and Parreñas illustrate the LBFM with a more contemporary film, Stanley Kubrick's *Full Metal Jacket* (1987):

> [T]he LBFM archetype represents the Southeast Asian prostitute whose femininity is characterized by a machine-like sexual drive and performance

> of eroticized poverty. This hypersexualized Southeast Asian figure comes alive in Stanley Kubrick's *Full Metal Jacket*, in which Papillon Soo portrays a Vietnamese prostitute who entices two American soldiers with the invitation "Well, baby, me so horny, me so horny. Me love you long time. You party?" In this now classic depiction of Asian women, she promises them cheap wanton sex of "me sucky sucky, me love you too much." These figures of Asian femininity have gone viral ... Their circulation across hemispheres and in various cultural productions perpetuates the century-old view of Asian women as dangerously hypersexual. (Hwang & Parreñas, 2021, p. 568)

A thousand other films illustrate racism and promote racist stereotypes. However, *Till* (2022) is one of the most powerful, intense, and gripping recent films to depict the violence associated with racism and hate. This biographical film depicts the life and murder of Emmitt Till (see Figure 48), a 14-year-old boy from Chicago who was visiting his cousins in Money, Mississippi, in 1955 when he was abducted, tortured, and murdered for allegedly flirting with a White woman, 20-year-old Carolyn Bryant. The woman's husband and brother took Till from his aunt's home, forced him to carry a cotton gin fan to the Tallahatchie River, beat him, gouged out one of his eyes, shot him in the head, and threw his body into the river, tied to the fan with barbed wire. The body was recovered 3 days later, bloated, and dirty. It was only possible to identify the body by a ring that was still on Till's finger.

Till's mother, Mamie Bradley, insisted that her son's body be returned to Chicago. She also insisted on an open casket, allowing *Jet* magazine to publish a photo. The story was picked up by the news media, and the incident helped inspire the civil rights movement in the United States.

An all-White jury in Mississippi deliberated for less than an hour before finding the defendants not guilty, citing uncertainty about the identity of the body. Protected by double jeopardy laws, the two murderers, Bryant and Milam, admitted to their crime in a 1956 interview with *Look* magazine. They were paid US $4,000 for their story. Seventy years after the murder, Carolyn Bryant recanted her testimony. These events became inflection points in the Civil Rights movement, and in March of 2022, President Joe Bided signed into law the Emmett Till Antilynching Act, making lynching a federal hate crime punishable by up to 30 years in prison.

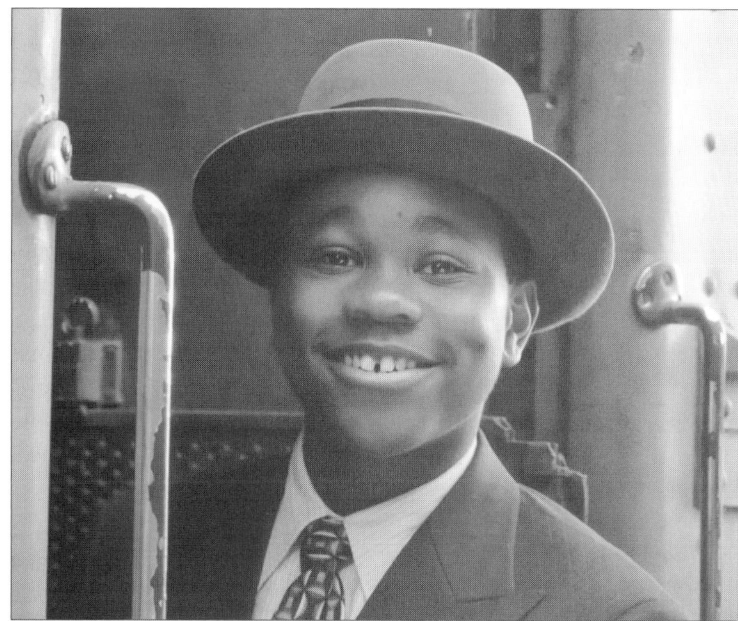

Figure 48.
Till (2022, Eon Productions, Frederick Zollo Productions, Metro-Goldwyn-Mayer, Orion Pictures, Whoop/One Ho Productions/Lil' Whoop Productions). Produced by Keith Beauchamp, Barbara Broccoli, Tina Broccoli, Chinonye Chukwu, Whoopi Goldberg, et al. Directed by Chinonye Chukwu.

Violence, Revenge, and *Kill Bill*

Beatrix Kiddo (aka "the bride," played by Uma Thurman) is not a typical prototype of a violent figure. She is a middle-aged woman who was in a relationship, does not abuse substances, and does not have a poor socioeconomic background. Research has shown repeatedly that substance abuse increases the likelihood of violent acts; other risk factors for violence include being young, male, single, and of lower socioeconomic status. Nevertheless, Thurman is engaging, fascinating, and compelling in her role as the vengeful character in *Kill Bill: Vol. 1* (2003) and *Kill Bill: Vol. 2* (2004), both of which involve dramatic depictions of violence (e.g., see Figure 49). Some viewers will argue these are two of the most artistic action films ever made. Others will see the violence as overly graphic and gratuitous. Still others will speak of the role of violence influencing today's culture and today's youth, and argue that despite the artistry, the violent imagery that defines these films cannot be beneficial for youths or adults. Others will speak to the glorification of murder and the purposeless nature of revenge. Some will say the violence is justified as it is always either in self-defense or directed solely at those individuals who killed her family and left her for dead. Finally, some will note the film is meant to be seen as entertainment, distraction, appreciation, and even inspiration (e.g., the theme of a woman's courage and bravery). Each of these perceptions is valid and at least partially accurate.

David Carradine (who played the character Bill) maintained that the essence of a Tarantino movie is not the violence, not the action but the inside look at the mind, the heart, of violent people. This insight emphasizes looking more deeply at all cinematic characters and looking beyond violent acts to better understand them. There are a variety of violent characters in the film; each is portrayed as unique, with diverse backgrounds, motivations, thought processes, and actions. Rather than one-dimensional "bad guys," Tarantino develops all of his characters, showing their flaws, strengths, nuances, and everyday interactions behind their violent presentation.

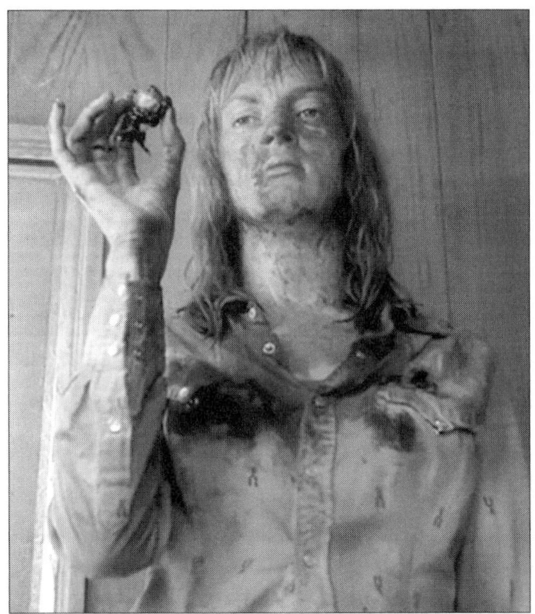

Figure 49. *Kill Bill: Vol. 2* (2004, Miramax Films, A Band Apart, Super Cool ManChu). Produced by Lawrence Bender, Yinchun Fang, Koko Maeda, Dede Nickerson, et al. Directed by Quentin Tarantino.

Some people will be offended by the frequency and intensity of the violence in these films. This is justified, for in many ways these are quintessential violent movies. Scores of people are killed, arms are chopped off, blood sprays, and eyes are ripped out of their sockets, at times in cartoonish ways. The bride is raped while in a coma, then buried alive, and other characters are tortured as the killer watches them suffer and die. One of the most violent sequences occurs in *Kill Bill: Vol. 1* and is presented completely in animation; this episode presents the traumatic history of an assassin, who as a girl watched her father and mother brutally murdered in front of her. Tarantino does not do this for gratuitous purposes – there is real depth to these characters, an intricate story to be told, and beautiful cinematic artistry to appreciate. The dramatic mixture of violence and cinematic genius is reminiscent of Stanley Kubrick's classic, *A Clockwork Orange* (1971), which was criticized for being overly violent and degrading women, neither of which was Kubrick's intent.

Many of Tarantino's other films involve similar themes and use violence as a communication medium: Examples include *Reservoir Dogs* (1992), *Pulp Fiction* (1994), and *Jackie Brown* (1997). He also wrote the screenplay for *From Dusk till Dawn* (1995). Most recently, Tarantino (along with Robert Rodriguez) wrote and directed two full-length horror films that were shown together as *Grindhouse* (2007) and were touted as a homage to gory exploitation films. Individually, these violent films are titled *Death Proof* and *Planet Terror*; they portray, respectively, a stunt race car driver (Kurt Russell) who stalks and kills women until he encounters a group of women who turn the tables on him, and an army of flesh-eating zombies created by a bioweapon mishap.

Most people reading *Movies and Mental Illness* will have an interest in films and be aware of the death of David Carradine in Bangkok, Thailand, on June 4, 2009. Carradine was found hanging by a rope in his hotel room closet, and speculation about his death has included suicide, murder by Kung Fu gangs he was investigating, and autoerotic asphyxiation. Two of Carradine's ex-wives have reported that he practiced erotic self-bondage. Whatever the cause of his death, he was a gifted actor who was perfectly cast in the *Kill Bill* films.

Is Violence Gratuitous?

In most current action and horror movies, the purpose of the violence is to stimulate, dazzle, and entertain the viewer for a brief period. This helps the viewer escape from their present reality and magically enter a more exciting world. The violence in this type of action film (usually a Hollywood product) is unrealistic, unnecessary, and/or gratuitous. It is merely a means to an end – the overriding purpose is to sell movie tickets, not to enhance the cinematic art, relay an important message to the viewer, or engender insights.

I have identified seven exceptions to this type of escapism violence, and I have grouped films around these thematic exceptions: namely, (1) depicting a particular reality, (2) showing the ridiculous and futile nature of violence, (3) revealing the psyche of violent people, (4) showing how violence is a cyclical trap, (5) projecting a dangerous future, (6) showing the potential danger of authority roles and group contagion, and (7) demonstrating obstacles people must face with courage and sacrifice. These at least begin an argument that violence in films can have a meaningful purpose. However, this does not mean that the purpose outweighs the negative effects associated with violence.

Depicting a Particular Reality

Often violence is the most succinct and honest way to portray the reality of a particular situation, problem, or conflict. In *Elephant* (2003), the reality of violence in schools is depicted. Director Gus Van Sant portrays the typical everyday life of several students who are unaware of the danger and violence about to take place. *Hotel Rwanda* (2004) depicts another terrible reality: the genocide that took place in Rwanda in which nearly 1 million Rwandans were killed. The film focuses on the heroic behavior of a hotel owner, Paul Rusesabagina, who saved well over 1,000 lives, and the multiple threats of violence he had to face to do so. *Till* (2022) does the same – it depicts real events with a horrifying impact for the viewer.

Rendition (2007) attempts to show the realities of politics. The film is a depiction of "extraordinary rendition" – the detaining of suspected terrorists with minimal evidence (e.g., a phone record) and interrogating and questioning them on foreign soil without judicial oversight. In this film, an Egyptian man traveling in South Africa to attend a conference is detained without due process of law and is then tortured by means of waterboarding and other methods. The film also portrays Islamic extremists, brainwashing, and the training of suicide bombers.

> **"Sometimes I wonder will God ever forgive us for what we've done to each other. Then I look around and I realize God left this place a long time ago."**
>
> **Realistic cynicism portrayed by Leonardo DiCaprio, in *Blood Diamond* (2006)**

Blood Diamond (2006) is an intense action film with a deeper purpose – to depict and raise awareness about "conflict diamonds." The film takes place in Sierra Leone in 1999, where a civil war has ravaged the country, leaving millions of refugees; the irony is they were fighting over diamond fields when most of them had never even seen a diamond. The film notes that whenever something of value is found in Africa, many innocent villagers end up dying – this was the case with ivory, rubber, gold, oil, and diamonds. It is further noted that the Americans who purchase two thirds of the world's diamonds are usually unaware of the violence associated with the diamonds they buy. As one character puts it: "In America, it's bling-bling but out here it's bling-bang." Leonardo DiCaprio gives a standout performance as a diamond smuggler who transforms and sacrifices himself to help the victims of the diamond trade. The film concludes by noting that 40 countries signed the Kimberley Process in January 2003 to stem the flow of conflict diamonds, and that it is up to the consumer to demand conflict-free diamonds. It also notes there are still 200,000 child soldiers living in Africa, and the viewer gets to see horrifying examples of their training.

Other films also portray actual historical events, e.g., *Schindler's List* (1993). War films depict not only historical events but can be generalized to illustrate the atrocities and violence of present-day wars. For example, *Saving Private Ryan* (1998) reveals the realities of war, deglamorizing it, while not denigrating the sacrifices made by the men involved. Antiwar films reveal similar realities emphasizing the futility of war. *No Man's Land* (2001), a film that won an Academy Award for Best Foreign Language Film, is a good example; likewise, Stanley Kubrick made three excellent antiwar films: *Paths of Glory* (1957), *Dr. Strangelove or: How I Learned to Stop Worrying and Love the Bomb* (1964), and *Full Metal Jacket* (1987).

Showing the Ridiculous and Futile Nature of Violence

The purpose of the film *Series 7: The Contenders* (2001) is to demonstrate the futility and folly of violence. The film is a tongue-in-cheek fictional reality television show where six people are randomly chosen from their government-issued numbers and forced to hunt and kill the others while cameras film them for the television audience. The narrator excitedly describes "real people, real murders" and states that "the rules are as simple as life and death." Dawn, a pregnant woman, is "the longest running contender;" she continues with each new episode enhancing the theme of "kill or be killed." Her success fails to impress her family, and her sister labels her as an "animal, whore, addict, murderer, and thief." A similar theme is found in *The Hunger Games* (2012) and all its sequels, dystopian films in which two children are selected to fight similar young couples from 11 other districts. Each couple must fight until they or their opponents die; the games are televised, and only one couple can be the final winner. Jennifer Lawrence stars in this film, and she comes across as frightened, but still confident and assured.

Revealing the Psyche of Violent People

As discussed earlier in the chapter, most of Quentin Tarantino's films embody theme of revealing the psyche of violent people. Serial killer movies (discussed in more detail in Chapter 13) sometimes attempt to attain this level, but they rarely succeed. In *American Psycho* (2000), assuming the violence is all in Patrick Bateman's mind, the purpose of the violence is to depict the inner psyche and violent fantasies of a disturbed man. The film illustrates a fundamental contradiction, as Bateman spends hours daydreaming about violent acts while his body, attire, job, business cards, selection of social outings, and overall presentation are virtually perfect. Thus, the film gets at what no one else in Bateman's world would be privy to - his mind. *Sweeney Todd: The Demon Barber of Fleet Street* (2007) is in part a musical, which allows the music to contain or "hold" the violence, almost sectioning it off from the rest of the film. The barber's (Johnny Depp) revenge and killings seem to reveal more about his psyche and deterioration than anything else.

The Act of Killing (2012) is a powerful documentary that lingers with the viewer long after they have seen the film. The movie deals with death squads in Indonesia that are reported to have killed more than a million people. Death squad leaders describe horrendous acts of torture and murder; these stories are told while their companions listen and laugh at the details of these accounts, all of which are viewed as heroic acts of bravery by the individuals relating the stories. The viewer is reminded of Hannah Arendt's comment about Otto Adolf Eichmann, after Eichmann was hanged for war crimes and crimes against humanity: "It was as though in those last minutes he was summing up the lesson that this long course in human wickedness had taught us - the lesson of the fearsome, word-and-thought-denying *banality of evil*" (Arendt, 2006, p. 365). Evil is a topic that has been recently addressed by many psychologists and social scientists (e.g., Baron-Cohen, 2011; Bartlett, 2005; Mikulincer & Shaver, 2012; Pinker, 2011; Taylor, 2009; Zimbardo, 2007).

Showing How Violence Is a Cyclical Trap

In *American History X* (1998), one of the purposes of the violence is to show its cyclical nature. This film relates the following sequence of events: A man gets involved in a violent group, he gets out of the group but not before the consequences of his involvement emerge, and he tries to challenge and resolve these new conflicts but must face the fact that it is too late and violence ensues, completing the circle. The message: Do not get involved with violence in the first place. Mel Gibson's *Apocalypto* (2006) is graphically violent depicting the self-destruction of the Mayan culture.

"I'm going to peel off his skin and make him watch me wear it."

A comment made by a violent Mayan in *Apocalypto* (2006)

A History of Violence (2005), directed by David Cronenberg, depicts Tom Stall (Viggo Mortensen), an everyday family man who owns a café in a small town. He is involved in a hold-up by two criminals; however, he instinctively springs to action, killing both men and saving all his customers and workers. The media proclaim him a hero, and this news attracts three thugs from Philadelphia who claim Tom has led a previous life filled with violence and that they have come to take him back. The film reinforces research that suggests a history of violence is the best predictor of future violent behavior. It also emphasizes that one can never fully escape one's past, and that once violence starts, it finds a way to cycle back. One of the comments Tom's wife makes after learning about his history illustrates a common misconception in films. She asks: "What are you, some multiple personality schizoid?!" She is confusing two mental disorders in her statement, and she assumes that violence must mean mental illness of some kind (in the case of Tom Stall, it does not).

No one can escape the shadow part of their character in *Crash* (2004). This Academy Award for Best Picture winner integrates several stories in an eclectic mix of races and ethnicities in Los Angeles that provides a meaningful look at the pain of racism, the dangers of discrimination, and the possibility of redemption. Even the Buddhist who practices nonviolence eventually resorts to highly violent and threatening acts. The film depicts the vicissitudes of the human condition and illustrates that violence leads to more violence, which can be verbal, emotional, or physical.

In Wim Wenders' *The End of Violence* (1997), Bill Pullman plays Mike Max, an action-violence film director who hides from society and starts a new life after he is almost murdered. While this character promotes violence in his movies, he also fears violence, as documented by his elevated level of paranoia, leading him to believe his enemies can come from anywhere - land, water, and sky. A contrasting character, Ray Bering (played by Gabriel Byrne) tries to prevent violence as a secret government officer working a program that oversees the city with thousands of cameras watching over every interaction. The cyclical nature of violence is evident both in the man who directs violent movies only to be attacked and thereby become a victim of violence, and in the man trying to prevent violence through spying, who is himself killed.

Projecting a Dangerous Future

The message associated with these films is clear: If society keeps heading in a particular direction, a dangerous future is inevitable. *A Clockwork Orange* (1971), in a very artistic way, speaks to this theme about youth violence, the role of the prison system, and the predominant psychological approach at the time, behaviorism. Rather than denigrating such a film and labeling it as offensive, it is more helpful to see the film as a message and motivator to promote change in the present. In *Sin City* (2005), the graphic, stylized violence and surreal settings created with computer animation present a violent and dangerous future. The violence and societal control seen in films such as *Equilibrium* (2002) and *The Island* (2005) clearly depict an unpleasant and dangerous future. Likewise, each of the films in the *Mad Max* series (1979, 1981, 1985, 2015) depict a dangerous apocalyptic world characterized by violence and dramatic car chases.

Showing the Potential Danger of Authority Roles and Group Contagion

Group contagion occurs when an individual's identity is merged with that of a group, and the individual begins to accept and conform to the values and beliefs of the group. This process of **deindividuation** can be linked with increases in aggressive behavior, as people feel more anonymous acting within a group rather than alone. These social psychology themes can clearly be seen in *A Clockwork Orange* (1971), *Fight Club* (1999), *Amores Perros* (2000), and gang-related movies such as *South Central* (1992). It also occurs in larger numbers in the persecution of religious figures, where crowds and major groups of people turn against Gandhi in *Gandhi* (1982) and against Jesus in *The Passion of the Christ* (2004).

These themes are also present with gang behavior, which is frequently portrayed in movies. *City of God* (2003), a Brazilian drama-documentary about a poor area of Rio de Janeiro, portrays how gangs can take over much of a major city through group violence, leaving young people with few options other than joining the drug lords or dying. In *South Central* (1992), the gangs portrayed take over the city at night, implement rules that allow them to keep their power, emphasize controlling the "hood" by killing, and enforce the idea that "nothing goes on without we saying so." The film emphasizes three alternatives to gang life: (1) kill the enemy; (2) turn against oneself and go crazy; or (3) change. The film also speaks to anger and hate in the lead character, Ali, who must change and influence others to break his own *hate cycle,* thus removing his *badge of shame*. This theme is also found in a nongang film, *Antwone Fisher* (2002), in which a young African American man must face his own anger about abuse that can be traced back to the time of slavery.

Gang-related films often explore issues of racism and the link between racism and violence; this is the case in *South Central* (1992) as well as in *8 Mile* (2002), which stars the rapper Eminem.

Gangs of violent skinheads promoting hate are depicted in four especially powerful films: *American History X* (1998), *The Believer* (2001), *MacArthur Park* (2001), and *Hate* (1995).

In the psychologically complex film *Fight Club* (1999), men gather to fight one-on-one against each other, physically and brutally until one of the combatants can no longer stand. An entirely underground fight club movement grows and moves from city to city. The violence is depicted as a way of expressing anger and repressed rage, as an alternative to the monotony of everyday life, as an antidote to consumerism and depression, and as a way of feeling "really alive."

Demonstrating Obstacles People Must Face With Courage and Sacrifice

The Sand Pebbles (1966) stars Steve McQueen confronting a violent Chinese mob and finding the courage to shoot and kill a Chinese shipmate to end the shipmate's torture by the mob. *Hotel Rwanda* (2004) depicts the courage of one man trying to cope with the violence that tore apart his nation. *To Kill a Mockingbird* (1962) illustrates the courage of attorney Atticus Finch confronting angry townspeople. Jesus and Gandhi look directly in the face of violent crowds in *The Passion of the Christ* (2004) and *Gandhi* (1982), respectively. Both show the enormous sacrifice and courage that is often necessary to confront oppression and defeat violence.

The Impact of Violence in Films

In the United States, children are exposed to an average of almost 11 hours of media viewing each day, and they spend more time learning from these experiences than they do learning from schoolteachers and in formal classes (Warburton, 2012). According to the American Academy of Pediatrics, the typical American youngster will have witnessed about 200,000 acts of violence on television by the age of 18 and is likely to have witnessed several thousand additional acts of violence in films such as *The Hunger Games: Catching Fire* (2013) or any of the many *Halloween* films. Contemporary films and television programs are replete with violence, and it is difficult to avoid violence in the media or to briefly catalogue the most egregious examples of violence in recent films.

Several studies have examined the role of violence in television and movies and explored its impact on aggression, attitudes, and behavior. Likewise, hundreds of articles have emphasized the impact of movie violence on children and adolescents, and authors often attempt to link this violence with violent acts committed by teens. However, while viewing violent movies does appear to contribute to increases in acts of aggression, the degree of influence is unclear, as many other factors are involved (e.g., video games, parental upbringing, level of poverty, education level, etc.) Bushman et al. (2015) surveyed media psychologists, pediatricians, and parents and discovered that all three groups agreed that exposure to media violence can increase aggression in children, with the highest ratings for video games and movies. They note that most researchers believe violent media increases violence in children.

Often the person committing the violent act in movies is mentally ill, and as many as 70% of movie characters with mental illness are dangerous. This certainly contributes to the misconception that all people with mental disorders are violent. Some films can appropriately make the distinction between violence and mental illness, such as Roman Polanski's *Repulsion* (1965), Martin Scorsese's *Taxi Driver* (1976; Figure 50) and *Raging Bull* (1980) (Zimmerman, 2003).

Horror Movies and Violence

Violence is a staple feature of all horror films, and there are numerous examples of films in which one or more characters in a horror film is

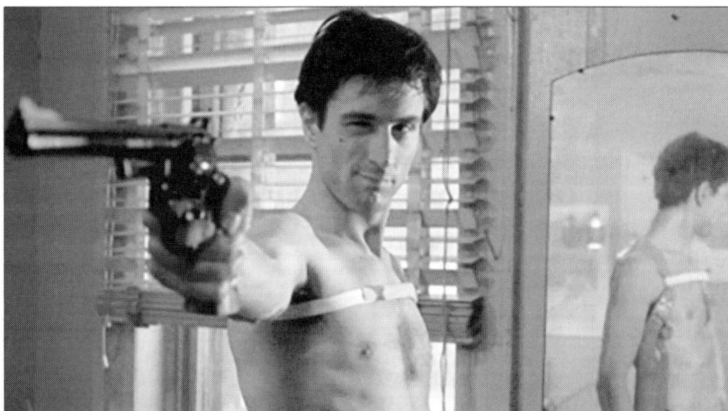

Figure 50.
Taxi Driver (1976, Columbia Pictures, Bill/Phillips, Italo/Judeo Productions). Produced by Phillip M. Goldfarb, Julia Phillips, and Michael Phillips. Directed by Martin Scorsese.

a person with a mental illness, perpetuating the myth that people with mental illnesses are dangerous and unpredictable. Prominent examples include Norman Bates in *Psycho* (1960), Leatherface in *Texas Chainsaw Massacre* (1974), Michael Meyers in *Halloween* (1978), Jack Torrance in *The Shining* (1980), Freddy Krueger in *A Nightmare on Elm Street* (1984), and Hannibal Lecter in *The Silence of the Lambs* (1991). Two films are particularly noteworthy.

Midsommar (2019, Swedish), is a gripping horror film directed by auteur Ari Aster. It portrays a group of young people who travel to a remote Swedish village to study a cult and their midsummer rituals in a festival that only occurs once every 90 years. One of the characters is completing an anthropology dissertation on the cult. The protagonist takes Ativan, a benzodiazepine, to cope with her anxiety, partly due to the murder-suicide of her sister and parents. She eventually is lionized and celebrated by the cult, but only after all of her fellow travelers have all been murdered. Critic Matthew Rozsa, reviewing the film in *Salon*, described the film as "a masterpiece of the horror genre and a parable about the struggles of living with mental illness" (Rozsa, 2019).

Hereditary (2018), by the same director, is an equally compelling film, in which an old woman, Annie, suffers from a DID (complicated by the fact that she is also a witch); her husband suffered from psychotic depression and starved himself to death, and her son has schizophrenia. The vehicular decapitation of her granddaughter, herself a victim of epilepsy, is an unforgettable scene. The protagonist, Annie, attends a grief support group, but lies to her husband and claims she is only going out to watch movies. She knows that there is a rich and complex history of mental illness in her family, and she worries about her own mental health and that of her children. Both *Midsommar* and *Hereditary* deal with the common familial concern that mental illness is inherited and unavoidable.

"Can I tell you a secret? ... I think she likes you. I mean, she's attracted to you. She says that's not true, but it is, I'm sure. And, to be honest, I think you're perfect for each other. You'd make a great couple. She's got a great body. You've seen it for yourself. She lost weight and she has a really great figure."

Martin tries to fix up his mother and a married cardiologist, in *The Killing of a Sacred Deer*

The Killing of a Sacred Deer (2017) is a film starring Colin Farrell and Nicole Kidman and directed by Yorgos Lanthimos who also directed *The Lobster (2015)* and *Dogtooth* (2009). This gripping horror story involves a young man whose father died on the operating table after an operation performed by Dr. Steven Murphy (Colin Farrell), a renowned and prosperous cardiologist married to a successful ophthalmologist, Anna (Nicole Kidman). Steven and Anna and their two children seem to have a perfect life, but their life becomes much more complicated after Dr. Murphy befriends the son of the man who died during surgery. The two develop an odd relationship, one characterized by sexual innuendo. At one point, the boy invites Dr. Murphy over for dinner, encouraging him to have sex with his mother, who seems receptive to the idea ("I won't let you leave until you've tasted my tart"). The terror of the film doesn't become clear until the conclusion of the movie, and there is a surprising and unforgettable ending reminiscent of *Sophies Choice* (1982).

In *Old Man* (2022), Stephen Lang's character, a paranoid loner, must face and confront his violent past. He does so in the context of unknowingly meeting a character (who turns out to be himself at a much younger age) in his cabin in the Smoky mountains.

The book *Monsters, Demons and Psychopaths: Psychiatry and Horror Film* (Forcen, 2016) discusses the genre of the horror film from a psychodynamic perspective, and the book "whets the appetite of the horror fan, of the mental health enthusiast, and of lay readers alike" (Schlozman, 2017). Schlozman is the author of *The Zombie Autopsies: Secret Notebooks from the Apocalypse* (Schlozman, 2011).

Jeffrey Bullins (2017) has written a chapter devoted to the meme of escaped (male) mental patients in American horror films, using John Carpenter's *Halloween* (1978) as an exemplar film. It is described as a good example of the slasher subgenre, "movies that feature killers stalking babysitters, campers, sorority girls, and so on" (p. 13). *Halloween* was one of the most successful independent films of all time, and introduced the iconic masked killer, Michael Myers.

War and Mass Murder

Numerous films have been devoted to the problems of genocide or mass murder. Some of the most compelling are *The Diary of Anne Frank* (1959), *Judgment at Nuremberg* (1961), *Little Big Man* (1970), *The Killing Fields* (1984), *The Official Story* (1985), *Salvador* (1986), *The Mission* (1986), *Natural Born Killers* (1994), *Welcome to Sarajevo* (1997), *Windhorse* (1998), *City of God* (2002), *The Last Samurai* (2003), *Hotel Rwanda* (2004), *The Last King of Scotland* (2005), *God Grew Tired of Us* (2006), *Pinochet's Last Stand* (2006), *Defiance* (2008), *Darfur Now* (2008), *Shake Hands with the Devil* (2007), *Katyn* (2007), *We Need To Talk About Kevin* (2011), *Avatar* (2009), and *The Hunger Games* (2012). Some classic films depicting the horror of World War I include *All Quiet on the Western Front* (1932), *Gallipoli* (1981), *Johnnie Got His Gun* (1971) and *Paths of Glory* (1957). Mass murder is also portrayed in almost every film depicting World War II and the Holocaust; some salient examples include *The Shop on Main Street* (1966), *Sophie's Choice* (1982), *Europa Europa* (1990), *Schindler's List* (1993), *Life Is Beautiful* (1997), the documentary *The Last Days* (1998), *The Pianist* (2002), *The Boy in the Striped Pajamas* (2008), and *Inglorious Basterds* (2009). Films about the Vietnam War are also compelling indictments of the horror and futility of war; especially memorable films include the documentary *Hearts and Minds* (1974), *The Deer Hunter* (1978), *Coming Home* (1978), *Apocalypse Now* (1979), *Platoon* (1986), *Full Metal Jacket* (1987), *Casualties of War* (1989), *We Were Soldiers* (2002), and the documentary *Kim's Story* (1996) about the life of the 9-year-old child who was photographed running down a country road naked and in pain from napalm burns. The photograph won a Pulitzer Prize, and the film tells the story of Kim Phuc's life after the war ended.

The Hurt Locker (2008) was the surprise winner for the Oscar for Best Picture and depicts the impact of the Iraqi war on an elite team of soldiers as well as the deaths of numerous individuals during the war.

The Act of Killing (2012) is a chilling film that documents mass murders committed in Indonesia after a military coup in 1965. The death squad leaders who are interviewed appear proud and almost gleeful as they describe despicable atrocities and the murder of more than a million suspected communists. One of the military leaders depicts how he would decapitate his victims in Figure 51. The murderers are regarded as present-day heroes in Indonesia. This is a film you will not soon forget.

"We crushed their necks with wood. We hung them. We strangled them with wire. We cut off their heads. We ran them over with cars. We were allowed to do it ... we murdered people and were never punished. The people we killed, there's nothing to be done about it. They have to accept it. Maybe I'm just trying to make myself feel better, but it works: I've never felt guilty, never been depressed, never had nightmares."

A former military leader, in *The Act of Killing* (2012), proudly describing the murders he committed

Peter Jackson directed the war documentary *They Shall Not Grow Old* (2018). The film is technically brilliant; Jackson used original footage from World War I taken from the Imperial War Museum's archives. The clips were over 100 years old and included original interviews of soldiers who fought in the war. Jackson colorized the clips and added sound effects. The movie is dedicated to his grandfather, who fought in World War I, and it gives viewers a sense of both the horror and the futility of war.

School Shootings

School shootings are now at their highest recorded levels. There was a marked decline in 2020 as schools shut down in response to the COVID-19 pandemic, but school shootings sharply increased in 2021, and they have continued to increase (Katsiyannis et al., 2023). Gun violence has become a massive public health crisis. Although shooters are always angry and troubled youths, there is scant evidence that these events result from mental illness, and ample evidence linking school shootings to the easy availability of guns. Edwards and Kotera (2022) note,

> Mental illness is not a predictor of gun violence. However, false assumptions of mental illness only reinforce the negative belief that individuals who have mental illness are dangerous and violent,

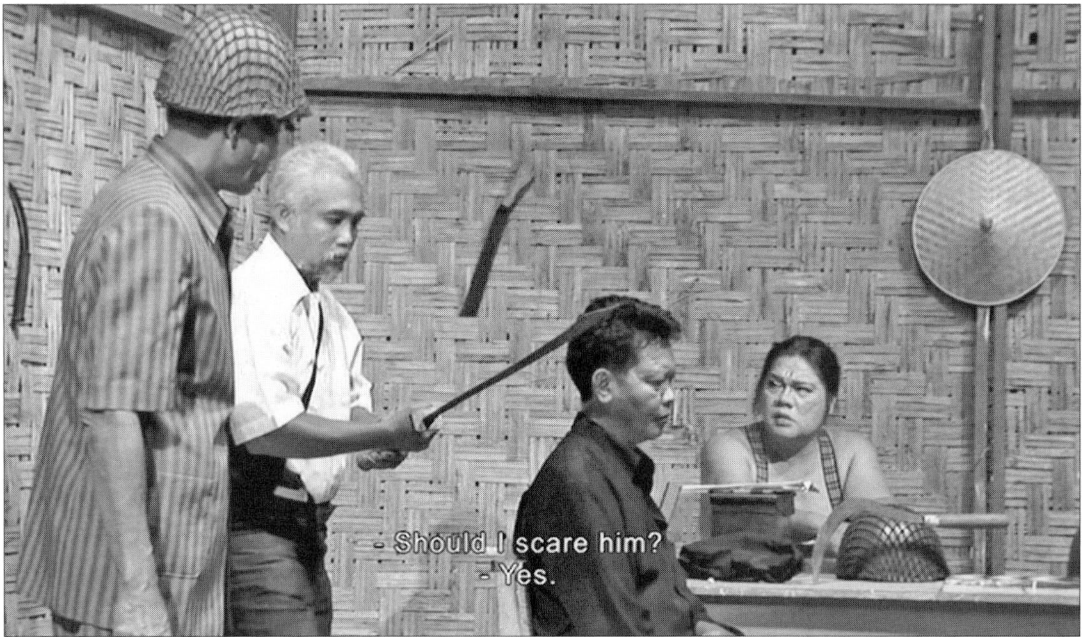

Figure 51. *The Act of Killing* (2012, Final Cut for Real, Piraya Film A/S, Novaya Zemlya, Spring Films). Produced by Christine Cynn, Torstein Grude, Werner Herzog, Maria Kristensen, et al. Directed by Joshua Oppenheimer and Christine Cynn.

> exacerbating the stigma already attached to those suffering from mental illnesses. Linking gun crime to mental illness is a barrier to seeking treatment and having a mental illness does not necessarily imply an individual will commit indiscriminate acts of violence. Research reports that most mental health symptoms were not related to gun violence, but easy access to firearms and other demographic variables were identified as the primary cause. (Edwards & Kotera, 2022)

Video games are frequently associated with school shootings carried out by White perpetrators. Markey et al. (2020) found that "participants who read a mock news story about a school shooting were more likely to blame video games when the shooter was White than when the shooter was Black" (p. 493). In a subsequent study reported in the same article, they examined over 200,000 news stories about 204 mass shootings committed in the US and found that when a shooting occurred at a school, video games were over 8 times more likely to be discussed when the shooter was White than when the shooter was Black.

Regrettably, there is an entire genre of films devoted to the topic of mass murders in US schools. One of the most compelling of these films is *We Need to Talk About Kevin* (2011), a film depicting a mother's attempt to love a child who is hateful and vicious, almost from birth. Kevin eventually kills his father and sister, along with several dozen classmates, sparing his mother because "you never want to kill your audience." Gus Van Sant deals with school shootings in his film *Elephant* (2003), and Michael Moore tries to make sense out of the 1999 Columbine High School shootings by Eric Harris and Dylan Klebold, in his film *Bowling for Columbine* (2002). Much of Moore's film is a formal accusation of lax gun control laws in the United States, and the film includes interviews with the late Charlton Heston, former president of the National Rifle Association.

Luckiest Girl Alive (2022) deals with double trauma: first a rape by a drunken college student, followed by a horrific school shooting a week later. Much of the film involves flashbacks experienced by Ani, a New York writer for a tabloid magazine who is engaged to be married to a handsome, wealthy man. She has everything, but the memories of her rape and the shooting continue to haunt her and make it impossible for her to experience a satisfying, normal sex life with her fiancé. Ani is confronted by a filmmaker making a documentary about the shooting, and she must deal with accusations made by her rapist who survived the shooting and suggested she helped plan the event to retaliate for her rape. The film takes place in 1999, the same year as the Columbine school shootings, and there are numerous parallels. *Elephant* is a much more powerful movie.

Paper Tiger (2020) is a powerful film that depicts the challenges faced by a widowed Chinese mother with terminal cancer who can't understand the odd behavior of her 17-year-old son, Edward. He is bullied at school, hallucinates his dead father, and is diagnosed with schizophrenia. Refusing to take his medication, Edward becomes increasingly ill. He is fascinated by Nazi memorabilia and spends time on the Web reading about school shootings. His mother, knowing she is dying and fearing what her son might do after her death, checks into a hotel with him and shoots him after he falls asleep.

Paper Tiger is based on a true story. In 2015, Lai Hang, a Laotian woman living near Los Angeles, was diagnosed with cancer. On the same day, she filled out the paperwork required to buy a handgun (see Figure 52) and began her 10-day waiting period. Lai had confided in a friend that her son was *seoi zai* – a wicked child. Like Edward in *Paper Tiger*, Lai's son was fascinated with mass shootings, and Lai believed he was planning such an attack. She checked herself and her son into a hotel room in Rosemead; when he fell asleep, she shot him twice in the chest before crawling into his bed and stroking his hair. Both the incident and the film raise important questions about parental responsibility for preventing violence and the reluctance of many Asian Americans to accept mental illness or seek treatment for it when it occurs (Balaraman et al., 2022).

Mass (2021) is the debut film of director Fran Kranz, and it centers on two sets of parents who

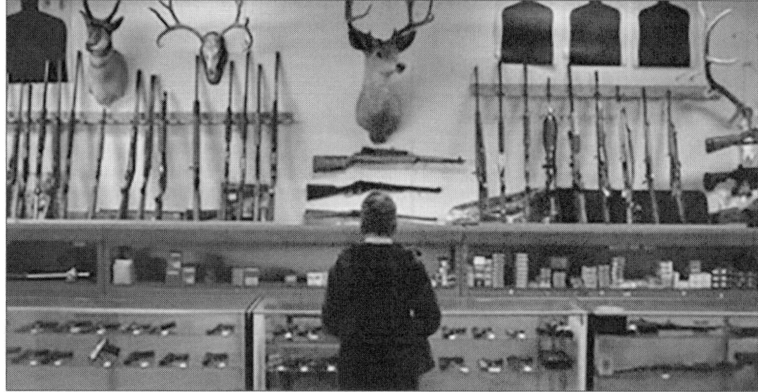

Figure 52.
Paper Tiger (2020, XRM Media). Produced by Bonnie Buckner, Sorel Carradine, Michael Y. Chow, Dawn DeVoe, et al. Directed by Paul Kowalski.

agree to meet in the basement of a church, both sets of parents hoping to get past their grief over the loss of a son. One pair are the parents of a school shooter who committed suicide after killing 10 of his fellow students; the other the parents of one of the children who was shot and killed. The parents of the victim wonder how the shooter's parents could have missed signs showing that their son was disturbed and dangerous. The parents of the victim argue that the shooter was sociopathic and evil, or he must have had a neurological anomaly of some sort; the parents of the shooter frame their understanding of what happened in terms of school bullying and the stress of adjusting to a new school. Almost the entire film is shot in a single room with each set of parents sitting across from each other, and the film's title has a double meaning: It refers to mass murder, but also to the Catholic mass and the redemption it offers. There is some rapprochement in the end.

Beautiful Boy (2010) is a film that depicts the difficulties a married couple faced after learning that their college age son had shot 17 professors and students before taking his own life. They eventually find a videotape their son had left for them with a simple message: "Mom and Dad, I'm sorry. Please don't hate me." (A 2018 film with Steve Carell has the same name but deals with methamphetamine addiction.)

A recent documentary, *Raising a School Shooter* (2021), has three parents telling their story: Sue Klebold, Jeff Williams, and Clarence Elliot. They are, respectively, the parents of Dylan Klebold, Andy Williams, and Nicholas Elliot. Dylan was one of the two students responsible for the Columbine High School shootings in 1999, one of the deadliest shootings in history. Dylan committed suicide after the shooting. Andy shot and killed two classmates and wounded 13 other students in 2001 when he was 15 years old. He is currently in prison. Nicholas killed one teacher and wounded another, and he is also in prison. The audio interviews play out while the subjects go about the quotidian tasks of daily life. This film is the third in a triology from Swedish husband-and-wife directors Frida and Lasse Barkfors; the other two are *Pervert Park* (2014), which examines the lives of sex offenders, and *Death of a Child* (2017), a film documenting the stories of parents who have been responsible for their own child's death.

"Do you bring a casserole to the house of somebody whose son has shot up a school?"

Sue Klebold, mother of Columbine shooter Dylan Klebold

The Fallout (2021) is the most recent film to address school shootings, and especially the aftermath of these awful events. The film trailer shows two girls casually chatting in a restroom when they hear shots. They hide in a toilet stall, standing on the toilet so their feet won't show. They are terrified, and the audience senses and shares their terror. Both girls survive, and the film focuses on how the two girls cope after the shooting, in part by using sex, alcohol, and drugs to dull their grief (see Figure 53). The film was written and directed by Megan Park, who recalled participating in active shooter drills when she was a student.

The murders at Robb Elementary School in Uvalde, Texas, in May 2022, were especially horrific, in part because of the ineptitude of law enforcement officers and their reluctance to put their own lives in danger to stop the killing of children. In marked contrast, in November 2022, officers arrived in 4 minutes after a 911 call during a school shooting in Saint Louis by a recent Performing Arts High School graduate who arrived with an AR-15 style rifle and 600 rounds of ammunition. Only two people were killed because the gunman's rifle jammed after his second murder. Undoubtedly, dozens more would have been killed if the shooter's gun had not malfunctioned. The shooter left a note that read,

> I don't have any friends. I don't have any family. I never had a girlfriend. I never had a social life. I've been an isolated loner my entire life. This was the perfect storm for a mass shooter.

Along with the note, there was a list of school shootings that had occurred around the country, noting how many people had been killed at each site, and there was a detailed map of the school. The Saint Louis shooter was Black; this is an outlier event, insofar as school shooters in the past have been predominately White, and most weapons have been legally owned (Jewett et al., 2022).

It seems likely that future films will follow the Uvalde shooting, much like the Columbine shootings were the stimulus for Gus Van Sant's *Elephant* (2003). Anyone interested in tracking the frequency and magnitude of mass public shootings in the United States since 1966 can find detailed data on The Violence Project website. This database documented 191 shootings and over 1,369 deaths as of September 2023. According to the database, 68.6% of these shootings involved a perpetrator who was mentally ill, although differentiating between mental illness and evil continues to bedevil those of us who are mental health professionals.

Physical and Sexual Abuse in Films

Domestic Violence and Films

Domestic violence is a serious, ubiquitous, and underreported problem in our society. Violence sufficient to cause death or severe injury will occur in about one in 25 families, and hitting, slapping, or punching will occur in approximately one in four families. It is unfortunate that some men feel that marriage gives them special license to hit, hurt, or rape their spouse. (Whether or not a man can be charged with raping his wife is one of the themes explored in the 1959 film *Anatomy of a Murder*.) Two out of three

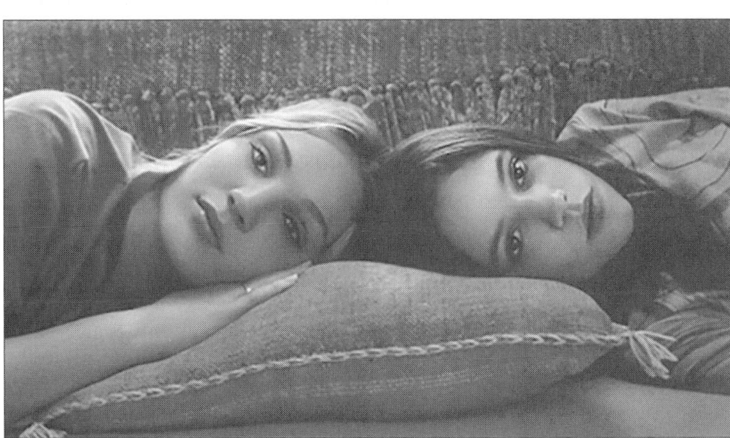

Figure 53.
The Fallout (2021, SSS Entertainment, Good Pals, SSS Film Capital, 828 Productions, Clear Horizon). Produced by Mark Andrews, Colin Bates, David Brown, Julia Buffone, et al. Directed by Megan Park.

female victims of violence know their attackers; however, they frequently will not report their abuse because they desire to protect their assailants or because they fear reprisals (White et al., 2011).

The film *Personal Velocity* (2002) studies three quite different, vulnerable, and courageous women, each in separate segments. One segment addresses issues of domestic violence; it stars Kyra Sedgwick as Delia, a woman who is physically abused by her husband. She is slapped hard in the face at the kitchen table in front of her children for saying the wrong thing, and she is frequently beaten. Delia develops enough motivation to leave when she realizes the pain of what her children are going through; this helps her to "break through the inertia." When speaking to her children, she says she stayed with her husband because he needed her more; this speaks to the irrational self-sacrificing of the victim. In looking back, Delia admits that she and her husband never talked about their problems. In a later scene, a memory of her husband triggers a catharsis. Delia struggles to create a new life, depending on compassionate people, such as a counselor at a women's shelter and an old acquaintance who houses Delia and her children.

One type of domestic violence that does not get a lot of attention due to its often-intangible nature is that of psychological-emotional abuse. Psychological-emotional abuse is a common phenomenon depicted in films that would be too extensive in number to list here. One poignant example that illustrates emotional abuse occurs in the film *Waitress* (2007). Jeremy Sisko portrays Earl, the husband of Jenna (Keri Russell). Earl is an extraordinarily needy and psychologically abusive husband. He controls her every move, does not allow Jenna to have a car, collects her tip money as soon as he sees her, and watches her every action with suspicion. He sometimes tells her he will pick her up from work and then decides to simply leave her waiting for hours, while at other times he greets her by honking his car's horn, embarrassing her in front of her coworkers. He is fueled by significant jealousy and becomes upset when she tells him she is pregnant, fearing the baby will take away her attention; he subsequently insists she verbally admit that she will put him ahead of the baby and prioritize taking care of him (he, of course, is fully capable of taking care of himself). He also forces her to repeat verbatim sentences on several occasions - usually involving her proclaiming her dedication and allegiance to caring for him - to produce a temporary sense of reassurance. He forces himself upon her sexually but only cares about his personal gratification. Jenna eventually confronts Earl in a classic scene that should not be missed.

Rape and Films

Rape is included in this section rather than in the chapter on sexual and gender identity disorders because rape is an act of violence and an act of sexual abuse, *not* an act of sexual passion.

The statistics on rape are sobering. The United States has one of the highest rates of rape in the world - 4 times higher than Germany, 13 times higher than England, and 20 times higher than Japan. It is estimated that one out of three women will be sexually assaulted in her lifetime, and one out of seven will be raped by her husband. Among rape victims, 61% are under the age of 18, and 78% know their attacker. One in four college women have either experienced rape or have been exposed to attempted rape, and most men and women involved in acquaintance rape had been drinking or using drugs at the time of the rape. About a third of the victims of rape develop a rape-related PTSD sometime in their lifetime. Only about 16% of rapes are reported to the police in the United States, usually because women feel that nothing can be done or because they feel it is a private matter between them and their assailants. When compared with women who have not experienced rape, rape victims are found to be more than 9 times more likely to attempt suicide.

Rohypnol (flunitrazepam), a powerful benzodiazepine often referred to as the "date rape drug" is about 10 times more powerful than diazepam (Valium). It is used to treat insomnia and to take the edge off the crash that accompanies withdrawal from binge use of other drugs. Women who have passed out after unwittingly taking Rohypnol have found that the profound sedation and memory impairment that accompany its use have made it difficult for them to prosecute their assailants. Rohypnol is used to facilitate a rape in the film *Virgin* (2003); the rape has horrific consequences for the woman.

Rape has been a recurrent theme in contemporary American films. There were significant rape scenes in *A Clockwork Orange* (1971), Ken Russell's *The Devils* (1971), and *My Old Man's Place* (1972). Paul (Marlon Brando) rapes a passive and indifferent Jeanne (Maria Schneider) in *Last Tango in Paris* (1973). There is a vicious and unforgettable rape scene in *Blue Velvet* (1986). Farrah Fawcett takes control of the situation and exacts revenge on a rapist in *Extremities* (1986); Dustin Hoffman gets revenge following his wife's graphic rape in Sam Peckinpah's violent film *Straw Dogs* (1971); and two independent women inadvertently kill a man who tries to rape one of them in *Thelma & Louise* (1991). Vietnamese women are raped in several of the Vietnam War films, most notably in *Casualties of War* (1989). Harrison Ford is wrongly accused of rape in *Presumed Innocent* (1990). Date rape occurs in the 1995 film *Higher Learning*; gang rape is portrayed in *Last Exit to Brooklyn* (1989); and there are homosexual rapes in *Deliverance* (1972) and *American History X* (1998). A nun is raped in *The Bad Lieutenant* (1992), but the nun forgives her assailant and refuses to press charges against him. Two children play a game of rape in *Welcome to the Dollhouse* (1996). Ingmar Bergman takes up the theme of the rape of innocence in *The Virgin Spring* (1959), and two rapes occur in the gritty Dutch film *Antonia's Line* (1995), one of which involves a man who rapes his sister, a woman with an intellectual disability. *Dead Man Walking* (1995) presents the viewer with difficult choices about the appropriateness of capital punishment in a case of rape and murder, and we are forced to think about whether drug intoxication is a mitigating circumstance in this case and others like it. The character playing Russell Crowe's wife is raped and killed in Ridley Scott's *Gladiator* (2000).

Attempted rape of a man by a woman is discussed extensively in the film adaptation of Michael Crichton's novel, also titled *Disclosure* (1994). When Tom Sanders (Michael Douglas) rebuffs Meredith Johnson (Demi Moore), the new female boss, she lies and manipulatively accuses her new subordinate of sexual harassment. A Black man is wrongfully accused of rape in *To Kill a Mockingbird* (1962), and the routine rape of slave women in the antebellum South is vividly portrayed in *12 Years a Slave* (2013).

Promising Young Woman (2020) is a powerful film about a medical school dropout who spends her evenings pretending to be drunk and picking up men, punishing them when they try to take advantage of her inebriation (see Figure 54). She does this in part to avenge the rape and death of a medical school classmate years before. When she returns to her medical school and brings up the girl's history of rape, the dean nonchalantly remarks, "Things like this happen all the time." The film has a surprising and unforgettable ending.

Alison Hatch (2017) estimates that one out of every five women and one out of every 20 men experience sexual assault on campus. Survivors are often blamed for their assaults, and when perpetrators are found guilty, punishments are often trivial or nonexistent.

The recent film *She Said* (2022) details the investigations of two New York Times reporters into the sexual assault charges levied against Miramax mogul Harvey Weinstein. The reporting led to the #MeToo movement and a national condemnation of sexual abuse, harassment, and rape culture. Some of the women who spoke out against Weinstein included Gwyneth Paltrow, Ashley Judd, Jennifer Lawrence, Angelina Jolie, and Uma Thurman. Ashley Judd plays herself in the film. More than 100 women have accused Weinstein of sexual abuse. He was found guilty in 2020 and sentenced to 23 years in prison, and he has been expelled from the Academy of Motion Picture Arts and Sciences.

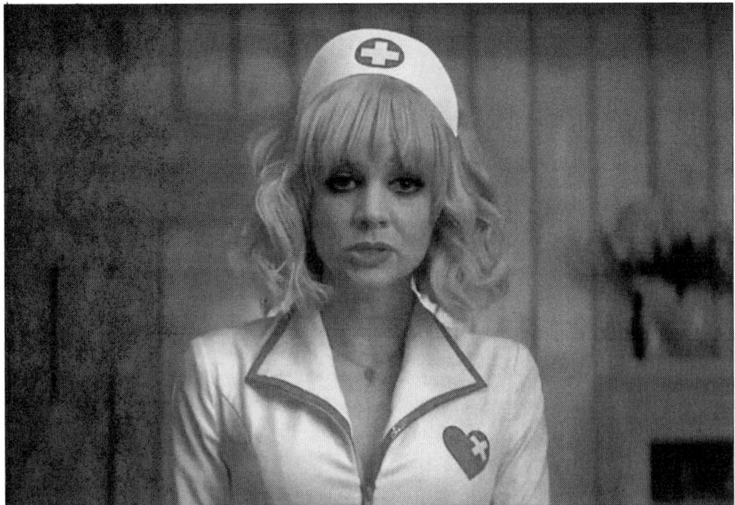

Figure 54.
Promising Young Woman (2020, FilmNation Entertainment, Focus Features, LuckyChap Entertainment). Produced by Tom Ackerley, Glen Basner, Ben Browning, Alison Cohen, et al. Directed by Emerald Fennell.

Victims of Physical and Sexual Abuse

Every act of violence or abuse has both a perpetrator and a victim. Both are depicted in films, but for emphasis of story, character development, or artistic integrity, one is often emphasized over the other. The cultural phenomenon *Slumdog Millionaire* (2008), which received eight Academy Awards (including for Best Picture, Best Director, and Best Adapted Screenplay), depicts abuse and torture of children and of the protagonist as an adult. This film is a classic underdog story in which the protagonist overcomes several adversities in his quest for love.

In *Precious* (2009), Gabourey Sidibe portrays Claireece (Precious) Jones, an illiterate, obese, African American, 16-year-old, who is pregnant for the second time by her father. She lives in Harlem with her viciously abusive and dangerous mother, and Precious struggles to cope with constant degradation and abuse (physical, psychological, and emotional) from her mother through fantasies and dissociation. She gradually builds self-esteem through the help of a teacher at an alternative school.

Peter Jackson's film *The Lovely Bones* (2009), based on the bestselling novel, is about a young teenage girl who is raped and murdered by a pedophile in her neighborhood. The focus in the film is on the perpetrator's chilling acts of violence, his subsequent cover-up behaviors, his craving, obsession, intent, plan to kill again, and the impact of the death on the girl's family.

In the psychological film *Doubt* (2008), Philip Seymour Hoffman portrays Father Brendan Flynn, a priest accused of sexual misbehavior by the school's superior, Sister Aloysius Beauvier (Meryl Streep). As a study of the psychology of doubt, the film is remarkable, as it gives no clear answer as to the priest's innocence or culpability, and the viewer leaves the theater with doubt. The film is included in this section not for its depiction of abuse, but because it illustrates the issues underlying the accusation of abuse.

In the intense, realistic film *Mysterious Skin* (2004), two boys are sexually molested by their coach, and their lives go in completely different directions. Brian, as a child, has nightmares, nosebleeds, blackouts, and enuresis, along with nervous, skittish behavior as he enters adolescence. He realizes he has lost time and believes it is linked with a UFO experience. He is described as asexual. Neil, on the other hand, is hypersexual, and likes the attention and grooming of his coach, and he sets up other children to be groomed by the coach. As an adolescent, he cruises parks, has sex with men for money, and takes pride in being written about on dirty bathroom stalls. He has minimal sexual boundaries, uses drugs, gets a sexually transmitted disease, and becomes the victim of severe violence during one of his tricks. *Antwone Fisher* (2002) is based on the true story of a young man, Antwone Fisher (Derek Luke), who enlists in the Navy and begins to have problems with anger and assault. He is sent to a Navy psychiatrist (Denzel Washington) and eventually opens his traumatic past, which includes a history of significant physical and sexual abuse.

Pedro Almodóvar's *Bad Education* (*La Mala Educación;* 2004, Spain) addresses sexual abuse by Catholic priests. A young boy, Ignacio, is seduced by a pedophile priest, and the movie suggests this seduction led to Ignacio's adult homosexuality and transvestitism. Reviewing this film for *PsycCRITIQUES*, Joanne Crawford (2006) noted,

> The movie has very unambiguous homosexual scenes throughout. Oral and anal sex are depicted graphically. If not explicit, these scenes are realistic. Though lurid, *Bad Education* is about consequences and emotions rather than about sex itself, or its perversion. The themes of violence and sexuality, though intertwined, are played out with great sensuality and finesse, and are laced with humor. (Crawford, 2006)

Some films depict entire groups, cultures, or ethnicities that are victims of physical or sexual abuse. *The Magdalene Sisters* (2002), based on a true story, depicts the lives of a large group of young girls sent away for behavior problems who are forced to endure daily physical hardships, abuse, and humiliation. Each adolescent sent to this Catholic workhouse is abused by nuns who seem oblivious to the pain they inflict.

Another type of abuse not often discussed is harassment. Charlize Theron portrays Josey Aimes, a woman who attempts to support her children by working in a blue-collar mining job in *North Country* (2005). She and the other women experience significant harassment (verbal, physical, emotional, and sexual) by the men, including finding semen on her clothes in her locker, confronting words written with feces on the walls in the woman's locker room, and the placement of a vibrator in her lunch pail. Other depictions of violence in the film include rape and physical abuse by one's partner.

Mystic River and Sexual Abuse

In *Mystic River* (2003), director Clint Eastwood depicts three boyhood friends (Sean Penn as Jimmy, Tim Robbins as Dave, and Kevin Bacon as Sean) who reunite following the death of Jimmy's daughter. At the film's onset, the three boys are approached by a man in a car who intimidates them and identifies himself as a cop. Only Dave gets in the car with the man who turns out to be a pedophile. Dave is sexually abused and escapes from his abductor after 4 days. The story moves ahead about 30 years, and the viewer sees the adult Dave, now married with a son. Dave has never fully recovered from the abduction.

Tim Robbins, who won an Academy Award for Best Supporting Actor for his role as Dave, provides a stunning portrayal of a sexual abuse survivor. Dave is passive, timid, unassuming, and unemotional, yet appears to have a happy family life. In what can be viewed as an unfortunate consequence, Dave sees a man abusing a young boy, and his own abuse history is triggered; trying to free the boy and (metaphorically) himself, Dave snaps, kills the man and allows the boy to escape. Consequently, Dave is plagued with confusion and pain that he is unable to share with his wife; he tells her a different story, and he becomes a suspect in the murder of Jimmy's daughter who had died the same night. Dave becomes more distant (thus appearing more guilty), increasingly quirky, and begins to talk to himself. In one dramatic scene, he seems to hallucinate, hearing voices in his head.

The Accused and Rape

The Accused (1988) is based on a true story of gang rape on a pool table in a blue-collar bar. The crime was especially despicable as far as more than a dozen spectators stood by clapping and cheering while a woman was repeatedly raped. No one attempted to stop the rape or assist the victim. The complacency of the bystanders in the film is in part attributed to the fact that Sarah Tobias (Jodie Foster) had been drinking heavily and smoking pot earlier in the evening, had openly flirted with one of the men, was provocatively dressed, and had engaged in a sensuous dance immediately before being raped. Her defense is weakened further by the fact that she had jokingly referred to one of the men earlier in the evening, telling her girlfriend, "I should take him home and fuck his brains out." The attorneys for the defense argue that Tobias is simply "trailer park trash" who was an enthusiastic and willing participant in everything that occurred.

Some of the most vivid scenes in the film occur during an insensitive gynecological examination by a woman doctor who asks detailed questions about Sarah's sexual history ("Have you ever made love to more than one man at a time?") and recent experiences. The insensitivity is compounded by the questions of the assistant district attorney, who wants to know how Sarah was dressed and when was the last time she experienced intercourse before the rape.

Tobias loses the first legal round, when the three rapists are convicted but have their sentences reduced from rape to "reckless endangerment." However, she is eventually successful in convicting several of the men who witnessed the rape and did nothing. The film concludes with two sobering facts: (1) in the United States, a rape is reported every 6 minutes, and (2) one out of every four rape victims is attacked by two or more assailants.

"Raped? She fucked a bar full of guys then she turns round and blames them for it? Listen lady, she loved it, she had an audience, she did the show of her life!"

Blaming the victim in *The Accused*

Neglect and Abandonment

An interesting portrayal of an attempt to resolve neglect can be found in Ben Affleck's directorial debut, *Gone Baby Gone* (2007). In this multilayered, complex film, a young girl, who is the neglected child of a cocaine addict, is missing. As the plot develops, we learn that a retired police captain (Morgan Freeman) has kidnapped the girl, rationalizing it by arguing that he is trying to give her a better life and that she was otherwise destined for a terrible future. We also learn that the captain has a personal agenda in that his only child was murdered years ago. The girl seems to be treated exceptionally well, and she has a happy life with her new caretakers. The film concludes with the girl and the protagonist watching television and the camera shifts so that they are then watching the viewer – leaving the viewer with the question of how best to handle a situation in which there are multitudes of parents who neglect their children and potentially high-quality parents who would like to have children but cannot.

International Films: Violence and Physical and Sexual Abuse

Violence

Rashomon (1950, Japan) is a classic Akira Kurosawa film in which a bandit, a wife, and a samurai tell three conflicting stories about the rape of the wife and the murder of her husband. The film is considered a classic and is often shown in both film studies programs and social psychology classes. The German director Werner Herzog commented that *Rashomon* was "as close to perfect as a film can get."

Osama (2003, Afghanistan) is based on a true story, and it is the first movie made in Afghanistan after the fall of the Taliban. It depicts the heavy discrimination, violence, and oppression of women under Taliban rule. Violence is also depicted in the everyday reality of everyone living in a poor section of Rio de Janeiro in *City of God* (2003, Brazil). Gangs and drugs are a normal part of existence for these children. This type of film is often a shock to viewers who live a very different life and are unaware of the daily poverty and dangers other people face. The Oscar-winning film *The White Ribbon* (2009, Germany) depicts themes surrounding the abuse and oppression of children. The film depicts not only secrecy, group contagion, and innocence transgressed but also a variety of reactions from the children to the abuse (e.g., denial, trance states, flat affect, automaton behavior, protecting the perpetrator, group bonding, etc.)

The film *2LDK* (2003, Japan) demonstrates the ridiculous and futile nature of violence. A competition develops between two girls rooming together following an audition for an acting role. Growing anger, resentment, and negative and hateful thoughts develop in each girl. These emotions are artfully shown as the girls speak and act one way, with voice-overs revealing their true but opposite thoughts. Eventually they come face-to-face and exchange physical assaults in the forms of electrocution, cleaning fluid, and attacks with a fire extinguisher. Violence is used to reveal the psyche of a violent thief in Peter Greenaway's *The Cook, the Thief, His Wife, & Her Lover* (1989, France/UK). In addition to being intensely controlling, the thief is revealed to be psychotic.

Das Experiment (2001, Germany) illustrates the potential dangers associated with authority roles and group contagion. This film depicts a research study in a prison setting in which subjects are divided into either *prisoners* (who waive their civil rights) or *guards* who are instructed to maintain peace and order. This film bears some initial structural similarity to one of the most well-known psychological experiments ever conducted, Philip Zimbardo's Stanford Prison Experiment. However, the depiction of violence goes well beyond what occurred in Zimbardo's study. The violence in this film, though at times exaggerated, is used to show the danger of group contagion and the power of the authority role. Shortly into the study, the guards collude and decide they need to humiliate the prisoners to regain control. Prisoners are stripped, ridiculed, called names, denigrated, urinated on, and even beaten and left to bleed to death. One guard captures and rapes a female psychologist. The prisoners experience depression, extreme helplessness, psychosis, and panic attacks. It is difficult for anyone from the United States to see this film and not be reminded of the shocking reports of prisoner abuse that occurred at Abu Ghraib prison in Baghdad or at the detention facility at Guantanamo Bay, Cuba.

A Prophet (2009, France/Italy) is an intense film that reveals the culture of prison and the subgroups, often based on racial divides, one finds in prison settings. Malik, 19, is an Arab sent to a French prison where he becomes a mafia kingpin. In the prison system, violence is the method of communication, of payment, of respect, of control, and of redemption.

The Warrior (2001, UK/France/Germany) takes places in feudal India. A warrior, working for a lord as an executioner, destroys entire villages and kills the defenseless and the poor on behalf of the lord. The film illustrates the challenges associated with breaking the vicious cycle of violence.

The Snowtown Murders (2011, Australia) is a gripping and graphic film based on the true story of John Blunting, who led a small group of men who committed mass murder in the grisliest killings to ever occur in Australia. Bunting is now serving consecutive life sentences for 11 murders. Many of his victims' bodies were deposited in barrels in an abandoned bank vault, and many had been tortured prior to being killed. Roger Ebert described Bunting's portrayal in this film as "the most frightening film about a psychopath I've seen" (Ebert, 2012).

Parasite (2019, Korea) was the first foreign film to win an Academy Award as best picture. It is a remarkable movie that highlights class differences, social distance, and wealth inequality, as well as the most negative aspects of capitalism. There is considerable violence, especially in the last 15 minutes of the film, and director Bong Joon Ho seems to suggest the violence is the logical endpoint for a social system that leaves the rich with so very much and the poor with so very little.

> **"If I had all this, I would be kinder."**
>
> **Comment by a poor wife cleaning a rich woman's home in *Parasite* (2019)**

Abuse

Men who abuse their wives are also likely to abuse their children. Domestic violence can be found in the intriguing film *3-Iron* (2004, South Korea). Alcohol or other drugs are commonly involved in cases of domestic violence, and this relationship is clearly present in *Once Were Warriors* (1994, New Zealand). This remarkable film documents the life of a New Zealand Māori family and the devastating effects of alcoholism and domestic violence on every member of the family, including the husband–father–perpetrator. The film is especially effective in portraying the effects of domestic violence on the children in the family: One son responds by returning to his Māori roots, while a sensitive, poetry-writing daughter responds by committing suicide.

Some of the most troubling portrayals of rape occur in those films in which rape is presented as a woman's fantasy, or in those films in which a woman who is being raped becomes aroused by the experience or attracted to the rapist. These themes are found in two otherwise remarkable movies, Pedro Almodóvar's *Tie Me Up! Tie Me Down!* (1990, Spain) and Lina Wertmuller's *Swept Away* (1974, Italy).

If there was ever a character who is a victim of abuse, it would be Lilya in *Lilya 4-Ever* (2002). This poignant Danish/Swedish film develops the character of Lilya, a 16-year-old girl who encounters every form of abuse and exploitation a person can experience. She is lied to and abandoned by her mother, rejected by her family, manipulated, and sold into prostitution by a man she had hoped to live with, gang raped, physically and sexually abused, and forced to work as an unpaid prostitute. She is completely tossed away by society, as the viewer clearly sees at the onset of the film when Lilya is depicted walking the streets, bloodied, and beaten up, with no safe place or person to turn to. Nevertheless, Lilya does not take on the victim role of helplessness and fear, but instead pushes forward. Her resiliency is commendable and inspirational, but she eventually reaches a breaking point and begins to contemplate suicide.

The impact of sexual abuse in childhood on adult life is portrayed in two excellent films, *The Celebration* (1998, Denmark/Sweden) and *Don't Tell* (2005, Italy/UK/France/Spain). The former depicts a dramatic announcement and confrontation of the father–perpetrator during his 60th birthday celebration in the presence of a host of extended family members. This film was done according to a film movement and style called **Dogme 95**, popularized and set forth by Lars von Trier, in which filmmakers abide by certain rules for a purer film, such as no nondiegetic sound (sound that is added after filming) and no special effects. *Don't Tell* is a powerful depiction of the secrecy and shame surrounding sexual abuse, the role of secrets, and the horror that lies behind facades of normalcy. The film also depicts the enabling role of a spouse: "It's a vice. He doesn't want to hurt you. He's sick" (says the mother as she enables her abusing spouse and rationalizes his behavior).

> **Christian: "I've just never understood why you did it."**
> **Father: "It was all you were good for."**
>
> **Christian, referring to his father's sexual abuse, and the father's arrogant reaction, in *The Celebration* (1998)**

5x2 (2004, France) explores the relationship of a couple in five stages, beginning at their divorce and flashing backward to when they first met. There are two ambiguous rape scenes in the film; however, most viewers would dismiss the ambiguity and clearly regard the behaviors depicted as rape. One occurs when the couple meets up after having been separated for a year and go to a hotel room to have sex. She is reluctant and passive, and he is animalistic; she wants him to stop after they begin, but he continues and rapes her. In another scene, immediately following his neglect of her on their wedding night, she meets a stranger who after some pleasant dialogue forces himself on her and prevents her from getting away, and she gives in to him. A classic cycle of violence is experienced by the *femme fatale* in the quirky film, *Terribly Happy* (2008, Denmark).

Many films depict the neglect of children by their parents. One particularly striking film in which neglect plays a key role is the Russian film *The Return* (2003). Two boys are abandoned and neglected by their father for 12 years, then suddenly and without warning the father returns. He is quick to leave them again for business, but then changes plans and takes his sons on a trip. The boys are pushed physically and emotionally to survive his challenges (e.g., they are left to do the work of figuring out how to set up a tent, push a car out of the mud, and row a boat in challenging waters) and continued abandonment (e.g., one boy is left in the middle of nowhere in the pouring rain because he asked too many questions about fishing). The father is an enigma throughout the film: Taciturn in speech with comments of "get in" and "get out," cryptic in his behavior, and secretive about his occupation. Among many other themes, one theme is clear: Many issues arise from abandonment and neglect by a parent, and one cannot simply return and expect everything to be normal. A mother neglecting her children due to her mental illness and her desperate quest for a man appears in *Something Like Happiness* (2005, Czech Republic).

Nobody Knows (2004, Japan) is based on real events concerning four children (the oldest being 12) who are abandoned by their mother and left to raise themselves. This is one of the most detailed depictions of the realities and struggles of abandonment in cinema history.

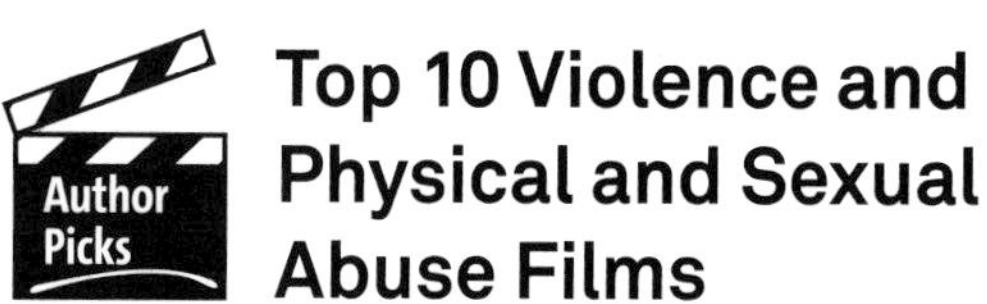

Top 10 Violence and Physical and Sexual Abuse Films

Rashomon (1950)
Schindler's List (1993)
Once Were Warriors (1994)
American Psycho (2000)
City of God (2003)
Kill Bill: Vol. 1 and Vol. 2 (2003, 2004)
Hotel Rwanda (2004)
Once Upon a Time in Hollywood (2019)
Parasite (2019)

Chapter 16

Treatment

She was fifteen years old, going on thirty-five, Doc, and she told me she was eighteen, she was plenty willing, I practically had to take to sewing my pants shut ... I don't think it's crazy at all and I don't think you do either. No man alive could resist that ... and that's why I got into jail to begin with. And now they're telling me I'm crazy over here because I don't sit there like a goddamn vegetable. Don't make a bit of sense to me. If that's what being crazy is, then I'm senseless, out of it, gone-down-the-road, wacko. But no more, no less, that's it.

Randle P. McMurphy responds
during a psychiatric interview,
in *One Flew Over the Cuckoo's Nest* (1975)

Treatment Modalities Portrayed in Films

Individual Psychotherapy

Individual psychotherapy is the most common treatment modality depicted in movies. Sometimes it is quite accurate; at other times, it is preposterous. Gabbard and Gabbard (1999) estimated that through 1998, over 450 films dealing with psychiatry had been created; from the films we have viewed, we conclude that most of these involve the modalities and topics discussed in this chapter.

There are many misconceptions regarding psychologists and mental health professionals that are perpetrated by films. We have previously outlined several of these cinematic biases and errors that confuse the public (for a fuller discussion of these, see Niemiec & Wedding, 2006). I believe US cinema has shown some improvement in each of these over the past 20 years. However, films are still replete with misconceptions. Seven of these are:

1. Psychiatrists are the main professionals who perform psychotherapy.
2. Psychoanalysis is the dominant practice in psychotherapy.
3. Psychologists are patently unethical.
4. Psychologists are cavalier about boundary violations.
5. Almost all therapists are men.
6. Almost all therapists are White.
7. Research is of little value.

Harriet Schultz (2005) discussed the ways in which women therapists are portrayed in film, with a particular focus on the portrayal of psychologists. She notes that most cinematic portrayals of psychotherapists present the therapist as a psychiatrist, and someone who does psychotherapy rather than manage medication, even though there are many more psychologists than there are psychiatrists, and many psychiatrists have abandoned the practice of psychotherapy (Crocker & Brenner, 2021). However, Petriceks (2021) has observed that many psychiatrists "are galvanized by the potential for long, deep conversations with suffering people, and the possibility of addressing such suffering through those conversations" (p. 238).

Trachsel et al. (2021) have provided the most recent and most trenchant analysis of psychotherapy ethics, and a chapter by Tobias Eichinger (2021) discusses the ways in which the ethical challenges associated with psychotherapy are presented in movies. Eichinger notes that "the quartet of stereotypical images of the crazy ("dippy"), the bad ("evil"), the good ("wonderful") and the sexually suggestive ("horny") therapist ... constitutes an index of ethical misconduct" (p. 1027).

Otto Wahl and his colleagues (2018) trained volunteers to code films with characters identified as psychotherapists, and then analyzed 22 films in which a therapist character appeared on screen for at least 15 minutes. They found that,

> Therapists were predominantly Caucasian, male, and between ages 40 and 60 years. Their most common characteristics were generally positive – intelligent, caring, knowledgeable, and compassionate. [However, more] than half were portrayed as unethical, and more than one-third as manipulative. Therapists were also commonly shown as touching clients in some way, disclosing client information without permission, and becoming involved in social relationships with clients. In addition, it was often unclear whether clients benefitted from their engagement in therapy. (Wahl et al., 2018, p. 238)

The most frequently portrayed theoretical orientation continues to be psychoanalysis, though it is only one of many approaches to therapy. Both the frequency of cinematic depictions of psychotherapy and many of the stereotypes can be credited to director Woody Allen, who has portrayed psychoanalysts in dozens of his films. Interestingly, the psychologist portrayal in the film *Anything Else* (2003) is one of his most stereotypical (e.g., he is a therapist who refuses to respond to important patient questions). One of the least stereotypic portrayals occurred the previous year when Allen directed *Hollywood Ending* (2002), a film about a man hired to direct a picture being produced by his ex-wife. The protagonist develops a case of psychosomatic blindness, and his therapist is portrayed as someone who accurately diagnoses the conversion disorder and offers helpful suggestions.

Almost all of Woody Allen's films present ethical and moral challenges, often in the context of therapy. For example, in *Another Woman* (1988), Marion Post (Gena Rowlands) is a philosopher and a college professor who rents a private office so she can focus on writing a book. Her new office is adjacent to the office of a psychiatrist, and she discovers that she can overhear therapy sessions through an office vent. She initially successfully blocks the sound, but she soon discovers that eavesdropping is seductive, and she becomes particularly intrigued by therapy sessions with Hope (Mia Farrow), a pregnant woman whose marriage is on the rocks. Listening in on Hope's therapy session, Marion begins to examine and understand her own life and her refusal to embrace it fully. In *Deconstructing Harry* (1997), Allen pays homage to Ingmar Bergman's *Wild Strawberries* (1957). It is his most autobiographical film, and it presents multiple examples of therapy boundary violations. For example, Harry's psychotherapist (Joan, played by Kirstie Alley) discharges Woody Allen's character (Harry Block – a blocked writer) so she can become his lover. Joan later marries Harry and has a son with him. She sees therapy patients in her home office, and one comic episode involves her screaming and berating her philandering husband (who is in an adjoining room) while trying to conduct therapy with a troubled client who is simply wondering if he should continue working at a dead-end job. Writing about this film, Miguel Floriano (2008) notes,

> In one of the most memorable scenes ... we see Joan (Kirstie Alley) arguing with her husband Harry because he has slept with one of her twenty-year old patients who has subsequently spilt the beans in a therapy session. The affronted wife is trying to strangle him, screaming that she is going to kill him, when a patient arrives for a consultation. Suddenly, she says she is sorry and gets up. The camera remains on the patient who, horrified, hears voices from off the set. "You fucked-up fuck! I can't believe you did this! Fucking asshole! You fucked my patient – You don't fuck somebody's patient! Fuck you!" Then she returns to the office, sits down and begins to write in her notebook. She asks poor Mr. Farber to pick up where they had left off but while he is trying to do this, she struggles to open a bottle of pills. She jumps up again and carries on with the argument at full volume "And with my patient! That is a sacred trust! My patient!" Harry attempts to defend himself: "But who else do I meet?" Joan sits down again and asks Mr. Farber to continue, but before he can she screams to the other end of the house, "Get your shit and your goddam clothes and get the fuck out of here! ... And I mean tonight, motherfucker." This is when Mr. Farber bursts into tears like a child. (Floriano, 2008, p. 22)

Other orientations illustrated by films include a humanistic and supportive approach in *Lantana* (2001), and what appears to be **transactional analysis** in *Good Will Hunting* (1997). (Note the titles of the books in Maguire's study when Sean Maguire [Robin Williams] pins Will Hunting [Matt Damon] to the wall.) Interestingly, one of the most widely used, popular, and empirically validated approaches, **cognitive behavior therapy**, is rarely depicted in films.

"My father was an alcoholic. Mean fuckin' drunk. He'd come home hammered, looking to wail on somebody. So, I had to provoke him so he wouldn't go after my mother and little brother."

Will Hunting describing his childhood, in a therapy session in *Good Will Hunting* (1997)

Antwone Fisher (2002) depicts multiple sessions of individual psychotherapy. Antwone (Derek Luke) and his psychiatrist, Dr. Jerome Davenport (Denzel Washington), slowly work through the topics of anger, physical abuse, sexual abuse, and trauma. The film is framed around the psychotherapy sessions, and the plot deepens whenever Antwone opens in a deeper way. The sessions can be divided into phases of resistance and exploration: At first Antwone refuses to share anything; later he begins to open up, sharing his physical abuse, next his sexual abuse, and finally his feelings as he witnessed the murder of his best friend. These five therapy phases are appropriately juxtaposed with relevant narrative components.

The psychiatrist is also influenced by the therapy sessions with this patient. Dr. Davenport had not realized the full extent of his isolation, and he was not aware of how he also needed to change. Davenport is humble enough to recognize his own weaknesses as he watched his patient's courage and resilience grow.

In addition to those in *Antwone Fisher*, other balanced individual psychotherapy portrayals can be seen in *Good Will Hunting* (1997), as just mentioned; *K-Pax* (2001); *The Sixth Sense* (1999); *Gothika* (2003); and *Elling* (2002); while unbalanced individual psychotherapy portrayals can be seen in *Normal* (2003); *Lantana* (2001); and *Vanilla Sky* (2001); see Niemiec and Wedding (2006). A particularly good albeit brief portrayal of an Asian American therapist whose suggestions are the catalyst for a major turning point in an adolescent's life can be seen in *The Squid and the Whale* (2005).

Successful individual treatment is seen in films such as *Sybil* (1976) and *Ordinary People* (1980). In *Ordinary People*, Conrad Jarrett (Timothy Hutton), following the accidental death of his brother, begins therapy with a psychiatrist (played by Judd Hirsch) who demonstrates warmth and caring and allows his patient to examine painful family relationships within the safety of individual therapy. In *Equus* (1977), Richard Burton plays a psychiatrist who treats a very disturbed young man played by Peter Firth. During psychotherapy, the true depth of the psychological disturbance is revealed. In some instances, as in *Best Boy* (1979), a rehabilitation program is portrayed.

David and Lisa (1962), a film based on a novel by psychiatrist Theodore Isaac Rubin, is a dated but still sensitive portrayal of a young man with a severe case of what is likely OCD and a phobia about being touched; he becomes curious about Lisa, a young woman who presents as autistic (displaying repetitive behaviors, limited communication, sing-song responses with rhymes). The film presents David's parents in stereotypical roles (e.g., the mother is overly enmeshed in her son's life, while the father is cold and distant), and the ending is trite. These concerns aside, this film is still worth viewing, and it portrays mental health professionals, and especially Dr. Swinford (Howard Da Silva), in a sympathetic light.

Films frequently present images of mental health professionals behaving unethically. For example, breaches in confidentiality are evident in *Equus* (1977), and sexual relationships between clients and mental health professionals are depicted in *Prince of Tides* (1991), *Mr. Jones* (1993), *Tin Cup* (1996), *Deconstructing Harry* (1997), and *Bliss* (1997). A psychiatrist rapes his son's best friend in Todd Solondz's *Happiness* (1998).

I have taught ethics to both psychology students and medical students, and I found *Prince of Tides* (1991) to be a springboard for lively class discussions. The movie portrays a psychiatrist treating a troubled woman who has made multiple suicide attempts. The woman's brother helps the psychiatrist understand family dynamics – but by the end of the film, the psychiatrist and the brother (who is married) have fallen in love, and this is clearly a boundary violation ... but what if it was a second cousin helping with therapy or a next-door neighbor? Creativity researcher James Kaufman noted,

> The film [*Prince of Tides*] also perpetuates the myth that therapy is miraculous as long as you remember some type of bad thing from the past. In reality, it's usually an ongoing process with small and meaningful insights that lead to progress. (Stringer, 2016)

The relationship between a psychologist and her patient in *Numb* (2007) is especially troubling because the boundary violations are so patently wrong (e.g., the therapist calls her patient at home, meets with him in a restaurant, is inappropriately self-disclosing, and proclaims her love for him in a crowded restaurant).

In *Prime* (2005), Meryl Streep plays Lisa Metzger, a Jewish social worker who discovers that her client Rafi Gardet (Uma Thurman) has taken a younger lover – who is identified later in therapy as Lisa's son, played by Bryan Greenberg. Rafi describes her sexual life with David in lurid detail, at one point describing his penis as "beautiful." Streep knows she should reveal this obvious dual relationship but postpones doing so because she is intrigued and fascinated by what she is learning about her son (Norcross & Norcross, 2006).

Kevin Spacey plays psychologist Henry Carter, in *Shrink* (2009). Carter is a flawed character who is addicted to marijuana (see Chapter 11), which he routinely smokes before sessions with clients and between sessions. He eventually quits smoking, and he can make a meaningful impact in therapy with a young adolescent girl who has experienced a significant loss in her life.

Mumford (1999) is a Lawrence Kasdan film that depicts a man named Mumford with dubious credentials who sets up shop as a psychologist in a small town – also named Mumford. It turns out that Mumford is a former IRS agent and cocaine addict, and he is an imposter pretending to be a psychologist. He commits numerous boundary violations such as going for long walks with a patient whom he finds especially attractive and telling other townspeople intimate details about the lives of his patients; however, the movie also suggests that psychotherapy is primarily "the purchase of friendship," and that credentials and training really are not all that important if one is a sympathetic listener.

> **"What kind of doctor are you?"**
> **"PhD. Psychologist."**
> **"Oh, not a real doctor."**
> **"That's right. The fake kind."**
>
> **Mumford responding with sarcasm to a common misconception, in *Mumford* (1999)**

Stutz (2022) is a documentary film in which director and actor Jonah Hill interviews his therapist, psychiatrist Phil Stutz (see Figure 55). Stutz has worked with numerous Hollywood actors in addition to Hill. Stutz has Parkinson's, but he is mentally alert and still practices psychotherapy. The film introduces him and his belief that life involves three fundamental challenges: pain, uncertainty, and the need for constant work. He also shares his belief in the importance of radical acceptance, gratitude, and the need for processing loss through nonattachment. Therapists will find the film interesting; Stutz hardly practices evidence-based therapy, but he is someone who has helped hundreds of people along the way.

Group Psychotherapy

Manic (2003) depicts group psychotherapy on an inpatient unit for adolescents. It is accurate

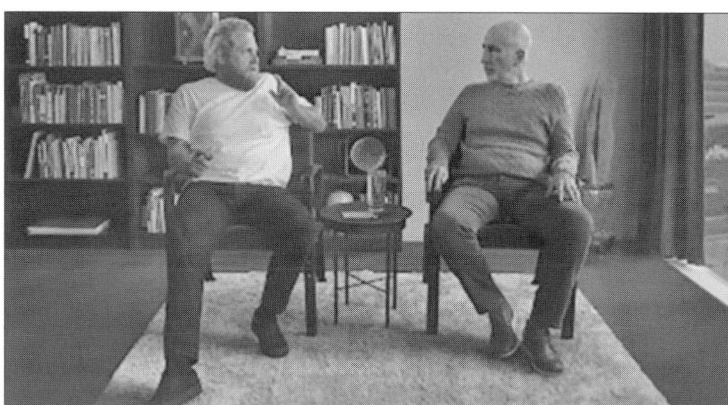

Figure 55.
Stutz (2022, Netflix). Produced by Chelsea Barnard, Diane Becker, Matt Dines, Alison Goodwin, et al. Directed by Jonah Hill.

and appropriate as a portrayal of group intervention, helped by the inclusion of some actual psychiatric patients. The psychiatrist (Don Cheadle) has his hands full with severely depressed individuals; patients who are self-injurious, threatening, and violent; and patients with explosive personalities. He attempts to include everyone in group discussions, and he cleverly reframes patient experiences in a positive, balanced way. In stark contrast, the group therapy sessions portrayed in the film *Wilbur Wants to Kill Himself* (2002) are disappointing and unrealistic. One of the psychiatrists is overly supportive, obsequious, and flirtatious with patients, while the other psychiatrist smokes during sessions, sets himself apart from the group, and makes jokes about not wanting to be there.

One Flew Over the Cuckoo's Nest

One of the great joys associated with teaching abnormal psychology and related courses and using *Movies and Mental Illness* as a text is the opportunity to introduce a new generation of students to films we watched – and loved – as college students. *One Flew Over the Cuckoo's Nest* (1975) is one of those films; two others are *Psycho* (1960) and *A Clockwork Orange* (1971).

Films such as *One Flew Over the Cuckoo's Nest* attempt to show the human injustices that existed and are occasionally still found in the mental health system. In this classic film, once McMurphy moves from the prison system into the mental health system, he loses all civil rights, such as his right to refuse treatment. The issues addressed by the film are not the usual problems of large institutions such as lack of facilities, of cleanliness, of staff, or of organizational communication. Instead, the film addresses fundamental issues of autonomy and paternalism. The treatment team has ultimate control over McMurphy's treatment and discharge. A rigid, controlling nurse, Nurse Ratched, widely regarded as one of the greatest

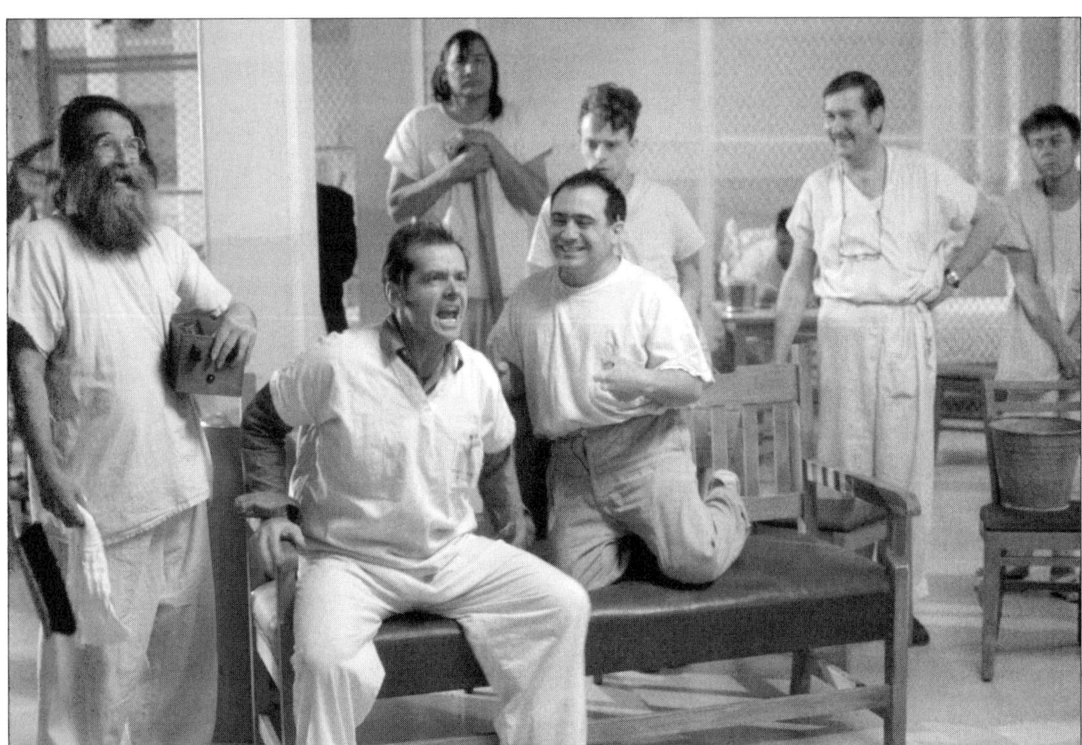

Figure 56. *One Flew Over the Cuckoo's Nest* (1975, Fantasy Films, Bryna Productions, N. V. Zvaluw). Produced by Michael Douglas, Martin Fink, and Saul Zaentz. Directed by Miloš Forman.

villains in cinema history, engages in an ongoing power struggle with a patient whom she perceives as a threat to her control of the unit. She uses her position and knowledge of the system to gain control over McMurphy. McMurphy's lobotomy is the ultimate abuse of psychiatric power. The relative power of doctors, nurses and patients is underscored in the film, as illustrated in Figure 56.

Will Sampson, a six-foot-seven Muscogee Indian, had never acted in a film before. He was selected for the role of Chief Bromden because he was the only Native American the casting department could find who matched the character's incredible size, and he is magnificent in the role. Louise Fletcher (who played Nurse Ratched) died in 2022 at the age of 88. She had steady work in a number of minor roles after *Cuckoo's Nest*, but never overcame "Oscar's curse" after she won the Academy Award for Best Actress in a Leading Role. In her obituary in the *Guardian*, Ryan Gilbey notes,

> She was 40 at the time and had only recently returned to acting after a long break. She auditioned repeatedly for the role, unaware that the producers were courting and being rebuffed by actors including Jane Fonda, Angela Lansbury, and Ellen Burstyn. The director Miloš Forman envisaged the part as "the personification of evil," but revised his opinion after casting Fletcher: "I slowly started to realize that it would be much more powerful if she doesn't know that she's evil. She, as a matter of fact, believes that she's helping people." (Gilbey, 2022)

Fletcher's parents were both deaf, and after accepting her Oscar, Fletcher ended her speech in sign language to thank her parents. (Her mother had become deaf after a childhood illness, and her father became deaf after being struck by lightning at age 4.)

Psychiatric Hospitalization

Mental health treatment settings are most often portrayed in films as capacious institutions, and their depiction is almost always negative. Psychiatric hospitals are usually filmed as dark, gloomy, and unwelcoming places with considerable background noise (often screaming), staff nurses dressed in white, and patients with nothing to do other than to walk the halls of the institution acting odd. It is immediately obvious to the viewer when a movie scene takes place in such an institutional setting. From a cinematic perspective, this stereotyped presentation makes sense because the viewer is more likely to remember a majestic, foreboding hospital exterior than a simple clinical office. These hospitals typically have stunning architecture, curious corridors, and an interesting dayroom.

Most films that depict the treatment of a person with mental illness during a period predating the last 15–20 years show a psychiatric hospital. In most cases these institutions are dreary and foreboding, and these hospitals are certainly not places that one would seek out for care. Martin Scorsese's film *Shutter Island* (2010) offers this classic portrayal of a psychiatric institution. In this film (set in the 1950s), the sickest patients are treated, and some sordid aspects of the history of psychiatry are revealed, such as extreme isolation, allowing patients to lie in their own filth, and use of extensive restraints. Then, it is correctly noted that Thorazine, the first new and truly effective psychopharmacological agent, was introduced in the early 1950s. A psychiatrist, played by Ben Kingsley, explains that the role of the psychiatrist is to heal, to listen and to care for patients, and not to judge them.

"Which is best, to live as a monster or die as a good man?"

Teddy Daniels (Leonardo DiCaprio) asks before undergoing a lobotomy, in *Shutter Island* (2010)

Some movies with these dreary though memorable settings include *The Snake Pit* (1948), *One Flew Over the Cuckoo's Nest* (1975), *Don Juan DeMarco* (1994), *Twelve Monkeys* (1995), *Sling Blade*

(1996), *Instinct* (1999), *Girl, Interrupted* (1999), *A Beautiful Mind* (2001), *Analyze That* (2002), and *Asylum* (2005).

One Flew Over the Cuckoo's Nest (1975), as described in the previous section, is a classic film that depicts the violation of human rights in mental institutions, but it was certainly not the first. *The Snake Pit* (1948) was one of the earliest films to raise consciousness about the treatment of persons with mental illness. It depicted the institution metaphorically as a zoo in which patients were fenced in, and as a place for visitors to tour, and a place where patients were "herded" into their own cages (rooms). One crucial difference between the two films is that the character of Virginia in *The Snake Pit* is truly mentally ill, whereas Randle Patrick McMurphy in *One Flew Over the Cuckoo's Nest* is not. *Chattahoochee* (1989) also describes the plight of those who disagree with institutional authority and power, and *Nuts* (1987) portrays a woman's struggle not to be committed to an institution.

Ben Harris has analyzed the critical acclaim for *The Snake Pit* and argues that this film helped motivate reforms for people with mental disorders who were being housed in psychiatric institutions, often with little or no treatment (Harris, 2021).

Beautiful Dreamers (1990) is based on a true story from the life of Walt Whitman. Whitman was especially interested in the care of people with mental illness because he had a younger brother who was both physically and mentally ill. In the film, Rip Torn plays the role of Walt Whitman. Whitman visits a hospital in London, Ontario, where he is appalled by the treatment of the patients. He finds a sympathetic and congenial psychiatrist, Dr. Maurice Bucke, and the two of them work together to introduce more humane approaches to treatment. In real life, Dr. Bucke became Whitman's official biographer.

The film *K-Pax* (2001) moved away from some of the stereotypes of the psychiatric hospital environment. It depicts an institution in New York that has adequate light, numerous windows, and meaningful activities for both staff and patients. The patients contact and communicate easily with one other. Although the film loses this focus at times, such as when the patients begin to run about in a frenzy, their excitement is not "crazy" and random but grows out of support for one another. Overall, *K-Pax* portrays a less dehumanizing environment than did many older films.

As the closing of psychiatric hospitals continues, there will be fewer institutions to portray in films, and eventually the only portrayals of massive psychiatric institutions in movies will be in period films.

"Okay, I know you're thinking, 'What is this? Kid spends a few days in the hospital and all his problems are cured?' But I'm not. I know I'm not. I can tell this is just the beginning. I still need to face my homework, my school, my friends. My dad. But the difference between today and last Saturday is that for the first time in a while, I can look forward to the things I want to do in my life. Bike, eat, drink, talk. Ride the subway, read, read maps. Make maps, make art. Finish the Gates application. Tell my dad not to stress about it. Hug my mom. Kiss my little sister. Kiss my dad. Make out with Noelle. Make out with her more. Take her on a picnic. See a movie with her. See a movie with Aaron. Heck, see a movie with Nia. Have a party. Tell people my story. Volunteer at 3 North. Help people like Bobby. Like Muqtada. Like me. Draw more. Draw a person. Draw a naked person. Draw Noelle naked. Run, travel, swim, skip. Yeah, I know it's lame, but, whatever. Skip anyway. Breathe ... Live."

Craig contemplates life after he leaves the hospital, in *It's Kind of a Funny Story* (2010)

It's Kind of a Funny Story (2010) is about the psychiatric hospitalization of a teenage boy, Craig (Keir Gilchrist), who seeks help after seriously contemplating suicide by jumping off the Brooklyn Bridge. Because there are too few patients on the adolescent ward, Craig is assigned to an adult ward. While in the hospital he bonds

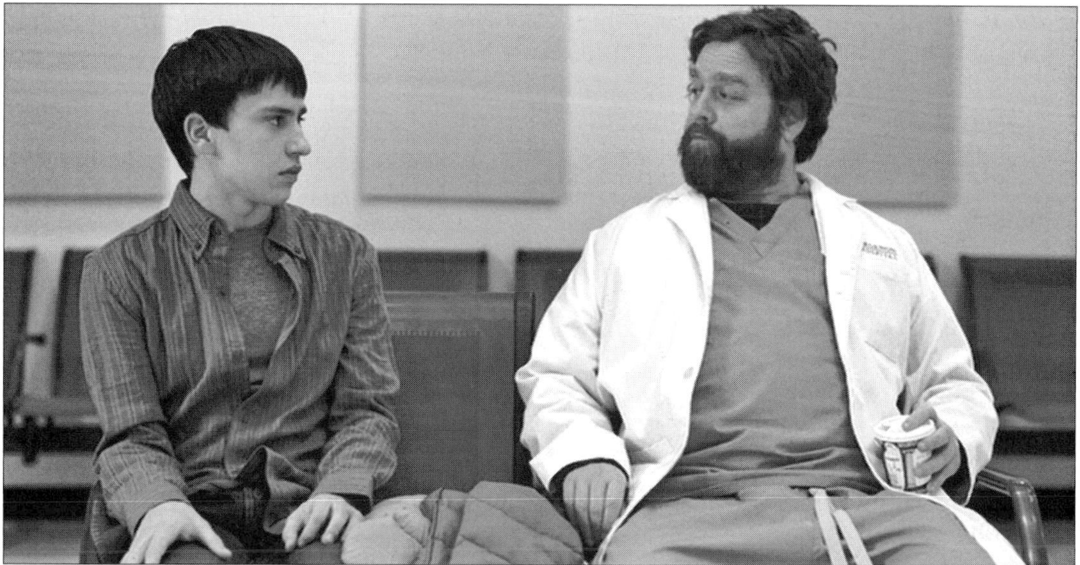

Figure 57. *It's Kind of a Funny Story* (2010, Focus Features, Wayfare Entertainment, Misher Films, Journeyman Pictures, Gowanus Projections, Start Media). Produced by Patrick Baker, Andy Berman, Ben Browning, Michael Maher, et al. Directed by Anna Boden and Ryan Fleck.

with other patients, and especially with Bobby (Zach Galifianakis), a man hospitalized because of a series of suicide attempts. Bobby becomes Craig's mentor, introducing him to the other patients and hospital life. The close and symbiotic relationship that develops between Craig and Bobby is illustrated in Figure 57.

Unit of Difficult Patients: What Future for the Criminally Insane? (2017) is a documentary telling the story of several patients involuntarily committed to a French hospital for the criminally insane. The film has English subtitles, and it will serve as an introduction to what life is like for providers who elect to work in similar settings. Viewers who are mental health professionals will be struck by the number of patients diagnosed with OCD, a diagnosis that would be rare in similar institutions in the United States serving the criminally insane.

Elephant Song (2014) depicts extended interactions between a Canadian psychiatrist and his patient, a complicated and manipulative man who killed his Cuban mother. A former psychiatrist who had been treating the young man goes missing, and another psychiatrist, an administrator, is pulled in to interrogate the patient. Mind games are played on both sides, and we see numerous ethical violations by both the physician and a ward nurse.

No Letting Go (2015) is a full-length film based on an award-winning short 2013 film titled *Illness*. The longer film was directed by Jonathan Bucari, and it is based on the true-life experiences of producer and screenwriter Randi Silverman. The movie portrays a typical family consisting of a father, mother, and three children living in a New York suburb. Timothy, the middle child, begins showing signs of mental illness at age 10; in the film, the parents first become aware of their son's anxiety problems when he refuses to participate in a school play. His illness grows progressively worse, and Timothy is moved from school to school as his parents try to help him. Treatment by a child psychologist, and later by a psychiatrist, proves to be of little benefit, and medications are ineffectual; a second psychiatrist is consulted who recommends long-term intensive treatment at a residential setting in Maine. Although Timothy suffers some setbacks (e.g., he runs away from the treatment center when he learns his mother is being treated for breast cancer), he responds well, learns more effective ways to cope with his bipolar disorder, and is eventually reunited with his family. It is interesting that Timothy at age 14 is played by Noah Silverman, the screenwriter's son, and the brother of the real-life inspiration for the film. *No Letting Go* is melodramatic, but it does an excellent job illustrating how difficult life can be for a family trying to raise a child with a serious mental illness.

A Clockwork Orange

Stanley Kubrick's *A Clockwork Orange* (1971) does not take place in a psychiatric institution, but instead at a specialized hospital running a research program for the prison system. This film remains a prototype in the cinematic exploration of the ethical issues associated with behavior therapy. In the film, Malcolm McDowell plays Alex, the leader of a vicious gang. Alex and his friends are psychopathic personalities: They thrive on violence and commit both rape and murder without any evidence of remorse. However, while audiences are repulsed by Alex's violence, they find themselves attracted by his high-spirited personality and his love of classical music.

Alex is captured after being set up by his friends, who have come to resent his authority. He is convicted of murder and sentenced to 14 years in prison; however, he is given the option of early release if he is willing to participate in a conditioning experiment. In scenes almost as horrifying as the earlier rape scenes, Alex is injected with a nausea-inducing drug and repeatedly forced to watch scenes depicting rape and violence while Beethoven symphonies are played in the background (Figure 58).

The conditioning proves to be successful, and Alex cannot even think about a violent incident without becoming ill. He is released from prison but finds himself unable to cope with life on the streets. He eventually attempts suicide. While he is recovering in the hospital, a reform movement occurs in the government, and Alex is portrayed as a guinea pig who was abused by the previous administration. The treatment is reversed, and Alex is once again able to fantasize happily about rape and murder. The film dramatically presents the conundrum faced by society as it contemplates treatments that attempt to improve society by limiting personal freedom (e.g., mandatory injections of drugs such as **Depo-Provera** that reduce testosterone levels and diminish sex drive in men convicted of sexual crimes).

Treatment Interventions

Hypnosis

It is interesting to discuss hypnosis in a book about movies, because the film viewer goes in and out of light trance states throughout the movie-viewing experience. However, we have

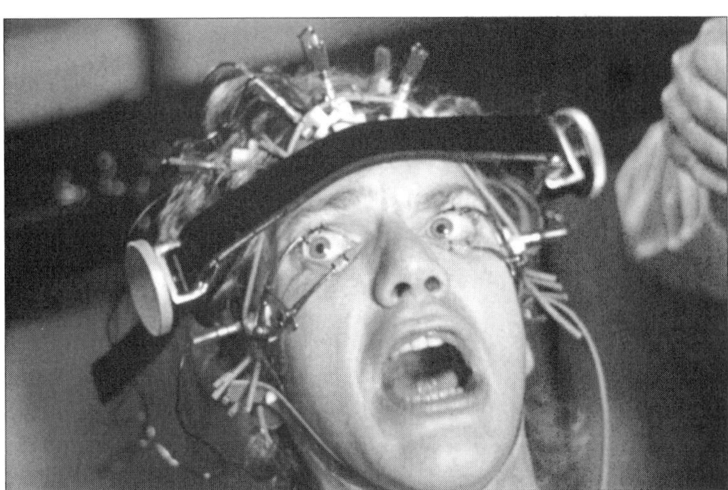

Figure 58.
A Clockwork Orange (1971, Warner Brothers, Polaris Productions, Hawk Films, Max L. Raab Productions, Si Litvinoff Production). Produced by Stanley Kubrick, Si Litvinoff, Max L. Rabb, and Bernard Williams. Directed by Stanley Kubrick.

grown so accustomed to the habit of viewing movies and television shows that we rarely realize when we have entered a trance state. Hypnosis has been portrayed in numerous films, but it is rarely given an accurate or realistic portrayal.

Hypnosis has remained a popular intervention for over 100 years and is an empirically validated intervention for many psychological and medical disorders. Hypnosis continues to fight a battle against public misconception, part of which unfortunately is perpetrated by movies (also by stage hypnotists).

The portrayal of hypnosis in films has a history as long as movies themselves. The portrayal, however, is a negative, stereotypical one. Barrett (2006) explored the role of hypnosis in over 230 films and found most of the portrayals to be negative, with hypnosis being applied to seduce the subject, to bring the subject to kill, to make the subject harm themselves, or to get the subject to commit a crime. She reports there are very few realistic portrayals – exceptions include *Mesmer* (1994, Austria/Canada), directed by Roger Spottiswoode; and *Equus* (1977, UK/US), directed by Sidney Lumet. In the latter film, an accurate explanation of hypnosis by a psychiatrist is depicted.

Robert Wiene's *The Cabinet of Dr. Caligari* (1920, Germany) is a classic silent film that portrays Dr. Caligari using hypnosis to control the life and behavior of a sleepwalker in a carnival sideshow who can predict the future. He accurately predicts the imminent death of one of the characters in the film. Like so many films, this movie erroneously suggests that hypnotists have absolute control over the people they hypnotize.

Torture and hypnosis are used in tandem to brainwash British scientists in *The Ipcress File* (1965); "Ipcress" stands for "Induction of Psycho-neuroses by Conditioned Reflex under strESS." Kenneth Branagh's *Dead Again* (1991) has Derek Jacobi playing an antique dealer who dabbles in hypnotherapy, using hypnosis to regress patients to the point that they can re-experience events from their past lives. Hypnosis also is used to treat the title character in *Donnie Darko* (2001). Life coach Tony Robbins uses hypnosis to help the character Hal appreciate real beauty rather than shallow outward appearances in the Farrelly brothers' film *Shallow Hal* (2001). Robbins also uses a trigger phrase when he decides Hal needs to "break out" of the hypnotic spell: "Shallow Hal wants a gal." The character Prot is hypnotized by Jeff Bridges' character, a psychiatrist, in *K-Pax* (2001).

When directing *Heart of Glass* (1976, Germany), Werner Herzog had almost all of the actors hypnotized so they could realistically play their roles as hypnotized subjects. In the movie *Good Will Hunting* (1997), the character of Will Hunting (Matt Damon) ridicules a therapist trying to hypnotize him, breaking into the song "Afternoon Delight" in the middle of a therapy session. (Will is eventually treated by Robin Williams' character – a community college psychology professor – who proves to be an effective therapist.)

In Chan-wook Park's remarkable film *Oldboy* (2003), a man who has kept the protagonist, Dae-su, imprisoned for 15 years uses hypnosis (and hypnotic "triggers" delivered over a smartphone) to get Dae-su and his daughter to become lovers (without ever realizing that they were related); when Dae-su discovers what has happened, he cuts out his tongue. Eventually he seeks out this same hypnotist to help him overcome his torment over his incestuous relationship with his daughter. Dae-su must communicate with the female hypnotist through writing because he can no longer speak. She treats Dae-su using a quick hypnotic induction to split him into two distinct personalities: "The beast," someone who remembers the incestuous relationship with the daughter, and an innocent Dae-su who remembers nothing. The hypnotist suggests that the beast walks away, growing older by 1 year with each step. At the age of 70, the beast is instructed to die. This happens, and the innocent Dae-su wakes up in the snow, remembering nothing.

A common misconception is that hypnosis represents a form of mind control through which a person can be programmed to do things against their will. This myth is perpetuated by films like *The Manchurian Candidate* (1952) and its 2004 remake. In the more recent film, a character, upon hearing the designated cue word, immediately comes under the hypnotist's spell (cinematically accompanied by changes in ambient light) and is at once fully controlled by the voice of the hypnotist. Through flashbacks, other characters are shown killing while in a trance. One character is depicted going fully against his own values when he smothers his long-time lover following a trance suggestion. Of course, this is cinematic nonsense.

"I was a damn good shrink. Nineteen years I worked with a lot of people through a lot of shit. OK, I slept with a patient or two. It's not like I didn't care about them. I loved being a doctor. I used to not charge half my patients. Then the fucking state comes along, they send in some bitch undercover, and I'm fucked. Life isn't fair, is it?"

Robin Williams reviews his life as a hypnotherapist, in *Dead Again* (1991)

In films like Kenneth Branagh's *Dead Again* (1991) and Woody Allen's *The Curse of the Jade Scorpion* (2001), hypnosis is used as a blatant form of manipulation for malevolent purposes. In the former film, a hypnotist (who is also an antiques dealer) takes advantage of vulnerable people by asking them questions in the trance state about where rare antiques can be found in their home or at their work sites; he then gives the suggestion that the person will have total amnesia for the experience. In the latter film, hypnosis is used to steal jewels; here too, subjects are told they will be totally amnestic for the hypnosis episode. Films like these convince viewers that hypnosis can be used to make people do things that are illegal, unethical, and immoral. Likewise, some films suggest that hypnosis may be painful and destructive. *The Butterfly Effect* (2003) perpetrates this misconception by having a young man replay his past under hypnosis; when he does, we see him squirming in pain, his nose bleeds, and he falls onto the floor only to become amnestic for the experience.

"Just think of your mind as a movie. You can pause, rewind or slow down any details you want."

A hypnotherapist's advice in *The Butterfly Effect* (2003)

Professionals are often depicted as incompetent in their use of hypnosis, such as the psychologist in *Donnie Darko* (2001) who uses hypnosis with a patient who has schizophrenia; this diagnosis would be a contraindication for hypnosis. The patient in *Donnie Darko* begins to masturbate while in a trance.

Even when the intent to use hypnosis is justified and well intentioned, it is most often depicted in an overly dramatic manner; for example, in many films the hypnotic technique of "age regression" is employed, and the patient is shown reliving very painful experiences or past traumatic events. The psychiatrist played by Jeff Bridges in *K-Pax* (2001) explains hypnosis, performs an induction, and begins to explore his patient's past. The patient screams in agony and nearly goes into shock. Hypnosis is very rarely this dramatic.

The film *Office Space* (1999) presents an interesting dilemma in which a psychologist induces a trance, deepens the trance – and then has a heart attack and dies before he can bring the patient out of the trance state. The trance would wear off shortly if not immediately, but since this is a comedy, the character stays in the trance for days.

In most of these films, the subject is depicted as helpless and under the control of the hypnotist. These depictions ignore the well-established therapeutic truism that "all hypnosis is self-hypnosis."

Medications

The first genuinely effective antipsychotic medication was **chlorpromazine** (Thorazine), first used as an antihistamine. Several compounds with comparable properties were also synthesized. Thorazine was believed to be a miracle drug that would empty all our mental hospitals. These medications did enable many patients to live once again in the community; unfortunately, they were often indiscriminately prescribed, and dosages were usually excessive. Because of a lack of knowledge about the drug and its consequences, excessive sedation, and **extrapyramidal side effects** (muscle cramps of the head and neck; restless pacing or fidgeting; and stiffening of muscular activity in the face, body, arms, and legs) were common. In *One Flew Over the Cuckoo's Nest* (1975), the patients receive excessive dosages of medications that sedate them and put them at high risk for debilitating side effects.

Today there are several different classifications of pharmacological agents. **Antipsychotic medications** are given to treat thought disorders, such as schizophrenia, and some mood and anxiety disorders. **Antidepressants** are given for mood disorders, and **mood stabilizers** such as **Depakote** and **lithium** are common medication choices for bipolar disorders. **Anxiolytic** (antianxiety) medications are carefully prescribed for patients with anxiety disorders. Some of these drugs, such as Xanax, Valium, and Librium, can be addictive. These drugs are also the ones most often used in combination with alcohol and recreational drugs. The 1982 movie *I'm Dancing as Fast as I Can* stars Jill Clayburgh as the award-winning TV producer Barbara Gordon, who becomes addicted to Valium but eventually recovers.

> **"You know, our bodies are capable of incredible things when they're subjected to anxiety and stress. I found my ex-best friend's cufflinks in my wife's purse one time. I couldn't get an erection for a year and a half."**
>
> **Inappropriate self-disclosure by a psychiatrist in *Garden State* (2004)**

In *Don Juan DeMarco* (1994), Marlon Brando plays a psychiatrist who wants to treat his patient (Johnny Depp) solely with psychotherapy; however, he is pressured by other physicians to treat Depp's character with psychotropic medications. David Cronenberg's *Dead Ringers* (1988) is a film about two identical twins who are gynecologists. They routinely switch roles at work without anyone knowing, and the more aggressive twin (Elliot) often shares his (unwitting) lovers with his timid brother (Beverly). The twins routinely take amphetamines to get up and barbiturates to come down, each prescribing medication for the other. Jeremy Irons brilliantly plays the role of each brother. Cronenberg coauthored the script and based the film on the true story of Stewart and Cyril Marcus, identical twins who were successful New York gynecologists and the authors of a leading textbook in gynecology. The brothers died in 1975 in their Manhattan apartment because of their attempts to withdraw from barbiturate addiction.

In the film *Garden State* (2004), the overly sedated protagonist, who has been taking various medications for a mood disorder for over a decade, decides on his own to discontinue taking medication after learning of the death of his mother. He prospers without the medication, meets a wonderful woman, learns to be assertive when dealing with his controlling psychiatrist father, and feels genuinely happy for the first time in years. While this film is meant to be inspirational and liberating, it also imparts an inappropriate and confusing message to countless people who are taking similar medications.

Electroconvulsive Therapy

In the 1950s, both electroshock and insulin shock became accepted treatment methods to induce seizures, and many psychiatrists were convinced that seizures could be used to protect patients from mental illness. By the 1960s, electrical stimulation, called **electroconvulsive therapy** (ECT), was well established as the safest way to induce seizures.

Originally, ECT was used for many psychiatric illnesses, including schizophrenia. However, more effective pharmacological approaches were developed for most of these disorders. Today, severe depression, mania, and occasionally some types of thought disorders are treated with ECT, but only when other approaches have failed. The procedure is accompanied by the administration of short-acting general anesthesia and muscle paralytic agents that prevent the muscle contractions associated with seizures. Then a very mild electrical stimulus is passed through the brain, which causes the seizure. A series of 8–10 treatments is usually administered before clinically meaningful results are obtained.

McDonald and Walter (2001) examined the portrayal of ECT in 22 American movies from the middle of the 20th century to the onset of the 21st century and concluded that ECT was initially portrayed as a severe but helpful treatment; however, it progressed to being represented as a negative and cruel treatment. In one study, after viewing ECT portrayed in movies, medical students were more likely to talk friends and family out of receiving ECT, and one third reported a decrement in their support for ECT (Walter et al., 2002).

In the past, ECT was used frequently and indiscriminately, often with excessive voltage. In films such as *One Flew Over the Cuckoo's Nest* (1975) and *An Angel at My Table* (1990), ECT is pictured as a painful, lengthy treatment, with the hapless patient strapped to a table by sadistic attendants. Contemporary use of ECT takes about 5–10 minutes from start to finish and rarely results in a visible seizure. There are also clear practice guidelines that help physicians identify when ECT is appropriate and when it is not. In *One Flew Over the Cuckoo's Nest,* ECT was used as punishment for patients who challenged the authority of Nurse Ratched. Its use was just as inappropriate when used to treat New Zealand novelist Janet Frame, as portrayed in *An Angel at My Table*. Another controversial film biography, *Frances* (1982), depicts the 1930s Hollywood actress Frances Farmer and her confinement in mental institutions for rebellious behavior. Frances, played by Jessica Lange, received both shock treatment and a lobotomy.

Pascal Sienaert (2016) analyzed how ECT is portrayed in international movies and TV programs, going back to 1948. Sienaert concluded,

> In most scenes (47/82; 57.3%) ECT is given without consent, and without anesthesia (59/82; 72%). Unmodified ECT is depicted more frequently in American scenes (48/64, 75%), as opposed to scenes from other countries (11/18; 64.7%). Bilateral electrode placement is used in almost all (89%, 73/82) scenes. The vast majority of movies (46/57, 80.7%) and TV programs (18/25, 72%) show a negative and inaccurate image of the treatment. ... In the majority of scenes, ECT is used as a metaphor for repression, mind and behavior control, and is shown as a memory-erasing, painful and damaging treatment, adding to the stigma already associated with ECT. Only a few exceptions paint a truthful picture of this indispensable treatment in modern psychiatry. (Sienaert, 2016, p. 882)

In *A Beautiful Mind* (2001), John Nash receives **insulin shock therapy** and not ECT, although many viewers do not make this distinction. When insulin shock therapy is used, insulin is injected, the body goes into a state of shock and convulsions ensue. *A Beautiful Mind* shows Nash receiving multiple treatments over several weeks.

Social Work and Films

Out of all the various mental health professions portrayed in films, the field of social work might be the one most often portrayed in a positive light. Valentine and Freeman (2002) studied 27 movies that include social workers – usually child welfare workers – across many settings. They found that social workers are most typically placed in one of three roles: advocate, supervisor, or clinician. All three of these roles can be seen in the social worker's role in *Elling* (2002, Norway). A social worker is assigned to two adults – one with social anxiety disorder and the other with intermittent explosive disorder – who have recently been released from a psychiatric hospital. The social worker supervises their progress, advocates for them, and counsels them as they integrate back into regular society. He is authoritarian at times but is also motivational and compassionate, helping them to connect with numerous community services. He uses exposure and systematic desensitization to help his clients face their anxiety. Another movie with a sympathetic portrayal of a social worker is *Strange Voices* (1987), a film that illustrates the short journey between serious mental illness and homelessness.

Social workers are also the group most likely to work in the field with people coping with mental illness or addictions, and along with coworkers they provide invaluable services for people living on the street. Social workers have a profound commitment to social justice, and they are especially well prepared to deal with the intersecting problems of poverty, racial disparities, homelessness, and marginalization (Trawver et al., 2019).

The movie *The Invisible Class* (2020) is a powerful and unforgettable documentary that addresses the rise of homelessness in the United States, and the damage it creates. Some of the most powerful images were filmed in San Francisco's tenderloin district. Reviewing this film in *Street Sense Media*, Will Schick (2019) wrote,

> Josh Hayes stumbled onto the subject of homelessness almost by accident. He was working on a photography project when he came upon a novel idea. Instead of taking thousands of photos of the Golden Gate Bridge like all his other classmates, Hayes thought he could focus his project on something slightly more challenging. For him, people as subjects seemed far more interesting.
>
> And so Hayes approached a man he saw who was homeless in a park and asked the man if it would be all right to photograph him in exchange for some money. The man agreed. They later had a talk that would change Hayes's life.
>
> What happened next is the subject of Hayes's new film, *The Invisible Class*. It is the result of eleven years of research and thousands of hours of taped video and audio interviews. The film takes place nationwide over the span of one 24-hour period to explain what Hayes says are the three major causes of homelessness (the lack of affordable housing, income inequality, and criminalization). (Schick, 2019)

Although not included on Hayes' top three list, there is good evidence that many of the half-million people experiencing homelessness on any given night in the United States are either addicted or mentally ill – or both (McGuire et al., 2021). In addition, veterans seem especially vulnerable. Nichter et al. (2022) analyzed a large dataset ($N = 4{,}069$) to examine the prevalence and correlates of homelessness in veterans. They found a lifetime prevalence of 10.2% for homelessness. Adverse childhood experiences (ACEs), trauma, household income, younger age, and drug use disorders emerged as the strongest correlates of homelessness. These veterans were also at significantly greater risk for suicide, suicide attempts, and suicidal ideation.

Treatment of Different Disorders

Treatment of Anxiety Disorders

There are numerous approaches to the treatment of anxiety, and all of them are at least partially efficacious. Education can be a critical first step in therapy, and it is often tremendously therapeutic for the patient with an anxiety disorder simply to realize that they are not going insane and that these disorders are commonplace and often readily respond to treatment. In addition, patients need to realize that their symptoms are not life-threatening, that they will not pass out or fall down no matter how bad they feel, and that many people experience similar symptoms but assign different labels (**attributions**) to these sensations (e.g., a tingling sensation in your stomach before you give a speech can be interpreted as anticipatory excitement and a signal that you are going to do a good job).

It is also critical to carefully assess a patient's prior use of alcohol or drugs as ways of coping with their anxiety symptoms. Many of these patients have learned to use substances to modulate their anxiety levels: For example, alcoholism is common in veterans with PTSD (as portrayed in *Born on the Fourth of July*). In addition, it is necessary to assess the consumption of coffee, soft drinks, and nicotine. All three exacerbate the symptoms of anxiety.

Psychotherapy may be helpful for some patients with anxiety. Behavior therapy appears to be the treatment of choice for many phobic disorders, and some patients have been helped by behavioral methods after years of insight therapy. Almost all behavior therapies will involve exposure to the feared stimulus or situation. **In vivo exposure with response prevention** is an empirically validated approach (and the treatment of choice for OCD and other anxiety disorders) involving a graduated exposure hierarchy of anxiety-arousing stimuli, where the patient is prevented from avoiding the stimulus and must use anxiety management coping skills instead. **Flooding** and **implosion** are related techniques that involve massive exposure to the feared stimuli. Niemiec and Ferland (2006) discuss how the film *Batman Begins* (2005) illustrates flooding; in this film, Bruce Wayne faces his fear of bats and takes on the name Batman, in part, to demonstrate his mastery of his fear. Mindfulness and hypnosis may also be used as adjunctive therapies in the treatment of anxiety.

VanDyke and Anderson (2013) argue that the popular, animated movie *The Croods* (2013) is a good model for illustrating key principles involved in the treatment of anxiety, such as fear acquisition and extinction, safety learning, avoidance, modeling, and the reevaluation of situations. Lee and Matlock (2022) have argued that the documentary film *UNSTUCK: An OCD Kids Movie* (2017) can be a useful tool for families, educators, and therapists working in pediatrics or family medicine settings where children with OCD are treated.

Movies themselves can be powerful stimuli when developing an **exposure hierarchy** for a person with an anxiety disorder. Movies can be tailored to the individual's fears, obsessions, and dysfunctional belief patterns. The individual will typically be asked to watch a film or a particular scene (often repeatedly) while practicing anxiety management techniques. For example, a person with a contamination fear of dirt might be asked to watch a war film where dirt, dust, and blood are prominent, such as *Saving Private Ryan* (1998), and the individual will be trained to use coping skills to manage their anxiety as it rises during parts of the film. The individual who is homophobic and afraid of contamination with the AIDS virus might be asked to watch *Kissing Jessica Stein* (2002) and *The Birdcage* (1995), and those afraid of getting in an accident or seeing an accident could watch action films containing multiple crashes such as the *Lethal Weapon* series (1987, 1989, 1992, 1998). Other films that could potentially be used for desensitization purposes include *Cast Away* (2000), *Philadelphia* (1993), and *Super Size Me* (2004), for fear of isolation, contamination, and throwing up in public, respectively. Children or adolescents afraid of being rejected might be asked to watch *A Bug's Life* (1998), *Shrek* (2001), or *Hercules* (1997), and those afraid of the dark might watch particular scenes from *Harry Potter and the Sorcerer's Stone* (2001) or its sequels. The use of films in therapy is explored further in Wedding and Niemiec (2003).

Cognitive therapy, including the practice of cognitive restructuring, is often used in treating anxiety disorders. Cognitive therapy helps patients identify and understand the internal statements and irrational thoughts that may trigger arousal in certain situations and settings (Beck & Emery, 1985). Medication may also be used as a treatment or, more commonly, as an adjunct to therapy. Widely used classes of drugs include **β-blockers** (often used to treat social phobias), **tricyclic antidepressants** (often used for panic disorder and agoraphobia), and **selective serotonin reuptake inhibitors** (SSRIs; for OCD and comorbid depression issues). **Benzodiazepines** are also widely used in the treatment of anxiety symptoms, and include diazepam (Valium), chlordiazepoxide (Librium), and alprazolam (Xanax). In addition, there is growing interest in the use of over-the-counter herbal remedies such as **kava-kava** (available from health food stores) and **valerian root** in the treatment of mild to moderate anxiety.

Treatment of Mood Disorders

Lithium carbonate is often the treatment of choice for bipolar disorders. This agent is a naturally occurring element that has been found to be effective in correcting the chemical imbalance associated with this illness. No one is sure how or why lithium works, but it is believed that it either alters the neurotransmitters or inhibits viruses that affect DNA. If lithium carbonate is not effective, other mood stabilizers can be used (e.g., **Depakote**).

Cognitive behavior therapy (CBT), which addresses a client's defective thinking process, is particularly helpful for patients with depression. This approach to psychotherapy forces the patient to examine the evidence for their negative beliefs, and the therapist encourages patients to reframe their beliefs based on the evidence presented in therapy. Once beliefs change, patients begin to perceive the world in a more balanced way, which has an impact on future behaviors. This technique has been highly successful and is believed to be as efficacious as antidepressants in the treatment of mild to moderate depression.

Side Effects (2013) is an interesting film that deals in part with the optimal treatment of depression using anxiolytic medications; the surprise ending suggests life – like therapy – is seldom as simple as we might like.

Treatment of Alcoholism

The first stage of treatment of alcoholism is **detoxification,** or "drying out." This process can vary from several days to a month in duration and is usually extremely unpleasant for the person involved. Vitamins are routinely prescribed in the treatment of addictions. At one time, tranquilizers (primarily Librium and Valium) were often administered to help an individual cope with the physiological distress that accompanies detoxification; however, this approach to treatment has always been controversial and is less common now.

Antabuse (disulfiram) blocks the metabolism of alcohol and may help some alcoholics avoid resumption of drinking after detoxification. An individual taking Antabuse will become violently ill if exposed to even a very small amount of alcohol and will experience nausea, vomiting, sweating, and accelerated respiration, and heart rate. Antabuse is most useful in the first months of sobriety, when the craving for alcohol is most intense.

Alcoholics Anonymous (AA), a self-help fellowship founded in 1935, is widely regarded as an important part of treatment for most alcoholics. More than a million people in the United States belong to this self-help group, and there are more than 1.5 million members worldwide. Every town of any size has a local chapter of AA, and many large cities have meetings in different chapters every evening of the week. These meetings involve self-disclosure, social support, and a commitment to the disease model of alcoholism. The well-known 12 steps of AA are presented in Table 11 in Chapter 11. The founding of AA is described in the film *My Name Is Bill W.* (1989).

"The last time I seen my father, he was blind and diseased from drinking. And every time he put the bottle to his mouth, he don't suck out of it, it sucks out of him until he shrunk so wrinkled and yellow even the dogs didn't know him."

Chief Bromden describes his father's alcoholism in *One Flew Over the Cuckoo's Nest* (1975)

Al-Anon is a related group for families and friends of alcoholics. The program is modeled on AA and also uses a 12-step model. **Alateen** is a similar affiliated group designed to serve teenage children of alcoholic parents.

Although most providers in the substance abuse community are quick to praise the excellent work done by AA, there is little empirical evidence supporting the program. In addition, some individuals find the quasireligious philosophy of the organization distasteful.

AA meetings have been portrayed in numerous films including *The Lost Weekend* (1945),

Days of Wine and Roses (1962), *Clean and Sober* (1988), *When a Man Loves a Woman* (1994), *Drunks* (1995), *28 Days* (2000), and *Flight* (2012). All of these films offer sympathetic portrayals of AA meetings and participants.

Participation in AA saves the life of Kate (Mary Elizabeth Winstead) in *Smashed* (2012). This film depicts Kate drinking in her car before going to teach her first-grade class; she throws up in front of her students and then feigns pregnancy as an excuse for vomiting. She starts each day with a beer in the shower, and in one episode she becomes enraged when she cannot buy beer or wine in a convenience store because of "Blue Laws"; she publicly urinates on the floor and then runs out of the store after stealing a bottle of wine. Her out-of-control behavior is clearly enabled by her husband who continues to drink heavily, even after Kate stops. We see Kate relapse after losing her job, but she eventually achieves sobriety, rejecting her ex-husband's request that she return to the life they once shared.

Treatment of Drug Addiction

Before treatment of drug addiction can begin, **detoxification** must occur. In general, the severity of detoxification from narcotic drugs depends on the health status of the addict and the purity of the drugs they have been taking. Withdrawal from barbiturates tends to be more serious than withdrawal from heroin, cocaine, or alcohol. Detoxification is potentially life threatening and should occur in a structured medical setting. The film *Quitting* (2001) depicts the challenges and pain of detoxifying outside of a structured hospital environment. Anxiolytics such as Valium, Librium, and Xanax are sometimes used to reduce the severity of the effects of detoxification.

Methadone is a synthetic narcotic that is taken orally rather than injected. It is administered daily, usually in an outpatient setting. The drug itself is addicting; however, it is longer lasting, and with daily use the addict can avoid the symptoms of withdrawal that typically occur a few hours after use of drugs such as heroin. In addition, the drug blocks the reinforcing effects of other narcotics. With methadone treatment, there is a reduction in intravenous drug use and a concomitant reduction in crime. In addition, the likelihood of needle sharing, and AIDS is dramatically reduced. Despite these benefits, methadone maintenance programs remain controversial, and there are some clear disadvantages to methadone maintenance therapy, including the development of a large underground market for methadone, the fact that many people drop out of methadone treatment because of side effects (sweating, impotence, constipation, and insomnia), and the fact that many people are philosophically offended by the idea of giving addicts another addictive drug in the name of treatment.

Some programs have used **narcotic antagonists** such as **naloxone** or **naltrexone** to treat opioid addiction. These drugs block the reinforcing effects of narcotics; in effect, the addict may still take drugs, but they no longer produce a high. However, because of the potential for precipitating withdrawal reactions, these programs are complex and costly and require medical supervision.

Programs such as **Narcotics Anonymous** (NA), modeled after AA, advocate total abstinence from drugs. These programs are often associated with therapeutic communities in which a highly structured program and frequent group therapy are core components of treatment. Former addicts who serve as powerful role models for residents often staff these programs. Therapy is often confrontational and may involve spouses and significant others. The film *Clean and Sober* (1988) presents an excellent example of the kind of treatment that occurs in a **therapeutic community**, with Morgan Freeman in the role of a recovered addict and counselor.

Antidepressant medications are sometimes used to help treat amphetamine or cocaine addiction. However, in general, all treatment programs for stimulant addiction have unimpressive success records. Methamphetamine addiction is explored in *Spun* (2002), *The Salton Sea* (2002), and *Winter's Bone* (2010). This last film is especially effective in documenting the relationship between rural poverty in the Ozarks and the proliferation of underground methamphetamine labs.

The success of smoking cessation programs has been more notable. Nicotine gum and transdermal nicotine patches hold considerable promise as important aids in comprehensive treatment packages. Behavior modification and hypnosis are two other techniques that have helped many individuals overcome their addiction to nicotine.

Despite the success of some treatment programs, the only real solution to the drug problem is prevention. Prevention will involve limiting the flow of drugs to the United States and educating the public about the deleterious effects of drug use.

Using Films in Therapy

Lampropoulos et al. (2004), in a dated but still useful article, surveyed 827 licensed practicing psychologists and found that 88% considered movies to be effective therapeutic tools, and only 1% viewed them as potentially harmful. They also asked therapists who had viewed films and used them in therapy to rank their value as therapeutic tools. The five films with the highest ratings, listed in rank order, were *Ordinary People, Philadelphia, The Great Santini, On Golden Pond,* and *Trip to Bountiful.* They also offer six general recommendations (with cautions) for therapists who want to integrate cinematherapy into their clinical practice. These include the following (p. 539): (1) Therapists should carefully consider who is and who is not a good candidate for the therapeutic use of motion pictures. (2) Therapists should choose the timing of the intervention and assign a movie that is appropriate for client's problems. (3) Movie selection criteria include choosing titles that clients enjoy or are familiar with and those recommended by other therapists. (4) Desirable movie characteristics include the ability to inspire and evoke emotions, the depiction of characters solving problems, and, generally, of appropriate role models. (5) Therapists should view a movie before assigning it to a client and have a clear rationale for doing so. (6) Therapists should process the exercise in a debriefing session and address any negative client responses.

More recently, Steven Schlozman, an academic psychiatrist and a cinephile, has written a book titled *Film* (2020) in which he describes how films or film clips can be incorporated into treatment regimens. For example, clips from *Charlotte's Web* (1973) were used to treat a 6-year-old girl with a spider phobia, and viewing *Adam* (2009) helped a high-functioning 16-year-old boy with a diagnosis of ASD learn to tell others about his diagnosis and ask for clarification in situations in which he became confused. Schlozman writes, "He literally learns the social cues that he understands come naturally for others, and he credits *Adam* for helping him to accept responsibility for these challenges" (Schlozman, 2020, p. 32). Numerous other examples are given, and Schlozman notes, "One of the wonderful things about art is the fact that it has therapeutic utility even in the absence of a formal therapeutic engagement with a clinician" (Schlozman, 2020, p. 41).

Ethical Issues and the Right to Humane Treatment

Movies illustrate the ongoing struggles for civil and human rights that have occurred in the mental health system. They also reflect the prevailing stigma that still affects persons with mental illness. Our language characterizes individuals with these illnesses as crazy, nuts, or wacky. The people who treat them are called shrinks, do-gooders, or bleeding hearts (Trachtenberg, 1986), and media often portray patients as clowns, buffoons, or harmless eccentrics (Hyler et al., 1991). In *The Dream Team* (1989) and *The Couch Trip* (1988), a little bit of freedom proves adequate to cure mental illness. Other films, such as *Psycho* (1960) and its remakes and sequels, depict individuals with mental illnesses as homicidal maniacs. In John Carpenter's *Halloween* film series, an escaped psychiatric patient serially kills teenagers who have engaged in sexual experimentation. When Tommy Lee Wallace directed *Halloween III* (1982), the central villain was portrayed as a madman toy maker who made wicked Halloween masks programmed to harm children. However, the original madman on the loose from a mental hospital returned in *Halloween IV* and *V* (1988, 1989). These films and others have misled the public about the dangerousness of psychiatric patients.

One Flew Over the Cuckoo's Nest was not the first movie to portray patients' lack of control over treatment. One of the first movies to address mental illness seriously was *The Snake Pit* (1948), a film directed by Anatole Litvak that stars Olivia de Havilland as Virginia Stuart Cunningham. The movie portrays a woman trying to overcome her illness in a crowded mental institution. The horrifying conditions portrayed in the film mobilized state legislators to improve the level of care provided in institutions. This movie was especially effective in portraying the lack of power women have traditionally had in inpatient psychiatric settings. In *The Snake Pit*, Virginia truly has a mental illness and is taken for treatment by a caring husband. However, many women who did not have mental illnesses were placed in psychiatric hospitals and kept there as a convenience for husbands who had grown tired of them (Geller & Harris, 1994). I once reviewed historical records for Saint Louis State hospital (formerly Saint Louis Lunatic Asylum, built in 1863), and I was shocked to see the reason for admission for one of the female patients simply was "refuses to do her chores." There was also a column in these record books for "exacerbating conditions," and one of the most common entries was "masturbation."

Another powerful film, *Chattahoochee* (1990), not only depicts the horrible conditions in a Florida state hospital during the 1950s but also one patient's campaign to change these conditions. In this film, Korean War veteran Emmett Foley (played by Gary Oldman) loses many of his rights because of his protests. This film, based on a true story, begins when Foley becomes depressed by unemployment and tries to provoke the police into killing him after he shoots up the neighborhood. He wants his wife to receive his life insurance (which she would be denied if he committed suicide). Instead, he is sent to Chattahoochee, a prison for people with mental illness. The conditions in Chattahoochee are deplorable. With the support of his friend Walker Benson (Dennis Hopper), he begins a letter-writing campaign to protest the abuse he has experienced. His writing privileges are taken away, and he starts writing in a Bible and surreptitiously slipping pages to his sister. A state commission is formed, hearings are held, and conditions improve as a result.

The Jacket (2005) stars Adrien Brody playing the role of Jack Starks, a veteran who sustains a head injury in the Iraq war, enters a coma, and is taken for dead; however, a hospital attendant notices eye movement, and eventually Brody's character comes out of his coma, although he still has a profound retrograde amnesia. He is wrongly accused of killing a police officer but is found to be not guilty by reason of insanity. He is sent to a psychiatric institute "for the criminally insane" run by Dr. Thomas Becker (Kris Kristofferson), a sadistic psychiatrist. Therapy consists of putting Brody in a wet, hot straitjacket and keeping him in a morgue-like setting to recreate the sensation of being in the womb. The hospital staff are presented as controlling and abusive, and the film perpetuates the myth that psychiatric hospitals are dangerous places run by inhumane and uncaring staff; in fact, the exact opposite is true, and the individuals who work in these settings are usually dedicated and caring.

Ian McKellen is masterful in his role as a sadistic psychiatrist, Dr. Peter Cleave, in *Asylum* (2005). The film is based on a Patrick McGrath novel and takes place in an old, gothic psychiatric hospital. A new psychiatrist, Dr. Max Raphael (Hugh Bonneville), has arrived to take over management of the hospital – the job Peter

Cleave craved – and his wife and young son accompany him. The son befriends a patient, a man who has been institutionalized because he murdered his wife; his diagnosis is "severe personality disorder with features of morbid jealousy." Natasha Richardson plays Stella, the boy's bored mother, and she is soon involved in a torrid affair with the patient. Although I liked the film, I was troubled by the subtext suggesting that psychiatric hospitals are dangerous places staffed by indifferent attendants and cruel professionals.

"I want you to understand what's going to happen next. The shock will wear off, and it will be replaced by devastating grief. In time, you will come to terms with what you have done, and you'll just be very, very sad. And that sadness will stay with you for the rest of your life."

Psychiatrist Max Raphael tells his wife what to expect after the accidental drowning of their son, in *Asylum* (2005)

---

55 Steps (2017, German/Belgian) is a Billy August film based on a true story that unfolded in San Francisco in 1985. Hilary Swank plays Colette Hughes, a civil rights attorney who had a previous career as a psychiatric nurse (see Figure 59). She becomes obsessed with defending Eleanor Riese, played by Helena Bonham Carter, a woman who is involuntarily committed and given multiple psychotropic drugs without her consent. The medications are given repeatedly, and they result in multiple serious medical problems. The physicians at Saint Mary's Hospital "lawyer up," insisting that doctors know better than patients about what treatment is best, and they minimize the side effects of the drugs they inject (weight gain, sedation, dystonia, bradykinesia, tremor, tardive dyskinesia, and neuroleptic malignant syndrome). They attempt to block their patient's right to consult with her attorney, but Hughes will have none of it. Told to "wait," she responds, "I'm going to wait five minutes – and then I'm going to call the state Board of Hospitals to tell them you refuse to let me see my client." Jeffrey Tambor plays Mort Cohen, a senior attorney who teaches constitutional law at

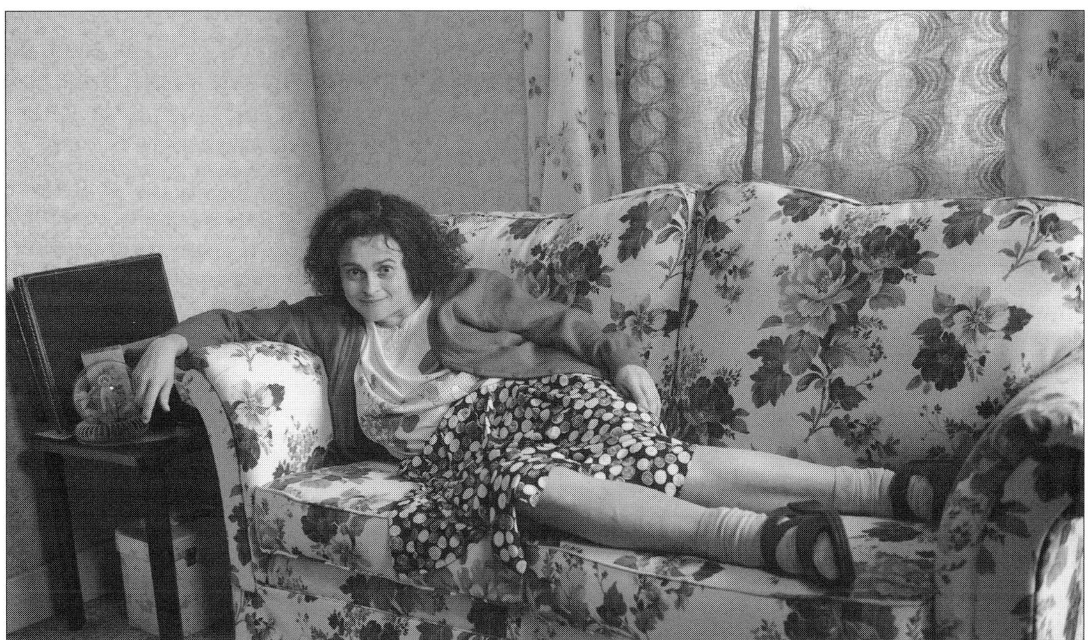

Figure 59. *55 Steps* (2017, Elsani Film, Aloe Entertainment, ChickFlicks Productions, MMC Movies, Mass Hysteria Entertainment, Potemkino Port). Produced by Mary Aloe, Stuart Berton, Helena Bonham Carter, Philip Borbély, et al. Directed by Bille August.

Golden Gate University; Cohen works with Hughes on a class action lawsuit that will eventually affect the lives of over 150,000 people. The film addresses core issues of individual autonomy, informed consent, justice, and beneficence; it also makes the point that competency is a legal term, not a medical term, and judges – not doctors – have the final say about a patient's competence. The case was appealed to the California Supreme Court, but Hughes and Cohen prevailed with the support of the ACLU. Colette Hughes died prematurely, and her death was attributed to the medications she was forced to take. The film ends by paying homage to the heroes in the case, showing photos of the real Colette Hughes, Eleanor Riese, and Mort Cohen.

Another film that portrays unethical treatment of inpatients is director Steven Soderbergh's *Unsane* (2018). The film revolves around the life of Sawyer Valentini, a woman being pursued by a stalker. She makes an appointment with a counselor at a local treatment center, assuming she was signing up for outpatient treatment. During her interview, she admits to occasionally having suicidal thoughts, and then unknowingly signs a statement agreeing to a 24-hour hold because she is a "danger to self or others." The 1-day involuntary hold turns into 1 week, and we see Sawyer repeatedly being sedated against her will. It is especially troubling when she discovers that her stalker has turned up at the hospital and now has a job passing out medications. The police come but leave once they see her signed release. She manages to get to another patient's smartphone by trading off a promise of fellatio for access. Sawyer calls her mother who attempts to intervene, but her mother winds up being killed by Sawyer's stalker. Sawyer attempts to get her stalker to have sex with another woman in Sawyer's presence so he will know what it feels like to love another woman, but he is unable to complete the act and winds up murdering the patient he brought to Sawyer's isolation room. We learn that the hospital is only being run for profit, and they discharge patients as soon as their insurance runs out. The film is unrealistic in many ways (e.g., psychiatric hospitals do not have men and women sharing open bay sleeping quarters), and it presents hospital staff as mercenary and uncaring. However, the suspense is genuine, and it is especially impressive that Soderbergh filmed the movie in 10 days using only an iPhone.

Hospital social workers are often in the best position to help patients refuse involuntary psychotropic medication. Mark Ruffalo (a social worker – not the actor) has written,

> Defending the psychiatric patient's right to refuse treatment falls squarely in the domain of the social worker who is uniquely qualified to address issues pertaining to ethicality as they relate to a client's position as a member of the broader society. Protecting a client's right to refuse medication requires no special training in psychopharmacology but, rather, knowledge and understanding of the rule of law and the application of professional ethics. The right of the individual to own his or her body and self, and thus refuse medication treatment with psychotropics, is a sacred right in our society, and the social worker must serve first and foremost as a defender of freedom and human dignity. (Ruffalo, 2016, p. 271)

An especially challenging issue arises in prisons when persons who are mentally ill have committed capital crimes that would normally result in the death penalty – *if* they were judged to be sane. In such circumstances, courts have vacillated about whether states or the federal government can force a prisoner to take psychotropic medications that would result in better mental health, leaving the prisoner competent enough to understand the charges brought against them, and sane enough to be executed.

International Films: Treatment

David Cronenberg's film *A Dangerous Method* (2011, UK/Germany) is a provocative and entertaining work of historical fiction that depicts the relationship between Sigmund Freud and Carl

Jung, as well as the early history of psychoanalysis. The film features Sabina, a psychosis patient, who was treated by Freud and Jung before becoming a respected physician and scholar. Jung is portrayed as a serious and curious clinician who interacts with patients in a calm, concerned, and deliberate way. He prioritizes work over family – in one scene he stops a conversation about his wife's pregnancy so he can describe his work. Freud is stereotyped as someone obsessed with dreams and sex, and he is frequently shown smoking cigars. The first meeting of these two men is reported to have lasted over 13 hours. Freud, the founder of psychoanalysis, interprets almost all dreams and conflicts in terms of sexuality. Jung challenges Freud's theories, especially his emphasis on sex, and suggests there are other ways to "peek" into the workings of the human mind, such as trying to determine the meaning behind "coincidences," which he later labeled **synchronicity**. The film addresses several topics that are of interest to mental health professionals interested in psychoanalysis or Jungian psychology: hysteria (a common diagnosis in psychiatry at the time), repression, aggression, suppression of instincts, anima/animus, the shadow, the pleasure principle, dream analysis, mysticism, and the rigors of science.

"Whatever you do, give up any idea of trying to cure them."

Freud's advice to Jung in *A Dangerous Method* (2011)

In the film, Jung has erotic, ecstatic, and sadomasochistic sex with Sabina. In his *PsycCRITIQUES* review of the film, Taylor (2012) notes,

> There is no evidence that any of the sexual scenes in the film actually ever happened. We have only Sabina's ravings to any and all that she and Jung were lovers. Cronenberg made sure that the statement that the most intimate, erotic parts of the movie remain "highly speculative" is buried deep in the credits at the end. (Taylor, 2012)

There is no doubt that movies are notorious for depicting psychologists and psychiatrists who cross boundaries, especially sexual ones. In fact, it is far easier to spot a psychotherapist who crosses boundaries than one who does not throughout an entire film, especially if the character is the protagonist.

King of Hearts (1966) is a charming French film that has achieved cult status. The movie stars a young Alan Bates as a Scottish soldier sent into a small French village during World War I to disarm a bomb. He discovers that the villagers have all fled, and the inmates of a local psychiatric hospital are running the town. While I enjoyed the film, it does perpetuate the myth that people with mental illness are simply harmless eccentrics.

House of Fools (2002, Russia/France) is a film reminiscent of *King of Hearts* but based on a true story. It takes place in a psychiatric institution in war-torn Chechnya. When the town is about to be taken over by the enemy, the staff evacuate, but the patients stay, and the soldiers find refuge in the hospital. The movie raises questions about the folly of war, and it uses the hospital as a metaphor for the insanity of a world at war.

Intimate Strangers (2004, France) is a film built around the idea that accountants and psychotherapists have a lot in common. A woman in a troubled marriage is looking for the office of a psychiatrist she is visiting for the first time when she mistakenly enters the office of a timid accountant just down the hall. She begins to share intimate details about her troubled marriage (e.g., her husband wants her to have sex with other men so he can watch), but the accountant initially does not interrupt – he is in a profession in which people needing tax advice about issues like divorce often reveal very personal facts about their private lives. After some time, it becomes clear that the woman believes she is confiding in a psychiatrist, but by this time the accountant is so intrigued by her story that he is loath to reveal his identity. When he does explain the misunderstanding, the patient is upset – but continues to come for therapy sessions because she is benefiting from them, and the patient and "therapist" have a good connection with one another. In their review of this film for *PsycCRITIQUES*, John C. Norcross and his son, Jonathan Norcross, remark,

> This film, drawing on the Freudian tradition, can be encountered on a number of levels. As a public portrayal of insight-oriented psychotherapy, the film fails miserably. The film inaccurately depicts psychoanalytic treatment ... and reinforces four pervasive stereotypes: That anyone can do psychotherapy; that psychotherapy largely consists of a patient's monologue with occasional open-ended questions from the psychotherapist; that an erotic transference will inevitably develop between an attractive female patient and a distinguished male therapist; and that ... commonsense methods are superior to psychoanalytic treatment in modifying behavior ... On the other hand, as a public representation of the intimacy of psychotherapy, the film succeeds admirably. *Intimate Strangers* provides a riveting example of the constructive power of (quasi) psychotherapy and ... the centrality of an affirming, empathic relationship to a successful outcome. Love heals both the patient and the psychotherapist. Moreover, the film underscores that therapy can be one rare and privileged place where people can gradually live without secrets and lies. (Norcross & Norcross, 2005)

The film *16 Years of Alcohol* (2003, Scotland) demonstrates the links between alcohol abuse and violence and hints at the genetics of alcoholism (e.g., one of the earliest and most vivid memories of the protagonist, Frankie, was watching his drunken father copulating with a woman he had met at a pub). *Candy* (2006, Australia) offers a compelling portrayal of heroin addiction and treatment. The title is both the name of the female lead (Abbie Cornish) and a euphemism for heroin. Candy is deeply in love with a bohemian poet named Dan (Heath Ledger, in his first role after *Brokeback Mountain*). Their addiction is supported and celebrated by a chemistry professor friend, Casper, played by Geoffrey Rush. Candy starts by snorting heroin with Dan, but soon moves to mainlining. She overdoses the first time she injects the drug, and almost dies in a bathtub. Dan and Candy's sexual and social lives suffer as they become increasingly involved with heroin, and Candy turns to prostitution to secure the money needed to support their habits. Candy becomes pregnant but miscarries because of her addiction. Both Candy and Don try methadone as a way of coping with their addiction, and eventually go cold turkey to overcome their habit, spending days lying on a dirty mattress. Both overcome their addiction, but Candy relapses after initiating an affair with a drug-using neighbor. Candy eventually tries to reunite with Dan, but he rejects her, knowing their relationship was only based on a mutual love of heroin. The film is divided into three distinct segments, named to describe the protagonists' descent into addiction: "Heaven," "Earth," and "Hell."

"They say for every ten years you've been a junkie; you'll have spent seven of them waiting. On the one hand it was nice having all that time to think. On the other, anxiety was a full-time job."

Dan (Health Ledger) reflects on life as an addict in *Candy* (2006)

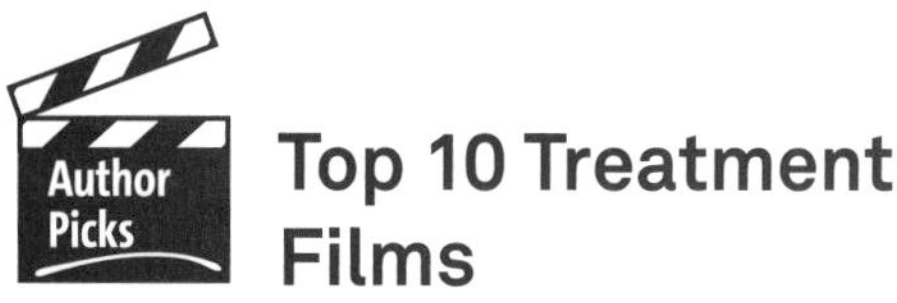

Top 10 Treatment Films

The Cabinet of Dr. Caligari (1920)
The Snake Pit (1948)
David and Lisa (1962)
One Flew Over the Cuckoo's Nest (1975)
Ordinary People (1980)
Good Will Hunting (1997)
Antwone Fisher (2002)
Intimate Strangers (2004)
Shutter Island (2010)
It's Kind of a Funny Story (2010)

References

Abbott, K. (2011, December 12). A chess champion's dominance – and madness. *Smithsonian Magazine.* https://www.smithsonianmag.com/history/a-chess-champions-dominanceand-madness-4307709/

abc News. (2010, December 20). *'Black Swan': Psychiatrists diagnose ballerina's descent.* https://abcnews.go.com/Health/Movies/black-swan-psychiatrists-diagnose-natalie-portmans-portrayal-psychosis/story?id=12436873

Agel, J. (1970). *The making of Kubrick's 2001.* New American Library.

Agrest, D. C. (2011). Suicide: Mar Adentro (The Sea Inside). In H. G. Colt, S. Quadrelli, & L. D. Friedman (Eds.), *The picture of health: Medical ethics and the movies* (pp. 441–449). Oxford University Press.

Akram, A., O'Brien, A., O'Neill, A., & Latham, R. (2009). Crossing the line – learning psychiatry at the movies. *International Review of Psychiatry, 21*(3), 267–268. https://doi.org/10.1080/09540260902746880

Alexander, M. (2009). The couple's odyssey: Hollywood's take on love relationships. *International Review of Psychiatry, 21*(3), 183–188. https://doi.org/10.1080/09540260902748092

Allen, J. G., & Smith, W. H. (1993). Diagnosing dissociative disorders. *Bulletin of the Menninger Clinic, 57,* 328–343.

Altman, W. S., Stein, L., & Westfall, J. E. (Eds.). (2017). *Essays from excellence in teaching* (Vol. XVI; pp. 1–4). Society for the Teaching of Psychology.

American Psychiatric Association. (1994). *Diagnostic and statistical manual of mental disorders* (4th ed.).

American Psychiatric Association. (2000). *Diagnostic and statistical manual of mental disorders* (4th ed., text revision).

American Psychiatric Association, DSM-5 Task Force. (2013). *Diagnostic and statistical manual of mental disorders: DSM-5* (5th ed.).

American Psychological Association, Working Group on Investigation of Memories of Childhood Abuse. (1998). Final conclusions of the American Psychological Association Working Group on Investigation of Memories of Child Abuse. *Psychology, Public Policy, and Law, 4*(4), 933–940.

Anand, S. (2017). Movies in mind: Pawn Sacrifice–Appreciating the anatomy of oddness. *Australian and New Zealand Journal of Psychiatry, 51*(3), 299–300. https://doi.org/10.1177/0004867417691148

Ansell, E. B., Wright, A. G. C., Markowitz, J. C., Sanislow, C. A., Hopwood, C. J., Zanarini, M. C., Yen, S., Pinto, A., McGlashan, T. H., & Grilo, C. M (2015). Personality disorder risk factors for suicide attempts over 10 years of follow-up. *Personality Disorders: Theory, Research, and Treatment, 6*(2), 161–167. https://doi.org/10.1037/per0000089

Appel, M., & Gnambs, T. (2022). Women in fiction: Bechdel-Wallace Test results for the highest-grossing movies of the last four decades. *Psychology of Popular Media.* Advance online publication. https://doi.org/10.1037/ppm0000436

Arango, C., Dragioti, E., Solmi, M., Cortese, S., Domschke, K., Murray, R. M., Jones, P. B., Uher, R., Carvalho, A. F., Reichenberg, A., Shin, J. I., Andreassen, O. A., Correll, C. U., & Fusar-Poli, P. (2021). Risk and protective factors for mental disorders beyond genetics: An evidence-based atlas. *World Psychiatry, 20*(3), 417–436.

Arendt, H. (2006). *Eichmann in Jerusalem: A report on the banality of evil.* Penguin Classics.

Arısoy, E., & Gökmen, E. (2021). Meaning of space in cinema: An analysis on Dogtooth. In M. N. Erdem, N. Kocabay-Sener, & T. Demir (Eds.), *Handbook of research on aestheticization of violence, horror, and power* (pp. 192–214). IGI Global. https://doi.org/10.4018/978-1-7998-4655-0.ch011

Armengol, J. M., & Varela-Manograsso, A. (2022). Pain and glory: Narrative (de)constructions of older gay men in contemporary Spanish culture and cinema. *Journal of Aging Studies, 63,* Article 101030. https://doi.org/10.1016/j.jaging.2022.101030

Arndt, W. B., Jr. (1991). *Gender disorders and the paraphilias.* International Universities Press.

Asnaani, A., Richey, J. A., Dimaite, R., Hinton, D. E., & Hofmann, S. G. (2010). A cross-ethnic comparison of lifetime prevalence rates of anxiety disorders. *Journal of Nervous and Mental Disease, 198*(8), 551–555. https://doi.org/10.1097/NMD.0b013e3181ea169f

Autism Key. (2020, July 30). *Anthony Hopkins reveals a late-in-life autism diagnosis.* https://www.autismkey.com/anthony-hopkins-autism-aspergers-diagnosis/

Aval, N. M. (2021). The effectiveness of transcranial direct current stimulation (tDCS) on improving the severity of stuttering and anxiety in school-aged children who stutter. *Journal of Practice in Clinical Psychology, 9*(3), 227–236.

Aviram, H. (2012). Review of Sex fiends, perverts, and pedophiles: Understanding sex crime policy in America [Review of the book Sex fiends, perverts, and pedophiles: Understanding sex crime policy in America, by C. Leon]. *Law & Society Review, 46*(4), 931–934.

Avni, S., Tolley, P., Tolley, C., & Iannantuono, A. (2011). Review of Tying Your Own Shoes: One film, four perspectives. *Journal on Developmental Disabilities, 17*(1), 83–92.

Badouk Epstein, O. (2019). Trauma work via the lens of attachment theory: Gaslight—Reality distortion by familiar attachment figures. In B. Huppert (Ed.), *Approaches to psychic trauma: Theory and practice* (pp. 347–363). Rowman & Littlefield.

Balaraman, K. K., Dan, S., Ortega, N., Srinivasan, M., Palaniappan, L., Singh, J., Chung, S., & Joshi, S. V. (2022). Psychological distress and mental health service utilization disparities in disaggregated Asian American populations, 2006–2018. *Asian American Journal of Psychology.* Advance online publication. https://doi.org/10.1037/aap0000294

Barnes, B. (2020, February 18). Ben Affleck tried to drink away the pain: Now he's trying honesty. *New York Times.*

Baron-Cohen, S. (2011). *The science of evil: On empathy and the origins of cruelty.* Basic Books.

Barranco, R. E., Rader, N. E., & Trinh, M. T. (2020). Ticket sales and violent content in popular movies. *Deviant Behavior, 41*(8), 1005–1017. https://doi.org/10.1080/01639625.2019.1596535

Barrett, D. (2006). Hypnosis in film and television. *American Journal of Clinical Hypnosis, 49,* 13–30. https://doi.org/10.1080/00029157.2006.10401549

Bartlett, S. J. (2005). *The first comprehensive psychology of human evil. The pathology of man: A study of human evil.* Charles C. Thomas.

Baumgartner, T., Lutz, K., Schmidt, C. F., & Jäncke, L. (2006). The emotional power of music: How music enhances the feeling of affective pictures. *Brain Research, 1075*(1), 151–164. https://doi.org/10.1016/j.brainres.2005.12.065

Baxendale, E., Roche, K., & Stephens, S. (2019). An examination of autoerotic asphyxiation in a community sample. *Canadian Journal of Human Sexuality, 28*(3), 292–303. https://doi.org/10.3138/cjhs.2018-0047

Beck, A. (1976). *Cognitive therapy and the emotional disorders.* Meridian.

Beck, A., & Emery, G. (1985). *Anxiety disorders and phobias: A cognitive perspective.* Basic Books.

Bedford, S. A., Hunsche, M., & Kerns, C. M. (2022). Co-occurrence of obsessive-compulsive disorder and autism spectrum disorder: Differentiation, assessment, and treatment. In E. A. Storch, J. S. Abramowitz, & D. McKay (Eds.), *Complexities in obsessive-compulsive and related disorders: Advances in conceptualization and treatment* (pp. 332–351). Oxford University Press.

Behun, R. J., & Owens, E. W. (2020). *Youth and internet pornography: The impact and influence on adolescent development.* Routledge; Taylor & Francis.

Bell, R. M. (2014). *Holy anorexia.* University of Chicago Press.

Bergsma, A., ten Have, M., Veenhoven, R., & de Graaf, R. (2011). Most people with mental disorders are happy: A 3-year follow-up in the Dutch general population. *Journal of Positive Psychology, 6*(4), 253–259. https://doi.org/10.1080/17439760.2011.577086

Bernstein, E. M., & Putnam, F. W. (1986). Development, reliability, and validity of a dissociation scale. *Journal of Nervous & Mental Disease, 174,* 727–735. https://doi.org/10.1097/00005053-198612000-00004

Bioglio, L., & Pensa, R. (2018). Identification of key films and personalities in the history of cinema from a Western perspective. *Applied Network Science, 3*(50). https://doi.org/10.1007/s41109-018-0105-0

Blanchard, R., & Hucker, S. J. (1991). Age, transvestism, bondage, and concurrent paraphilic activities in 117 fatal cases of autoerotic asphyxia. *British Journal of Psychiatry, 159,* 371–377. https://doi.org/10.1192/bjp.159.3.371

Blumer, Markie L. C. (2010). "And Action!" Teaching and learning through film. *Journal of Feminist Family Therapy, 22*(3), 225–235.

Botha, S., & Harvey, C. (2022). Disabling discourses: Contemporary cinematic representations of acquired physical disability. *Disability & Society.* Advance online publication. https://doi.org/10.1080/09687599.2022.2060801

Bouchard, M.-C., Jalbert, G., Bourassa, D., Bernier, N., & Côté, K. (2023). Production, envoi et retransmission de sextos chez les adolescents: Prévalence et facteurs associés [Production, sending and retransmission of sexting in adolescents: Prevalence and associated factors]. *Canadian Journal of Behavioural Science / Revue canadienne des sciences du comportement, 55*(3), 228–239. https://doi.org/10.1037/cbs0000321

Bouvet, L., Barbier, J.-E., Cason, N., Bakchine, S., & Ehrlé, N. (2017). When synesthesia and savant abilities are mistaken for hallucinations and delusions: Contribution of a cognitive approach for their differential diagnosis. *The Clinical Neuropsychologist, 31*(8), 1459–1473. https://doi.org/10.1080/13854046.2017.1288269

Bramesco, C. (2016, January 5). Film vs. digital: The most contentious debate in the film world, explained. *Vox.* https://www.vox.com/2016/1/5/10714588/film-digital-35mm-70mm-explainer

Brand, B., & Pasko, D. (2017). *Split* is based on myths about dissociative identity disorder [Review of the film *Split*, by M. N. Shyamalan, Dir.]. *PsycCRITIQUES, 62*(18). https://doi.org/10.1037/a0040801

Briere, J. (1989). University males' sexual interest in children: Predicting potential indices of "pedophilia" in a nonforensic sample. *Child Abuse and Neglect, 13,* 65–75. https://doi.org/10.1016/0145-2134(89)90030-6

Bring Change to Mind. (2022). *Schizo.* https://bringchange2mind.org/learn/psas/schizo

Brown, G. R. (1994). Women in relationships with cross-dressing men: A descriptive study from a nonclinical setting. *Archives of Sexual Behavior, 23*(5), 515–530. https://doi.org/10.1007/BF01541495

Bullins, J. (2017). The meme of escaped (male) mental patients in American horror films. In S. Packer (Ed.), *Mental illness in popular culture* (pp. 13–21). Praeger; ABC-CLIO.

Bushman, B. J., Gollwitzer, M., & Cruz, C. (2015). There is broad consensus: Media researchers agree that violent media increase aggression in children, and pediatricians and parents concur. *Psychology of Popular Media Culture, 4*(3), 200–214. https://doi.org/10.1037/ppm0000046

Butler, L. D., & Palesh, O. (2004). Spellbound: Dissociation in the movies. *Journal of Trauma & Dissociation, 5,* 61–87. https://doi.org/10.1300/J229v05n02_04

Byrne, B. (2009). Why psychiatrists should watch films (or what has cinema ever done for psychiatry?). *Advances in Psychiatric Treatment, 15,* 286–296. https://doi.org/10.1192/apt.bp.107.005306

Calhoun, A. J., & Gold, J. A. (2020). "I feel like I know them": The positive effect of celebrity self-disclosure of mental illness. *Academic Psychiatry, 44*(2), 237–241. https://doi.org/10.1007/s40596-020-01200-5

Canby, V. (1981, July 17). Review of Arthur [Review of the film Arthur]. *New York Times,* p. 10.

Cape, G. S. (2003). Addiction, stigma and movies. *Acta Psychiatrica Scandinavica, 107*(3), 163–169. https://doi.org/10.1034/j.1600-0447.2003.00075.x

Cape, G. (2009). Movies as a vehicle to teach addiction medicine. *International Review of Psychiatry, 21*(3), 213–217. https://doi.org/10.1080/09540260902747094

Capps, D. (2010). Identity with Jesus Christ: The case of Leon Gabor. *Journal of Religion and Health, 49*(4), 560–580. https://doi.org/10.1007/s10943-009-9317-z

Cardeña, E., & Reijman, S. (2010). [Review of the film Peacock, by M. Lander, Dir.]. *PsycCRITIQUES, 55*(51).

Cardeña, E., & Spiegel, D. (1993). Dissociative reactions to the Bay Area earthquake. *American Journal of Psychiatry, 150,* 474–478.

Carroll, D. W. (2013). Life challenges and life stories. In D. W. Carroll (Ed.), *Families of children with developmental disabilities: Understanding stress and opportunities for growth* (pp. 121–134). American Psychological Association.

Centers for Disease Control and Prevention. (2022). *Fast facts and fact sheets.* https://www.cdc.gov/Tobacco/data_statistics/fact_sheets/fast_facts/index.htm

Centerwall, B. S. (1992). Hiding in plain sight: Nabokov and pedophilia. *Texas Studies in Literature and Language, 32,* 468–484.

Chater, A. M. (2021). Does intentional asphyxiation by strangulation have addictive properties? *Addiction, 116*(4), 718–724. https://doi.org/10.1111/add.15247

Chaudhuri, S. (2006). *Feminist film theorists: Laura Mulvey, Kaja Silverman, Teresa de Lauretis, Barbara Creed* (Routledge Critical Thinkers). Routledge.

Chen, W., & Adler, J. L. (2019). *Assessment of screen exposure in young children,* 1997 to 2014. *JAMA Pediatrics, 173*(4), 391–393. https://doi.org/10.1001/jamapediatrics.2018.5546

Classen, C., Koopman, C., & Spiegel, D. (1993). Trauma and dissociation. *Bulletin of the Menninger Clinic, 57,* 178–194.

Close, J., Earley, P., & Close, G. (2015). *Resilience: Two sisters and a story of mental illness.* Hachette Audio.

CNN. (2017, August 20). *No one believed he would rape nursing home residents: Now he is going to prison.* https://edition.cnn.com/2017/08/20/health/nursing-home-aide-rape-trial-guilty/index.html

Coleman, D. (2014). *The bipolar express: Manic depression and the movies.* Rowman & Littlefield.

Convery, S. (2017, October 30). Kevin Spacey apologises after being accused of sexual advance on 14-year-old actor. *Guardian.* https://www.theguardian.com/us-news/2017/oct/30/kevin-spacey-anthony-rapp-apologises-accused-sexual-advance-14-year-old-boy

Corrigan, P. W. (2018). *The stigma effect: Unintended consequences of mental health campaigns.* Columbia University Press.

Crawford, C. J. (2006). [Review of the film Bad education, by P. Almodóvar, Dir.]. *PsycCRITIQUES, 51*(26).

Crawford, C. J. (2007). A Hollywood portrayal of the Special Olympics [Review of the film The ringer (2005), by B. W. Blaustein, Dir.]. *PsycCRITIQUES, 52*(14).

Crocker, E. M., & Brenner, A. M. (2021). Teaching psychotherapy. *Psychiatric Clinics of North America, 44*(2), 207–216. https://doi.org/10.1016/j.psc.2020.12.004

Datta, V. (2009). Madness and the movies: An undergraduate module for medical students. *International Review of Psychiatry, 21*(3), 261–266. https://doi.org/10.1080/09540260902748001

de Leo, D., & Heller, T. (2008). Social modeling in the transmission of suicidality. *Crisis: The Journal of Crisis Intervention and Suicide Prevention, 29,* 11–19. https://doi.org/10.1027/0227-5910.29.1.11

de Moura, A. C. M. L., Rodrigues, C. N., Costa, P. H. V., & Polese, J. C. (2020). The practices, orientation, satisfaction, and sexual response in men with spinal cord injury. *Sexuality and Disability, 38,* 615–623. https://doi.org/10.1007/s11195-020-09666-9

Denkinger, J. K., Rometsch, C., Murray, K., Schneck, U., Brißlinger, L. K., Azad, Z. R., Windthorst, P., Graf, J., Hautzinger, M., Zipfel, S., & Junne, F. (2022). Addressing barriers to mental health services: Evaluation of a psychoeducational short film for forcibly displaced people. *European Journal of Psychotraumatology, 13*(1), Article 2066458. https://doi.org/10.1080/20008198.2022.2066458

Denzin, N.K. (1991). *Hollywood shot by shot: Alcoholism in American cinema.* Aldine De Gruyter.

Desbuleux, J. C., & Fuss, J. (2023). The self-reported sexual real-world consequences of sex doll use. *Journal of Sex Research.* Advance online publication. https://doi.org/10.1080/00224499.2023.2199727

dickey, l. m., & Puckett, J. A. (2023). *Affirmative counseling with transgender and gender diverse clients.* Hogrefe.

Dickson, E. J. (2019, October 7). Deepfake porn is still a threat, particularly for K-Pop stars. *Rolling Stone.* https://www.rollingstone.com/culture/culture-news/deepfakes-nonconsensual-porn-study-kpop-895605/

Dimolareva, M., & Dunn, T. J. (2021). Animal-assisted interventions for school-aged children with autism spectrum disorder: A meta-analysis. *Journal of Autism and Developmental Disorders, 51*(7), 2436–2449. https://doi.org/10.1007/s10803-020-04715-w

Distractify. (2020, December 30). *Anthony Hopkins was diagnosed with Asperger's in 2014, which made him "a Loner."* https://www.distractify.com/p/is-anthony-hopkins-autistic

Drag, L. L., & Bieliauskas, L. A. (2019). Differential diagnosis of depression and dementia. In L. D. Ravdin & H. L. Katzen (Eds.), *Handbook on the neuropsychology of aging and dementia* (pp. 179–195). Springer Nature Switzerland AG. https://doi.org/10.1007/978-3-319-93497-6_12

Drobonikuv, M. J., & Mychailyszyn, M. P. (2021). Animal interaction affecting core deficit domains among children with autism: A meta-analysis. *Journal of Autism and Developmental Disorders, 51*(12), 4605–4620. https://doi.org/10.1007/s10803-021-04891-3

Ebert, R. (2012, March 14). *A psychopath using mind control.* https://www.rogerebert.com/reviews/the-snowtown-murders-2012

Edwards, E. R., Barnes, S., Govindarajulu, U., Geraci, J., & Tsai, J. (2021). Mental health and substance use patterns associated with lifetime suicide attempt, incarceration, and homelessness: A latent class analysis of a nationally representative sample of U.S. veterans. *Psychological Services, 18*(4), 619–631. https://doi.org/10.1037/ser0000488

Edwards, A.-M., & Kotera, Y. (2022). Commentary: Linking mass shootings with mental illness and stigma. *International Journal of Mental Health and Addiction.* Advance Online Publication. https://doi.org/10.1007/s11469-022-00787-0

Eichenberg, C., Khamis, M., & Hübner, L. (2019). The attitudes of therapists and physicians on the use of sex robots in sexual therapy: Online survey and interview study. *Journal of Medical Internet Research, 21*(8), Article e13853. https://doi.org/10.2196/13853

Eichinger, T. (2021). Psychotherapy ethics in film. In M. Trachsel, J. Gaab, N. Biller-Andorno, Ş. Tekin, & J. Z. Sadler (Eds.), *The Oxford handbook of psychotherapy ethics* (pp. 1027–1040). Oxford University Press.

Eisenberg, M. M., & Blank, M. B. (2013). "Just call me Hitch...": The enigma of Alfred Hitchcock [Review of the film Hitchcock, by S. Gervasi, Dir.]. *PsycCRITIQUES, 58*(6).

Ellis, A., & Ellis, D.J. (Collaborator). (2010). *All out! An autobiography.* Prometheus.

Esmail, S., Darry, K., Walter, A., & Knupp, H. (2010). Attitudes and perceptions towards disability and sexuality. *Disability and Rehabilitation: An International, Multidisciplinary Journal, 32*(14), 1148–1155. https://doi.org/10.3109/09638280903419277

Ettman, C. K., Abdalla, S. M., Cohen, G. H., Sampson, L., Vivier, P. M., & Galea, S. (2020). Prevalence of depression symptoms in US adults before and during the COVID-19 pandemic. *JAMA Network Open, 3*(9), e2019686. https://doi.org/10.1001/jamanetworkopen.2020.19686

Feist, G. J., Dostal, D., & Kwan, V. (2021). Psychopathology in world-class artistic and scientific creativity. *Psychology of Aesthetics, Creativity, and the Arts.* Advance online publication. https://doi.org/10.1037/aca0000440

Ferrari, A. (2021). The persistence of stigma reduction after teaching abnormal psychology using celebrity narratives. *Teaching of Psychology, 48*(3), 191–196. https://doi.org/10.1177/0098628320979886

Fitzpatrick, K. R. (2020, June 16). Our testament. *Los Angeles Review of Books.* https://lareviewofbooks.org/article/our-testament

Floriano, M. A. H. (2008). The cinema as therapy: Psychoanalysis in the work of Woody Allen. *Journal of Medicine and Movies, 4,* 17–26.

Forcen, F. E. (2017). *Monsters, demons and psychopaths: Psychiatry and horror film.* Routledge/Taylor & Francis Group.

Forcen, F. E., & Forcen, C. E. (2015). The practice of holy fasting in the late middle ages: A psychiatric approach. *Journal of Nervous and Mental Disease, 203*(8), 650–653. https://doi.org/10.1097/NMD.0000000000000343

Frances, A. (2013). *Saving normal: An insider's revolt against out-of-control psychiatric diagnosis, DSM-5, Big*

Pharma, and the medicalization of ordinary life. William Morrow.

Freckelton, I. (2013). Sexual surrogate partner therapy: Legal and ethical issues [Editorial]. *Psychiatry, Psychology and Law, 20*(5), 643–659. https://doi.org/10.1080/13218719.2013.831725

Frese, F. J. (2006). Another beautiful mind – with daughters [Review of the film Proof]. *PsycCRITIQUES, 51*(33).

Frese, F. J. (2013). Humanizing a twelve-step icon [Review of the media *Bill w*, by D. Carracino & K. Hanlon, Dir.]. *PsycCRITIQUES, 58*(38). https://doi.org/10.1037/a0034123

Fröber, K., & Thomaschke, R. (2021). In the dark cube: Movie theater context enhances the valuation and aesthetic experience of watching films. *Psychology of Aesthetics, Creativity, and the Arts, 15*(3), 528–544. https://doi.org/10.1037/aca0000295

Fullerton, C. S., Ursano, R. J., & Wang, L. (2004). Acute stress disorder, posttraumatic stress disorder, and depression in disaster or rescue workers. *American Journal of Psychiatry, 161*(8), 1370–1376. https://doi.org/10.1176/appi.ajp.161.8.1370

Gabbard, G. O. (2017). The day after. *Psychoanalytic Dialogues, 27*(3), 384–385. https://doi.org/10.1080/10481885.2017.1310529

Gabbard, K., & Gabbard, G. (1999). *Psychiatry and the cinema* (2nd ed.). American Psychiatric Press.

Gámez-Guadix, M., & Incera, D. (2021). Homophobia is online: Sexual victimization and risks on the internet and mental health among bisexual, homosexual, pansexual, asexual, and queer adolescents. *Computers in Human Behavior, 119,* Article 106728. https://doi.org/10.1016/j.chb.2021.106728

Garrisson, H., Scholey, A., Verster, J. C., Shiferaw, B., & Benson, S. (2022). Effects of alcohol intoxication on driving performance, confidence in driving ability, and psychomotor function: A randomized, double-blind, placebo-controlled study. *Psychopharmacology, 239*(12), 3893–3902. https://doi.org/10.1007/s00213-022-06260-z

Gates, Z. Y. (2022). What if LeBron James was a scientist? The influence of role models on Black male youth in STEM programs. In A. G. Robins, L. Knibbs, T. N. Ingram, M. N. Weaver, Jr., & A. A. Hilton (Eds.), *Young, gifted and missing: The underrepresentation of African American males in science, technology, engineering and mathematics disciplines* (pp. 115–128). Emerald. https://doi.org/10.1108/S1479-364420220000025009

Gauthier, S., Rosa-Neto, P., Morais, J. A, & Webster, C. (2021). *World Alzheimer Report 2021: Journey through the diagnosis of dementia.* Alzheimer's Disease International.

Geller, J., & Harris, M. (Eds.). (1994). *Women of the asylum: Voices from behind the walls, 1840–1945.* Doubleday.

Gerritsen, D. L., Kuin, Y., & Nijboer, J. (2014). Dementia in the movies: The clinical picture. *Aging & Mental Health, 18*(3), 276–280. https://doi.org/10.1080/13607863.2013.837150

Geymonat, G. G. (2019). Disability rights meet sex workers' rights: The making of sexual assistance in Europe. *Sexuality Research & Social Policy, 16*(2), 214–226. https://doi.org/10.1007/s13178-019-0377-x

Ghaziuddin, M., & Ghaziuddin, N. (2021). Bipolar disorder and psychosis in autism. *Psychiatric Clinics of North America, 44*(1), 1–9. https://doi.org/10.1016/j.psc.2020.11.001

Ghiselli, N. & Davis, G. (2011). Stuttering: Fact or fiction [Review of the film *The King's Speech*, by T. Hooper, Dir.]. *PsycCRITIQUES, 56*(13). https://doi.org/10.1037/a0023604

Ghoshal, N., & Wilkinson, P. O. (2017). Flowers for Algernon: The ethics of human experimentation on the intellectually disabled. *Psychiatria Danubina, 29*(Suppl 3), 194–195.

Gilbey, R. (2022, September 25). Louise Fletcher obituary. *Guardian.* https://www.theguardian.com/film/2022/sep/25/louise-fletcher-obituary

Gill, M. (2012). Sex can wait, masturbate: The politics of masturbation training. *Sexualities, 15*(3-4), 472–493. https://doi.org/10.1177/1363460712439655

Gius, C. (2022). Addressing the blurred question of 'responsibility': Insights from online news comments on a case of nonconsensual pornography. *Journal of Gender Studies, 31*(2), 193–203. https://doi.org/10.1080/09589236.2021.1892610

Goffman, E. (1986). *Frame analysis: An essay on the organization of experience.* Northeastern University Press.

Goodwin, R. D., Dierker, L. C., Wu, M., Galea, S., Hoven, C. W., & Weinberger, A. H. (2022). Trends in U.S. depression prevalence from 2015 to 2020: The widening treatment gap. *American Journal of Preventive Medicine, 63*(5), 726–733. https://doi.org/10.1016/j.amepre.2022.05.014

Grady, M. D., & Levenson, J. S. (2021). Prevalence rates of adverse childhood experiences in a sample of minor-attracted persons: A comparison study. *Traumatology, 27*(2), 227–235. https://doi.org/10.1037/trm0000273

Grandin, T. (2020). Job preparation and how to help people on the spectrum have successful employment. In R. Bédard & L. Hecker (Eds.), *A spectrum of solutions for clients with autism: Treatment for adolescents and adults* (pp. 149–156). Routledge; Taylor & Francis. https://doi.org/10.4324/9780429299391-19

Grandin, T., Fine, A. H., O'Haire, M. E., Carlisle, G., & Bowers, C. M. (2015). The roles of animals for individuals with autism spectrum disorder. In A. H. Fine (Ed.), *Handbook on animal-assisted therapy: Foundations and guidelines for animal-assisted interventions* (pp. 225–236). Elsevier Academic Press. https://doi.org/10.1016/B978-0-12-801292-5.00016-X

Graser, M. (2013, November 12). Epic fail: How Blockbuster could have owned Netflix. *Variety*. https://variety.com/2013/biz/news/epic-fail-how-blockbuster-could-have-owned-netflix-1200823443/

Greenberg, H. R. (1993). *Screen memories: Hollywood cinema on the psychoanalytic couch*. Columbia University Press.

Guillen, M. (2009, January 10). *Waltz with Bashar: Interview with Ari Folman*. https://screenanarchy.com/2009/01/waltz-with-bashirinterview-with-ari-folmon.html

Gundgurthi, A., Kharb, S., Dutta, M. K., Pakhetra, R., & Garg, M. K. (2012). Insulin poisoning with suicidal intent. *Indian Journal of Endocrinology and Metabolism, 16*(Suppl 1), S120–S122.

Hacker, K., Collins, J., Gross-Young, L., Almeida, S., & Burke, N. (2008). Coping with youth suicide and overdose: One community's efforts to investigate, intervene, and prevent suicide contagion. *Crisis: The Journal of Crisis Intervention and Suicide Prevention, 29*, 86–95. https://doi.org/10.1027/0227-5910.29.2.86

Hall, R. C. W., & Friedman, S. H. (2015). Psychopathology in a galaxy far, far away: The use of Star Wars' dark side in teaching. *Academic Psychiatry, 39*(6), 726–732. https://doi.org/10.1007/s40596-015-0337-6

Hallam, J., & Shaw, L. (Eds.). (2020). *Movies, music and memory: Tools for wellbeing in later life*. Emerald. https://doi.org/10.1108/9781839091995

Hanevik, H., Hestad, K. A., Lien, L., Joa, I., Larsen, T. K., & Danbolt, L. J. (2017). Religiousness in first-episode psychosis. *Archive for the Psychology of Religion, 39*(2), 139–164. https://doi.org/10.1163/15736121-12341336

Hare, R. D. (2006). Psychopathy: A clinical and forensic overview. *Psychiatric Clinics of North America, 29*, 709–724. https://doi.org/10.1016/j.psc.2006.04.007

Hariyanto, T. I., Putri, C., Arisa, J., Situmeang, F. V., & Kurniawan, A. (2021). Coronavirus disease-2019 in older people with cognitive impairment. *Archives of Gerontology and Geriatrics, 93*, 104299.

Harper, C. A., Lievesley, R., & Wanless, K. (2023). Exploring the psychological characteristics and risk-related cognitions of individuals who own sex dolls. *Journal of Sex Research, 60*(2), 190–205. https://doi.org/10.1080/00224499.2022.2031848

Harrington, A. (2019). *Mind fixers: Psychiatry's troubled search for the biology of mental illness*. W. W. Norton.

Harris, B. (2021). The Snake Pit: Mixing Marx with Freud in Hollywood. *History of Psychology, 24*(3), 228–254. https://doi.org/10.1037/hop0000188

Hart, K.-P. R., & Cutler-Broyles, T. (Eds.). (2021). *Kink and everyday life: Interdisciplinary reflections on practice and portrayal*. Emerald Publishing.

Hatch, A. E. (2017). *Campus sexual assault: A reference handbook*. ABC-CLIO.

Heath, E. (2019). *Mental disorders in popular film: How Hollywood uses, shames, and obscures mental diversity*. Lexington Books; Rowman & Littlefield.

Hediger, K., Wagner, J., Künzi, P., Haefeli, A., Theis, F., Grob, C., Pauli, E., & Gerger, H. (2021). Effectiveness of animal-assisted interventions for children and adults with post-traumatic stress disorder symptoms: A systematic review and meta-analysis. *European Journal of Psychotraumatology, 12*(1), Article 1879713. https://doi.org/10.1080/20008198.2021.1879713

Heider, F., & Simmel, M. (1944). An experimental study of apparent behavior. *American Journal of Psychology, 57*, 243–259. https://doi.org/10.2307/1416950

Hesse, M., Schliewe, S., & Thomsen, R. R. (2005). Rating of personality disorder features in popular movie characters. *BMC Psychiatry, 5*, 45. https://doi.org/10.1186/1471-244X-5-45

Hodapp, R. M., & Fidler, D. J. (2021). Down syndrome. In L. M. Glidden, L. Abbeduto, L. L. McIntyre, & M. J. Tassé (Eds.), *APA handbook of intellectual and developmental disabilities: Foundations* (pp. 123–150). American Psychological Association.

Hodges, F. M. (2005). The antimasturbation crusade in antebellum American medicine. *Journal of Sexual Medicine, 2*, 722–731. https://doi.org/10.1111/j.1743-6109.2005.00133.x

Holt, R. W. (2023). You can have too much sex? The line between sexual expression and addiction. In A. M. Schubert & M. Pope (Eds.), *Handbook for human sexuality counseling: A sex positive approach* (pp. 357–376). American Counseling Association.

Huntjens, R. J. C., Rijkeboer, M. M., & Arntz, A. (2019). Schema therapy for Dissociative Identity Disorder (DID): Rationale and study protocol. *European Journal of Psychotraumatology, 10*(1), Article 1571377. https://doi.org/10.1080/20008198.2019.1571377

Huntington, C., Willoughby, B., & Rhoades, G. (2022). Associations of adolescents' pornography viewing with their romantic relationship skills and behaviors. *Journal of Sex Research*. Advance online publication. https://doi.org/10.1080/00224499.2022.2096844

Huta, V., & Hawley, L. (2010). Psychological strengths and cognitive vulnerabilities: Are they two ends of the same continuum or do they have independent relationships with well-being and ill-being? *Journal of Hap-*

piness Studies, 11(1), 71–93. https://doi.org/10.1007/s10902-008-9123-4

Huxley, A. (1954). *Doors of perception*. Harper and Brothers.

Hwang, M. C., & Parreñas, R. S. (2021). The gendered racialization of Asian women as villainous temptresses. *Gender & Society, 35*(4), 567–576. https://doi.org/10.1177/08912432211029395

Hyler, S.E. (1988). DSM-III at the cinema: Madness in the movies. *Comprehensive Psychiatry, 29,* 195–206. https://doi.org/10.1016/0010-440X(88)90014-4

Hyler, S.E., & Bujold, A.E. (1994). Computers and psychiatric education: The "Taxi Driver" mental status examination. *Psychiatric Annals, 24,* 13–19. https://doi.org/10.3928/0048-5713-19940101-07

Hyler, S.E., Gabbard, G.O., & Schneider, I. (1991). Homicidal maniacs and narcissistic parasites: Stigmatization of mentally ill persons in the movies. *Hospital and Community Psychiatry, 42,* 1044–1048.

Iaccino, J.F., & Dondero, J.E. (2013a). Technology can be deadly: A female serial killer for the new age [Review of the film Scream 4]. *PsycCRITIQUES, 57*(50). https://doi.org/10.1037/a0031286

Iaccino, J.F., & Dondero, J.E. (2013b). Edgar Allan Poe matches with one of the first identified serial killers! [Review of the film The Raven]. *PsycCRITIQUES, 59*(2). https://doi.org/10.1037/a0035401

Iati, M. (2023, May 11). "The Good Doctor" memes go viral, reigniting debate about autism portrayal. *The Washington Post*. https://www.washingtonpost.com/lifestyle/2023/05/11/good-doctor-memes-autism/

Innala, S.M., & Ernulf, K.E. (1992). Understanding male homosexual attraction: An analysis of restroom graffiti. *Journal of Social Behavior and Personality, 7,* 503–510.

Jackson, E. (2006). A stutter's perspective: A stutter's challenge. *Journal of Stuttering, Advocacy & Research, 1*(3), 114–118.

Jacobson, J. A. (2011). Consent, competence, and capacity: A Beautiful Mind. In H. G. Colt, S. Quadrelli, & L. D. Friedman (Eds.), *The picture of health: Medical ethics and the movies* (pp. 61–65). Oxford University Press.

James, W. (1936). *The varieties of religious experience*. Modern Library.

Jamison, K.R. (1993). *Touched with fire: Manic-depressive illness and the artistic temperament*. Free Press.

Jewett, P. I., Gangnon, R. E., Borowsky, I. W., Peterson, J., Areba, E. M., Kiragu, A., & Densley, J. (2022). US mass public shootings since Columbine: Victims per incident by race and ethnicity of the perpetrator. *Preventive Medicine, 162,* 1–8. https://doi.org/10.1016/j.ypmed.2022.107176

Johnson, M. (2021). Psychopath, sociopath, or autistic: Labeling and framing the brilliance of Sherlock Holmes. In M. Johnson & C. J. Olson (Eds.), *Normalizing mental illness and neurodiversity in entertainment media: Quieting the madness* (pp. 83–95). Routledge; Taylor & Francis.

Johnson, M., & Walker, T. (2021). Introduction: Why depictions of mental illness matter. In M. Johnson & C. J. Olson (Eds.), *Normalizing mental illness and neurodiversity in entertainment media: Quieting the madness* (pp. 1–10). Routledge; Taylor & Francis.

Kalra G. (2011). Teaching diagnostic approach to a patient through cinema. *Epilepsy & Behavior, 22*(3), 571–573. https://doi.org/10.1016/j.yebeh.2011.07.018

Kashdan, T.B. (2009). *Curious? Discover the missing ingredient to a fulfilling life*. William Morrow.

Katsiyannis, A., Rapa, L. J., Whitford, D. K., & Scott, S. N. (2023). An examination of US school mass shootings, 2017–2022: Findings and implications. *Advances in Neurodevelopmental Disorders, 7*(1), 66–76. https://doi.org/10.1007/s41252-022-00277-3

Katz, D. A. (2022). *Questions raised by the controversy over recovered memories of incest (Lief,* 2003). *Psychodynamic Psychiatry, 50*(1), 114–115. https://doi.org/10.1521/pdps.2022.50.1.114

Kavanagh, C., & Cavanna, A. E. (2020). James Bond villains and psychopathy: A literary analysis. *Journal of Psychopathology, 26*(4), 273–283.

Kazğan, A., Yildiz, S., Korkmaz, S., & Atmaca, M. (2021). Borderline kişilik bozukluğunda oto-vampirizm: Olgu sunumu [Auto-vampirism in borderline personality disorder: A case report]. *Klinik Psikiyatri Dergisi: Journal of Clinical Psychiatry, 24*(2), 265–269.

Kertesz, J., Lenahan, P., & Tran, R. (2005). Post-traumatic stress disorder. In M. Alexander, P. Lenahan, & A. Pavlov (Eds.), *Cinemeducation: A comprehensive guide to using film in medical education* (pp. 75–79). Radcliffe.

Kieseppa, T., Partonen, T., Haukka, J., Kaprio, J., & Lonnqvist, J. (2004). High concordance of bipolar I disorder in a nationwide sample of twins. *American Journal of Psychiatry, 161*(10), 1814–1821. https://doi.org/10.1176/ajp.161.10.1814

Killian, K. D. (2023). An analysis of Black Widow (2021): Marvel's most feminist film features powerful sisters and an attenuated male gaze. *Journal of Feminist Family Therapy, 35*(1), 106–113. https://doi.org/10.1080/08952833.2022.2139926

King, C. K., & Rings, J. A. (2022). Adolescent sexting: Ethical and legal implications for psychologists. *Ethics & Behavior, 32*(6), 469–479. https://doi.org/10.1080/10508422.2021.1983818

Kinsey, A. C., Pomeroy, W. B., & Martin, C. E. (1948). *Sexual behavior in the human male*. Saunders.

Kinsey, A. C., Pomeroy, W. B., Martin, C. E., & Gebhard, P. H. (1953). *Sexual behavior in the human female*. Saunders.

Konca, A. S. (2022). Digital technology usage of young children: Screen time and families. *Early Childhood Education Journal, 50*(7), 1097–1108. https://doi.org/10.1007/s10643-021-01245-7

Kuhnigk, O., Schreiner, J., Reimer, J., Emami, R., Naher, D., & Harendza, S. (2012). Cinemeducation in psychiatry: A seminar in undergraduate medical education combining a movie, lecture, and patient interview. *Academic Psychiatry, 36*(3), 205–210. https://doi.org/10.1176/appi.ap.10070106

Kuo, W. H., Gallo, J. J., & Eaton, W. W. (2004). Hopelessness, depression, substance disorder, and suicidality: A 3-year community-based study. *Social Psychiatry Psychiatric Epidemiology, 39*(6), 497–501. https://doi.org/10.1007/s00127-004-0775-z

Lachmann, F. M. (2016). Some reflections on Shame, the film. *Psychoanalytic Psychology, 33*(2), 371–377. https://doi.org/10.1037/a0036559

Lampropoulos, G. K., Kazantzis, N., & Deane, F. P. (2004). Psychologists' use of motion pictures in clinical practice. *Professional Psychology: Research and Practice, 35*(5), 535–541. https://doi.org/10.1037/0735-7028.35.5.535

Latzman, N. E., Casanueva, C., & Dolan, M. (2017). *Understanding the scope of child sexual abuse: Challenges and opportunities.* RTI Press Publication No. OP-0044-1711. RTI Press. https://doi.org/10.3768/rtipress.2017.op.0044.1711

Lazarus, R. S. (1999). *Stress and emotion: A new synthesis.* Springer.

Lee, R. L., & Matlock, S. R. (2022). Review of UNSTUCK: An OCD kids movie [Review of the film Unstuck: An OCD kids movie]. *Families, Systems, & Health, 40*(3), 422–423. https://doi.org/10.1037/fsh0000722

Lefebvre, A.-A., Audet, A., Savard, M., Mackay, M. C., Brassard, A., Daspe, M.-È., Lussier, Y., & Vaillancourt-Morel, M.-P. (2022). A contemporary exploration of the relationship between attachment and sexual satisfaction: The role of technology-mediated sexual interaction. *Sexual and Relationship Therapy.* Advance online publication. https://doi.org/10.1080/14681994.2022.2130231

Leitner, L. M. (2008). [Review of the film Lars and the Real Girl, by C. Gillespie, Dir.]. *PsycCRITIQUES, 53*(35).

Leitner, L. M., & Imai, H. (2011). Many people labeled mentally ill have broken hearts [Review of the film Crooked beauty]. *PsycCRITIQUES, 56*(10).

Leon, C. (2011). *Sex fiends, perverts, and pedophiles: Understanding sex crime policy in America.* NYU Press.

Liao, S. (2011). Personhood and the ethics of dementia: Iris. In H. G. Colt, S. Quadrelli, & L. D. Friedman (Eds.), *The picture of health: Medical ethics and the movies* (pp. 463–467). Oxford University Press.

Lilienfeld, S. O., & Berg, J. M. (2012). A psychological urban legend with disastrous consequences. *PsycCRITIQUES, 57*(20).

Lipoff, J. (2020, May 14). *Alfred Hitchcock, COVID-19, and the MacGuffin.* https://www.kevinmd.com/blog/2020/05/alfred-hitchcock-covid-19-and-the-macguffin.html

Loftus, E. F. (1996). The Myth of Repressed Memory and the realities of science. *Clinical Psychology: Science and Practice, 3*(4), 356–362. https://doi.org/10.1111j.1468-2850.1996.tb00089.x

Loftus, E., & Ketcham, K. (1994). *The myth of repressed memory: False memories and allegations of sexual abuse.* St. Martin's Press.

Lucas, K. T. (2022). Deepfakes and domestic violence: Perpetrating intimate partner abuse using video technology. *Victims & Offenders, 17*(5), 647–659. https://doi.org/10.1080/15564886.2022.2036656

Ludwig, A. M. (1998). Method and madness in the arts and sciences. *Creativity Research Journal, 11,* 93–101 https://doi.org/10.1207/s15326934crj1102_1

Lutfiyya, Z. M., Schwartz, K. D., & Hansen, N. (2009). False images: Reframing the end-of-life portrayal of disability in Million Dollar Baby. In S. Shapshay (Ed.), *Bioethics at the movies* (pp. 225–241). Johns Hopkins University Press.

Maenner, M. J., Shaw, K. A., Baio, J., Washington, A., Patrick, M., DiRienzo, M., Christensen, D. L., Wiggins, L. D., Pettygrove, S., Andrews, J. G., Lopez, M., Hudson, A., Baroud, T., Schwenk, Y., White, T., Rosenberg, C. R., Lee, L. C., Harrington, R. A., Huston, M., ... Dietz, P. M. (2020). Prevalence of autism spectrum disorder among children aged 8 years – Autism and Developmental Disabilities Monitoring Network, 11 Sites, United States, 2016. *MMWR Surveillance Summaries, 69*(4), 1–12.

Mallers, M. H., Claver, M., & Lares, L. A. (2014). Perceived control in the lives of older adults: The influence of Langer and Rodin's work on gerontological theory, policy, and practice. *The Gerontologist, 54*(1), 67–74. https://doi.org/10.1093/geront/gnt051

Manning, M. J. (2017). How traditional holiday TV movies depict mental illness. In S. Packer (Ed.), *Mental illness in popular culture* (pp. 137–146). Praeger; ABC-CLIO.

Marcantonio E. R. (2017). Delirium in hospitalized older adults. *The New England Journal of Medicine, 377*(15), 1456–1466. https://doi.org/10.1056/NEJMcp1605501

Markey, P. M., Ivory, J. D., Slotter, E. B., Oliver, M. B., & Maglalang, O. (2020). He does not look like video games made him do it: Racial stereotypes and school shootings. *Psychology of Popular Media, 9*(4), 493–498. https://doi.org/10.1037/ppm0000255

McCabe, P. (1992). *The butcher boy.* Picador.

McDonald, A., & Walter, G. (2001). The portrayal of ECT in American movies. *Journal of ECT, 17,* 264–274. https://doi.org/10.1097/00124509-200112000-00006

McGoldrick, K. D. (2017). Tourette's and tic disorders. In S. Goldstein & M. DeVries (Eds.), *Handbook of DSM-5 disorders in children and adolescents* (pp. 417–430). Springer International; Springer Nature. https://doi.org/10.1007/978-3-319-57196-6_21

McGuire, M., Bell, S. K., Wilson, M., & Llorente, M. D. (2021). Why persons with serious mental illness end up homeless. In E. C. Ritchie & M. D. Llorente (Eds.), *Clinical management of the homeless patient: Social, psychiatric, and medical issues* (pp. 151–168). Springer Nature Switzerland AG. https://doi.org/10.1007/978-3-030-70135-2_10

McIntyre, R. S., Berk, M., Brietzke, E., Goldstein, B. I., López-Jaramillo, C., Kessing, L. V., Malhi, G. S., Nierenberg, A. A., Rosenblat, J. D., Majeed, A., Vieta, E., Vinberg, M., Young, A. H., & Mansur, R. B. (2020). Bipolar disorders. *Lancet, 396*(10265), 1841–1856. https://doi.org/10.1016/S0140-6736(20)31544-0

McIntyre, S., Goldsmith, S., Webb, A., Ehlinger, V., Hollung, S. J., McConnell, K., Arnaud, C., Smithers-Sheedy, H., Oskoui, M., Khandaker, G., & Himmelmann, K. (2022). Global prevalence of cerebral palsy: A systematic analysis. *Developmental Medicine & Child Neurology, 64*(12), 1494–1506. https://doi.org/10.1111/dmcn.15346

Mehlum, L. (2000). The Internet, suicide, and suicide prevention. *Crisis: The Journal of Crisis Intervention and Suicide Prevention, 21,* 186–188. https://doi.org/10.1027//0227-5910.21.4.186

Middleton, W. (2013). *Parent–child incest that extends into adulthood: A survey of international press reports,* 2007–2011. *Journal of Trauma & Dissociation, 14*(2), 184–197. https://doi.org/10.1080/15299732.2013.724341

Mikulincer, M., & Shaver, P. R. (Eds.). (2012). *The social psychology of morality: Exploring the causes of good and evil.* American Psychological Association. https://doi.org/10.1037/13091-000

Mitchell, W. J. T. (2020). *Mental traveler: A father, a son, and a journey through schizophrenia.* University of Chicago Press. https://doi.org/10.7208/chicago/9780226696096.001.0001

Mondragon, N. I., Munitis, A. E., & Txertudi, M. B. (2022). The breaking of secrecy: Analysis of the hashtag #MeTooInceste regarding testimonies of sexual incest abuse in childhood. *Child Abuse & Neglect, 123,* Article 105412. https://doi.org/10.1016/j.chiabu.2021.105412

Morales, E., Gauthier, V., Edwards, G., & Courtois, F. (2016). Masturbation practices of men and women with upper limb motor disabilities. *Sexuality and Disability, 34*(4), 417–431.

Mori, C., Park, J., Temple, J. R., & Madigan, S. (2022). Are youth sexting rates still on the rise? A meta-analytic update. *Journal of Adolescent Health, 70*(4), 531–539. https://doi.org/10.1016/j.jadohealth.2021.10.026

Nagata, J. M., Chu, J., Ganson, K. T., Murray, S. B., Iyer, P., Gabriel, K. P., Garber, A. K., Bibbins-Domingo, K., & Baker, F. C. (2023). Contemporary screen time modalities and disruptive behavior disorders in children: A prospective cohort study. *Journal of Child Psychology and Psychiatry, 64*(1), 125–135. https://doi.org/10.1111/jcpp.13673

Najdowski, C. J. (2017). Legal responses to nonconsensual pornography: Current policy in the United States and future directions for research. *Psychology, Public Policy, and Law, 23*(2), 154–165. https://doi.org/10.1037/law0000123

Nathan, D. (2011). *Sybil exposed: The extraordinary story behind the famous multiple personality case.* Free Press.

National Institute on Alcohol Abuse and Alcoholism. (2000). *Alcohol Alert. Children of alcoholics: Are they different?* (NIH Publication Number 09-PH 288). https://www.niaaa.nih.gov/publications/aa09.htm

National Institute of Mental Health. (2003). *In harm's way: Suicide in America* (NIH Publication Number 03-4594). https://www.nimh.nih.gov/publicat/NIMH-harmsway.pdf

National Institutes of Health. (2019, April 30). *Crisis and suicide prevention services struggle with demand after celebrity suicides* [News release]. https://www.nih.gov/news-events/news-releases/crisis-suicide-prevention-services-struggle-demand-after-celebrity-suicides

Neimeyer, G. J. (2013). On the origin of the specious: The evolution of the DSM-5 [Review of the books Diagnostic and Statistical Manual of Mental Disorders: DSM-5 (5th ed.), Desk Reference to the Diagnostic Criteria From DSM-5, & The Pocket Guide to the DSM-5 Diagnostic Exam, by American Psychiatric Association, American Psychiatric Association, & A. M. Nussbaum]. *PsycCRITIQUES, 58*(45).

Nelson, S. M., Griffin, C. A., Hein, T. C., Bowersox, N., & McCarthy, J. F. (2022). Personality disorder and suicide risk among patients in the veterans affairs health system. *Personality Disorders: Theory, Research, and Treatment, 13*(6), 563–571. https://doi.org/10.1037/per0000521

Nemeroff, C. B., & Craighead, W. Edward (2001). *The Corsini encyclopedia of psychology and behavioral science.* Wiley.

Nichter, B., Tsai, J., & Pietrzak, R. H. (2022). Prevalence, correlates, and mental health burden associated with homelessness in U.S. Military veterans. *Psychological*

Medicine. Advance online publication. https://doi.org/10.1017/S0033291722000617

Niederkrotenthaler, T., & Till, B. (2020). Effects of awareness material featuring individuals with experience of depression and suicidal thoughts on an audience with depressive symptoms: Randomized controlled trial. *Journal of Behavior Therapy and Experimental Psychiatry, 66,* Article 101515. https://doi.org/10.1016/j.jbtep.2019.101515

Niemiec, R. M. (2020). Character strengths cinematherapy: Using movies to inspire change, meaning, and cinematic elevation. *Journal of Clinical Psychology, 76*(8), 1447–1462. https://doi.org/10.1002/jclp.22997

Niemiec, R. M., & Ferland, D. (2006). The layers of transformation [Review of the film Batman Begins]. *PsycCRITIQUES, 51*(2).

Niemiec, R. M., & Wedding, D. (2006). The role of the psychotherapist in movies. *Advances in Medical Psychotherapy and Psychodiagnosis, 12,* 73–83.

Niemiec, R. M., & Wedding, D. (2014). *Positive psychology at the movies: Using films to build character strengths and wellbeing* (2nd ed.). Hogrefe.

NIMH. (2023, July 31). *Health statistics.* https://www.nimh.nih.gov/health/statistics

Noland, C. (2020). Communication and sexual self-help: Erotica, kink and the Fifty Shades of Grey phenomenon. *Sexuality & Culture: An Interdisciplinary Quarterly, 24*(5), 1457–1479

Norcross, J. C., & Norcross, J. (2005, October 2). A distant look at psychotherapeutic intimacy [Review of the film Intimate strangers]. *PsycCRITIQUES, 50*(41). https://doi.org/10.1037/05188711

Norcross, J. C., & Norcross, J. (2006, May 24). Psychotherapist conundrum: My son is sleeping with my patient [Review of the film *Prime*]. *PsycCRITIQUES, 51*(21). https://doi.org/10.1037/a0002505

Norden, M. (1994). *The cinema of isolation.* Rutgers University Press.

Norja, R., Karlsson, L., Antfolk, J., Nyman, T., & Korkman, J. (2021). How old was she? The accuracy of assessing the age of adolescents based on photos. *Nordic Psychology, 74*(1), 70–85. https://doi.org/10.1080/19012276.2021.1887752

North, C. S. (2015). The classification of hysteria and related disorders: Historical and phenomenological considerations. *Behavioral Sciences (Basel, Switzerland), 5*(4), 496–517. https://doi.org/10.3390/bs5040496

Oatley, K., & Niemiec, R. M. (2011). A view from the interior [Review of the media *Black Swan*, by D. Aronofsky, Dir.]. *PsycCRITIQUES, 56*(17). https://doi.org/10.1037/a0023595

Ogun, S. A., Arabambi, B., Oshinaike, O. O., & Akanji, A. (2022). A human calculator: A case report of a 27-year-old male with hypercalculia. *Neurocase, 28*(2), 158–162. https://doi.org/10.1080/13554794.2022.2046781

O'Hara, M. (2017). Hitchcock: Master of suspense and mental illness. In S. Packer (Ed.), *Mental illness in popular culture* (pp. 55–64). Praeger; ABC-CLIO.

Olver, M. E., Stockdale, K. C., & Wormith, J. S. (2011). A meta-analysis of predictors of offender treatment attrition and its relationship to recidivism. *Journal of Consulting and Clinical Psychology, 79*(1), 6–21. https://doi.org/10.1037/a0022200

Oppenheimer, R. (1956). Analogy in science. *American Psychologist, 11*(3), 127–135. https://doi.org/10.1037/h0046760

Orchowski, L. M., Spickard, B. A., & McNamara, J. R. (2006). Cinema and the valuing of psychotherapy: Implication for clinical practice. *Professional Psychology: Research and Practice, 37,* 506–514. https://doi.org/10.1037/0735-7028.37.5.506

Otgaar, H., Dodier, O., Garry, M., Howe, M. L., Loftus, E. F., Lynn, S. J., Mangiulli, I., McNally, R. J., & Patihis, L. (2022). Oversimplifications and misrepresentations in the repressed memory debate: A reply to Ross. *Journal of Child Sexual Abuse: Research, Treatment, & Program Innovations for Victims, Survivors, & Offenders, 32*(1), 116–126. https://doi.org/10.1080/10538712.2022.2133043

Owen, P. (2007). Dispelling myths about schizophrenia using film. *Journal of Applied Social Psychology, 37,* 60–75. https://doi.org/10.1111/j.0021-9029.2007.00147.x

Owen, P. R. (2012). Portrayals of schizophrenia by entertainment media: A content analysis contemporary movies. *Psychiatric Services, 63*(7), 655–659. https://doi.org/10.1176/appi.ps.201100371

Ozcakir, A., & Bilgel, N. (2014). Educating medical students about the personal meaning of terminal illness using the film, "Wit." *Journal of Palliative Medicine, 17*(8), 913–917. https://doi.org/10.1089/jpm.2013.0462

Packer, S. (Ed.). (2017). *Mental illness in popular culture.* Praeger; ABC-CLIO.

Pappas, S. (2020). What do we really know about kids and screens? *Monitor on Psychology, 51*(3), 42.

Park, N., & Peterson, C. (2009). Character strengths: Research and practice. *Journal of College and Character, 10*(4), np. https://doi.org/10.2202/1940-1639.1042

Pellecchia, M., Dickson, K. S., Vejnoska, S. F., & Stahmer, A. C. (2021). The autism spectrum: Diagnosis and epidemiology. In L. M. Glidden, L. Abbeduto, L. L. McIntyre, & M. J. Tassé (Eds.), *APA handbook of intellectual and developmental disabilities: Foundations* (pp. 207–237). American Psychological Association. https://doi.org/10.1037/0000194-009

Peters, B. C., Wood, W., Hepburn, S., & Moody, E. J. (2022). Preliminary efficacy of occupational therapy in an equine environment for youth with autism spectrum disorder. *Journal of Autism and Developmental Disorders, 52*(9), 4114–4128. https://doi.org/10.1007/s10803-021-05278-0

Peterson, C., & Seligman, M. E. P. (2004). *Character strengths and virtues: A handbook and classification.* American Psychological Association.

Petriceks, A. H. (2021). Comment on "Psychotherapy and the professional identity of psychiatry in the age of neuroscience." *Academic Psychiatry, 45*(2), 238–239. https://doi.org/10.1007/s40596-020-01266-1

Pinker, S. (2011). *The better angels of our nature: Why violence has declined.* Viking.

Piper, A., & Merskey, H. (2004). The persistence of folly: A critical examination of dissociative identity disorder: Part I: The excesses of an improbable concept. *Canadian Journal of Psychiatry, 49*(9), 592–600. https://doi.org/10.1177/070674370404900904

Pirkis, J., Blood, R. W., Francis, C., & McCallum, K. (2006). On-screen portrayals of mental illness: Extent, nature, and impacts. *Journal of Health Communication, 11*(5), 523–541. https://doi.org/10.1080/10810730600755889

Pizzo, A., Drobinin, V., Sandstrom, A., Zwicker, A., Howes Vallis, E., Fine, A., Rempel, S., Stephens, M., Howard, C., Villars, K., MacKenzie, L. E., Propper, L., Abidi, S., Lovas, D., Bagnell, A., Cumby, J., Alda, M., Uher, R., & Pavlova, B. (2020). Active behaviors and screen time in offspring of parents with major depressive disorder, bipolar disorder and schizophrenia. *Psychiatry Research, 285*, Article 112709. https://doi.org/10.1016/j.psychres.2019.112709

Ponterotto, J. G. (2012). *A psychobiography of Bobby Fischer.* Charles C. Thomas.

Potts, S. (2015). Review of The Bipolar Express: Manic depression and the movies [Review of the book The Bipolar Express: Manic depression and the movies, by D. Coleman]. *British Journal of Psychiatry, 206*(6), 525. https://doi.org/10.1192/bjp.bp.114.161810

Preyde, M., Parekh, S., & Heintzman, J. (2022). Electronic device utilization, bullying, school experiences, and discharge destination of youth admitted to an inpatient unit for psychiatric Illness. *Residential Treatment for Children & Youth, 39*(3), 261–277. https://doi.org/10.1080/0886571X.2021.1899883

Putnam, F. (1985). Multiple personality disorder. *Medical Aspects of Human Sexuality, 19,* 59–74.

Raffard, S., Bayard, S., Eisenblaetter, M., Tattard, P., Attal, J., Laraki, Y., & Capdevielle, D. (2023). Diminished capacity to make treatment decision for covid-19 vaccination in schizophrenia. *European Archives of Psychiatry and Clinical Neuroscience, 273*(2), 511–515. https://doi.org/10.1007/s00406-022-01413-9

Rahman, T., Grellner, K. A., Harry, B., Beck, N., & Lauriello, J. (2013). Infanticide in a case of folie à deux. *The American Journal of Psychiatry, 170*(10), 1110–1112. https://doi.org/10.1176/appi.ajp.2013.13010027

Raskin, J. (2021, January 4). *Medium.* https://repraskin.medium.com/statement-of-congressman-jamie-raskin-and-sarah-bloom-raskin-on-the-remarkable-life-of-tommy-raskin-f93b0bb5d184

Raskin, J. (2023). *Unthinkable: Trauma, truth, and the trials of American democracy.* HarperCollins.

Raskin, J. D., Maynard, D., & Gayle, M. C. (2022). Psychologist attitudes toward DSM-5 and its alternatives. *Professional Psychology: Research and Practice, 53*(6), 553–563. https://doi.org/10.1037/pro0000480

Rasmussen, C. E., & Jiang, Y. V. (2019). Judging social interaction in the Heider and Simmel movie. *Quarterly Journal of Experimental Psychology, 72*(9), 2350–2361. https://doi.org/10.1177/1747021819838764

Rastogi, M. (2011). Hurt people, hurt people [Review of the film Greenberg]. *PsycCRITIQUES, 56*(35).

Ratner, C. (2021). When "Sweetie" is not so sweet: Artificial intelligence and its implications for child pornography. *Family Court Review, 59*(2), 386–401. https://doi.org/10.1111/fcre.12576

Recupero, P. R., Rumschlag, J. S., & Rainey, S. E. (2021). The mental status exam at the movies: The use of film in a behavioral medicine course for physician assistants. *Academic Psychiatry, 46*(3), 325–330. https://doi.org/10.1007/s40596-021-01463-6

Reiss, D. M. (2017). [Review of the film The business of amateurs, by B. DeMars, Dir.]. *PsycCRITIQUES, 62*(37).

Ressler, R.K., Burgess, A.W., Souglas, J.E., Hartman, C.R., & D'Agostino, R.B. (1986). Sexual killers and their victims: Identifying patterns through crime scene analysis. *Journal of Interpersonal Violence, 1,* 288–308. https://doi.org/10.1177/088626086001003003

Rezaei-Fard, M., Lotfi, R., Rahimzadeh, M., & Merghati-Khoei, E. (2019). Effectiveness of sexual counseling using PLISSIT model to promote sexual function of women with spinal cord injury: A randomized controlled trial. *Sexuality and Disability, 37*(4), 511–519. https://doi.org/10.1007/s11195-019-09596-1

Riddle, K., & Martins, N. (2022). A content analysis of American primetime television: A 20-year update of the National Television Violence Studies. *Journal of Communication, 72*(1), 33–58. https://doi.org/10.1093/joc/jqab043

Roberston, L., Twenge, J. M., Joiner, T. E., & Cummins, K. (2022). Associations between screen time and internalizing disorder diagnoses among 9- to 10-year-olds. *Journal of Affective Disorders, 311,* 530–537. https://doi.org/10.1016/j.jad.2022.05.071

Rokeach, M. (1964). *Three Christs of Ypsilanti.* Knopf.

Rosenfarb, I. F. (2016). Are people with bipolar disorder merely eccentric? [Review of the film Infinitely Polar Bear, by M. Forbes, Dir.]. *PsycCRITIQUES, 61*(23).

Ross, C. (2022). False memory researchers misunderstand repression, dissociation and Freud. *Journal of Child Sexual Abuse, 31*(4), 488–502. https://doi.org/10.1080/10538712.2022.2067095

Rothman, E. F. (2021). *Pornography and public health.* Oxford University Press. https://doi.org/10.1093/oso/9780190075477.001.0001

Rozsa, M. (2019, July 15). *The real horror of the Midsommar ending.* https://www.salon.com/2019/07/15/the-real-horror-of-the-midsommar-ending/

Ruffalo, M. L. (2016). The social worker, psychotropic medication, and right to refuse. *Social Work, 61*(3), 271–272. https://doi.org/10.1093/sw/sww027

Sabbadini, A. (2015). The (mis)representation of psychoanalysis in film. In L. Huskinson & T. Waddell (Eds.), *Eavesdropping: The psychotherapist in film and television* (pp. 15–27). Routledge; Taylor & Francis.

Saint-Georges, C., Mahdhaoui, A., Chetouani, M., Cassel, R. S., Laznik, M.-C., Apicella, F., Muratori, P., Maestro, S., Muratori, F., & Cohen, D. (2011). Do parents recognize autistic deviant behavior long before diagnosis? Taking into account interaction using computational methods. *PLoS ONE, 6*(7), Article e22393. https://doi.org/10.1371/journal.pone.0022393

Sampogna, G., Elkholy, H., Baessler, F., Coskun, B., Pinto da Costa, M., Ramalho, R., Riese, F., & Fiorillo, A. (2022). Undergraduate psychiatric education: current situation and way forward. *BJPsych International, 19*(2), 34–36. https://doi.org/10.1192/bji.2021.48

Saunders, E.B., & Awad, G.A. (1991). Male adolescent sexual offenders: Exhibitionism and obscene phone calls. *Child Psychiatry and Human Development, 21*(3), 169–178. https://doi.org/10.1007/BF00705902

Savoie, V., Quayle, E., & Flynn, E. (2021). Prevalence and correlates of individuals with sexual interest in children: A systematic review. *Child Abuse & Neglect, 115,* Article 105005. https://doi.org/10.1016/j.chiabu.2021.105005

Schick, W. (2019, October 16). *Review: Josh Hayes's The Invisible Class is a film meant to inform, not entertain.* https://streetsensemedia.org/article/movie-review-homeless-video/

Schlozman, S. (2011). *The zombie autopsies: Secret notebooks from the apocalypse.* Grand Central.

Schlozman, S. (2017). [Review of the book Monsters, Demons and Psychopaths: Psychiatry and Horror Film, by F. E. Forcen]. *PsycCRITIQUES, 62*(25).

Schlozman, S. (2020). *Film.* Emerald.

Schultz, H. T. (2005). Hollywood's portrayal of psychologists and psychiatrists: Gender and professional training differences. In E. Cole & J. H. Daniel (Eds.), *Featuring females: Feminist analyses of media* (pp. 101–112). American Psychological Association. https://doi.org/10.1037/11213-007

Scott, A. O. (2011, November 10). Bride's mind is on another planet. *New York Times.* https://www.nytimes.com/2011/11/11/movies/lars-von-triers-melancholia-review.html

Seto, M. C. (2018). *Pedophilia and sexual offending against children: Theory, assessment, and intervention* (2nd ed.). American Psychological Association. https://doi.org/10.1037/0000107-000

Shand, J. P., Friedman, S. H., & Forcen, F. E. (2014). The horror, the horror: Stigma on screen. *The Lancet Psychiatry, 1*(6), 423–425. https://doi.org/10.1016/S2215-0366(14)00014-5

Shapiro, P., Tobia, A., & Aziz, R. (2018). Is the film Unbreakable really about PTSD with dissociation? *Academic Psychiatry, 42*(6), 871–872. https://doi.org/10.1007/s40596-018-0979-2

Shen, Y.-J. (2015). Cultivating multiculturally competent counselors through movies. *Journal of Creativity in Mental Health, 10*(2), 232–246. https://doi.org/10.1080/15401383.2014.959679

Shin J. H. (2022). Dementia epidemiology fact sheet 2022. *Annals of Rehabilitation Medicine, 46*(2), 53–59. https://doi.org/10.5535/arm.22027

Shriver, T. (2008, August 11). What Tropic Thunder thinks is funny. *Washington Post.* https://stopsayingretard.org/2008/08/12/what-tropic-thunder-thinks-is-funny/

Sieff, E.M. (2003). Media frames of mental illnesses: The potential impact of negative frames. *Journal of Mental Health, 12,* 259–269. https://doi.org/10.1080/0963823031000118249

Sienaert, P. (2016). Based on a true story? The portrayal of ECT in international movies and television programs. *Brain Stimulation, 9*(6), 882–891. https://doi.org/10.1016/j.brs.2016.07.005

Simonton, D.K. (2009). Teaching creativity: Current findings, trends, and controversies in the psychology of creativity. *Teaching of Psychology, 39*(3), 217–222. https://doi.org/10.1177/0098628312450444

Sontag, S. (1996, February 25). The decay of cinema. *The New York Times.* https://archive.nytimes.com/www.nytimes.com/books/00/03/12/specials/sontag-cinema.html?module=inline

Speck, L. G., Schöner, J., Bermpohl, F., Heinz, A., Gallinat, J., Majić, T., & Montag, C. (2019). Endogenous oxytocin response to film scenes of attachment and loss is pronounced in schizophrenia. *Social Cognitive and Affective Neuroscience, 14*(1), 109–117. https://doi.org/10.1093/scan/nsy110

Spirituality & Practice. (n.d.). *September 11: Directed by various directors*. https://www.spiritualityandpractice.com/films/reviews/view/6248?id=6248

Sprott, R. A., & Berkey, B. (2015). At the intersection of sexual orientation and alternative sexualities: Issues raised by Fifty Shades of Grey [Review of the film Fifty shades of grey, by S. Taylor-Johnson, Dir.]. *Psychology of Sexual Orientation and Gender Diversity, 2*(4), 506–507.

Stack, S., & Bowman, B. (2012). *Suicide movies: Social patterns 1900–2009*. Hogrefe.

Starkey, A. (2022, August 13). *How Alfred Hitchcock influenced Brian De Palma*. https://faroutmagazine.co.uk/how-alfred-hitchcock-influenced-brian-de-palma/

Steinberg, M. (1991). The spectrum of depersonalization: Assessment and treatment. In A. Tasman, & S. Goldfinger (Eds.), *Review of psychiatry* (Vol. 10; pp. 223–247). American Psychiatric Press.

Stern, S. C., & Barnes, J. L. (2019). Brief report: Does watching The Good Doctor affect knowledge of and attitudes toward autism? *Journal of Autism and Developmental Disorders, 49*(6), 2581–2588. https://doi.org/10.1007/s10803-019-03911-7

Steuer, J. (2015). The kids are not alright [Review of the media *The skeleton twins*, by C. Johnson, Dir.]. *PsycCRITIQUES, 60*(13). https://doi.org/10.1037/a0038596

St. Louis, K. O. (2020). Comparing and predicting public attitudes toward stuttering, obesity, and mental illness. *American Journal of Speech-Language Pathology, 29*(4), 2023–2038. https://doi.org/10.1044/2020_AJSLP-20-00038

Stringer, H. (2016). Therapy on camera. *Monitor on Psychology, 47*(11), 44–46. https://www.apa.org/monitor/2016/12/therapy-camera

Stringer, R. J. (2022). Waiting for the stop sign to turn green: Contemporary issues on drug and alcohol impaired driving policy. *American Journal of Criminal Justice, 47*, 735–748. https://link.springer.com/article/10.1007/s12103-022-09705-5#citeas

Stuart, H. (2003). Violence and mental illness: An overview. *World Psychiatry, 2*, 121–124.

Suskind, R. (2014a). *Life, animated: A story of sidekicks, heroes, and autism*. Kingswell.

Suskind, R. (2014b, March 9). Reaching my autistic son through Disney. *New York Times Magazine*. https://www.nytimes.com/2014/03/09/magazine/reaching-my-autistic-son-through-disney.html

Swan, A. B. (2021). From the box office to the classroom: Using films to explore psychological concepts. In H. Scherschel & D. S. Rudmann (Eds.), *Teaching tips: A compendium of conference presentations on teaching, 2020–21* (pp. 91–92). Society for the Teaching of Psychology.

Swenson, L.P., & Schwartz-Mette, R.A. (2011). Heists and heartbreak: Social pressures in the town [Review of the film The town]. *PsycCRITIQUES, 56*(28).

Szasz, T.S. (1974). *The myth of mental Illness: Foundations of a theory of personal conduct* (Revised ed.). Harper Row.

Szasz, T.S. (1977). *Psychiatric slavery: When confinement and coercion masquerade as cure*. Free Press.

Szmigiero, K. (2022). "We all go a little mad sometimes:" Representations of insanity in the films of Alfred Hitchcock. *Culture, Medicine, and Psychiatry, 47*(1), 152–175. https://doi.org/10.1007/s11013-022-09789-y

Tahira, A. C., Verjovski-Almeida, S., & Ferreira, S. T. (2021). Dementia is an age-independent risk factor for severity and death in COVID-19 inpatients. *Alzheimer's & Dementia, 17*(11), 1818–1831. https://doi.org/10.1002/alz.12352

Taylor, E. (2012). Did Jung really sleep with Sabina? [A review of the film A dangerous method]. *PsycCRITIQUES, 57*(16).

Taylor, K. (2009). *Cruelty: Human evil and the human brain*. Oxford University Press.

Taylor, T., & Hsu, M. (2003). *Digital cinema: The Hollywood insider's guide to the evolution of storytelling*. Michael Wiese.

Temko, J. E., Grigorian, A., Barrios, C., Lekawa, M., Nahmias, L., Kuza, C. M., & Nahmias, J. (2020). Race, age, and lack of insurance increase risk of suicide attempt in trauma patients. *Archives of Suicide Research*, 26(2), 846–860. https://doi.org/10.1080/13811118.2020.1838370

Tenenbaum, E. J., Carpenter, K. L. H., Sabatos-DeVito, M., Hashemi, J., Vermeer, S., Sapiro, G., & Dawson, G. (2020). A six-minute measure of vocalizations in toddlers with autism spectrum disorder. *Autism Research, 13*(8), 1373–1382. https://doi.org/10.1002/aur.2293 https://doi.org/10.1002/aur.2293

Thibault, R. T., Dahl, L., & Raz, A. (2019). Why neuroimaging can't diagnose autism. In A. Raz & R. T. Thibault (Eds.), *Casting light on the dark side of brain imaging* (pp. 79–82). Elsevier Academic Press. https://doi.org/10.1016/B978-0-12-816179-1.00012-8

Till, B., Tran, U. S., Voracek, M., Sonneck, G., & Niederkrotenthaler, T. (2014). Associations between film preferences and risk factors for suicide: An online survey. *PLoS ONE, 9*(7), Article e102293. https://doi.org/10.1371/journal.pone.0102293

Trachsel, M., Biller-Andorno, N., Gaab, J., Sadler, J.Z., & Tekin, Ş. (Eds.). (2021). *The Oxford handbook of psychotherapy ethics*. Oxford University Press. https://doi.org/10.1093/oxfordhb/9780198817338.001.0001

Trachtenberg, R. (1986). Destigmatizing mental illness. *The Psychiatric Hospital, 17*, 111–114.

Trawver, K. R., Oby, S., Kominkiewicz, L., Kominkiewicz, F. B., & Whittington, K. (2019). Homelessness in America: An overview. In H. Larkin, A. Aykanian, & C. L. Streeter (Eds.), *Homelessness prevention and intervention in social work: Policies, programs, and practices* (pp. 3–39). Springer Nature Switzerland AG. https://doi.org/10.1007/978-3-030-03727-7_1

Treffert, D. A. (2009). The savant syndrome: An extraordinary condition. A synopsis: past, present, future. Philosophical Transactions of the Royal Society of London. *Series B, Biological Sciences, 364*(1522), 1351–1357. https://doi.org/10.1098/rstb.2008.0326

Uva, J. L. (1995). Autoerotic asphyxiation in the United States. *Journal of Forensic Sciences, 40*(4), 574–581. https://doi.org/10.1520/JFS13828J

Valentine, D., & Freeman, M. (2002). Film portrayals of social workers doing child welfare work. *Child and Adolescent Social Work Journal, 19*(6), 455–471. https://doi.org/10.1023/A:1021145713542

VanDyke, M. M., & Anderson, V. H. (2013). Acquiring fear, learning safety, and modeling growth: The Croods flourish [Review of the film The Croods]. *PsycCRITIQUES, 59*(6). https://doi.org/10.1037/a0035402

Van Roost, K., Horn, M., & Koski, A. (2022). Child marriage or statutory rape? A comparison of law and practice across the United States. *Journal of Adolescent Health, 70*(3, Suppl), S72–S77.

VA Office of Mental Health and Suicide Prevention. (2020). *2019 National veteran suicide prevention annual report.* VA Office of Mental Health and Suicide Prevention, Department of Veterans Affairs. https://www.mentalhealth.va.gov/docs/data-sheets/2022/2022-National-Veteran-Suicide-Prevention-Annual-Report-FINAL-508.pdf

Vassar, M., Mazur, A., Hillier, S., Wilson, R., Demand, A., Lu, K., & Peyok, D. (2020). Evaluation of accuracy of portrayals of posttraumatic stress disorder in popular war movies. *Journal of Nervous and Mental Disease, 208*(7), 579–580. https://doi.org/10.1097/NMD.0000000000001167

Vera-Gray, F., McGlynn, C., Kureshi, I., & Butterby, K. (2021). Sexual violence as a sexual script in mainstream online pornography. *British Journal of Criminology, 61*(5), 1243–1260. https://doi.org/10.1093/bjc/azab035

von Krafft-Ebing, R. (1898). *Psychopathia sexualis: A medico-jegal study.* F. A. Davis Co.

Wahl, O. (1995). *Media madness: Public images of mental illness.* Rutgers University Press.

Wahl, O. F. (2009). Depictions of mental illnesses in children's media. *Journal of Mental Health, 12*(3), 249–258. https://doi.org/10.1080/0963823031000118230

Wahl, O., Reiss, M., & Thompson, C. A. (2018). Film psychotherapy in the 21st century. *Health Communication, 33*(3), 238–245. https://doi.org/10.1080/10410236.2016.1255842

Walker, E. F., Grimes, K. E., Davis, D. M., & Smith, A. J. (1993). Childhood precursors of schizophrenia: Facial expressions of emotion. *The American Journal of Psychiatry, 150*(11), 1654–1660. https://doi.org/10.1176/ajp.150.11.1654

Walker, E. F., Savoie, T., & Davis, D. (1994). Neuromotor precursors of schizophrenia. *Schizophrenia Bulletin, 20*(3), 441–451. https://doi.org/10.1093/schbul/20.3.441

Walter, G., McDonald, A., Rey, J., & Rosen, A. (2002). Medical student knowledge and attitudes regarding ECT prior to and after viewing ECT scenes from movies. *Journal of ECT, 18*(1), 43–46. https://doi.org/10.1097/00124509-200203000-00012

Warburton, W. (2012). Growing up fast and furious in a media saturated world. In W. Warburton & D. Braunstein (Eds.), *Growing up fast and furious: Reviewing the impacts of violent and sexualised media on children* (pp. 1–33). Federation Press.

Ward, O. (1999). John Langdon Down: The man and the message. *Down Syndrome Research and Practice*, *6*(1), 19–24. https://doi.org/10.3104/perspectives.94

Watters, E. (2010). *Crazy like us: The globalization of the American psyche.* Free Press.

Wedding, D. (2000). Cognitive distortions in the poetry of Anne Sexton. *Suicide & Life-Threatening Behavior, 30,* 150–154.

Wedding, D. (2001). The portrayal of alcohol and alcoholism in the western genre. *Journal of Alcohol & Drug Education, 46,* 3–11.

Wedding, D. (2017). Public education and media relations in psychology. *American Psychologist, 72*(8), 764–777. https://doi.org/10.1037/amp0000202

Wedding, D., & Niemiec, R. (2003). The clinical use of films in psychotherapy. *Journal of Clinical Psychology, 59*(2), 207–215. d https://doi.org/10.1002/jclp.10142

Wedding, D., Wongpakaran, N., & Wongpakaran, T. (2017). The use of films to enhance pedagogy in the psychology classroom. In G. J. Rich, U. P. Gielen, & H. Takooshian (Eds.), *Advances in cultural psychology: Constructing human development. Internationalizing the teaching of psychology* (p. 61–71). IAP Information Age.

Wehmeyer, M. L., Buntinx, W. H. E., Lachapelle, Y., Luckas-son, R. A., Schalock, R. L., Verdugo, M. A, Borthwick-Duffy, S., Bradley, V., Craig, E. M., Coulter, D. L., Gomez, S. C., Reeve, A., Shogren, K. A., Snell, M. E., Spreat, S., Tassé, M. J., Thompson, J. R., & Yeager, M. H. (2008). The intellectual disability construct and its relation to human functioning. *Intellectual and Developmental Disabilities, 46,* 311–318.

Werner, A. (2005). American Prometheus: The Triumph and Tragedy of J. Robert Oppenheimer [Book Review]. *The American Journal of Psychiatry, 162*(12), 2402–2402. https://doi.org/10.1176/appi.ajp.162.12.2402

West, L. (2023, March 10). The Whale is not a masterpiece – It is a joyless, harmful fantasy of fat squalor. *The Guardian.* https://www.theguardian.com/film/2023/mar/10/lindy-west-on-the-whale

White, J.W., Koss, M.P., & Kazdin, A.E. (Eds.). (2011). *Violence against women and children: Vol. 1: Mapping the terrain.* American Psychological Association.

Wilson, A. H., Blake, B. J., Taylor, G. A., & Hannings, G. (2013). Cinemeducation: Teaching family assessment skills using full-length movies. *Public Health Nursing, 30*(3), 239–245. https://doi.org/10.1111/phn.12025

Wilson, N., Heath, D., Heath, T., Gallagher, P., & Huthwaite, M. (2014). Madness at the movies: Prioritised movies for self-directed learning by medical students. *Australasian Psychiatry, 22*(5), 450–453. https://doi.org/10.1177/1039856214545550

World Health Organization. (1992). *ICD-10 classifications of mental and behavioural disorder: Clinical descriptions and diagnostic guidelines.*

World Health Organization. (2022). *Dementia.* https://www.who.int/news-room/fact-sheets/detail/dementia

World Population Review. (2022, October 10). *Age of consent by country,* 2022. https://worldpopulationreview.com/country-rankings/age-of-consent-by-country

Xie, H., Ainsworth, A., & Caldwell, L. (2021). Grandparent(s) coresidence and physical activity/screen time among Latino children in the United States. *Families, Systems, & Health, 39*(2), 282–292. https://doi.org/10.1037/fsh0000601

Young, L. R. (2011). [Review of the film Love and other drugs, by E. Zwick, Dir.]. *PsycCRITIQUES, 56*(37).

Zhang, L., Ravdin, L.D., Relkin, N., Zimmerman, R.D., Jordan, B., Lathan, W.E., & Ulug, A.M. (2003). Increased diffusion in the brain of professional boxers: A preclinical sign of traumatic brain injury. *American Journal of Neuroradiololgy, 24*(1), 52–57.

Zimbardo, P. (2007). *The Lucifer effect: Understanding how good people turn evil.* Random House.

Zimmerman, J.N. (2003). *People like ourselves: Portrayals of mental illness in the movies.* Scarecrow Press.

Appendices

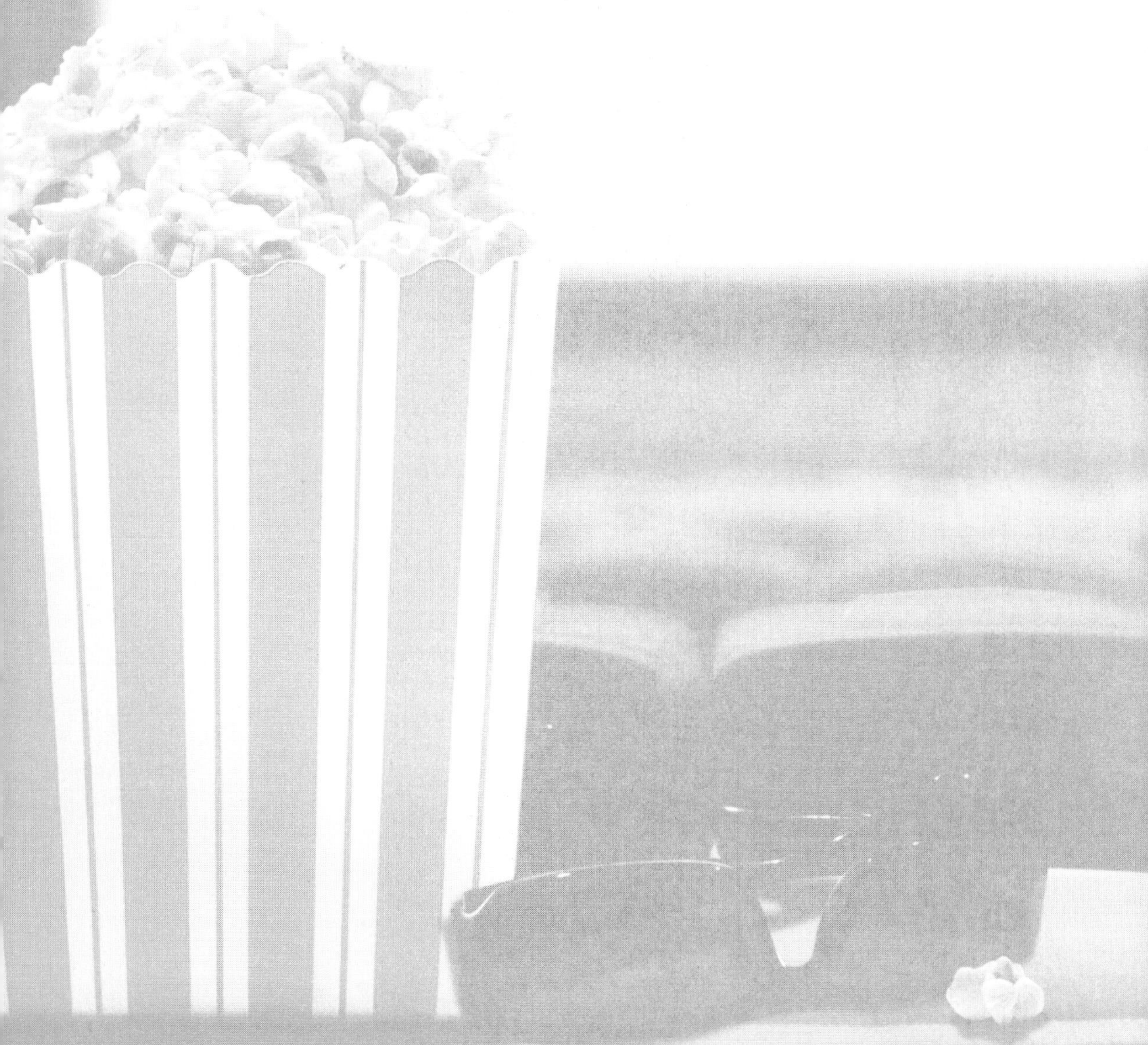

The American Film Institute's Top 50 Heroes and Villains

Heroes

1. **Atticus Finch**
   To Kill a Mockingbird
2. **Indiana Jones**
   Raiders of the Lost Ark
3. **James Bond**
   Dr. No
4. **Rick Blaine**
   Casablanca
5. **Will Kane**
   High Noon
6. **Clarice Starling**
   The Silence of the Lambs
7. **Rocky Balboa**
   Rocky
8. **Ellen Ripley**
   Aliens
9. **George Bailey**
   It's a Wonderful Life
10. **T. E. Lawrence**
    Lawrence of Arabia
11. **Jefferson Smith**
    Mr. Smith Goes to Washington
12. **Tom Joad**
    The Grapes of Wrath
13. **Oskar Schindler**
    Schindler's List
14. **Han Solo**
    Star Wars
15. **Norma Rae Webster**
    Norma Rae
16. **Shane**
    Shane
17. **Harry Callahan**
    Dirty Harry
18. **Robin Hood**
    The Adventures of Robin Hood
19. **Virgil Tibbs**
    In the Heat of the Night
20. **Butch Cassidy and the Sundance Kid**
    Butch Cassidy and the Sundance Kid
21. **Mahatma Gandhi**
    Gandhi
22. **Spartacus**
    Spartacus
23. **Terry Malloy**
    On the Waterfront
24. **Thelma Dickerson & Louise Sawyer**
    Thelma & Louise
25. **Lou Gehrig**
    The Pride of the Yankees
26. **Superman**
    Superman
27. **Bob Woodward & Carl Bernstein**
    All The President's Men
28. **Juror #8**
    12 Angry Men
29. **General George Patton**
    Patton
30. **Luke Jackson**
    Cool Hand Luke
31. **Erin Brockovich**
    Erin Brockovich
32. **Philip Marlowe**
    The Big Sleep
33. **Marge Gunderson**
    Fargo
34. **Tarzan**
    Tarzan the Ape Man
35. **Alvin York**
    Sergeant York
36. **Rooster Cogburn**
    True Grit
37. **Obi-Wan Knobi**
    Star Wars
38. **The Tramp**
    City Lights
39. **Lassie**
    Lassie Come Home
40. **Frank Serpico**
    Serpico

41. **Arthur Chipping**
    Goodbye Mr. Chips
42. **Father Edward**
    Boys Town
43. **Moses**
    The Ten Commandments
44. **Jimmy "Popeye" Doyle**
    The French Connection
45. **Zorro**
    The Mark of Zorro
46. **Batman**
    Batman
47. **Karen Silkwood**
    Silkwood
48. **Terminator**
    Terminator 2: Judgment Day
49. **Andrew Beckett**
    Philadelphia
50. **General Maximus Decimus Meridus**
    Gladiator

Villains

1. **Dr. Hannibal Lecter**
   The Silence of the Lambs
2. **Norman Bates**
   Psycho
3. **Darth Vader**
   The Empire Strikes Back
4. **The Wicked Witch of the West**
   The Wizard of Oz
5. **Nurse Ratched**
   One Flew Over the Cuckoo's Nest
6. **Mr. Potter**
   It's a Wonderful Life
7. **Alex Forrest**
   Fatal Attraction
8. **Phyllis Dietrichson**
   Double Indemnity
9. **Regan MacNeil**
   The Exorcist
10. **The Queen**
    Snow White and the Seven Dwarfs
11. **Michael Corleone**
    The Godfather: Part II
12. **Alex De Large**
    Clockwork Orange
13. **HAL 9000**
    2001: A Space Odyssey
14. **The Alien**
    Alien
15. **Amon Goeth**
    Schindler's List
16. **Noah Cross**
    Chinatown
17. **Annie Wilkes**
    Misery
18. **The Shark**
    Jaws
19. **Captain Bligh**
    Mutiny on the Bounty
20. **Man**
    Bambi
21. **Mrs. John Iselin**
    The Manchurian Candidate
22. **Terminator**
    The Terminator
23. **Eve Harrington**
    All About Eve
24. **Gordo Gekko**
    Wall Street
25. **Jack Torrance**
    The Shining
26. **Cody Jarrett**
    White Heat
27. **Martians**
    The War of the Worlds
28. **Max Cady**
    Cape Fear
29. **Reverend Harry Powell**
    The Night of the Hunter
30. **Travis Bickle**
    Taxi Driver
31. **Mrs. Danvers**
    Rebecca
32. **Clyde Barrow & Bonnie Parker**
    Bonnie and Clyde
33. **Count Dracula**
    Dracula
34. **Dr. Szell**
    Marathon Man

35. **J. J. Hunsecker**
Sweet Smell of Success
36. **Frank Booth**
Blue Velvet
37. **Harry Lime**
The Third Man
38. **Caesar Enrico Bandello**
Little Caesar
39. **Cruella De Vil**
One Hundred and One Dalmatians
40. **Freddy Krueger**
A Nightmare on Elm Street
41. **Joan Crawford**
Mommie Dearest
42. **Tom Powers**
The Public Enemy
43. **Regina Giddens**
The Little Foxes
44. **Baby Jane Hudson**
Whatever Happened to Baby Jane?
45. **The Joker**
Batman
46. **Hans Gruber**
Die Hard
47. **Tony Montana**
Scarface
48. **Verbal Kint**
The Usual Suspects
49. **Auric Goldfinger**
Goldfinger
50. **Alonzo Harris**
Training Day

Note. Reprinted with permission from "AFI's 100 Greatest Heroes and Villains," by The American Film Institute. https://www.afi.com/afis-100-years-100-heroes-villians/

Syllabus for a Sample Course in Abnormal Psychology That Integrates Films

Movies and Mental Illness: Understanding Psychopathology

Course Description

This course focuses on the portrayal of mental illness in films. Representations of psychopathological states in films will be examined within the context of contemporary social issues such as stigma and discrimination. Major mental disorders will be highlighted.

Objectives

Upon completion of this course, the student will be able to:

- discuss the social influence of films;
- discuss the significance of film in the public perception of mental illnesses;
- compare behavioral symptoms of major mental disorders;
- identify discrimination and stigma associated with mental disorders;
- analyze the portrayal of various mental illnesses in films.

Required Text

Wedding, D. (2024). *Movies and mental illness: Using films to understand psychopathology* (5th ed.). Hogrefe.

Learning Experiences

Seminar, Dyad Presentation, Videos, and Written Papers

Students should watch all of the films outside of class, preferably in small groups. All films selected are well known and will be easily available through DVD rental outlets or on the Internet. Please come to class prepared to discuss whether each week's film presented an accurate portrayal of the condition being discussed. In addition to the assigned film, each student will be required to view a second film discussed in each week's relevant chapter; come to class prepared to give a 5-minute synopsis of the film and your opinion about the accuracy of the disorder being portrayed. Sign up before each session on the class homepage to avoid duplicate selections.

(a) Tuesdays 10 a.m.–12	(b) Thursdays 10 a.m.–12	Topic	Readings and films to view before coming to class
Sep 2	Sep 4	(a) Introduction to the class (b) Films and psychopathology	(b) Chapter 1: Films and Psychopathology
Sep 9	Sep 11	(a & b) Neurodevelopmental disorders	(a) Chapter 2: Neurodevelopmental Disorders (b) *Crip Camp* (2020)
Sep 16	Sep 18	(a & b) Schizophrenia spectrum and other psychotic disorders	(a) Chapter 3: Schizophrenia Spectrum and Other Psychotic Disorders (b) *Horse Girl* (2020)
Sep 23	Sep 25	(a & b) Bipolar and depressive disorders	(a) Chapter 4: Bipolar and Depressive Disorders (b) *Touched With Fire* (2015)
Sep 30	Oct 2	(a & b) Anxiety and obsessive-compulsive disorders	(a) Chapter 5: Anxiety and Obsessive-Compulsive Disorders (b) *The Aviator* (2004)
Oct 7	Oct 9	(a & b) Trauma- and stressor-related disorders	(a) Chapter 6: Trauma- and Stressor-Related Disorders (b) *The Fallout* (2021)
Oct 14	Oct 16	(a & b) Dissociative disorders	(a) Chapter 7: Dissociative Disorders (b) *Psycho* (1960)
Oct 21	**Oct 23**	**(a) Review session** **(b) Midterm examination**	**No readings or film**
Oct 28	Oct 30	(a & b) Somatic symptom, feeding, eating, elimination, and sleep–wake disorders	(a) Chapter 8: Sleep–Wake, Eating, and Somatic Symptom Disorders (b) *To the Bone* (2017)
Nov 4	Nov 6	(a & b) Sexual dysfunctions and gender dysphoria	(a) Chapter 9: Gender Dysphoria and Sexual Dysfunctions (b) *Good Luck to You, Leo Grande* (2022)
Nov 11	Nov 13	(a & b) Disruptive, impulse-control, and conduct disorders	(a) Chapter 10: Disruptive, Impulse-Control, and Conduct Disorders (b) *We Need to Talk About Kevin* (2011)
Nov 18	Nov 20	(a & b) Substance-related and addictive disorders	(a) Chapter 11: Substance-Related and Addictive Disorders (b) *Winter's Bone* (2010)
Nov 25	Nov 27	(a & b) Neurocognitive disorders	(a) Chapter 12: Neurocognitive Disorders (b) *The Father* (2020)

(a) Tuesdays 10 a.m. – 12	(b) Thursdays 10 a.m. – 12	Topic	Readings and films to view before coming to class
Dec 2	Dec 4	(a & b) Personality disorders and paraphilic disorders	(a) Chapters 13 & 14: Personality Disorders; Paraphilic Disorders (b) *No Country for Old Men* (2007)
Dec 9	Dec 11	(a & b) Violence, physical and sexual abuse, and treatment	(a) Chapters 15 & 16: Violence and Physical and Sexual Abuse; Treatment (b) *Till* (2022)
Final Exam			

Note. Adapted from the syllabus Danny Wedding used in an abnormal psychology course he taught at Yonsei University in Seoul, Korea, where he was the 2008–2009 Fulbright-Yonsei Distinguished Scholar.

Recommended Websites

Movies in General

Internet Movie Database (the largest movie database)
https://www.imdb.com

Movie Review Query Engine (over 76,000 movie titles; over 748,000 reviews)
https://www.mrqe.com

American Film Institute
https://www.afi.com

Independent Movies
https://www.indiewire.com

Other Recommended Movie Databases

Rotten Tomatoes (movie database)
https://www.rottentomatoes.com

Literature, Arts, and Medicine Database
https://medhum.med.nyu.edu

AMC Film site
https://www.filmsite.org

Films Featuring Mental Disorders
https://en.wikipedia.org/wiki/List_of_films_featuring_mental_disorders

Films Involving Disabilities
https://iris.peabody.vanderbilt.edu/resources/films/

Cinematherapy.com
https://www.cinematherapy.com

Hollywood Entertainment Corporation
https://www.reel.com (coming soon)

Internet Movie Network
https://www.movieweb.com

Twelve Misconceptions About Mental Illness and Mental Health Professionals Perpetuated by Movies

Misconception	Film examples
Love alone conquers mental illness.	*Benny & Joon* (1993) *Mozart and the Whale* (2005) *Stateside* (2004) *Wilbur Wants to Kill Himself* (2002) *Matchstick Men* (2003)
People with mental illness are violent.	*Keane* (2004) *Edmond* (2005) *The Killing of John Lennon* (2006) *Nixon* (2004) *Peacock* (2010) *Nightmare on Elm Street* (1984) *The Adopted One* (2020)
People with mental illness are wild and crazy.	*Michael Clayton* (2007) *Mozart and the Whale* (2005) *Blake Snake Moan* (2006) *The Big White* (2005) *I'm a Cyborg, But That's OK* (2007)
People called delusional or psychotic are telling the truth and being mentally healthy and grounded.	*Flightplan* (2005) *K-Pax* (2001) *Happy Accidents* (2000) *The Jacket* (2005)
Parents cause schizophrenia, autism, etc. (the myth of the schizophrenogenic parent).	*Clean, Shaven* (1993) *Shine* (1996)
All mental illness has a traumatic etiology.	*The Fisher King* (1991) *The Snake Pit* (1948) *The Three Faces of Eve* (1957) *K-Pax* (2001) *Nurse Betty* (2000)
Schizophrenia is the same as dissociative identity disorder, gender identity disorder, etc.	*Me, Myself & Irene* (2000) *Dressed to Kill* (1980)

Misconception	Film examples
Psychiatric hospitals are dangerous places, or at least unhelpful; the patients are not sick, they are harmlessly eccentric or misdiagnosed.	*One Flew Over the Cuckoo's Nest* (1975) *Asylum* (2005) *The Jacket* (2005) *King of Hearts* (1966) *House of Fools* (2002)
Psychiatric treatment (e.g., ECT, medications) blocks creativity and intelligence.	*A Beautiful Mind* (2001) *A Clockwork Orange* (1971)
It is liberating to discontinue psychiatric treatment on one's own (e.g., medications).	*Garden State* (2004)
The treatment of mental illness involves boundary violations by a therapist (these are usually sexual).	*The Prince of Tides* (1991) *Final Analysis* (1992) *Mr. Jones* (1993) *Tin Cup* (1996) *Numb* (2007) *A Dangerous Method* (2011)
Psychological diagnoses are routinely made up by psychologists and patients, and touted as a standard condition.	*Me, Myself & Irene* (2000) Advanced delusionary schizophrenia with involuntary narcissistic rage *Asylum* (2005): Severe personality disorder with features of morbid jealousy *The Ringer* (2005): Highly functioning developmental disability

Portrayals of Psychotherapists in Movies

For more details see Niemiec & Wedding (2006), The role of the psychotherapist in movies, *Advances in Medical Psychotherapy and Psychodiagnosis, 12*, 73–83.
* = Both balanced and unbalanced portrayals are found in this film.

Balanced Portrayals

A Beautiful Mind (2001)
Another Year (2010)
Antwone Fisher (2003)
David and Lisa (1962)
Don Juan DeMarco (1994)
Donnie Darko (2001)
Elling (2002)
Equus (1977)
Girl, Interrupted (1999)
Good Will Hunting (1997)
Gothika (2003)*
Hope Springs (2012)
Hollywood Ending (2002)
Identity (2003)
Intimate Strangers (2004)
K-Pax (2001)
Klepto (2003)
Lars and the Real Girl (2007)
Life Itself (2018)
Manic (2003)
Ordinary People (1980)
Psycho (1960)
Stateside (2004)
Transamerica (2005)*
What Happens in Vegas (2008)
Three Christs (2020)

Unbalanced Portrayals

Analyze This (1998)
Antichrist (2009)
Anything Else (2003)
Asylum (2005)
Basic Instinct 2 (2006)
Batman Begins (2005)
Bliss (1997)
Changeling (2008)
The Chorus (2004)
A Dangerous Method (2011)
Deconstructing Harry (1997)
The Departed (2006)
Dirty, Filthy Love (2004)
Final Analysis (1992)
The Great New Wonderful (2005)
Happiness (1998)
Happy Accidents (2000)
Harvey (1950)
High Anxiety (1977)
I Am Sam (2001)
The Island (2005)
Jesus of Montreal (1989)
Mr. Jones (1993)
Normal (2003)
Numb (2007)
One Flew Over the Cuckoo's Nest (1975)
Prime (2005)
Shrink (2009)
Shutter Island (2010)
Stay (2005)
Temple Grandin (2010)
The Adopted One (2020)
The Silence of the Lambs (1991)
The Snake Pit (1948)
Twelve Monkeys (1995)
Vanilla Sky (2001)
What About Bob? (1991)
Wilbur Wants to Kill Himself (2002)

Films Illustrating Psychopathology

Contents

Key to Ratings

ΨΨΨΨΨ	A must-see film that combines artistry with psychological relevance
ΨΨΨΨ	Highly recommended both as art and as professional education
ΨΨΨ	A good film that will interest almost any mental health professional
ΨΨ	Mildly interesting and somewhat educational; possibly worth your time
Ψ	Description provided for your information only; don't bother with the film

Neurodevelopmental Disorders

Adam (2009) Drama-Romance ΨΨΨΨ
Beth gradually falls in love with Adam, a high-functioning man with autism spectrum disorder, but she eventually decides she can't make a permanent commitment to him. The film is sympathetic in its portrayal of Adam and is genuinely helpful in illustrating some of the challenges faced by highly intelligent people coping with autism spectrum disorder.

Antonia's Line (1995) Comedy ΨΨΨΨ
A film with unforgettable characters, including Loony Lips and Dede, two people with intellectual disabilities who fall in love and get married. The film is a joyful celebration of life and family.

Any Day Now (2012) Drama ΨΨΨ
Two gay men in a loving, committed relationship must fight to maintain custody of the special needs son they adopt. Based on a true story.

Being There (1979) Comedy ΨΨΨΨ
Peter Sellers plays the role of a gardener with borderline IQ who finds himself caught up in a comedy of errors in which his simple platitudes are mistaken for wisdom. This film is a precursor to *Forrest Gump*.

Ben X (2007) Drama ΨΨΨ
A young man with an autism spectrum disorder loses himself in videogames while plotting revenge on his classmates who torment him.

Best Boy (1979) Documentary ΨΨΨΨ
Ira Wohl's moving tribute to his cousin (a man with an intellectual disability) examines the options facing the young man when his father dies, and his aging mother is no longer able to care for him. This film won an Academy Award for Best Documentary film.

Best Man: "Best Boy" and All of Us Twenty Years Later (1997) Documentary ΨΨΨ
A sequel to the 1979 film, *Best Boy*, documenting that director Ira Wohl's cousin has a rich, full, and meaningful life, despite his cognitive limitations.

Beyond Borders (2009, Belgium) Drama ΨΨΨ
A short film that interweaves three stories - those of a boy with an intellectual disability (Down syndrome), a woman with multiple sclerosis, and a blind man. The common theme that binds them is the importance of positive relationships.

Big White, The (2005) Drama/Crime Ψ
Black comedy starring Robin Williams, Holly Hunter, Giovanni Ribisi, and Woody Harrelson. Margaret (Hunter) is diagnosed with Tourette's disorder (although it doesn't match DSM-5 criteria); she has little self-control over her verbal outbursts.

Bill (1981) Biography ΨΨ
Mickey Rooney won an Emmy for playing a man with an intellectual disability who was forced to leave an institution after 46 years in this made-for-TV movie.

Black Balloon, The (2008, Australia) Drama-Romance ΨΨΨΨ
A teenage boy in a dysfunctional family copes with the challenges of caring for his brother with autism spectrum disorder while his mother is bedridden because of pregnancy. The film provides excellent illustrations of the combined stresses of adolescence and caregiving.

Boy Who Could Fly, The (1986) Fantasy ΨΨ
Love story about the affection that develops between a teenage girl whose father has just committed suicide and a new neighbor who is autistic.

Breaking and Entering (2006) Drama ΨΨΨ
A Bosnian boy robs an architect who secretly follows the young thief home and eventually becomes involved with the boy's mother. The architect and his live-in girlfriend are raising her adolescent daughter who has a pervasive developmental disorder, but the stress of caring for the child interferes with the adults' relationship. The film also depicts seasonal affective disorder.

Charly (1968) Drama ΨΨΨ
Cliff Robertson won an Oscar for his role as a man with an intellectual disability who is transformed into a genius, only to find himself eventually returning to his previous level of disability. (Compare this film with *Molly* [1999] and *Flowers for Algernon* [2000].)

Charlie Bartlett (2007) Ψ
A teenage boy is diagnosed with ADHD and prescribed Ritalin. He eventually teams up with another boy to begin selling the drug to his classmates.

Child Is Waiting, A (1963) Drama ΨΨ
Burt Lancaster and Judy Garland star in this film about the treatment of children with intellectual disabilities living in institutions.

City of Lost Children, The (1995, France) Fantasy-Drama ΨΨΨ
A mad scientist is aging prematurely so he tries to capture children to steal their dreams. The circus strongman

named One (Ron Perlman), who has a developmental disability, teams up with a bold, bright young girl to save the children.

Crip Camp (2020) Documentary ΨΨΨΨΨ
A wonderful film about the development and history of Camp Jened, a summer camp in the Catskills for young people with various disabilities. The history of the disability rights movement is beautifully documented.

"There was a romance in the air if you wanted to experience it. I never dated outside of camp. But at Jened, you could have make-out sessions behind the bunks and different places like that."

Judith Heumann, a disability right activist, describing life at *Crip Camp*

Dangerous Woman, A (1993) Drama ΨΨ
Debra Winter plays a woman with a mild intellectual disability who becomes involved with an itinerant alcoholic.

Day in the Death of Joe Egg, A (1972) Comedy ΨΨ
British black comedy that examines the issue of mercy killing.

Dead Mother, The (1993, Spain) ΨΨΨ
Drama-Thriller
Child with characteristics of autism and a developmental disability witnessed her mother's murder by a petty thief who kidnaps the child, now a woman, 2 decades later.

Dodes'ka-den (Clickety-Clack) (1970, Japan)
Drama ΨΨΨ
Akira Kurosawa film about a boy with an intellectual disability living in the slums of Tokyo. This was Kurosawa's first color film. Although now regarded as a classic, this film was not well received by the public or by critics when it was released, and its failure led to Kurosawa's attempt to commit suicide by slashing his wrists in 1971. Kurosawa survived the suicide attempt, and eventually died at age 88 in Tokyo.

Dominick and Eugene (1988) Drama ΨΨΨΨ
This is a coming-of-age film about two brothers. Eugene, who is finishing medical school, is the primary caregiver for his brother Dominick who has an intellectual disability and works as a Pittsburgh trash collector. Dominick's income supports the brothers, but Eugene needs to move to California for his residency.

Extremely Loud and Incredibly Close (2011) ΨΨΨΨ
Drama
An 11-year-old boy with what might be an autism spectrum disorder searches for meaning after his father dies in the 9/11 bombings of the World Trade Center.

Flowers for Algernon (2000) Drama ΨΨ
A made-for-TV movie about an intellectually challenged man and the changes that occur in his life when he undergoes surgery to enhance his IQ. The surgery is successful, but there are unanticipated consequences.

Forrest Gump (1994) Fantasy ΨΨΨΨΨ
Traces the life of Forrest Gump (Tom Hanks), who triumphs in life despite an IQ of 75 and a deformed spine. The film will make you examine your stereotypes about intellectual disability.

Forrest Gump: "Lieutenant Dan, what are you doing here?"
Lieutenant Daniel Taylor: "I'm here to try out my sea legs."
Forrest Gump: "But you ain't got no legs, Lieutenant Dan."

***Forrest Gump* (1994)**

Front of the Class (2008) Drama ΨΨΨΨ
This film is based on the life of Brad Cohen; it deals with his courage as a child dealing with Tourette's disorder and an ignorant and unsympathetic father. Cohen later went on to become a gifted and award-winning teacher.

Girlfriend (2010) Drama ΨΨΨ
A young man with Down syndrome inherits money and uses it to pursue a single mother he has loved since high school.

Harvie Krumpet (2003) Animation-Comedy ΨΨΨ
A short film about a character who faces innumerous tragedies and challenges, including Tourette's disorder. Geoffrey Rush narrates the film.

Her Name Is Sabine (2007, France) ΨΨΨΨ
Documentary
Striking documentary depicting the impact of a psychiatric institution on a woman with autism.

Horse Boy, The (2009) Documentary ΨΨΨΨ
A family travels to Mongolia to find a shaman who can help their son who has an autism spectrum disorder. Compare this film with *Lighthouse of the Whales* (2016).

House of Cards (1993) Drama Ψ
Tommy Lee Jones is wasted in an insipid movie about a young girl who becomes autistic and withdrawn.

Hyde Park on Hudson (2012) Biography ΨΨ
This film portrays a weekend in the life of FDR (Bill Murray) and depicts his romantic involvement with a distant cousin, played by Laura Linney, despite his need for a wheelchair.

I Am Sam (2001) Drama ΨΨΨ
Sean Penn portrays a man with a mild intellectual disability who fights for custody rights for his daughter.

I Think We're Alone Now (2008) Documentary ΨΨ
This documentary profiles two individuals in love with the pop singer Tiffany. One of the two is identified as someone with Asperger's syndrome; the other is a hermaphrodite from Denver.

Intelligent Lives (2018) Documentary ΨΨΨΨΨ
Chris Cooper narrates this thoughtful documentary about the limits of intellectual assessment and the stigma that results from labels like mental retardation. Cooper and his wife insisted that their son, Jesse, born with cerebral palsy, be educated in public schools. Jesse became a successful student, sadly dying when he was 17.

Importance of Tying Your Own Shoes, The (2011) ΨΨ
A troubled young man becomes the leader of a theater troupe whose members all have some form of intellectual disability.

Jack Goes Boating (2010) Drama ΨΨΨ
Philip Seymour Hoffman directs and plays the role of Jack, a limo driver with limited intellectual ability and social skills, who becomes romantically involved with Connie and learns to swim so he can take her on a boat ride.

Jefftowne (1998) Documentary ΨΨ
A man with Down syndrome lives with his 93-year-old adoptive parent and spends his time socializing.

Junebug (2005) Comedy-Drama ΨΨ
An autistic painter has a minor but highly stereotypic role in an otherwise good film.

King's Speech, The (2010) Drama ΨΨΨΨΨ
Colin Firth plays the role of Bertie (George VI) who must accept the responsibilities of being King of the United Kingdom when his older brother abdicates the throne. His role as national leader is complicated by his childhood-onset fluency disorder (stuttering), a problem treated successfully by speech therapist Lionel Logue (Geoffrey Rush).

King George VI: "If I'm King, where's my power? Can I form a government? Can I levy a tax, declare a war? No! And yet I am the seat of all authority. Why? Because the nation believes that when I speak, I speak for them. But I can't speak."

Bertie contemplates his dilemma as a leader, in *The King's Speech* (2010)

Larry (1974) Biography ΨΨ
Dated but still interesting film about a man discharged from a psychiatric hospital and forced to cope with the outside world. The film suggests the patient himself isn't ill but still acts strange because he has grown up in a world where everyone acts a little odd.

Life, Animated (2016) Documentary ΨΨΨΨΨ
A must-see film for any mental health professional or educator. Ron Suskind documents the life journey of his son, Owen, a seemingly normal boy until age 3 when he was diagnosed with autism. He displays stereotyped movements and echolalia but seems to be helped by watching endless Disney films and identifying with the characters.

Lighthouse of the Whales (*El Faro de Las Orcas*; 2016, Spain) Drama ΨΨΨ
An anxious mother travels from Madrid to Argentina after seeing a documentary about the therapeutic value of whales.

Love and Other Drugs (2010) Drama-Romance ΨΨ
A sexual relationship between a pharmaceutical salesman with attention deficit disorder (ADD) and a woman with Parkinson's grows into love. Jake Gyllenhaal and Anne Hathaway star, and there are lots of Viagra jokes.

Magic Life of V (2019, Finland) Documentary ΨΨΨΨ
A young woman learns how to cope with a history of childhood trauma by helping her intellectually disabled brother. The film will introduce viewers to live action role playing (LARP).

Mary and Max (2009) Animation-Comedy-Drama ΨΨΨΨ
Philip Seymour Hoffman provides the voice of Max, a morbidly obese 44-year-old man living in Manhattan,

who develops an unlikely but lasting friendship with Mary, an 8-year-old girl living in Melbourne. Max is a man with autism spectrum disorder who functions at a very high level.

Me, Too (2009, Spain) Drama ΨΨΨΨ
Daniel has Down syndrome and graduates from a university. After he begins a new job, he promptly falls in love with Laura, a coworker whose life is very different from Daniel's.

Memory Keeper's Daughter, The (2008) Drama ΨΨ
A physician's wife has twins, one of whom has Down syndrome. He instructs the nurse to put the child in an institution for the feeble-minded; she ignores his instructions and raises the child on her own.

Monica and David (2009) Documentary ΨΨΨΨ
Two young people with Down syndrome marry and live together with her parents and create a meaningful life.

Mozart and the Whale (2005) Comedy/Drama ΨΨ
Based on a true story about two high-functioning people with autism spectrum disorder who meet and develop a lifelong relationship.

Molly (1999) Drama Ψ
This film tries hard to be another *Rain Man,* with a female autistic character (Elisabeth Shue), but ends up being highly stereotypic, unrealistic, and not at all helpful in educating the public about autism.

Motherless Brooklyn (2019) Drama ΨΨΨ
Ed Norton directed this film and stars in it as Lionel Essrog, a detective with Tourette's syndrome. It is a dramatic but accurate depiction of the disorder and a useful introduction for someone who has never been around anyone with Tourette's.

My Left Foot (1989, Ireland/UK) ΨΨΨΨ
Drama-Biography
Based on the true story of Christy Brown, a successful artist-author who triumphed over cerebral palsy. Brown grew up as part of a large, poor, working class Irish family. At that time, the world was ill-equipped to understand or care for people with cerebral palsy. A "prisoner in his own body," Brown never gave up. He painted and wrote several novels and books of poetry.

My Name is Khan (2010, India) Drama ΨΨΨΨ
In a film that represents a new perspective in Bollywood filmmaking, a man with autism spectrum disorder travels across the United States with a message for the president that although he is routinely discriminated against, he is not a terrorist. The portrayal of high-functioning autism spectrum disorder (formerly Asperger's disorder) is accurate and engaging.

Niagara, Niagara (1998) Drama ΨΨ
Two teenagers on the lam encounter multiple problems on the road. Reminiscent of *Bonnie and Clyde*, the film is chiefly memorable because it is one of the few films in which Tourette's disorder is sympathetically and realistically portrayed.

Of Mice and Men (1992) Drama ΨΨΨ
John Malkovich stars as Lenny, a farmhand with an intellectual disability. This is a wonderful film but see the 1939 original as well, starring Burgess Meredith and a young Lon Chaney.

"He's a nice fella. You don't need no sense to be a nice fella."

A comment on Lenny's personality, in *Of Mice and Men* (1992)

Other Sister, The (1999) Comedy ΨΨ
This film portrays a young woman's struggles to be an independent adult and to distance herself from an overly protective family. She is successful in her special school, enters the local community college against her father's wishes, and develops friendships.

Pauline and Paulette (2001, Belgium) ΨΨΨΨ
Following the death of their older sister, Martha, two sisters unwillingly become responsible for their sister Pauline who has a developmental disability.

Peanut Butter Falcon, The (2019)
Comedy/Drama ΨΨΨΨ
A 22-year-old man with Down syndrome escapes from an assisted living facility and bonds with a small-time crook. The unlikely duo are tracked by a social worker who ultimately joins with them in escaping to Florida, after Zak, the protagonist, gets to visit a wrestling school run by his longtime hero, "Salt Water Redneck." The film's title comes from Zak's wrestling persona.

Praying With Lior (2007)
Documentary/Biography ΨΨΨ
A young man with Down syndrome prepares for his Bar Mitzvah. The ceremony is especially important because the boy's father is a rabbi.

Pushing Tin (1999) Drama/Comedy ΨΨ
John Cusack portrays an air traffic controller with adult attention deficit disorder.

Radio (2003) Drama ΨΨΨ
Cuba Gooding Jr. plays a man with a developmental disability who, when given a chance by the coach (Ed Harris) of the local football team, inspires and influences many lives. A tad sentimental, but the pros outweigh the cons in this heart-warming, true story.

Rain Man (1993) Drama ΨΨΨΨ
Dustin Hoffman plays Raymond, an autistic man who is also a savant, initially exploited by an older brother (played by Tom Cruise). Hoffman read widely about autism and worked with autistic people when preparing for this role. In the film, Raymond recites statistics about airline crashes, mentioning that only Qantas had a perfect record. All airlines cut this section of the film for inflight viewing – except Qantas!

Charlie: "He's not crazy, he's not retarded, but he's here."
Dr. Bruner: "He's an autistic savant. People like him used to be called idiot savants. There's certain deficiencies, certain abilities that impair him."
Charlie: "So he's retarded."
Dr. Bruner: "Autistic. There's certain routines, rituals that he follows."
Charlie: "Rituals, I like that."
Dr. Bruner: "The way he eats, sleeps, walks, talks, uses the bathroom. It's all he has to protect himself. Any break from this routine leaves him terrified."

Charlie Babbitt learns about autism spectrum disorder, in *Rain Man* (1993)

Rainman Twins, The (2008) ΨΨΨΨ
Documentary/Biography
A 1-hr *Extraordinary People* episode that introduces viewers to the world's only known identical twin autistic savants. The two girls have remarkable memory abilities, and they have both developed an extraordinary devotion to TV personality Dick Clark.

Ringer, The (2005) Comedy ΨΨ
A man desperate for money decides to fix the Special Olympics by entering to beat the reigning champion.

Rudely Interrupted (2009, Australia)
Documentary ΨΨΨΨ
A popular rock band from Australia made up of musicians with a variety of disabilities – Asperger's, Down syndrome, blindness, and deafness – go on a world tour.

Sessions, The (2012) ΨΨΨΨ
A joyous film based on a true story about a student at Berkeley who spends much of his life in an iron lung. He is determined to experience intercourse, and hires a sexual surrogate played by Helen Hunt to teach him what he doesn't know. The film makes the point that people with disabilities want and need a sex life, just like everyone else.

Shorty (2003) Documentary ΨΨΨΨ
A 55-year-old man with Down syndrome who is passionate about football is about to be inducted into the Hampden-Sydney College Athletic Hall of Fame.

Silent Fall (1994) Drama ΨΨΨ
A retired child psychiatrist works with a boy with autism who witnessed his parent's murder.

Sling Blade (1996) Drama ΨΨΨΨΨ
Billy Bob Thornton wrote the screenplay, directed the film, and played the lead in this remarkable film, which examines the life of a 37-year-old man with an intellectual disability who has been incarcerated in a mental hospital for the past 25 years after killing his mother and her lover. The fact that the protagonist winds up committing a third murder after being released perpetuates the misconception that people with developmental disabilities are potentially dangerous, but the film is well worth your time.

"I don't reckon you have to go with women to be a good daddy to a boy. You been real square-dealin' with me. The Bible says two men ought not lay together. But I don't reckon the Good Lord would send anybody like you to Hades. ... You take good care of that boy."

Karl accepts a gay man as a stepfather for his young friend, in *Sling Blade* (1996)

Snow Cake (2006) Drama ΨΨ
Sigourney Weaver portrays a high-functioning woman with autism spectrum disorder. This film received an "honorable mention" at the Voice Awards.

Somersault (2004, Australia) Drama Ψ
A small part of this coming-of-age tale involves a young boy with an autism spectrum disorder.

Temple Grandin (2010) Biography ΨΨΨΨΨ
This engaging film introduces the viewer to Temple Grandin, a woman with autism spectrum disorder who also has a PhD in animal husbandry. Although Temple

Grandin is extraordinary and atypical, the film conveys a tremendous amount of information about autism spectrum disorder.

"Trust me. We know how different she is." "Different, but not less."

A teacher and mother having a conversation about a young Temple Grandin

---

There's Something About Mary (1998) Comedy ΨΨ
Ted (Ben Stiller) tries to track down and rekindle love with Mary (Cameron Diaz). Mary has a brother with a developmental disability who plays a significant role in the story.

This Is Nicholas – Living With Autism (2019) Documentary ΨΨΨΨΨ
A lovely short film that chronicles the life of the film's director, Nicholas Ryan-Purcell, from age 13 to age 28. The film beautifully illustrates the importance of community in supporting a child on the autism spectrum.

Tim (1979) Drama ΨΨ
In this Australian film, an older woman has an affair with a man with an intellectual disability.

Thumbsucker (2005) Comedy/Drama ΨΨΨ
An adolescent boy self-soothes by secretly sucking his thumb. He is unable to stop and is diagnosed with attention deficit disorder. His life is transformed after he begins treatment with stimulant medication.

To Be and To Have (2005, France) Documentary–Drama ΨΨΨΨΨ
A creative teacher adapts his style to children of different ages, learning levels, and types of problems, including autism spectrum disorders, communication disorders, and ADHD.

Unforgotten: 25 Years After Willowbrook (1996) Documentary ΨΨΨΨΨ
Geraldo Rivera follows up on the original Willowbrook State School exposé and contrasts the grim reality of institutional life with the current success of some survivors, including Bernard Carabello, a man abandoned by his parents at age 3 because he had cerebral palsy. Bernard spent 18 years at Willowbrook.

Up Syndrome (2000) Documentary ΨΨΨ
A film about a young man with Down syndrome who deals with the struggles all young people confront: finding meaningful work, finding someone to love, and establishing purpose in life.

Village, The (2004) Drama–Suspense Ψ
Director M. Night Shyamalan's film about a village surrounded by forest containing the highly feared "those we don't speak of." One character with a developmental disability is believed to be especially dangerous.

What's Eating Gilbert Grape? (1993) Drama ΨΨΨ
Johnny Depp stars in this interesting portrayal of the dynamics of a rural Iowa family and small-town America. Depp's character's life revolves around the care of his brother (who has an autism spectrum disorder) and his morbidly obese mother.

Where the Crawdads Sing (2022) Mystery ΨΨ
A young girl is abandoned by her alcoholic father at age 10, and she raises herself in the marshland of North Carolina. She acquires normal language skills from her parents and siblings, but initially has few social skills, and she is ill-prepared to deal with puberty, sexuality, or the challenges that occur when she is charged with murder.

Schizophrenia Spectrum and Other Psychotic Disorders

11'09"01 – September 11 (2002) Drama ΨΨΨ
Eleven renowned directors from around the world look to their own cultures to create a short film in tribute to the tragedy of September 11, 2001. This fascinating collection of short films includes an allegory from Japanese director Shohei Imamura about a man who returns from war believing he is a snake.

12 Monkeys (1995) Science Fiction–Suspense ΨΨ
Terry Gilliam film about a time traveler (Bruce Willis) trying to save the world from a deadly plague. Brad Pitt costars as a character with paranoid schizophrenia. At times, the film seems to take on a cinematic representation of a nightmare.

13 Moons (2002) Drama ΨΨ
Three priests, a bail bondsman, a musician, and two clowns cross paths on nighttime city streets. One character, a drug addict needing an organ transplant, is blatantly psychotic throughout the film.

Adopted One, The (2020) Drama Ψ
A child kills his adoptive parents, is diagnosed with schizophrenia, and then spends 30 years in an institution. After the patient colludes with a psychiatrist to escape, he uses a hammer to bludgeon and kill dozens of victims. This is an awful film devoid of either pedagogical or artistic value.

Aguirre, the Wrath of God (1972, West Germany/Peru/Mexico) Adventure ΨΨΨΨ
Werner Herzog film about Spanish conquistadors searching for the mythic treasure of El Dorado deep into Peru's Amazon. The narcissistic leader (Klaus Kinski) deteriorates into psychosis, and dreams of founding an incestuous dynasty with his daughter.

Alone in the Dark (1982) Suspense Ψ
A psychotic patient besieges a psychiatrist's family during a citywide blackout.

Amadeus (1984) Biography-Musical ΨΨΨ
The film opens with the court composer Salieri, now old, mad, and suicidal, wondering if he murdered Mozart. Salieri is obsessed with the genius of Mozart and can never forgive his rival for his talent - or himself for his mediocrity.

Angel at My Table, An (1990) Biography-Drama ΨΨΨΨΨ
Jean Campion's biography of New Zealand novelist Janet Frame, who was misdiagnosed with schizophrenia and mistreated with electroconvulsive therapy (ECT).

Angel Baby (1995, Australia) Drama ΨΨΨ
Two mentally ill people who meet in an outpatient clinic, fall in love, and try to face life together. Unfortunately, their lives fall apart because of an ill-fated decision to mutually discontinue their medication. The film illustrates the fear experienced by a woman, already paranoid, who must deal with pregnancy and childbirth.

Angels of the Universe (2000, Iceland) Biography-Drama ΨΨΨ
Paul is a musician and artist in love with a woman from a different social stratum; when she leaves him, he becomes psychotic and is hospitalized. The scriptwriter based the film (and his book on which the film is based) on his experiences with his brother, a man coping with the challenge of mental illness.

Assassination of Richard Nixon, The (2004) Biography-Drama ΨΨΨ
Sean Penn portrays Sam Bicke, an aloof, taciturn, delusional furniture salesman who attempted to kill President Nixon. The film promotes the misconception that people with mental illness are frequently dangerous.

Asylum (2005) Thriller-Drama ΨΨ
A husband takes a job at a psychiatric institution and his wife begins to have an affair with a dangerous patient. The film perpetuates the misconception that patients in psychiatric hospitals are violent.

Bee Season (2005) Drama Ψ
A father (Richard Gere) becomes overinvolved in his daughter's spelling bee competitions and looks to Jewish mysticism for support.

Benny & Joon (1993) Comedy ΨΨΨ
A generally sympathetic portrayal of schizophrenia, with a vivid example of decompensation on a city bus; this otherwise good film trivializes the problem of schizophrenia by suggesting love alone is enough to conquer the problem. Watching Johnny Depp perform a Buster Keaton routine is reason enough to see the film.

Berlin Alexanderplatz (1980) Drama ΨΨΨΨΨ
This film, a 15-hr Fassbinder masterpiece, traces the gradual moral and mental disintegration of a man who leaves prison resolved to live a good life. The film explores exploitation of women, violence, homosexuality, and mental illness.

Betrayed (1988) Political-Thriller Ψ
Debra Winger plays an undercover agent who falls in love with a seemingly simple farmer who turns out to be a right-wing, paranoid fanatic.

Betty Blue (1986) Drama ΨΨΨ
Artistic, erotic French film about two young lovers and their passions that lead from poverty to violence and destruction. One particularly shocking scene depicts self-mutilation resulting from psychosis.

Bill of Divorcement, A (1932) Comedy ΨΨ
A mentally ill man is discharged from a psychiatric hospital and returns home to his wife and daughter. The movie marks Katharine Hepburn's debut as a film actress.

Birth (2004) Drama-Mystery ΨΨΨ
A rare depiction of shared psychotic disorder (*folie à deux*), featuring Nicole Kidman.

Black Swan (2010) Drama-Mystery-Thriller ΨΨΨΨΨ
Natalie Portman won an Academy Award for Best Actress in a Leading Role for her performance as a troubled ballerina who becomes obsessed with her dual role as both the white and black swan in Tchaikovsky's *Swan Lake*. The film depicts bulimia and anorexia and presents a differential diagnosis challenge because of a plot that includes fantasies, delusions, hallucinations, mother-daughter conflict, seduction by a director, a lesbian encounter, ecstasy abuse, and possible murder.

Boxing Helena (1994) Drama ΨΨ
An eminent surgeon is rebuffed by a beautiful woman. His obsessions turn delusional as he captures her and

eventually amputates her arms and legs while paradoxically fawning over her. This film was the directorial debut of Jennifer Chambers Lynch, daughter of filmmaker David Lynch.

Bubba Ho-Tep (2002) Comedy-Thriller Ψ
Two rest home residents who believe they are Elvis Presley and John F. Kennedy team up to fight evil. It is a silly movie.

Bug (2006) Drama-Horror ΨΨΨΨ
A William Friedkin film that offers a nice example of a shared delusional disorder (in this case the belief that the government implanted microscopic insects underneath her boyfriend's skin).

Butcher Boy, The (1997) Comedy ΨΨΨΨ
Dark comedy about a boy with schizophrenia, Francie Brady, living in Ireland in the 1960s. Francie's behavior ranges from absurd and humorous to delusional and dangerous.

"He took me, with the stink of filthy roadhouse whiskey on his breath, and I liked it. I liked it! With all that dirty touching of his hands all over me. I should've given you to God when you were born, but I was weak and backsliding, and now the devil has come home."

Francie Brady's mother laments her past, in *The Butcher Boy* (1997)

Camille Claudel (1988) Biography ΨΨΨ
Biographical film of the mistress of Rodin, who spent the last 30 years of her life in an asylum.

Canvas (2006) Drama ΨΨΨΨΨ
A remarkable portrayal of schizophrenia and its impact on the family, starring Marcia Gay Harden. This film won a Voice Award for its outstanding depiction of mental illness.

Caveman's Valentine, The (2001) Crime-Drama ΨΨ
Samuel L. Jackson plays the role of a homeless composer with schizophrenia living in a cave in New York City who takes on the job of hunting down a killer.

Clean, Shaven (1995) Mystery ΨΨΨΨ
A man with schizophrenia is released from a psychiatric hospital and returns home in search of his daughter. Vivid and realistic portrayal of the kinds of auditory hallucinations found in schizophrenia.

Peter Winter: "I was in a hospital bed, and I had been operated on. And they had put a small receiver in the back of my head and a transmitter in my finger. You know what they are?"
Nicole Winter: "A radio?"
Peter Winter: "Yeah, a radio. Anyway, to get at the transmitter, I had to take my fingernail off."

Peter explains to his daughter why he cut out his fingernail, in *Clean, Shaven*

Confessions of a Superhero (2007) ΨΨΨ
Documentary
A film that explores the lives of four individuals trying to make a living by posing as superheroes on Hollywood's Walk of Fame; the primary characters in the film impersonate Batman, Superman, Wonder Woman, and The Hulk.

Dangerous Method, A (2011, UK) ΨΨΨ
Biography-Drama
This David Cronenberg film documents the early days of psychoanalysis and some of the interactions between Freud and Jung. The film also features Sabina, a patient with psychosis, who prior to becoming a physician and scholar was treated by both Freud and Jung. In the film, Jung has sadomasochistic sex with Sabina.

Dead Man on Campus (1998) Comedy Ψ
Two roommates try to find a roommate who is likely to commit suicide so that they can have their flailing grades excused. The film perpetrates misconceptions that people with mental illness are violent, that people with mental illness are always psychotic, and that those who are paranoid are the most likely to commit suicide.

Dead of Night (1945) Horror ΨΨΨΨ
Five short episodes loosely linked together. The last of these, "The Ventriloquist's Dummy," stars Michael Redgrave, who must be hospitalized after he becomes convinced that he and his dummy are exchanging personalities.

Delusions of Grandeur (1973) Comedy Ψ
In 17th-century Spain, a wily servant saves his king from a tax collector.

Derailroaded (2005) Documentary-Biography ΨΨΨ
Portrays the music and life of cult-rock icon "Wild Man Fischer," a man with schizophrenia; the film is both funny and informative, and it is not exploitative.

Deranged (2012, Korea) Drama ΨΨ
A parasite infects the residents of Seoul, causing them to commit suicide, while a pharmaceutical salesman searches for a cure. Not to be confused with a far inferior horror film by the same name released the same year.

Dogtooth (2009, Greece) Drama ΨΨΨ
An intriguing film about a bizarre family in which the parents teach their children a unique language and prevent them from having any contact with the outside world. The film features brother–sister incest and depicts extensive psychological abuse of children.

Don Juan DeMarco (1995) Drama ΨΨΨ
Marlon Brando plays a compassionate psychiatrist working with Johnny Depp's character, someone who thinks he is the legendary Don Juan.

Donnie Darko (2001) Drama ΨΨΨ
Although this movie about a delusional high school student who frequently hallucinates a "demon bunny" instructing him that the end of the world is near sounds trivial, the film is complex with important commentary about fear, the pain of mental illness, and the nature of reality. It is a cult classic.

Don't Say A Word (2001) Suspense–Mystery ΨΨ
Michael Douglas plays a psychiatrist whose daughter is kidnapped for the ransom of a 6-digit code locked in the brain of a very disturbed psychiatric patient.

Dressed to Kill (1980) Thriller ΨΨ
Popular film in which Michael Caine plays Angie Dickinson's psychiatrist. The film confuses transsexuality and schizophrenia, and it is engaging, albeit not always accurate.

Edmond (2005) Thriller ΨΨΨ
Interesting and memorable story about a man (William H. Macy) who slowly loses touch with reality and never fully returns.

Entertainer, The (1960) Drama Ψ
This film, starring Laurence Olivier and Albert Finney, portrays Olivier's character as a third-rate vaudevillian whose delusions of grandeur alienate people around him.

Face to Face (1976, Sweden) Drama ΨΨΨΨ
Two psychiatrists are portrayed, one of whom (Liv Ullmann) is depressed, delusional, and suicidal, and a brief affair with another physician doesn't help. The poster for the film shows two faces superimposed on a strikingly realistic Rorschach plate.

Fan, The (1982) Horror Ψ
A Broadway star played by Lauren Bacall is terrorized by an embittered fan.

Fan, The (1996) Drama Ψ
Robert De Niro and Wesley Snipes are wasted in this tired film about a baseball fan who is obsessed with a Giants center fielder.

Final (2001) Drama ΨΨΨ
Well-acted performance by Denis Leary who plays Bill in this Campbell Scott film. Bill awakens from a coma in an isolated, bright room of a psychiatric hospital. He has frequent paranoid delusions, anger outbursts, and hallucinations as his therapist helps him remember flashbacks of his car accident and his father's death. Interesting portrayal of the doctor–patient relationship, presenting many questions about boundaries, ethics, and relational dynamics.

Fisher King, The (1991) ΨΨΨ
Drama–Fantasy–Comedy
Terry Gilliam film in which Robin Williams plays a homeless, mentally ill man who is befriended by a disillusioned former disc jockey. The movie is funny but confusing, and it misleads the public, suggesting that it is common for schizophrenia to result from trauma.

Flightplan (2005) Suspense–Drama ΨΨ
While on a long flight, a woman (Jodie Foster) frantically claims she has lost her child; however, other passengers do not remember a child traveling with her. For much of the film, the viewer is left questioning whether Jodie Foster has a psychotic disorder. The film suggests that individuals referred to as delusional or psychotic are telling the truth, and their delusions may well be reality-based.

Frailty (2001) Drama–Suspense ΨΨΨ
Bill Paxton plays a serial killing, religious zealot with a delusional disorder who believes he's on a mission from God to fight off demons (his human victims).

Gaslight (1944). Drama–Suspense ΨΨΨ
Charles Boyer, Ingrid Bergman, and Joseph Cotton star in this film about a young woman married to a duplicitous man who convinces her she is going mad when she notices missing pictures, hears mysterious footsteps in the night, and notices gaslights that dim without any reason. Bergman received an Academy Award for Best Actress for her role in the film, the first of her three Oscars. Watch for an 18-year-old Angela Lansbury in her screen debut. The term "gaslighting" is now widely used to refer to deliberate psychological manipulation to make victims question their memory or judgment.

Gothika (2003) Suspense ΨΨ
Halle Berry plays Dr. Miranda Grey who works to unravel the mystery of her patient's (Penélope Cruz) psychopathology and is confronted by disturbing secrets and the supernatural.

Goya in Bordeaux (1999, Spain) ΨΨΨ
Drama–Biography
Spanish film, depicting the famous painter Francisco de Goya on his deathbed, who recalls major events of his life, hallucinates, and experiences severe migraines. The film addresses themes of psychosis and creativity, integrity versus despair, and the interrelationship of life and death.

Grizzly Man (2005) Documentary ΨΨΨ
Werner Herzog film about Timothy Treadwell, a well-known naturalist who lived with grizzly bears for 13 summers. The viewer wonders about Treadwell's diagnosis as he becomes increasingly wild, and his behavior increasingly bizarre.

Happy Accidents (2000) Romance–Sci-Fi ΨΨ
A man states he is from the future – the year 2470. Marisa Tomei's character must decide if he is delusional or real.

He Loves Me, He Loves Me Not (*À La Folie... Pas Du Tout;* 2002, France) Drama ΨΨΨΨΨ
A must-see film for depiction of delusional disorders that is so extraordinary that it could only be done cinematically. First, the viewer sees reality from the young woman's perception and flashes back to the beginning, giving the viewer the vantage point of the man she loves. This French film stars *Amélie*'s Audrey Tautou.

Holy Blood (*Santa Sangre;* 1989, Mexico) ΨΨΨΨ
Horror–Thriller
A disturbing Alejandro Jodorowsky film about a young man forced to witness the mutilation of his mother and the suicide of his father. We never know if these events are real or simply delusions of a patient. The film is complex and visually stunning.

Horse Girl (2020) Drama ΨΨΨΨ
Alison Brie plays the role of Sarah, a young woman who would almost certainly be diagnosed as someone with schizophrenia. There is a strong family history of mental illness, she is delusional, and Sarah believes in alien abduction. She spends almost every evening watching the TV series *Purgatory*. A potentially promising romantic relationship goes sour when Sarah's new boyfriend finds her behavior, initially quirky and charming, simply too bizarre for him to handle.

House of Fools (2002) Drama ΨΨΨΨ
Based on a true story: the staff in a mental institution flee due to conflicts in Chechnya, leaving the patients to fend for themselves. Soon soldiers occupy the hospital, and the viewer is left with various questions of war, politics, mental health treatment, and who is really "crazy." Loaded with psychopathology examples, including a fire starter, and patients with all of the subtypes of schizophrenia.

Housekeeping (1987) Drama ΨΨΨΨ
An eccentric aunt comes to care for two sisters in the Pacific Northwest after the suicide of their mother. The girls can't decide if their aunt is simply odd or seriously mentally ill. The viewer confronts a similar dilemma.

I'm a Cyborg, But That's OK (2006, South Korea) Drama–Romance ΨΨΨ
Despite the odd title, this is a fascinating film about a psychotic woman who believes she is a cyborg and is admitted to a psychiatric hospital.

I Never Promised You a Rose Garden (1977) Drama ΨΨΨΨ
Accurate rendition of the popular book by the same name. The patient has command hallucinations that tell her to kill herself. There is a sympathetic portrayal of psychiatry and treatment; a breakthrough occurs when the protagonist first realizes she can feel pain.

Images (1972) Drama ΨΨΨ
Robert Altman's examination of the confused life of a woman with schizophrenia. A difficult film, but interesting, with a heuristic presentation of hallucinations.

Inner Senses (2002, Korea)
Horror–Thriller ΨΨ
A psychotic woman is treated by a psychologist who falls in love with her and who soon comes to share her hallucinations.

Julien Donkey-Boy (1999) Drama ΨΨ
Director Harmony Korine has made an interesting film about the horrors of schizophrenia, based on and dedicated to his uncle, whom he wanted to take out of a psychiatric institution to be in the film. The film is sometimes shocking and insightful and at other times comedic. Werner Herzog plays the role of an abusive father who contributes to his son's illness.

Keane (2004) Mystery–Thriller ΨΨΨΨ
An engaging depiction of a man who begins to mentally deteriorate because he believes his daughter is missing. The film leaves the viewer wondering what is real and

what is psychosis. Unfortunately, a powerful scene in which the protagonist randomly chases and attacks another man will stick out in the viewer's mind as a terrifying link between violence and mental illness.

Killing of John Lennon, The (2006, UK) ΨΨΨ
Biography-Drama
Inside look into the mind of the delusional Mark Chapman leading up to the day he murdered John Lennon. Chapman was obsessed with Holden Caulfield from *The Catcher in the Rye* and believed he was the protagonist; he read from the book at the murder scene and subsequent trial. This film promotes the misconception that people with mental illness are violent, and that Salinger's classic work somehow had something to do with Lennon's murder.

King of Comedy, The (1983) Drama ΨΨΨΨ
Martin Scorsese film about a fan who develops a delusional relationship with a talk show host after the two of them are forced to share a taxicab.

K-Pax (2001) Drama ΨΨΨΨ
Multilayered film in which Kevin Spacey plays Prot, a man claiming he's from a faraway planet who can give convincing evidence for his case to astrophysicists. The viewer is left to hypothesize whether the character has schizophrenia, dissociative fugue, or is an enlightened spiritual being; whichever is the case, the portrayal and diagnostic criteria are convincing for each.

La Dolce Vita (1960, Italy) Drama ΨΨΨ
Vintage Fellini film with an interesting vignette in which hundreds of Roman citizens develop a mass delusion following reports of a sighting of the Virgin Mary.

Lars and the Real Girl (2007) ΨΨΨΨ
Comedy-Drama
Lars is a gentle man who purchases a mail-order doll on the Internet, creates a history and an identity for her, and begins to introduce her to his friends. His community supports his fantasy, and through their support he begins to heal. Although there are schizotypal features, Lars would likely be diagnosed as someone with a delusional disorder.

Lighthouse, The (2019) Drama ΨΨΨΨ
A dramatic Robert Eggers film starring Robert Pattinson and Willem Dafoe as two "wickies" (lighthouse keepers) who respond to protracted isolation and situational intimacy by slowly becoming insane. Both men share secrets and drunken homoerotic moments, and both become delusional. Pattinson's character becomes increasingly paranoid and begins to hallucinate, at one point having sex with a mermaid and another time seeing the severed head of the lighthouse keeper he had come to replace.

Love Object (2004) Thriller Ψ
A young man dealing with work stress copes by purchasing a $10,600 lifelike, silicone doll that he begins to believe is subtly torturing him as he deteriorates into psychosis.

Lucy in the Sky (2019) Drama ΨΨ
Natalie Portman stars in a story loosely based on the life of Lisa Nowak, an astronaut who had flown to the International Space Station on the shuttle *Discovery*. Nowak became involved in a love triangle after her mission ended and she had returned to earth. She drove 900 miles to the Orlando airport with a knife, mallet, rubber tubing, and a BB gun. Once there, she confronted another astronaut who had been sleeping with Nowak's lover. She was subsequently arrested and charged with attempted murder. Numerous diagnoses have been offered to account for Nowak's behavior, but delusional disorder, erotomanic type seems to be the best fit.

Lunatics: A Love Story (1992) Comedy ΨΨΨ
A former mental patient spends 6 months hidden away in his apartment. The lead character has been described in reviews as agoraphobic, but a more serious diagnosis seems appropriate, especially considering the patient's delusions and hallucinations.

Lust for Life (1956) Biography ΨΨΨΨ
Kirk Douglas as Vincent van Gogh and Anthony Quinn as Paul Gauguin. The film portrays the stormy relationship of the two men and van Gogh's hospitalization and eventual suicide. Contrast with *Vincent* (1987) and Robert Altman's *Vincent & Theo* (1990). There are scenes in which van Gogh is feverishly painting that suggest bipolar disorder.

Madness of King George, The (1994) ΨΨΨ
Historical Biography
Nigel Hawthorne as King George III in an adaptation of a stage play examining the reactions of the court and family as the king becomes increasingly demented (due to porphyria, a genetic metabolic disorder).

> **"One may produce a copious, regular evacuation every day of the week and still be a stranger to reason."**
>
> **An observation by a court doctor, in *The Madness of King George* (1994)**

Magic (1978) Thriller ΨΨ
Anthony Hopkins' talents are largely wasted in this Richard Attenborough film about a ventriloquist obsessed with his dummy. Not nearly as good a film as the 1945 movie *Dead of Night*.

Man From Earth, The (2007) Drama-Sci-Fi Ψ
A mysterious, successful professor attempts to convince his friends he can live forever and that he has met a variety of historical figures (e.g., Buddha).

May (2002) Thriller Ψ
Macabre psychological study of an isolated, socially awkward girl who sinks into psychosis as she tries to make a "best friend" by assembling the best parts of other people's bodies after murdering them. The film promotes the misconception that people with mental illness are violent.

Misery (1990) Horror ΨΨ
Kathy Bates plays a delusional woman who becomes convinced she is justified in capturing a novelist and forcing him to rewrite his latest novel to meet her tastes.

Montenegro (1981) Drama ΨΨ
A Dusan Makavejev film about a bored housewife slowly becoming psychotic. She becomes sexually liberated and then murders her lover. Despite its psychopathological theme, the film is really about politics and social class.

Nightmare on Elm Street (1984) Horror ΨΨ
Director Wes Craven introduces us to Freddy Kruger in a film that has become a cult classic. The original film is superior to all the sequels.

Number 23, The (2007) Drama Ψ
A dogcatcher becomes obsessed with the number 23. Jim Carrey's considerable talents are largely wasted in this film, a movie that disappoints both artistically and pedagogically. The movie conflates obsessive-compulsive disorder, paranoia, paranoid personality disorder, and sexual sadism.

Observe and Report (2009) Ψ
Comedy-Drama
A mall security guard with bipolar disorder abuses drugs and is noncompliant with his medication. He is grandiose and delusional, believing that he is going to be able to solve the mall's problems of theft and "flashing."

Oil on Water (2007, South Africa) ΨΨΨ
Drama/Romance
An interesting examination of the ways in which a relationship is affected by schizophrenia.

Out of the Shadow (2004) ΨΨΨΨ
Documentary
Realistic and moving depiction of schizophrenia and its impact on the family.

Outrageous! (1977) Comedy ΨΨ
Canadian film about a gay hairdresser and a woman with schizophrenia who is pregnant.

People Say I'm Crazy (2003) ΨΨΨ
Documentary
Cinema verite-styled documentary of the daily life of a man with paranoid schizophrenia. Interesting for discussions on differentiation of schizophrenia, schizoaffective disorder, and mood disorders. Deeply honest, enlightening, and inspiring.

"I cannot trust my own perceptions."

John Cadigan, who directs and plays himself in *People Say I'm Crazy* (2003)

Perfect Strangers (2003) ΨΨ
Drama-Suspense
A mysterious man (Sam Neill) invites a woman he has just met to his private island home and then kidnaps her. The two become romantically involved, and she nurses him back to health after he is injured. His obsessions transfer to the woman who frequently hallucinates after her lover dies.

Pi (1988) Drama ΨΨΨΨ
Darren Aronofsky's first film features an eccentric and misanthropic mathematician who has built a supercomputer in his apartment, which he hopes to use to make predictions about the stock market. Max is paranoid and experiences delusions; however, he is also being pursued by both Wall Street business spies, and Hasidic Jews who plan to use Max's genius to find hidden meaning in the Torah.

Possessed (1947) Drama ΨΨΨ
Joan Crawford stars in a suspenseful film depicting catatonic schizophrenia with examples of waxy flexibility and numerous other symptoms of severe mental illness.

Professor and the Madman, The (2019) ΨΨΨ
History-Drama
Mel Gibson plays Prof. James Murray who sets to work to compile the *Oxford English Dictionary*. He is assisted by a physician who turns out to be a psychiatric inpatient. The two men collaborate effectively, despite Dr. Minor's (played by Sean Penn) delusions. The book by Simon

Winchester is a delightful read, and better than the movie it inspired.

Promise (1986) Drama ΨΨ
A made-for-TV movie, starring James Garner, about a man who honors a commitment made to his mother to care for his brother with schizophrenia. Excellent illustrations of the symptoms of schizophrenia.

Proof (2005) Drama ΨΨΨ
Gwyneth Paltrow portrays the daughter of a famous mathematician (Anthony Hopkins). She begins to develop symptoms of schizophrenia similar to those shown by her father as she attempts to solve a rare proof that has baffled other mathematicians.

Rampo Noir (2005, Japan) Horror Ψ
Four short, surreal horror films that are adaptations and tributes to the Japanese poet Rampo. Portrayals of hell, mental illness, and psychosis.

Red Dragon (2002) Thriller–Drama Ψ
Ralph Fiennes, as the serial killer in this prequel to *The Silence of the Lambs*, deepens in his delusional state as he becomes convinced he is a dragon. In one scene, he eats a painting of a dragon to internalize it.

Repulsion (1965) Horror ΨΨΨΨΨ
Powerful film about sexual repression and psychotic decompensation. Memorable examples of hallucinations (e.g., arms reaching out from walls); the film culminates in an unforgettable murder scene. This was Roman Polanski's first English-language film.

Revolution #9 (2001) Thriller–Drama ΨΨΨΨΨ
A psychological drama about a man coping with paranoid schizophrenia. Michael Risley's character is paranoid and delusional (e.g., he thinks the director of a perfume commercial is controlling his thoughts). The film offers an accurate and unflinching portrayal of how relationships are affected by a disease like schizophrenia.

Ruling Class, The (1972) Comedy ΨΨΨΨ
Brilliant British black comedy in which a member of the House of Lords inadvertently commits suicide and leaves his fortune and title to his son who is delusional and schizophrenic (Peter O'Toole). The son at first believes he is Jesus and later Jack the Ripper.

Saint of Fort Washington, The (1993) Drama ΨΨΨ
A man with schizophrenia is evicted from his home and winds up in a shelter, where a streetwise Vietnam veteran befriends him. Good portrayal of the life of people who are both mentally ill and homeless.

Save the Green Planet (2003, Korea) ΨΨ
Drama–Thriller
A young man pursues individuals he perceives are aliens from Andromeda, to keep them from destroying the planet.

Scissors (1991) Suspense Ψ
The paranoid delusions of a traumatized young woman take on a frightening reality when she finds her assailant dead.

Scotland, PA (2001) Comedy ΨΨ
Dark comedy and a subtle parody of Macbeth, about greed, power, love, and "going crazy." A young couple who take over the work at a restaurant after killing the owner, begin to deteriorate with rumination, guilt, and poor coping, as a police detective (Christopher Walken) investigates the murder case.

Shine (1996) Biography–Drama ΨΨΨΨΨ
True story of David Helfgott, an Australian musical prodigy whose brilliant career is interrupted by the development of an unspecified mental illness that is probably schizophrenia. The film not so subtly suggests that David's domineering father was directly responsible for his mental illness and conveys the misleading but endearing message that love and hope are sufficient to conquer mental illness.

> **"David, if you go you will never come back to this house again. You will never be anybody's son. The girls will lose their brother. Is that what you want? ... You want to destroy the family.... if you love me, you will stop this nonsense."**
>
> **David Helfgott's father admonishes him about leaving home, in *Shine* (1996)**

Shining, The (1980) Drama ΨΨΨΨ
Jack Nicholson is a recovering alcoholic who becomes a caretaker for an off-season Colorado resort. He gradually descends into psychosis and attempts to kill both his wife and his son.

Shock Corridor (1963) Drama ΨΨ
Journalist feigns insanity to get a story from a man admitted to a psychiatric hospital; later the journalist begins to lose touch with reality.

Shutter Island (2010) Drama ΨΨΨ
A Martin Scorsese film starring Leonardo DiCaprio as Teddy Daniels, a federal marshal investing a missing

person case at a hospital for the criminally insane in 1954. Although an interesting and intriguing film, it teaches the viewer little about mental illness.

Sixth Sense, The (1999) Drama ΨΨΨ
Bruce Willis plays a Philadelphia child psychologist treating a boy who sees himself surrounded by dead people. If this child were seen at a clinic, he would probably be diagnosed with childhood schizophrenia. The film has a surprise ending and offers some insight into a troubled marriage, but it offers little to help us understand child psychopathology.

Child: "We were supposed to draw a picture, anything we wanted. I drew a man who got hurt in the neck by another man with a screwdriver."
Psychologist: "You saw that on TV, Cole?"
Child: "Everyone got upset. They had a meeting. Mom started crying. I don't draw like that anymore."
Psychologist: "How do you draw now?"
Child: "Draw ... people smiling, dogs running, rainbows. They don't have meetings about rainbows."

A child figures out how to work the system, in *The Sixth Sense* (1999)

Snake Pit, The (1948) Drama ΨΨΨΨ
One of the first films to document the treatment of patients in a mental hospital.

Soloist, The (2009) Drama-Biography ΨΨΨΨΨ
Outstanding portrayal of schizophrenia in which Jamie Foxx portrays a brilliant, isolated musician, Nathaniel Ayers. The film focuses on the development of his friendship with an LA Times reporter, played by Robert Downey Jr.

Some Voices (2000, UK) Comedy ΨΨ
Ray has just been released from a psychiatric hospital, and he is cared for by his restaurateur brother. The film depicts the difficulties Ray experiences when he stops taking his medication.

Something Like Happiness (2005, Czech Republic) Comedy-Drama ΨΨ
Three adults who have been friends from childhood support one another as they try to find happiness along different paths; one is admitted to a psychiatric hospital.

Sophie's Choice (1982) Drama ΨΨΨ
Meryl Streep won an Academy Award for her portrayal of a concentration camp survivor infatuated with Nathan, who is described as having paranoid schizophrenia but who may suffer from a bipolar disorder exacerbated by alcohol abuse. Based on William Styron's novel with the same name.

Special (2006) Drama-Mystery ΨΨ
A man obsessed with comic books decides to take an experimental drug. The medication suppresses self-doubt, and the man quickly believes he has superpowers – including telepathy, the ability to go through walls, and superhuman crime fighting.

Spider (2002) Drama ΨΨΨΨΨ
Ralph Fiennes plays a patient with schizophrenia, disorganized type, who is released from the hospital to a group home. It's a dark, bleak, psychologically complex film and a brilliant portrayal of the isolation and inner world of schizophrenia. Directed by David Cronenberg.

Spiderman (2002) Fantasy-Drama ΨΨ
Sam Raimi classic based on the Marvel comic book series. The Green Goblin (Willem Dafoe) hears voices and seems to be mentally ill. The film perpetuates the myth that people who are mentally ill are also violent.

Stateside (2004) Drama ΨΨ
A young, spoiled, rich man turns his life around after he joins the Marines and falls in love with a woman with schizophrenia. Winner of a Voice Award.

Stay (2005) Mystery-Suspense Ψ
Ewan McGregor portrays a psychiatrist who tries to prevent one of his patients (Ryan Gosling) from committing suicide.

Story of Adèle H., The (1975, France) Biography ΨΨ
François Truffaut story about the sexual obsession of the daughter of Victor Hugo for a young soldier she can never marry.

Strange Voices (1987) Drama ΨΨΨ
A made-for-TV movie that shows the disintegration of a happy family when a college-bound daughter is diagnosed with schizophrenia.

Stroszek (1977, West Germany) Comedy ΨΨ
Offbeat Werner Herzog comedy about three Germans who come to America in search of the American dream. They fail to find it in Railroad Flats, Wisconsin. One of the three has schizophrenia.

Summer of Sam (1999) Drama-Documentary ΨΨΨ
This Spike Lee film succeeds artistically and presents interesting insights into ethnic dynamics and the process

of scapegoating; however, it provides little insight into the motives or the mental illness that drove serial killer David Berkowitz, the highly publicized "Son of Sam," to commit multiple murders. The emphasis is on the fear and psychological trauma of people living in New York City who know a serial killer is still on the loose.

Sweetie (1989) Comedy ΨΨΨΨ
Director Jane Campion paints a memorable and realistic picture of a woman with schizophrenia and the difficulties her illness presents for her and her family.

Sylvia and the Phantom (1945) Drama ΨΨΨ
French film about a young woman who must distinguish between reality and fantasy, love and illusion. Her many seducers include a narcissist, a lover, a criminal, and a phantom.

Synecdoche, New York (2008) Comedy/Drama ΨΨΨ
Interesting mix of delusion, physical illness, and existential angst in Charlie Kaufman's surrealistic film starring Philip Seymour Hoffman.

Take Shelter (2011) Drama-Thriller ΨΨΨΨ
An Ohio farmer named Curtis (Michael Shannon) develops a delusional disorder and hallucinates about an impending disaster. He assumes his symptoms signify the onset of mental illness because his mother was diagnosed with paranoid schizophrenia at age 30.

Tarnation (2003) Documentary ΨΨΨΨ
Poignant, disturbing, dramatic, and realistic film chronicles the life of a family plagued by mental illness. *Tarnation* illustrates schizophrenia and depersonalization disorder as well as the effects of brain damage and traumatic abuse. The film integrates home movies, photographs, short videos, diaries, and pop culture artifacts into striking visceral experience. If you can find this independent film, you should watch it.

Taxi Driver (1976) Drama ΨΨΨΨΨ
Robert De Niro becomes obsessed with Jodie Foster and determines to rescue her from prostitution. A classic film.

> **"Someday real rain will come and wash all the scum off the streets."**
>
> ***Taxi Driver*** **(1976)**

Tenant, The (1976) Horror ΨΨΨ
Roman Polanski film about an ordinary clerk who moves into an apartment in which the previous owner committed suicide. The new owner assumes the personality of the old owner, becomes paranoid, and commits suicide in the same way as the previous owner.

Three Christs (2017) History-Drama ΨΨ
Three patients, all of whom are diagnosed with paranoid schizophrenia, each believe themselves to be Jesus Christ. Richard Gere plays a college professor who leaves the academy to treat these patients with group therapy rather than electroshock.

Through a Glass Darkly (1962) Drama ΨΨΨΨΨ
Powerful and memorable Bergman film about a recently released mental patient who spends the summer on an island with her husband, father, and younger brother. This movie won an Academy Award for Best Foreign Language Film.

Truman Show, The (1998) Drama ΨΨΨΨ
This Peter Weir film stars Jim Carrey as Truman Burbank, who unbeknownst to him, has had his entire life broadcasted on a popular television show in which all of the people in his life are actors and his home and town are part of an elaborate production studio. This film provides a fascinating setup for a discussion of delusional disorders.

They Might Be Giants (1971) Comedy ΨΨ
George C. Scott stars in a film about a man who copes with his grief after his wife's death by developing the delusion that he is Sherlock Holmes. He becomes romantically involved with his psychiatrist (Joanne Woodward). The title is taken from Don Quixote's comment to Sancho Panza after sighting windmills.

Virgin (2003) Drama Ψ
A 17-year-old is raped by a man she is infatuated with, and subsequently she is ostracized, engages in kleptomania, and experiences delusions.

> **"Now that we're through with Humiliate the Host ... and we don't want to play Hump the Hostess yet ... how about a little round of Get the Guests?"**
>
> ***Who's Afraid of Virginia Woolf?*** **(1966)**

Who's Afraid of Virginia Woolf? (1966) ΨΨΨΨ
Drama
A Mike Nichols film, with Elizabeth Taylor and Richard Burton, who appear to have a shared psychotic disorder involving a son who never really existed; the film also portrays alcoholism and interpersonal cruelty. Elizabeth Taylor and Sandy Dennis both won Academy Awards for their performances in this film.

Wonder, The (2022, Ireland) Drama ΨΨΨΨ
Florence Pugh plays a 19th-century British nurse who is brought to Ireland to examine a child who is alleged to not have eaten for 4 months. The film is dramatic and engaging, and it is replete with psychopathology, including incest, anorexia, parental abuse, and a shared delusional disorder.

World Traveler (2001) Drama ΨΨ
Julianne Moore has a supporting role as an alcoholic with a delusional disorder.

Zebraman (2004, Japan) Drama-Crime Ψ
A passive teaching supervisor becomes the superhero Zebraman to escape his miserable, mundane life. The more he accepts his character, the stronger his powers become.

Bipolar and Depressive Disorders and Suicide

Adam (2020) Biography-Drama ΨΨ
A high-powered mortgage broker gets drunk, dives into shallow water, and suffers a spinal cord injury. Somewhat formulaic but based on a true story. Adam overcomes his depression by starting a relationship with a Russian nurse.

American Splendor (2003) Comedy-Drama-Documentary-Animation ΨΨΨΨ
Small-time comic book writer and curmudgeon, Harvey Pekar, reaches cult status including several appearances on the David Letterman Show. This film integrates a narrative about a depressed couple trying to get along and manage life's stressors, comic book animation, and documentary of the real Harvey Pekar.

Anna Karenina (1935) Drama ΨΨΨΨ
Greta Garbo leaves her husband (Basil Rathbone) and son to follow a new love (Fredric March); when she sees him kissing another woman, she commits suicide by stepping into the path of an oncoming train. Based on a novel by Tolstoy.

Another Year (2010, UK) Drama ΨΨΨΨ
Mary is a depressed woman who cannot sleep and who uses wine to cope. Her unhappiness is contrasted with the happy life of her friends Tom (Jim Broadbent) and Gerri (Ruth Sheen), a psychotherapist. Mary's problems only worsens when she tries to seduce Tom and Mary's attorney son, Joe, who simply isn't interested.

Art of Failure: Chuck Connelly, The (2008) Documentary ΨΨ
This is the story of a quirky, neo-expressionist painter of the 1980s, inspired by Andy Warhol and Jackson Pollock. The film depicts an agitated depression, but it also presents a caricature of the "troubled artist."

Assessment and Psychological Treatment of Bipolar Disorder (2011) ΨΨΨΨ
Victor Yalom interviews Kay Redfield Jamison who discusses the genetics, heritability and family history of bipolar disorder. Jamison discusses her own bipolar disorder, and the grief she experienced when her husband died.

À Tout de Suite (2004 , France) Drama ΨΨ
A naïve teenager runs away from home with her Moroccan boyfriend who has just killed a man in a bank robbery. She winds up abandoned in Morocco, depressed and exploited.

Beaver, The (2011) Drama ΨΨΨ
Mel Gibson plays the role of Walter Black, a profoundly depressed and suicidal man in a dysfunctional family, who uses a beaver puppet as an alter ego. Eventually he cuts off his arm to rid himself of the puppet, reunite his family, and put together a meaningful life. This film was nominated for a PRISM Award but lost out to *Take Shelter* and *Shame.*

Bell Jar, The (1979) Biography Ψ
An unsuccessful attempt to capture the spirit of Sylvia Plath's autobiographical novel *The Bell Jar*. Plath eventually committed suicide by putting her head inside an oven and turning on the gas.

Bipolar (2014) Drama Ψ
An awful film that presents a distorted and highly misleading portrayal of bipolar disorder.

Biutiful (2010, Spain) Drama ΨΨΨΨ
Javier Bardem portrays a flawed character who struggles to find meaning despite anxiety and depression due to a general medical condition (prostate cancer).

"You take water, for example. Sometimes it's water, sometimes it's ice. Sometimes it's steam, vapor. It always the same old H2O. It only changes its properties. Your mother's like that. She's like water."

Hank (Tommy Lee Jones) commenting on his bipolar wife's erratic behavior, in *Blue Sky* (1994)

Blue Sky (1994) Drama ΨΨΨΨ
Jessica Lange won an Academy Award for her role as a military wife with a bipolar disorder.

Broken Flowers (2005) Drama ΨΨ
Bill Murray is a depressed Lothario who moves from one casual affair to the next until he gets a letter telling him that he has a 19-year-old son, and he begins a quest to find the anonymous former girlfriend who wrote the letter.

Boy Interrupted (2009) Documentary ΨΨΨΨ
Two filmmakers tell the story of their son, Evan, a gifted child with bipolar disorder who committed suicide by jumping from the window of a skyscraper after leaving a note to his parents. This is a sensitive and moving film, and one hopes that producing the movie helped the parents at least partially heal after the loss of their son.

Cache (2005, France), Mystery–Thriller ΨΨ
A married couple begins to receive videotapes at their doorstep that depict surveillance of their house. The film provides an interesting commentary on the psychology of guilt.

Crooked Beauty: Navigating the Space Between Beauty and Madness (2010) ΨΨΨΨ
Documentary
Director and producer Ken Paul Rosenthal mixes photographs, interviews, and music to tell the story of activist and artist Jacks Ashley McNamara, a woman coping with depression and bipolar disorder. The film is recommended for therapists, and anyone interested in mental illness.

Crossover (1983) Drama Ψ
A male nurse is plagued by self-doubts after a psychiatric patient commits suicide.

Cure for Terminal Loneliness, A (2007) Drama ΨΨ
A short film about a lonely and depressed man who discovers that the cure for loneliness is reaching out to love another person.

Death in Venice (1971) Drama ΨΨΨ
A depressed older composer becomes infatuated with a young boy; the film is based on the novel by Thomas Mann.

Devil and Daniel Johnston, The (2005) ΨΨΨΨ
Documentary–Biography
Portrait of a musical genius who vacillates between madness and brilliant creativity. The film will be especially interesting for viewers interested in the relationship between mental illness and creativity.

Don McKay (2009) Drama ΨΨ
A depressed school janitor receives a letter from a high school friend telling him she is dying from cancer, and he returns to the small town he left years earlier to confront the past he left behind.

Eye of God (1997) Drama ΨΨ
Some of the scenes in this film address a boy who witnesses his mother's suicide, experiences acute stress disorder, and kills himself at age 14.

Eyes Upon Waking (2022) Biography–Drama ΨΨ
A recent film based on the director's personal history of multiple suicide attempts and her experience in a psychiatric hospital.

Faithless (2000) Drama ΨΨΨΨ
Liv Ullmann directed this film about a woman who has an affair with a deeply depressed man.

February's Dog (2022, Canada) ΨΨΨ
Two oil field workers are laid off on the same day. The film traces their anxiety and depression, and their despair is exacerbated by alcoholism and marital difficulties.

Field, The (1990) Drama ΨΨΨ
Dramatic presentation of the suicide by drowning of a young man who finds he cannot live up to his father's expectations.

Flying Scotsman, The (2006, Germany/UK) ΨΨΨ
Drama
Champion cyclist who constructed his bike out of pieces of washing machines suffers with depression and suicidal thoughts. This film received an Honorable Mention at the Voice Awards.

Fox and His Friends (1975) Drama ΨΨΨΨ
Werner Fassbinder's scathing indictment of capitalism revolves around the life of a poor gay circus performer who wins money, only to lose it through the exploitation of those he assumes are his friends. He responds by committing suicide.

Garden State (2004) Drama–Comedy ΨΨΨ
A young man flies to his hometown in New Jersey for his mother's funeral. He has been estranged from his family for several years. When he stops taking his bipolar medication, he begins to experiment with life and finds love.

Good Morning, Vietnam (1987) Comedy/Drama/War ΨΨ
Robin Williams as an Air Force radio announcer in Vietnam. Williams has a funny, frenetic style that could be described as hypomanic. One can't watch films like this without becoming sad thinking about the suicide of Robin Williams who suffered from bipolar disorder and Lewy body dementia.

Hairdresser's Husband, The (1992) Comedy-Drama ΨΨΨ
A woman chooses to commit suicide rather than face the incremental loss of love that she believes will accompany aging. This is a beautiful movie, despite the somewhat grim ending.

Harold and Maude (1971) Comedy ΨΨΨ
An acting-out teenager and an iconoclastic old woman bond and support one another's eccentricities, including Harold's repeated feigned suicide attempts.

Helen (2008) Drama ΨΨΨ
A music professor (Ashley Judd) is plagued by suicidal depression, and she finds comfort from another woman coping with her own problems.

Hello Ghost (2010, Korea) Drama ΨΨ
Ghosts plague a man after a series of failed suicide attempts; by letting the ghosts occupy his body to clear up unfinished business, he gets them to leave him alone, and he learns about himself in the process. Adam Sandler is reported to have bought the rights to remake this Korean film, but it has not yet been released.

Henry Poole Is Here (2008) Comedy-Drama ΨΨ
A depressed, isolated, and alcoholic man receives a terminal diagnosis and moves to the suburbs to wait to die; however, his life becomes complicated – and richer – after the face of Jesus appears on the stucco wall of his house, and a mute child begins to speak after touching the image.

Hitchhiker's Guide to the Galaxy, The (2005) Comedy ΨΨ
One of the major characters, a robot, exhibits several symptoms of depression.

Horse Feathers (1932) Comedy ΨΨ
Groucho Marx plays a manic college president who displays flight of ideation and pressured speech.

Hospital, The (1971) Comedy-Drama ΨΨΨ
George C. Scott is first rate as a disillusioned and suicidal physician despondent in part because of the ineptitude he sees everywhere about him. There is an especially memorable scene in which Scott is interrupted as he is about to commit suicide by injecting potassium into a vein. "People are sicker than ever. We cure nothing. We heal nothing."

House of Sand and Fog (2003) Drama ΨΨΨΨΨ
Jennifer Connelly and Sir Ben Kingsley play opposite one another in a gripping and deeply poignant story about two seemingly very different people, each with a legitimate claim to ownership of the same house. The film accurately portrays depression, alcohol abuse, suicide attempts, and suicide.

Hours, The (2002) Drama ΨΨΨΨΨ
Well-acted and well-crafted tapestry integrating three stories from different times – Nicole Kidman as the renowned novelist, Virginia Woolf, struggling to write her novel *Mrs. Dalloway*; Julianne Moore, who is reading the novel decades later; and Meryl Streep who embodies many of Mrs. Dalloway's characteristics. Each of the four main characters (the three women and Ed Harris) struggles with some form of mood disorder.

"Dearest, I feel certain that I am going mad again. I feel I can't go through another one of these terrible times and I shan't recover this time. I begin to hear voices and can't concentrate so I am doing what seems to be the best thing to do. You have given me the greatest possible happiness. You have been in every way all that anyone could be. I know that I am spoiling your life and without me you could work, and you will, I know. You see I can't even write this properly. What I want to say is that I owe all the happiness of my life to you. You have been entirely patient with me and incredibly good. Everything is gone from me but the certainty of your goodness. I can't go on spoiling your life any longer. I don't think two people could have been happier than we have been. Virginia"

Virginia Woolf's suicide note

Imaginary Heroes (2004) Drama ΨΨ
A young boy commits suicide by shooting himself, and each member of the family responds to the tragedy in a different way.

Infinitely Polar Bear (2014) ΨΨΨΨ
Comedy, Drama, Romance
Mark Ruffalo plays the role of a man recently released from the hospital who is forced by life's circumstances

to take over responsibility for his two daughters. It is a highly engaging film and an accurate depiction of the ways in which bipolar disorder can affect the family of someone with the disorder.

> **"My father was diagnosed manic depressive in 1967. He'd been going around Cambridge in a fake beard calling himself Jesus John Harvard. When he got better, he started working in public television in Boston. He met my mother there. He walked up and took her picture. On their first date, he took her on a driving tour of New England and told her all about his nervous breakdowns."**
>
> **A daughter describes her parents, in *Infinitely Polar Bear* (2015)**

Informant, The (2009) Drama Comedy ΨΨ
Steven Soderbergh film based on a true story about a bipolar whistleblower.

Inside Moves (1980) Drama ΨΨ
A man who has failed in a suicide attempt makes new friends in a bar and retains the will to live. Mainly notable as the comeback film for Harold Russell, the double amputee from *The Best Years of Our Lives* (1946).

Into the Wild (2007) Biography ΨΨΨΨ
Sean Penn directed this film that is based on a true story about an Emory student who graduates, gives away the money he had saved for law school, and moves to Alaska. It is a useful pedagogical exercise to speculate about potential diagnoses for this man.

It's a Wonderful Life (1946) Drama ΨΨΨ
A Christmas tradition. The film presents Jimmy Stewart as a complex character who responds to the stress of life in Bedford Falls by attempting suicide.

I've Loved You So Long (*Il Y a Longtemps Que Je T'aime;* 2008, France) Drama ΨΨΨΨ
A female physician moves in with her sister after serving a 15-year prison sentence for killing her own son. The two women struggle with learning to love one another and reunite as a family, and details about the boy's death only come clear at the end of the film.

Jellysmoke (2005) Drama–Romance ΨΨΨ
A young man with bipolar disorder is released from a psychiatric institution and struggles to adapt to his new life. Winner of a Voice Award.

> **"You see, George, you've really had a wonderful life. Don't you see what a mistake it would be to throw it away?"**
>
> **Clarence in *It's A Wonderful Life* (1946)**

Juliet of the Spirits (1965) Drama ΨΨΨ
Frederico Fellini film about a bored, lonely, depressed, and menopausal homemaker who hallucinates about the life of the exotic woman next door.

Last Days (2005) Drama ΨΨΨ
Slow-moving Gus Van Sant film depicting the final days of Nirvana singer–guitarist Kurt Cobain. Various manic and depressive symptoms are displayed.

Last Days of Disco, The (1998) Drama Ψ
One of the characters has bipolar disorder and is stereotyped as "looney" and "crazy"; however, he is depicted as compliant with lithium treatment, and his life is stable and balanced. Interesting contrast to the frequently portrayed stereotypes of bipolar disorder.

Last Picture Show, The (1971) Drama ΨΨΨΨ
Peter Bogdanovich adaptation of Larry McMurtry's novel describing the events - and personalities - involved in the closing of the town's only movie theater. There is a striking presentation of the symptoms of depression in the coach's wife.

Life Itself (2018) Drama ΨΨ
This film presents several stories that span continents and decades, stitching them together in the end and making the viewer appreciate how our lives connect with others in ways we don't fully understand. While not a critical success, anyone reading *Movies and Mental Illness* will be especially interested in the depiction of Will (Oscar Isaac) as a hopeless figure unable to deal with the loss of his wife early in the movie. Will dramatically commits suicide in the office of his therapist (Annette Bening).

Life Upside Down (1964, France) Drama ΨΨΨ
French film about an ordinary young man who becomes increasingly detached from the world. He is eventually hospitalized and treated, but with little success.

Lincoln (2013) Biography–Drama–History ΨΨΨΨ
Steven Spielberg directs Daniel Day-Lewis in the title role. Lincoln's well-documented clinical depression is apparent in many of the scenes, as is the challenge of life with Mary Todd Lincoln, played by Sally Field. The film provides numerous examples of Lincoln's depressed affect.

Little Miss Sunshine (2006) Comedy ΨΨΨ
Steve Carell plays a renowned gay Proust scholar who has just been released from the hospital after a suicide attempt.

Lonely Guy, The (1984) Comedy Ψ
Steve Martin plays a depressed and suicidal New Yorker.

Lonesome Jim (2006) Drama ΨΨΨ
Steve Buscemi directed this engaging film about a depressed and discouraged writer who returns to his childhood home in Indiana after failing to find success in New York City.

Maborosi (1995, Japan) Drama ΨΨΨΨ
A Japanese film about the effects of a man's seemingly irrational suicide on the wife who is left behind to care for their 3-month-old infant.

Maddened by His Absence (2012, France) Drama ΨΨΨ
A man returns to France for the funeral of his father and attempts to reunite with his wife, someone he left 9 years earlier, after the death of their child in an auto accident.

Manchester by the Sea (2016) Drama ΨΨΨΨ
Casey Affleck plays a man whose life becomes defined by grief following the death of his children in a house fire.

Manic (2003) Drama-Action ΨΨΨ
An adolescent inpatient unit has patients with intermittent explosive disorder, disorder, major depression, self-injurious behavior, and night terrors.

Me Before You (2016, UK) Romance-Drama ΨΨ
A wealthy banker becomes paralyzed and terrorizes a series of caretakers before falling in love with one. Ultimately, he follows through on his plans to fly to Switzerland for euthanasia. The movie was criticized and boycotted by the disability rights community in Britain.

Meet Bill (2007) Comedy-Drama ΨΨ
Aaron Eckhart portrays a man whose depression worsens when he discovers his wife is having an affair.

Melancholia (2011, Denmark) Drama ΨΨΨΨΨ
A memorable Lars von Trier film starring Kirsten Dunst playing the role of Justine, a profoundly depressed woman who has just been married. She and her husband attend an elaborate but unhappy wedding reception; that evening Justine spurns her husband's sexual overtures; she leaves him and later in the evening has sex with a coworker on a golf course. Meanwhile, the end of civilization approaches as the planet Melancholia draws close.

Melinda and Melinda (2004) Comedy-Drama ΨΨ
This Woody Allen film alternates between two versions of a story, one tragic, one comic. In the tragic version, we find a depressed and suicidal Melinda.

Michael Clayton (2007) Drama ΨΨΨΨ
Tom Wilkinson plays the role of a brilliant attorney whose bipolar-manic episodes make it almost impossible for him to function as an attorney.

Michael Clayton: "You are the senior litigating partner of one of the largest, most respected law firms in the world. You are a legend."
Arthur Edens: "I'm an accomplice!"
Michael Clayton: "You're a manic-depressive!"
Arthur Edens: "I am Shiva, the God of death."

George Clooney reasons with a bipolar Tom Wilkinson, in *Michael Clayton* (2007)

Mind the Gap (2004) Drama ΨΨΨ
The lives of five isolated, lonely and desperate people are intertwined in complex ways: eventually each live intersects with the other four. One poignant segment portrays a suicidal African American man who gets life-saving advice from a priest.

Mishima: A Life in Four Chapters (1985) Biography ΨΨΨ
A fascinating film about one of the most interesting figures in contemporary literature, Yukio Mishima. Mishima, a homosexual, traditionalist, and militarist, committed ritual suicide *(seppuku)* before being beheaded by a companion.

Monsieur Ibrahim (2003) Drama-Comedy ΨΨΨ
An elderly widower and troubled teen form a unique friendship while living in Paris in the 1960s. A secondary character, the boy's father, suffers from agitated, masked depression, and eventually abandons his son (who had already been abandoned by his mother) and commits suicide.

Monster's Ball (2002) Drama ΨΨΨΨ
Emotionally jarring film about two lost, self-hating people who begin to experience emotion and face their pain through their relationship. The film stars Billy Bob Thornton and Halle Berry (the latter won an Academy Award for Best Actress for her role in this film).

Morning (2010) Drama ΨΨΨΨ
A Seattle couple grieves the loss of their child to drowning.

Mosquito Coast, The (1986) Adventure ΨΨΨ
Harrison Ford is an eccentric American inventor who flees the United States for Central America because of his paranoia. His diagnosis is never clearly stated, but Ford appears to be bipolar (although almost continually manic in the film).

My First Wife (1984) Drama ΨΨ
A moving and well-directed Australian film about a man who falls apart after his wife decides to leave him.

Network (1976) Drama ΨΨΨ
A veteran anchorman who has just been told he is being fired announces on national TV that he will commit suicide on the air in 2 weeks. Ratings soar. He eventually reneges on his promise but becomes the leader of a national protest movement.

> **"...I'm as mad as hell, and I'm not going to take this anymore!"**
>
> **Newscaster Howard Beale, in *Network* (1976)**

Nightmare Alley (1947) Crime ΨΨ
Tyrone Power's favorite film. Power plays a carnival huckster who teams up with an unethical psychologist to dupe the public. Memorable carnival "geek" scenes include biting the heads off chickens.

Nightmare Alley (2021) ΨΨΨ
Guillermo del Toro's remake of the 1947 classic of the same name. This version stars Bradley Cooper and Cate Blanchett. Both the original and the remake are highly recommended (as art, not pedagogy).

Nine Lives (2005) Drama ΨΨΨ
This film is directed by Rodrigo Garcia, the son of the novelist Gabriel Garcia Marquez. It consists of nine relatively brief vignettes about the lives of nine women, one of whom is suicidal.

No Letting Go (2015) Drama ΨΨΨΨ
This film is based on the real-life experiences of Randi Silverman, the producer and screenwriter. The movie accurately depicts the way a child with a serious mental illness can affect family dynamics. The protagonist is shown at two points in his life, ages 10 and 16; he initially presents with anxiety symptoms but is eventually diagnosed as a person with bipolar disorder. The film may be useful to help parents understand the challenges they will confront when raising a child with a serious mental illness.

Of Two Minds (2012) Documentary ΨΨΨ
This engaging film documents the lives and struggles of three individuals living with bipolar disorder. Each person in the film describes the highs and the lows associated with the illness, and the life challenges their disorder has presented.

Off the Map (2003) Drama ΨΨΨ
Sam Elliott plays Charley, a veteran living in New Mexico with his wife and 11-year-old daughter. The family is eccentric (e.g., the wife tends her garden in the nude) but happy until Charley develops a crippling depression.

Oppenheimer (2023) Drama/Biography ΨΨΨΨΨ
Christopher Nolan's depiction of the life and work of J. Robert Oppenheimer, known as the father of the atomic bomb. The film depicts Oppenheimer's depression while at Cambridge, his multiple affairs, and his growing concern that he was personally responsible for the deaths of thousands of Japanese citizens.

Outcry, The (1957) Drama ΨΨΨ
Antonioni film about a man who becomes depressed and confused when he is rejected by his lover.

Perks of Being a Wallflower (2012) Drama ΨΨΨΨ
In a film that effectively captures the *angst* of high school, Logan Lerman plays Charlie, a lonely high school student. He is depressed until he makes friends with two other students. Charlie becomes suicidal and is hospitalized; while in the hospital his depression is traced to a history of sexual abuse by his aunt.

Pollock (2000) Drama ΨΨΨ
Ed Harris portrays the troubled painter Jackson Pollock, who struggles with alcoholism and bipolar disorder. Pollock died from a car crash while drunk in 1956. He was 44 years old. The film will interest anyone studying the relationship between bipolar disorder and creativity.

Prozac Nation (2001) Drama ΨΨΨ
A dramatic and realistic portrayal of depression and borderline personality disorder in a Harvard undergraduate.

Rabbit Hole (2010) Drama ΨΨΨΨ
Nicole Kidman stars in this powerful drama about a couple trying to cope with the loss of their 4-year-old son who was killed when he chased his dog into the street. Group therapy seems to provide little solace for the couple, and their relationship is clearly threatened by their loss. Kidman's character copes with her grief by starting an affair with the young man who was driving the car that killed her son.

"God had to take her. He needed another angel." "Why didn't he just make one? Another angel? I mean, he's God, after all. Why didn't he just make another angel?"

Nicol Kidman's character responds to an insensitive remark in a group therapy session, in *Rabbit Hole* (2010)

Rain (2001) Drama ΨΨ
Coming-of-age New Zealand film about a young girl whose mother is a depressed alcoholic.

Reason to Live (2009) Documentary ΨΨΨ
A film with first-person accounts by young people who are suicidal and who have made suicidal attempts, with commentary by their parents.

Respiro (2002) Drama ΨΨΨ
An Italian film about a woman with a serious bipolar disorder who must flee and hide in a cave to avoid coerced psychiatric treatment.

Running with Scissors (2006) Biography ΨΨ
Annette Bening plays the role of a bipolar mother who turns over her son's life to her psychiatrist.

Rust and Bone (2012, France) Drama ΨΨΨΨ
A whale trainer loses her legs and becomes profoundly depressed; the film offers a dramatic illustration of the ways in which an accident of this sort can trigger despair and withdrawal from the world, and the ways in which a relationship can buffer the pain of loss.

Scent of a Woman (1992) Drama ΨΨΨ
Al Pacino plays Colonel Slade, a depressed, blind veteran who seems to have lost all meaning in his life until he is challenged by a younger man.

September (1987) Drama ΨΨ
A Woody Allen film in which Mia Farrow plays a depressed woman recovering from a suicide attempt.

Seven Pounds (2008) Drama ΨΨΨΨ
Will Smith plays a character who attempts to use his suicide to gain redemption for an accident he caused that resulted in the deaths of seven people.

Seventh Veil, The (1945) Drama ΨΨ
Psychological drama about a gifted musician who loses the ability to play the piano and becomes depressed and suicidal. Hypnotherapy makes it possible for Ann Todd to play again, as well as to sort out her complex interpersonal relationships.

Shawshank Redemption, The (1994) ΨΨΨΨΨ
Drama
An outstanding film, memorable in part because of the suicide of one character who finds himself unable to adjust to life outside an institution.

Shopgirl (2005) Drama ΨΨ
A depressed salesgirl learns about the meaning of love through an affair with a much older man (played by Steve Martin, who also wrote the screenplay and the novella upon which the film was based).

Sherlock Holmes (2009, 2011) Action-Adventure ΨΨ
Robert Downey Jr. portrays the infamous detective but with significant periods of mania and some symptoms of depression.

Silver Linings Playbook (2012) ΨΨΨΨΨ
Drama-Comedy
Pat Solatano (Bradley Cooper) is struggling with bipolar disorder. His wife has left him, he has lost his job, he has just been discharged from a psychiatric hospital, and he is living with his parents. His life changes for the better after he meets Tiffany (Jennifer Lawrence), a woman with problems of her own (possibly borderline personality disorder).

"The world will break your heart ten ways to Sunday. That's guaranteed. I can't begin to explain that. Or the craziness inside myself and everyone else. But guess what? Sunday is my favorite day again. I think of what everyone did for me, and I feel like a very lucky guy."

Pat appreciates that he is making progress in his recovery from bipolar disorder, in *Silver Linings Playbook* (2012)

Single Man, A (2009) Drama ΨΨΨ
Colin Firth plays the role of a depressed gay man living alone and contemplating suicide after the death of his lover.

Skeleton Twins, The (2014) Comedy-Drama ΨΨ
Two estranged twins (Maggie and Milo) reunite after Milo survives a suicide attempt.

Son's Room, The (2001, Italy) ΨΨΨ
A psychoanalyst and his wife and daughter all grieve in their own way following the loss of the man's son in a scuba diving accident. The film is a good illustration of the way grief affects families.

Spanglish (2004) Comedy Ψ
An offbeat comedy about a talented cook and his manic wife who hires a Latina housekeeper.

Station Agent, The (2003) Drama-Comedy ΨΨΨΨ
Heartwarming, honest story of three lonely and disparate characters who form a unique friendship with one another. The three characters are a schizoid dwarf whose only desire is isolation, a woman who has repeated conflicts with her husband and attempts suicide, and a talkative man from New Jersey. Good mix of both healthy and unhealthy coping approaches to loneliness and depression.

Step Forward, A (2019, Japan) Documentary ΨΨΨ
A film that documents the efforts of a priest to save the lives of people who have come to the Sandanbeki cliffs to commit suicide.

Stronger (2017) Biography-Drama ΨΨΨ
The film is based on a true story, and stars Jake Gyllenhaal as Jeff Bauman, a man who loses his legs after the Boston marathon bombing.

Suicide Club (2002, Japan) Drama-Suspense ΨΨΨ
Fifty-four young girls collectively jump in front of an oncoming subway train, which triggers individual and group suicides around the country. This mysterious Japanese film raises questions of cause, documenting links between suicide and adolescence, violence, and consumerism, and it illustrates the contagion effect.

Suicide Room (2011, Poland) Drama ΨΨΨΨ
Dominik kisses another boy while drunk, and he is relentlessly tormented via social media as a result. He withdraws from school and begins to self-mutilate, tutored by a girl he meets in an online chat room devoted to suicide.

Summer Wishes, Winter Dreams (1973) Drama Ψ
Joanne Woodward is a bored, depressed housewife searching for meaning and purpose in her life. The film includes dreams that may be hallucinations, and a possible somatoform disorder.

Sunset Limited (2011) Drama ΨΨΨ
A depressed and suicidal college professor (Tommy Lee Jones) is rescued by a deeply religious blue collar worker (Samuel Jackson), and the two men discuss life's meaning and purpose. The college professor exhibits classic signs of depression.

Sylvia (2003) Drama ΨΨ
Gwyneth Paltrow portrays the life of respected American poet, Sylvia Plath, who committed suicide in 1963. The film focuses on the relationship between Plath and her husband, poet Ted Hughes.

"Sometimes I dream the tree, and the tree is my life. One branch is the man I shall marry, and the leaves my children. Another branch is my future as a writer, and each leaf is a poem. Another branch is a good academic career. But as I sit there trying to choose, the leaves bring to turn brown and blow away, until the tree is absolutely bare."

Sylvia Plath (Gwyneth Paltrow) contemplates her life, in *Sylvia* (2003)

Taste of Cherry (1997) Drama ΨΨΨΨ
An Iranian film about a man who wants to commit suicide but who can't find anyone to help him.

Three Identical Strangers (2018) Biography ΨΨΨΨΨ
Identical triplets are deliberately separated at birth by an unethical Yale psychologist and adopted by three different families. They have a chance encounter in 1980 and discover each other. All three deal with mental health issues, and in 1995, one brother committed suicide after a long struggle with depression.

Marco: "So Emily, can I ask you what your full fake name is?"
Carla: "Emily Lowell."
Marco: "Is that Emily Dickinson and Robert Lowell? Those are good poets. Do you know they were both bipolar?"

Marco flirts with another patient poet, in *Touched With Fire*

Touched With Fire (2015) ΨΨΨΨΨ
A Paul Dalio film about two patients with bipolar disorder who meet in a psychiatric hospital and begin an affair. The film accurately portrays the symptoms of bipolar disorder.

Two Lovers (2008) Drama ΨΨΨ
Joaquin Phoenix and Gwyneth Paltrow star in this film about a troubled, depressed, and suicidal man who is torn between his love for two women. The film begins and ends with suicide attempts.

Umberto D. (1952) Drama ΨΨΨΨΨ
Classic Vittorio De Sica film about an indigent old man in Rome who is being evicted and must face the prospects of homelessness and isolation. The old man fails a suicide attempt and finds a reason for living through his devotion to his dog.

Vincent (1987) Biography-Documentary ΨΨΨ
An interesting examination of the life of Vincent van Gogh. The focus is on the artist's work rather than his mental illness.

Vincent & Theo (1990) Biography ΨΨΨ
This Robert Altman film deals sensitively with van Gogh's troubled relationships with Gauguin and Theo, the incident with the prostitute and his ear, his hospitalization, and finally his suicide.

Virgin Suicides, The (1999) Drama ΨΨ
Sofia Coppola's directorial debut, about a repressed family with five daughters, who in response to their mother's control, repression, and forced isolation, decide to commit suicide.

Visioneers (2008) Drama Ψ
Zach Galifianakis is the protagonist in a drab film about office workers who explode because their lives lack meaning and purpose.

Visitor, The (2007) Drama ΨΨΨΨ
This film illustrates the apathy and indifference that can sometimes accompany depression. Richard Jenkins plays the role of Prof. Walter Vale, a man trying unsuccessfully to cope after the death of his wife.

Walking Man (2015) Documentary ΨΨΨ
After three high school students commit suicide in a rural Missouri school, a father and son, both of whom have bipolar disorder, walk across the state to educate others about the needs of people with mental illness.

War Within, The (2005) Drama Ψ
An examination of the motives behind the behavior of a suicide bomber.

Wilbur Wants to Kill Himself (2002)
Drama-Comedy ΨΨ
Disappointing and highly stereotypic movie of both suicide and boundary-crossing psychotherapists. Perpetrates the misconception that love can conquer mental illness (in this case, multiple and severe suicide attempts).

Winter Passing (2005) Drama ΨΨ
A depressed young woman living in New York City uses alcohol, drugs, and casual sex to cope. She travels to the Upper Peninsula of Michigan to visit her father, an alcoholic novelist, to see if she can obtain copies of the letters he wrote to her recently deceased mother years earlier.

Wit (2001) Drama ΨΨΨΨΨ
Emma Thompson portrays an English professor who has devoted her entire life to the work of John Donne. She develops ovarian cancer and reflects on the personal meaning of death as she undergoes aggressive medical treatment. The film will be useful for students learning about death, dying, and palliative care.

Woman Under the Influence, A (1974)
Drama ΨΨΨΨ
A John Cassavetes film in which Gena Rowlands plays a homemaker who must be hospitalized because of a mental illness that appears to be bipolar disorder. Peter Falk plays her mystified husband.

Wristcutters: A Love Story (2006) Fantasy ΨΨ
A young man commits suicide and then finds himself in purgatory, surrounded by other individuals who have all committed suicide in one way or another.

Wrong Man, The (1956) Drama-Crime ΨΨΨ
Hitchcock film in which a man and his wife (Henry Fonda and Vera Miles) become depressed in response to an unjust accusation of murder.

You're Not You (2014) Drama ΨΨ
Hilary Swank plays a concert pianist with ALS who ultimately decides to stop treatment and let herself die.

Anxiety and Obsessive-Compulsive Disorders

40 Year Old Virgin, The (2005) Comedy ΨΨ
Screwball comedy depicting issues relevant to those suffering from social phobia, such as fear of embarrassment, dating and sex fears, social inadequacy, and avoidance behavior.

Adaptation (2002) Comedy-Action ΨΨΨΨ
Multilayered Spike Jonze film in which Nicholas Cage plays twin brothers, one of whom is a neurotic screenwriter struggling to write a story based on a book about orchids.

Analyze That (2002) Comedy-Action ΨΨ
The follow-up film to *Analyze This*, in which a panic-disordered mob boss (Robert De Niro) malingers to get

released from prison, tries to maintain an ordinary job, and is convinced to return to the mob while stringing along his psychiatrist (Billy Crystal).

Analyze This (1999) Comedy-Action ΨΨ
The original Billy Crystal and Robert De Niro comedy in which De Niro plays the lead thug in a New York mafia group who develops panic attacks. De Niro sees a psychiatrist (Billy Crystal) for treatment.

Arachnophobia (1990) Comedy-Horror ΨΨ
A story about a doctor with a paralyzing fear of spiders. (Actually, the spiders in this film are intimidating, and fear appears to be a perfectly reasonable response.)

As Good As It Gets (1997) Romance ΨΨΨΨ
Jack Nicholson won his third Academy Award for Best Actor for this film, in which he portrays a homophobic, racist novelist with an obsessive-compulsive disorder.

Aviator, The (2004) Drama-Biography ΨΨΨΨΨ
Directed by Martin Scorsese, this film depicts Howard Hughes Jr.'s (Leonardo DiCaprio) early years (1920-1940s) and the progression of his obsessive-compulsive disorder. Winner of five Academy Awards and a Voice Award.

Katharine Hepburn: "What's that on the steering wheel?"
Howard Hughes: "Cellophane. If you had any idea of the crap that people carry around on their hands."
Katharine Hepburn: "What kind of crap?"
Howard Hughes: "You don't wanna know."

Howard Hughes displays symptoms of OCD, in *The Aviator*

Batman Begins (2005) Action-Drama ΨΨΨΨΨ
Sophisticated Christopher Nolan film telling the story of Bruce Wayne, a young boy with a phobia who watches his wealthy parents being murdered and subsequently becomes a superhero. Wayne's phobia of bats is conquered through systematic exposure. The movie demonstrates the importance of facing up to what one fears the most.

Broken English (2007) ΨΨ
Comedy-Drama-Romance
Parker Posey portrays an organizer-secretary-event planner who is bored and passes each day searching for a lover on the Internet. She chooses men who are unavailable, because of her fear of commitment. When she gets close to a genuine commitment herself, she has panic attacks.

Bubble (2005) Crime-Drama ΨΨ
Minimalist Steven Soderbergh project about three characters in a poor town, working at a factory. One suffers from anxiety and panic attacks.

Cars that Ate Paris, The (1974, Australia) Comedy Ψ
Early Peter Weir film that takes place in a secluded town in rural Paris, Australia, where the main source of income is the revenue from salvaged valuables from car wrecks. Panic attacks and exposure are depicted.

Casualties of War (1989) War ΨΨΨ
Brian De Palma film about five GIs who kidnap, rape, and murder a young Vietnamese girl. The film deals with themes of guilt, stress, violence, and, most of all, the dehumanizing aspects of war.

Cat Ladies (2009) Documentary ΨΨ
This film will introduce you to four ladies who share their lives with numerous cats. The film is a good introduction to a special subset of hoarding disorder: animal hording.

Columbus Circle (2010) Drama ΨΨ
A wealthy agoraphobic woman is forced to confront her fears when new neighbors move in.

Copycat (1995) Suspense-Thriller ΨΨ
Sigourney Weaver plays a criminal psychologist who struggles with agoraphobia symptoms as she helps police track down a serial killer (Harry Connick Jr.).

Coyote Ugly (2000) Comedy-Drama ΨΨ
A young woman moves to New York City to try to make it as a songwriter. She takes a job as a "coyote" bartender (dancing on the tables and flirting with customers) at a wild, interactive bar; the experience helps her overcome her social anxiety.

Creepshow (1982) Horror ΨΨ
A man with an insect phobia winds up being eaten alive by cockroaches. Directed by George Romero, who also directed the classic film *Night of the Living Dead*. Stephen King wrote the screenplay, and the film is better than it sounds.

Croods, The (2013) Animation ΨΨΨ
A family living in a cave assuages their anxiety by adopting a strict and restrictive set of rules; when they are forced to leave their cave, they learn to cope with the world by facing their fears and relying on each other.

Cyrano de Bergerac (1990, France) Romance ΨΨΨ
Gerard Depardieu stars as the inimitable Cyrano, a man obsessed with the size of his nose and convinced it makes him forever unlovable.

Da Vinci Code, The (2006) Drama-Mystery ΨΨ
This is a Ron Howard film about a murder inside the Louvre. Clues in Da Vinci's paintings lead to the discovery of a religious mystery protected by a secret society for 2,000 years – which could shake the foundations of Christianity. Tom Hanks' character experiences somatic anxiety symptoms including shortness of breath and discomfort in social situations.

Departed, The (2006) Crime-Drama-Mystery ΨΨ
Engaging Martin Scorsese film starring Leonardo DiCaprio, Matt Damon, Jack Nicholson, and Martin Sheen portraying Irish mafia, undercover detectives, and corrupt federal agents. DiCaprio's character experiences panic attacks, and anxiolytics are prescribed.

Devil (2010) Horror Ψ
Five people are trapped on an elevator; one is claustrophobic, and another is the Devil.

Dirty, Filthy Love (2004, UK) ΨΨΨΨ
Drama-Comedy
An outstanding movie about Mark Furness whose life falls apart because of his affliction with obsessive-compulsive disorder and Tourette's disorder. Treatment, support groups, and severe symptoms of OCD and Tourette's are shown in the film.

Dummy (2002) Comedy-Drama ΨΨ
A predictable film starring Adrian Brody as Steven, an aspiring ventriloquist, who is unemployed, naïve, passive, and socially awkward until he finds meaning and social support through his "dummy." Interesting metaphor of the socially phobic person finding his "inner voice." All ventriloquism in the film is performed by Adrian Brody. The DVD features interviews and comic classes with champion ventriloquist Jeff Dunham.

Elling (2001) Drama ΨΨΨΨΨ
Norwegian film about two men released from a psychiatric hospital who must prove themselves capable of coping with everyday life. Oscar nominee for Best Foreign Language Film.

Everything Is Illuminated (2005) ΨΨ
Comedy-Drama
A young Jewish American travels to the Ukraine to find the woman who saved his grandfather from the Nazis. He stores everything in small plastic bags and claims to have a phobia of dogs but ends up sharing both the backseat of a car and then a bed with a dog.

Falling (2022) Drama ΨΨΨΨ
Two girls decide to climb a 2,000-foot TV tower in a rural, isolated area to help one of the girls overcome a fear of heights that resulted from the death of her husband from a climbing accident a year before. The climb goes horribly wrong, and one of the girls dies.

Feardotcom (2002) Thriller-Horror Ψ
Various characters access a deadly website that makes their deepest fears or phobias come true (e.g., one has a phobia of beetles and soon is covered by them).

Gigantic (2008) Drama Comedy Romance ΨΨ
A mattress salesman develops an obsession about adopting a Chinese child; however, his new love interest isn't convinced that it is a good idea. Watch for multiple references to the concept of learned helplessness.

High Anxiety (1977) Comedy ΨΨ
Mel Brook's spoof of Hitchcock classics about a psychiatrist who works at "The Psycho-Neurotic Institute for the Very, Very Nervous." The film is better if you've seen the Hitchcock films on which the parody builds, such as *Psycho*, *Dial M for Murder*, and *Vertigo*.

House of Games (1987) Crime ΨΨ
Lindsay Crouse plays a role as a psychiatrist who has just written an important book on obsessive-compulsive disorders. She becomes obsessed with confidence games and is slowly drawn into the criminal life.

In the Bedroom (2001) Drama-Suspense ΨΨΨΨ
Introspective film with a talented cast that examines grief, despair, and revenge after the murder of someone deeply loved. Marisa Tomei's character develops an acute stress disorder following the trauma. The film makes good use of silence; those scenes underscore the tension, unspoken feelings, and underlying pain associated with the death of a loved one.

Inside Out (1986) Drama ΨΨ
A little-known but interesting film in which Elliott Gould plays a man with agoraphobia. He can obtain food, sex, and haircuts in his home, but finds that he cannot meet *all* his needs without leaving his house.

Kissing Jessica Stein (2002) Comedy ΨΨΨ
Quality independent film about a neurotic, young woman who in exploring her sexuality and intrapersonal life is able to extend beyond her rigidity and generalized anxiety.

**"What does your therapist think of all this?"
"Oh, I would never tell my therapist."
"Why not?"
"Because it's private."**

Dialogue in *Kissing Jessica Stein* (2002)

Lady in a Cage (1964) Drama-Suspense ΨΨ
Olivia de Havilland plays an upper-class woman trapped inside her home elevator. The film melodramatically portrays claustrophobia and panic.

Macbeth (1971) Drama ΨΨΨ
Powerful Roman Polanski adaptation of Shakespeare's play. It is interesting to speculate about the obsessions of Lady Macbeth and to compare Polanski's version with an earlier Orson Welles' adaptation.

Matador, The (2005) Comedy ΨΨ
Pierce Brosnan plays a narcissistic, antisocial "hit man." He suffers from panic attacks (without agoraphobia) that affect his ability to work.

Matchstick Men (2003) Comedy ΨΨΨΨ
Nicholas Cage plays Roy Waller, a con man with OCD, agoraphobia with panic, tics, and antisocial personality, in this interesting Ridley Scott film. Upon meeting his estranged daughter, things begin to change for Waller.

"Look, Doc, I spent last Tuesday watching fibers on my carpet. And the whole time I was watching my carpet, I was worrying that I, I might vomit. And the whole time, I was thinking, 'I'm a grown man. I should know what goes on my head.' And the more I thought about it ... the more I realized that I should just blow my brains out and end it all. But then ... I start worrying about what that was going to do to my goddamn carpet. Okay, so, ah-he, that was a GOOD day, Doc. And, and I just want you to give me some pills and let me get on with my life."

Roy Waller in *Matchstick Men* (2003)

Nothing (2003) Comedy ΨΨΨ
A Vincenzo Natali film about two men who make things disappear by hating and wishing. The film is based on the relationship of two good friends, a travel agent who works from home and suffers from severe agoraphobia and a self-absorbed loser who is treated with contempt.

Obsession (1976) Thriller Ψ
Brian De Palma version of Hitchcock's *Vertigo*. The De Palma film doesn't live up to the original.

Open Water (2003) Suspense Ψ
A young couple on a scuba diving trip are left behind to fend for themselves. Sharks circle, distant boats do not see the divers, and fish bite at them. While the film depicts the terror someone would experience if abandoned in the open water, it is not a notable depiction of an anxiety disorder.

Panic Room (2002) Crime-Suspense Ψ
Jodie Foster plays a claustrophobic woman who becomes imprisoned in the panic room of her house when burglars enter.

Phobia (1980, Canada) Horror-Mystery Ψ
Canadian film about the systematic murders of phobic psychiatric patients.

Phoebe in Wonderland (2008) Drama ΨΨΨ
Felicity Huffman plays a young girl with an obsessive-compulsive disorder and Tourette's disorder who engages in repetitive handwashing; there is an unflattering portrayal of a psychiatrist in the film.

"You are all so ready to label, medicate, and move on as if a name means something, as if all the answers are in a bottle. I've seen that solution. I have seen it all around me, and it is a life of side effects and dulled minds. Your profession just doesn't like kids to be kids."

A mother berates a child psychiatrist, in *Phoebe in Wonderland* (2008)

Play It Again, Sam (1972) Comedy-Romance ΨΨΨ
Early Woody Allen film depicting social anxiety. A neurotic film critic's wife leaves him, and he is crushed. His hero is a tough guy (Humphrey Bogart) whose apparition begins showing up to give him advice. He tries dating again and is unsuccessful until he learns to relax.

Raiders of the Lost Ark (1981) Adventure ΨΨ
Steven Spielberg film with Harrison Ford as Indiana Jones, an anthropologist who is forced by the situational demands of heroism to overcome his snake phobia.

Red Eye (2005) Horror-Thriller Ψ
Wes Craven film portraying a character who hates to fly but finds herself on the red eye flight to Miami trapped with a villainous but charming middle-aged man in a plot to assassinate a Homeland Security official.

Roommate, The (2011) Drama-Thriller Ψ
A freshman at UCLA finds life gets complicated after her roommate becomes obsessed with her.

She's One of Us (2003, France) Drama ΨΨ
A socially awkward and anxious woman struggles in her social interactions. Watch for echoes of Dostoyevsky's "Dream of a Ridiculous Man."

Solitary (2009) Drama–Mystery ΨΨ
A low-budget film about an agoraphobic housebound woman who becomes convinced that her husband and her therapist are conspiring to drive her insane.

Something's Gotta Give (2003) Comedy ΨΨ
Jack Nicholson plays a 63-year-old man obsessed with younger women; he has a genuine heart attack that is followed by a series of panic attacks.

Stranger than Fiction (2006) Comedy ΨΨΨ
An IRS auditor (Will Ferrell) suddenly finds himself the subject of a novel being read by the author that only the auditor can hear. The narration affects his entire life – his work, relationships, living situation, and livelihood – including his obsessive behavior (e.g., counting toothbrush strokes).

Unmarried Woman, An (1978) ΨΨΨ
Drama–Comedy
Tender, sensitive, and funny film with Jill Clayburgh learning to cope with the stress of being a single parent after her husband abandons her. Her friends, a psychiatrist, and an affair with Alan Bates all help.

UNSTUCK: An OCD Kids Movie (2017) ΨΨΨ
Documentary
Six children with OCD share their stories about how they cope and what has worked for them.

> **"I have this acrophobia. I wake up at night and I see that man falling."**
>
> **John Ferguson describing his symptoms, in *Vertigo* (1958)**

Vertigo (1958) Thriller ΨΨΨΨΨ
Wonderful Hitchcock film in which James Stewart plays a character whose life is dominated by his fear of heights. He designs his own behavior modification program early in the film without success.

Waiting for Ronald (2003) Short Film–Drama ΨΨΨ
This short film about a man who leaves a supervised residence to live with a friend in the community depicts OCD and a handwashing compulsion.

War of the Worlds (2005) Action ΨΨ
Directed by Steven Spielberg and starring Tom Cruise, Dakota Fanning, and Tim Robbins, this film depicts the impact of an alien invasion on a blue-collar father and two children. Cruise's character responds to tragedy with shock; his daughter develops a phobia; and Robbins' character has a psychotic break.

What About Bob? (1991) Comedy ΨΨ
Bill Murray plays an anxious patient who cannot function without his psychiatrist, played by Richard Dreyfuss. Not a great film, but a fun movie that explores the doctor–patient relationship and the obsessive-compulsive personality.

Whole (2003) Documentary ΨΨΨ
Fascinating documentary about individuals who have a strong desire to have one of their limbs amputated, despite being totally healthy. Presents interesting differential diagnostic questions. Is this OCD, body dysmorphic disorder, an identity disorder, or self-mutilation? One psychiatrist, who interviewed 53 people with this condition, proposed the rubric *body integrity identity disorder.*

> **"As a four-limb person, I don't feel incomplete. It's more of a feeling that my body doesn't belong to me."**
> **"The relief from the 50 years of torment I had was indescribable."**
> **"I'm complete now."**
>
> **Comments from individuals who want or have had healthy limbs removed, in *Whole* (2003)**

Without a Paddle (2004) Drama–Comedy Ψ
Three friends go canoeing after the death of a friend. One is painfully neurotic with numerous phobias including fear of small spaces, the dark, and cellophane wrap. He copes with difficult situations by pretending he is a *Star Wars* character.

Woman, a Gun, and a Noodle Shop, A (2009, China/Hong Kong) Drama–Comedy ΨΨΨ
A Zhang Yimou film depicting several quirky characters, including one with severe anxiety.

Woman in the Window, The (2021) ΨΨΨ
Mystery–Thriller
Amy Adams plays an agoraphobic child psychologist who misuses prescription drugs and alcohol. She witnesses a violent crime, only to be told by many others that it never happened. The psychologist's therapist makes home visits.

Young Adult (2011) Drama ΨΨ
Charlize Theron plays a young woman who returns to her hometown, hoping to recapture her youth and her former

boyfriend (who is now married). Among other problems, Theron's character suffers from trichotillomania.

Zombieland (2009) Horror Comedy Ψ
Four people team up to avoid zombies on a trip to California. One character has multiple phobias including a fear of clowns and a fear of rags used to wipe off tables.

Trauma- and Stressor-Related Disorders

Alive (1993) Action-Adventure-Drama ΨΨ
The survivors of a plane crash in the Andes survive for more than 70 days by eating the passengers who died. The film is a vivid portrayal of traumatic stress and its consequences.

All Quiet on the Western Front (1930) Drama ΨΨΨΨΨ
This remarkable film illustrates the horror of war and celebrates pacifism as its only solution. The film poignantly documents that it is young men who fight our wars and shows the folly of jingoism and blind patriotism.

> **"Oh, God! why did they do this to us? We only wanted to live, you and I. Why should they send us out to fight each other? If they threw away these rifles and these uniforms, you could be my brother, just like Kat and Albert. You'll have to forgive me, comrade. I'll do all I can. I'll write to your parents."**
>
> **Paul attempts to comfort a man he has killed, in *All Quiet on the Western Front* (1930)**

All Quiet On the Western Front (*Im Westen Nichts Neues;* 2022, Germany) Drama ΨΨΨ
A German remake of the classic 1930 film, with English subtitles. Not nearly as powerful as the original, the film depicts young German students lying about their age to enlist and go to war.

Best in Show (2000) Comedy ΨΨ
A couple entering their beloved dog in a competitive dog show fight continuously; their fights escalate in response to the tension and anxiety associated with the show. They later cure themselves of their "adjustment" problem by blaming their dog for being self-deprecating and purchase a new dog who does not mind watching them have sex.

Best Years of Our Lives, The (1946) Drama ΨΨΨΨ
Sam Goldwyn film about servicemen adjusting to civilian life after the war. One of the sailors has lost both hands.

Big Parade, The (1925) Romance-War ΨΨΨΨ
This epic film about World War I gives the viewer a sense of the stress of combat and the trauma of returning to civilian life minus a leg or an arm.

Birdy (1984) Drama-War ΨΨΨΨ
Nicolas Cage tries to help his friend, Matthew Modine, who is a catatonic inpatient in a military hospital. Both men are Vietnam veterans, but Modine's problems seem to predate the war. The film illustrates catatonia.

Black Rain (1989) Drama ΨΨΨ
Black-and-white film by Japanese filmmaker Shohei Imamura about the aftermath of the bombing of Hiroshima and its long-term psychological effects.

Born on the Fourth of July (1989) Drama-War-Biography ΨΨΨΨ
Oliver Stone film about the anger, frustration, rage, and coping of paralyzed Vietnam veteran Ron Kovic (Tom Cruise). Kovic was thrown out of the 1972 Republican convention but went on to address the Democratic convention in 1976. The film has especially memorable VA hospital scenes.

> **"Who's gonna love me, Dad? Whoever's going to love me?"**
>
> **Ron Kovic in *Born on the Fourth of July* (1989)**

Boy and the Bus, The (2013, UK) Drama-Family ΨΨΨ
Short film about a boy coping with the loss of his mother and a new living environment. He takes up "racing" a bus by running across the land.

Brave One, The (2007) Crime-Thriller Ψ
Jodie Foster plays newlywed a radio talk show host. She survives a brutal attack that leaves her fiancé dead. Following the attack, she is extremely anxious, yet she forces herself to get revenge.

Brothers (2009) Drama ΨΨΨΨΨ
A powerful film in which one brother (Tobey Maguire) is tortured for months in Afghanistan and forced to beat another POW to death; when he returns to the states, his PTSD threatens to unravel his family, he develops symptoms of paranoia, and he becomes convinced that his wife has been having an affair with his brother.

Coming Home (1978) Drama–War ΨΨΨΨ
Jon Voigt plays a paraplegic veteran who becomes Jane Fonda's lover in this sensitive antiwar film. Fonda's Marine Corps husband winds up committing suicide. Interesting analysis of the various ways different people respond to the stress of war.

Deer Hunter, The (1978) War ΨΨΨΨΨ
Robert De Niro in an unforgettable film about how Vietnam affects the lives of three high school buddies. The Russian roulette sequences are among the most powerful scenes in film history. Psychopathology themes include drug abuse, PTSD, and depression. The movie won five Academy Awards, including one for Best Picture, and De Niro has described it as his finest film.

Dog (2022) Comedy ΨΨΨ
An Army veteran and a K9 corps dog, both scarred by combat, make a road trip that turns out to be healing for both. The movie will interest anyone interested in animal assisted interventions for PTSD. Compare with another story about a Marine and her dog, *Megan Leavey* (2017).

Dry Land, The (2010) Drama ΨΨΨ
An Iraq war veteran returns to his Texas home, only to discover that you can't go home again. The film presents a vivid and accurate picture of the symptoms of PTSD.

Enduring Love (2004) Drama–Mystery ΨΨΨ
Several men try to save a boy in a hot air balloon that is out of control. All but one let go and the one who hangs on dies; the resulting PTSD and a character with delusional disorder are portrayed.

Experiment, The (2010) Drama ΨΨΨ
This interesting film is a remake of *Das Experiment*, which was a 2001 film based on Philip Zimbardo's infamous Stanford Prison Experiment. Both films document the effects of stress and show how life in an abnormal environment affects human behavior. Watching the film may help you understand some of the more egregious abuses that occurred at Abu Ghraib. (Zimbardo testified as an expert witness for the defense and wrote a book, *The Lucifer Effect*, based on this experience.)

Falling Down (1994) Drama ΨΨΨ
Good presentation by Michael Douglas of the cumulative effects of stress on a marginal personality. The film does not give us enough information to clearly diagnose the character played by Douglas, but he does display significant symptoms of paranoia.

Fearless (1993) Drama ΨΨΨΨ
Jeff Bridges in an engaging film that portrays some of the symptoms of anxiety in airline crash survivors. Interesting vignettes show group therapy for PTSD victims.

Fever Pitch (2005) Comedy Ψ
Jimmy Fallon's character is obsessed with the Boston Red Sox and struggles to adjust to a new relationship that impacts his passion for baseball. American remake of the 1997 UK film of the same title, based on the Nick Hornby novel in which the main character (Colin Firth) is obsessed with the Arsenal soccer team.

Final Cut, The (2004) Drama–Thriller Ψ
Some PTSD symptoms are displayed in a man (Robin Williams) who creates "memories" for people at funerals using a microchip implanted in the people's heads while they were living.

Fisher King, The (1991)
Drama–Fantasy–Comedy ΨΨΨΨ
Jeff Bridges plays a former talk show personality who unwittingly encourages a listener to go on a shooting spree. Bridges' withdrawal, cynicism, and substance use can all be interpreted and understood in the context of PTSD. However, Robin William's character's vivid, well-formed hallucinations of a "red knight" are unrealistic.

Full Metal Jacket (1987) Drama ΨΨΨΨ
This Stanley Kubrick film captures the horror of war – but also the stress of basic training. The latrine homicide-suicide scene in which Private Pyle kills his drill sergeant and then himself is unforgettable.

"If you ladies leave my island, if you survive recruit training, you will be a weapon. You will be a minister of death praying for war. But until that day you are pukes. You are the lowest form of life on Earth. You are not even human fucking beings. You are nothing but unorganized pieces of amphibian shit! Because I am hard, you will not like me. But the more you hate me, the more you will learn. I am hard but I am fair. There is no racial bigotry here. I do not look down on niggers, kikes, wops or greasers. Here you are all equally worthless. And my orders are to weed out all non-hackers who do not pack the gear to serve in my beloved Corps. Do you maggots understand that?"

Gunnery Sergeant Hartman,
in *Full Metal Jacket* (1987)

Glengarry Glen Ross (1992) Drama ΨΨΨ
A hard-hitting and powerful presentation of job-related stress and interpersonal conflict in the real estate business. Wonderful cast, with Jack Lemmon playing a figure whose despair over his job is reminiscent of Willy Loman in Arthur Miller's *Death of a Salesman*.

Hamburger Hill (1987) War ΨΨ
A graphic presentation of the stress and horror of war.

Hammer, The (2011) Biography ΨΨΨ
Matt Hamill becomes the first deaf wrestler to win a National Collegiate Championship, but not without significant social struggles and duress.

Home of the Brave (2006) Action-Drama ΨΨΨ
Soldiers returning from the war in Iraq attempt to reintegrate back home but struggle with the memories and ramifications of having served in war. Winner of a Voice Award.

Hurt Locker, The (2008) Drama ΨΨΨΨΨ
A soldier who is an expert at dismantling improvised explosive devices (IEDs) in Iraq finds civilian life insipid and boring. The opening quotation captures the theme of the film: "The rush of battle is often a potent and lethal addiction, for war is a drug."

"You love playing with that. You love playing with all your stuffed animals. You love your Mommy, your Daddy. You love your pajamas. You love everything, don't ya? Yea. But you know what, buddy? As you get older... some of the things you love might not seem so special anymore. Like your Jack-in-a-Box. Maybe you'll realize it's just a piece of tin and a stuffed animal. And the older you get, the fewer things you really love. And by the time you get to my age, maybe it's only one or two things. With me, I think it's one."

Staff Sergeant James thinking about defusing bombs as he speaks to his young son, in *The Hurt Locker* (2008)

In Country (1989) Drama ΨΨ
Bruce Willis plays a Vietnam veteran with PTSD who is unable to relate meaningfully to the world around him until he visits the Vietnam memorial.

Invisible War, The (2012) Documentary ΨΨΨΨ
An examination of rape in the military, a problem of epidemic proportions. The film will help students appreciate the psychological sequelae of rape.

Jacob's Ladder (1990) Drama ΨΨ
Complex film about a Vietnam veteran who has dramatic hallucinations of indeterminate etiology (possibly the result of military exposure to experimental drugs).

Last Kiss, The (2006) Drama ΨΨΨ
Cautionary tale, particularly for those around age 30 about midlife issues, falling in love, rites of passage, fear of commitment, and the importance of honesty. The film also portrays adjustment disorder.

M*A*S*H (1970) Comedy-War ΨΨΨ
Wonderfully funny Robert Altman film about military surgeons and nurses who use alcohol, sex, and humor to cope with the stress of war. The portrayal of Hawkeye Pierce, half-drunk but always ready for surgery, is troubling for mental health professionals.

Manchurian Candidate, The (2004) ΨΨΨ
Drama-Suspense
The new version of this classic film stars Denzel Washington as a Gulf War veteran with PTSD, paranoia, and memories he cannot understand, which lead him to unravel a conspiracy involving brainwashing and political maneuvering.

Manchurian Candidate, The (1962) ΨΨΨ
Drama-Suspense
This original version stars Frank Sinatra as a veteran who experiences flashbacks and PTSD symptoms.

Martha Marcy May Marlene (2011) Drama ΨΨΨΨ
A woman disengages from her family and spends 2 years in a cult; she eventually becomes disenchanted, but when she manages to escape to her sister's house, she experiences an acute stress disorder and behaves oddly and inappropriately. A related short film, *Mary Last Seen,* depicts the ways in which cult members manipulate newcomers.

Melvin Goes to Dinner (2003) Comedy ΨΨΨ
Interesting dialogue film about an unplanned get-together between four people. They discuss religion, God, faith, ghosts, affairs, and sex. The character Melvin probably has an adjustment disorder.

Men, The (1950) Drama ΨΨΨ
Marlon Brando in his first film plays a paralyzed World War II veteran full of rage about his injury and his limitations.

Mother Ghost (2002) Drama ΨΨΨ
A man (Mark Thompson) begins to have significant adjustment problems after his mother's death (she died a

year before) resulting in marital conflict, increased alcohol use, and other personal problems. Interesting interaction and therapy with a radio psychologist (Kevin Pollack) on the air.

My House in Umbria (2003) Drama ΨΨ
A made-for-TV movie in which Dame Maggie Smith plays one of four survivors of a railway bombing

Ordinary People (1980) Drama ΨΨΨΨ
This film was Robert Redford's debut as a director. It deals with depression, suicide, and family pathology, and it presents a sympathetic portrayal of a psychiatrist, played by Judd Hirsch. Conrad, the protagonist, would meet DSM-5 criteria for PTSD as well as depression.

Outrage, The (1964) Drama ΨΨΨ
Three versions of the details of a rape and murder are related in this updated remake of Akira Kurosawa's *Rashomon*. Paul Newman plays the outlaw in the film.

Pan's Labyrinth (2006, Spain/Mexico) ΨΨΨΨΨ
The imaginative, young Ofelia manages the trauma of her situation and the tyrannical behavior of her stepfather by creating a world of fantasy.

Paths of Glory (1957) War ΨΨΨΨΨ
Kirk Douglas in an early Stanley Kubrick film about the horrors and stupidity of World War I. There is a memorable scene in which a general repeatedly slaps a soldier, trying without success to bring him out of his shell-shocked state. The scene was repeated in the 1970 film *Patton*.

Pawnbroker, The (1965) Drama ΨΨΨ
Rod Steiger plays a concentration camp survivor who watched his wife being raped and his children being murdered; he copes by becoming numb. Interesting flashback scenes. Steiger lost the 1965 Academy Award for Best Actor to Lee Marvin in *Cat Ballou*.

Patton (1970) War-Biography ΨΨΨΨ
George C. Scott is perfect in the role of the controversial general who was relieved of his command after slapping a crying soldier who had been hospitalized for combat fatigue, or what would now be called PTSD. The film won an Academy Award for Best Picture, and George C. Scott won the Oscar for Best Actor.

> **"I want you to remember that no bastard ever won a war by dying for his country. He won it by making the other poor dumb bastard die for his country."**
>
> **General George S. Patton Jr. in *Patton* (1970)**

Princess and the Warrior, The (2000) ΨΨΨΨ
Drama
A nurse at a psychiatric hospital is hit by a truck and saved by a crook who cuts a hole in her throat and breathes for her. Upon recovering, the nurse goes on a journey to find this man. A minor character has PTSD. One intensely graphic and chilling scene depicts a kind-hearted adolescent with **pica**; believing the nurse has rejected him, the teenager eats glass.

Raising a School Shooter (2021) ΨΨΨΨ
Documentary
Three parents of school shooters share their stories, noting that they can never again live normally, even as they go about the tasks of daily living. It is impossible to watch the film without wondering what could have been done differently. All three parents allude to the bullying their children underwent while in school.

Rust and Bone (2012) Drama ΨΨΨΨ
A woman who trains killer whales at a marine park becomes a double amputee after an accident. She is supported by her lover, a former boxer, and the film celebrates the love and sexual joy that links these two people.

San Francisco (1936) Romance-Disaster ΨΨΨ
This is one of the greatest disaster films ever made, and the special effects give the viewer some appreciation for the acute stress one would experience in a real earthquake. Clark Gable and Spencer Tracy have memorable roles in this film.

Secret Lives of Dentists, The (2002) Drama ΨΨ
A married couple, both dentists, is unable to adjust to both living and working together. One begins an affair while the other stews in anger.

Shoah (1985) Documentary ΨΨΨΨΨ
Widely praised 9-hr documentary about the Holocaust. The film offers some insight into the behavior of both the German officials and their victims and illustrates antisocial personalities and PTSD.

Story of Us, The (1999) Comedy-Drama ΨΨ
Bruce Willis and Michelle Pfeiffer star as a couple on the brink of separation after 15 years of marriage. Directed by Rob Reiner.

Stuck (2007) Horror ΨΨ
A nurse's aide driving home from a party is high on ecstasy when she hits a homeless man who becomes lodged in her windshield. She hides the man, still stuck, in her garage while she makes love with her boyfriend,

eventually deciding it is better to kill the victim than to risk a potential driving-under-the-influence charge.

Tennis, Anyone...? (2005) Comedy ΨΨ
Two small time actors cope with life and find meaning despite the significant stressors in their lives.

Testament (1983) Drama ΨΨΨΨ
Jane Alexander plays an ordinary Bay Area mother heroically struggling to care for her children during a nuclear holocaust. Watch for Kevin Costner in a minor role as a father carrying his daughter to be buried in a bureau drawer. This is the best and most realistic of films depicting the consequences of nuclear war.

Twelve O'clock High (1949) War ΨΨΨ
Gregory Peck in an interesting presentation of the stress of combat and the ways in which leaders can influence the behavior of those they lead.

Upside of Anger, The (2005) Comedy-Drama ΨΨΨ
Joan Allen portrays a woman with an adjustment disorder who discovers her husband has gone off to Sweden with another woman, leaving his home and family. She befriends a jovial alcoholic to cope with her anger and the family disruption.

Walking on Water (2002) Drama ΨΨ
Australian film about a man who becomes haunted by intrusive memories and deteriorates into self-destructive behavior after suffocating a gay friend who was dying of AIDS.

Dissociative Disorders

3 Women (1977) Drama ΨΨΨΨ
Strange but engaging Robert Altman film about California women who seem to exchange personalities.

Altered States (1980) Science Fiction ΨΨ
A less than satisfying film based in part on the sensory deprivation experiments of Dr. John Lilly. The scientist (William Hurt) combines isolation tanks with psychedelic mushrooms to induce altered states of consciousness. Good special effects.

Amateur (1994) Drama-Comedy ΨΨ
Hal Hartley film in which a man who is amnestic because of a traumatic head injury becomes involved with a nun who has left the convent to write pornographic novels. Almost every character in the film has a complex double identity and is uncertain about who they really are.

Anastasia (1956) Drama ΨΨΨΨ
Yul Brynner, Helen Hayes, and Ingrid Bergman star in this film about an amnestic woman who is believed to be the lost princess Anastasia, daughter of the last czar of Russia.

Black Friday (1940) Horror ΨΨ
Boris Karloff and Bela Lugosi star in this film about transplanting a gangster's brain into a college professor's cranium.

Butterfly Effect, The (2003) Drama-Suspense ΨΨ
A young man (Ashton Kutcher) tries to change his traumatic past with unpredictable and increasingly problematic consequences. When he reflects on blackouts, he enters the memory and can change it for the long term but must face the consequences of the change each time. The film attempts to depict chaos theory.

Dark Mirror, The (1946) Thriller Ψ
Olivia de Havilland plays both parts in a story of twin sisters, one of whom is a deranged killer.

Dead Again (1991) Mystery-Romance ΨΨΨ
Emma Thompson costars with her husband, Kenneth Branagh (who also directed the film). The movie illustrates traumatic amnesia and its treatment through hypnosis. The hypnotist, an antique dealer, is not the most professional of therapists!

Despair (1979) Drama ΨΨΨΨ
Fassbinder film based on a novel by Vladimir Nabokov. A Russian Jew émigré in Germany who runs a chocolate factory kills another man who looks like him and tries to pass it off as his own suicide. When his plan fails, he becomes psychotic.

Devils, The (1971) Drama-Historical ΨΨΨ
Ken Russell film adapted from Aldous Huxley's book *The Devils of Loundun*. The film traces the lives of 17th-century French nuns who experienced highly erotic dissociative states attributed to possession by the devil.

Double Life of Veronique, The (1991) Fantasy-Drama ΨΨ
The lives of two women turn out to be linked in complex ways the viewer never fully understands.

Double Life, A (1947) Crime ΨΨ
Ronald Coleman plays an actor who is unable to sort out his theatrical life (in which he plays Othello) and his personal life.

Dr. Jekyll and Mr. Hyde (1932) Horror ΨΨΨΨ
Fredric March in the best adaptation of Robert Louis Stevenson's classic story about the ultimate dissociative disorder. Stevenson was an alcoholic, and the mysterious liquid that dramatically transforms Jekyll's personality may be a metaphor for alcohol.

Exorcist, The (1973) Horror ΨΨ
Linda Blair stars as a 12-year-old girl possessed by the devil in William Friedkin's film based on the William Peter Blatty novel. One of the most suspenseful films ever made – it is wonderful, but it won't teach you much about mental illness.

Falling, The (2014, UK) Drama ΨΨΨ
Mass hysteria breaks out in a Catholic girls' school in Britain. The film depicts an agoraphobia mother and brother-sister incest and may be based on a true incident that occurred in Great Britain at a similar school in 1965. The film's cathartic ending, which involve the agoraphobic mother leaving the home to embrace her daughter who had just fallen from a tree, seems contrived.

Fight Club (1999) Drama-Suspense ΨΨΨΨ
A disillusioned, insomniac (Edward Norton) meets a dangerous, malcontent part of himself in the character of Brad Pitt. Norton then establishes "fight clubs" in which men can unload their aggressions onto one another.

> **"It's only after we've lost everything that we are free to do anything."**
>
> **A premise of *Fight Club* (1999)**

Forgotten, The (2004) Drama ΨΨ
A woman grieving over the loss of her 9-year-old son is told by her husband and her therapist that her son never existed, and that all her memories were created in response to a miscarriage. The mother doesn't believe what she is being told.

Frankie & Alice (2010) Drama ΨΨ
Halle Berry plays the role of Alice, a Los Angeles woman with DID and three personalities: (1) Francine L. Murdoch, Black woman, age 32, IQ 132; (2) Alice, White woman, age unknown, IQ 102. (3) Genius, Black female, age 8–12, IQ 156. The film is based on a true story.

Freud: The Secret Passion (1962) ΨΨ
Drama-Biography
John Huston pays homage to Sigmund Freud using a composite patient loosely based on the case of Anna O. Jean-Paul Sartre was involved in writing the initial draft, and Marilyn Monroe turned down the part of Anna out of respect for the Freud families' wishes. Mainly interesting for history buffs.

Girl Cut in Two, A (2007, France) Drama ΨΨΨ
A Claude Chabrol film about a weatherwoman who is being pursued by two suitors: an older, married novelist and the young heir to a pharmaceutical fortune. She falls in love with the older man who introduces her to sexual adventure, but she eventually marries the younger man.

Great Dictator, The (1940) Comedy ΨΨ
A satire of Adolph Hitler, with Charlie Chaplin in the role of a Jewish barber who suffers amnesia and eventually finds himself assuming the personality of Adenoid Hynkel, the dictator of Tomania.

Hereditary (2018) Horror ΨΨΨ
Put in this category because of a grandmother with DID, the film also involves a grandfather with psychotic depression (who starves himself to death), a son with schizophrenia, and various other characters with other disorders. Ari Aster directed this interesting film, and it is highly recommended, although none of the charters are especially good examples of the disorders they portray.

Identity (2003) Suspense-Thriller ΨΨΨ
A serial killer with a DID is at his final hearing before receiving the death penalty. This story juxtaposes this story with another tale of several people suddenly stuck at an isolated motel and living in terror as they are killed one by one. These two components are cleverly woven together as the people being killed represent DID alters.

Interpersonalities (2008) Mystery ΨΨΨ
Short film that depicts several characters, including a psychiatrist, all of whom are based on various alters of the protagonist's personality.

Last Temptation of Christ, The (1988) ΨΨΨ
Religious
Challenging and controversial Martin Scorsese film in which Jesus, while on the cross and in great pain, has a dissociative episode in which he imagines himself as an ordinary man who married Mary Magdalene and lived a normal life.

Lizzie (1957) Drama ΨΨ
Eleanor Parker, a woman with DID, is treated by psychiatrist Richard Boone.

Method (2003) Suspense-Thriller Ψ
An actress, studying and playing the role of a past serial killer, tries too hard to "feel her character," and she dissociates and takes on her character's behavior.

Mirage (1965) Drama ΨΨ
A scientist who makes an important discovery develops amnesia after viewing the death of a friend.

My Girl (1991) Drama-Comedy ΨΨ
The film centers on an 11-year-old girl whose mother has just died and whose grandmother has Alzheimer's disease. The child responds by developing a series of imaginary disorders. Strong performances by Dan Aykroyd and Jamie Lee Curtis.

Nurse Betty (2000) Drama-Mystery ΨΨΨΨ
Neil LaBute film about a woman (Renée Zellweger) who witnesses a traumatic event and develops a dissociative fugue. She travels to Los Angeles to find a character in a soap opera. Zellweger's character presents an interesting springboard for a debate about the differences between dissociative fugue and delusional disorder.

Numb (2007) Drama ΨΨ
Matthew Perry portrays a character who develops a depersonalization disorder that he overcomes by falling in love.

Overboard (1987) Comedy ΨΨ
Goldie Hawn plays a haughty millionaire who develops amnesia and is claimed by an Oregon carpenter as his wife and forced to care for his children.

Paris, Texas (1984) Drama ΨΨΨ
Wim Wenders film about a man found wandering in the desert with no personal memory. He eventually reunites with his brother and his wife and begins to put his life together.

Peacock (2009) Drama ΨΨΨΨ
A timid and unassuming bank clerk is found to be living a double life when a train crashes into his home. Cillian Murphy is extraordinary, playing both the male and female personalities.

Persona (1966) Drama ΨΨΨΨΨ
Complex, demanding, and fascinating Bergman film starring Liv Ullmann as an actress who suddenly stops talking after one of her performances. A nurse treats Ullmann, and the two women appear to exchange "personas."

Piano, The (1993) Drama ΨΨΨΨΨ
Jane Campion film about a woman who had voluntarily stopped speaking as a child. She communicates with written notes and through playing the piano, a pleasure forbidden to her by her New Zealand husband. There are scenes of extraordinary sensuality between characters played by Harvey Keitel and Holly Hunter, as well as a dramatic suicide attempt.

"The voice you hear is not my speaking voice – but my mind's voice. I have not spoken since I was six years old. No one knows why – not even me. My father says it is a dark talent, and the day I take it into my head to stop breathing will be my last. Today he married me to a man I have not yet met. Soon my daughter and I shall join him in his own country. My husband writes that my muteness does not bother him – and hark this! He says, 'God loves dumb creatures, so why not I?' Twere good he had God's patience, for silence affects everyone in the end."

Ada's thoughts at the beginning of *The Piano* (1993)

Poison Ivy (1992) Drama Ψ
A newcomer into a pathological family plans to take over the role of wife and mother. The father is an alcoholic and the mother is a hypochondriac.

Prelude to a Kiss (1992) Comedy-Romance ΨΨ
The ultimate example of a dissociative disorder. A beautiful young woman and a sad old man kiss on her wedding day and exchange bodies. The film makes this extraordinary event seem almost plausible.

Primal Fear (1996) Drama ΨΨΨ
Richard Gere stars in this suspenseful drama about a man (Ed Norton) who commits heinous crimes, ostensibly because of a dissociative disorder. The film raises useful questions about the problem of malingering and differential diagnosis.

Psycho (1960) Horror-Thriller ΨΨΨΨΨ
Classic Hitchcock film starring Anthony Perkins as Norman Bates, who vacillates between his passive, morbid personality, and his alter ego as his dead mother. In the final minutes of the film, a psychiatrist offers a somewhat confusing explanation for Bates's behavior. The shower scene is one of the most famous scenes in film history.

"When he met your sister, he was touched by her... aroused by her. He wanted her. That set off the 'jealous mother' and 'mother killed the girl'! Now after the murder, Norman returned as if from a deep sleep. And like a dutiful son, covered up all traces of the crime he was convinced his mother had committed."

Psychiatrist Fred Richmond explains the aberrant behavior of Norman Bates, in *Psycho* (1960)

Raising Cain (1992) Thriller-Drama Ψ
Confusing De Palma film about a child psychologist with multiple personalities who begins to kill women and steal their children to be subjects in his experiments.

Return of Martin Guerre, The (1982) ΨΨΨ
Historical
Gerard Depardieu as a 16th-century peasant who returns to his wife after a 7-year absence. His true identity is never made clear. This film, the basis for the American movie *Sommersby,* was based on a true story.

Secret Window (2004) Drama-Suspense ΨΨΨ
Mort Rainey (Johnny Depp) finds his wife cheating on him in a motel; the film jumps forward 6 months to a scene in which Mort is an isolated writer in a house in the woods and now separated from his wife. He is visited and threatened by an odd psychopath (John Turturro). Based on the Stephen King short story, "Secret Window, Secret Garden."

Sisters (1973) Thriller-Horror ΨΨ
De Palma film about Siamese twins separated as children; one is good, the other quite evil. The use of Siamese twins is a Hitchcock-like twist on the theme of multiple personality.

Sommersby (1993) Drama ΨΨ
Richard Gere returns to wife Jodie Foster after a 6-year absence during the Civil War. Gere is remarkably changed, so much so that it appears he is a different man. (Also see *The Return of Martin Guerre.*)

Spellbound (1945) Thriller ΨΨΨΨ
Ingrid Bergman and Gregory Peck star in this Hitchcock thriller. Peck is an amnestic patient who believes he has committed a murder; Bergman is the psychiatrist who falls in love with him and helps him recall the childhood trauma responsible for his dissociative state. Hitchcock loved linking childhood and repressed childhood memories with adult psychopathology (also see *Marne*).

> **"Our story deals with psychoanalysis, the method by which modern science treats the emotional problems of the sane. The analyst seeks only to induce the patient to talk about his hidden problems, to open the locked doors of his mind. Once the complexes that have been disturbing the patient are uncovered and interpreted, the illness and confusion disappear ..."**
>
> **Opening Screen for *Spellbound* (1945)**

Steppenwolf (1974) Drama ΨΨ
Film adaptation of Herman Hesse's remarkable novel about Harry Haller (played by Max von Sydow), a misanthropic protagonist who wrestles with the competing forces of good and evil within himself.

Stigmata (1999) Suspense-Horror Ψ
A beautician begins to have episodes of visions, seizures, and stigmata wounds on her body after her mother sends her a sacred rosary from Brazil.

Suddenly, Last Summer (1959) Drama ΨΨΨ
Adaptation of a Tennessee Williams story about an enmeshed and pathological relationship between a mother (Katharine Hepburn) and her homosexual son and a dissociative amnesia in a cousin who witnessed the son's death. Among its other virtues, the film includes a fascinating discussion of the benefits of lobotomy.

> **"He-he was lying naked on the broken stones ... It looked as if-as if they had devoured him! ... As if they'd torn or cut parts of him away with their hands, or with knives, or those jagged tin cans they made music with. As if they'd torn bits of him away in strips!"**
>
> ***Suddenly, Last Summer* (1959)**

Sullivan's Travels (1941) Comedy-Drama ΨΨΨΨ
Joel McCrea plays a movie director who goes out to experience life as it is lived outside a Hollywood studio. He winds up getting a head injury, becoming amnestic, and being sentenced to 6 years on a chain gang.

Sybil (1976) Drama ΨΨΨ
Made-for-TV movie in which Joanne Woodward, the patient in *The Three Faces of Eve,* plays a psychiatrist treating a woman with 16 different personalities.

Thérèse: The Story of Saint Thérèse of Lisieux (2004) Drama ΨΨΨ
The story of Saint Thérèse, the Carmelite nun who wrote *Story of a Soul*, and suffered from numerous somatic symptoms. She eventually died from tuberculosis.

Three Faces of Eve, The (1957) Drama ΨΨΨΨ
Joanne Woodward won an Academy Award for her portrayal of a woman with three personalities (Eve White, Eve Black, and Jane); based on a 1954 book by Thigpen and Cleckley. Lee J. Cobb is Eve's therapist, and he helps her with hypnosis.

Unknown White Male (2005) Drama ΨΨΨΨ
An excellent exploration of the fugue state based on a true story about a man who discovers himself on a Coney Island subway with no recollection of who he is or how he got there.

> **Narrator: "How much of our past lives, the thousands of moments we experience, helps to make us who we are? If you took all these remembrances, these memories, away, what would be left? How much is our personality, our identity, determined by the experiences we have, and how much is already there – pure 'us'"?**
>
> **A question about who we are without memories, in *Unknown White Male***

Voices Within: The Lives of Truddi Chase (1990) Drama ΨΨ
Made-for-TV movie about a woman with multiple personality disorder (DID); based on the bestselling book *When Rabbit Howls.*

Whatever Happened to Baby Jane? (1962) Drama ΨΨΨ
Bette Davis and Joan Crawford star as two elderly sisters who were formerly movie stars. Jane (Bette Davis) had been a child star, but her fame was eclipsed by the renown of her talented sister, now confined to a wheelchair. Jane torments her sister and experiences a dramatic dissociative episode in the final scene in the movie.

Woman With 15 Personalities (2010) Documentary ΨΨΨΨ
A 46-year-old social work student presents to a psychiatrist with symptoms of severe DID. Her first alter came out at age 5 as a way of escaping physical and sexual abuse. One of the alters is sexually promiscuous; one is suicidal and has made several suicide attempts. The film depicts EEG changes that occur as different alters emerge. The movie will be a good starting place for a classroom discussion about the reality of the disorder.

X-Men: The Last Stand (2006) Action-Science Fiction ΨΨ
Superheroine mutant Jean Grey is portrayed as someone with DID; the actress playing the role researched DID to make her character more realistic.

Zelig (1983) Comedy ΨΨ
Quasidocumentary about Woody Allen as Zelig, a human chameleon whose personality changes to match that of whomever he is around. He is treated by psychiatrist Mia Farrow, whom Zelig eventually marries. Watch for Susan Sontag, Saul Bellow, and Bruno Bettelheim.

Sleep–Wake, Eating, and Somatic Symptom Disorders

Note: Physical illnesses, diseases, and deformities are also depicted in movies in this section.

2 Days in Paris (2007) Romance ΨΨΨ
Julie Delpy film about a couple, each with distinct psychological problems – he has a somatic symptom disorder and she has an intermittent explosive disorder.

3 Needles (2005) Drama Ψ
Brutal and disturbing film depicting the transmission of HIV and the misconceptions that arise (e.g., the belief that having sex with a virgin will cure the disease).

12 Angry Men (1957) Drama ΨΨΨΨΨ
Henry Fonda stars in this fascinating courtroom drama that illustrates social pressure, the tendency toward conformity in social settings, and the stress associated with noncompliance with societal norms.

50/50 (2011) Comedy-Drama ΨΨΨ
Based on a true story about a man who has a rare cancer with a 50% survival rate. Psychology students will appreciate the interactions between the patient and his neophyte therapist, with whom he becomes romantically involved.

61 (2001) Biography-Drama Ψ
Billy Crystal film with a subplot focused on the impact of stress on the body of Roger Maris during his quest to beat Babe Ruth's home run record.

Agnes of God (1985) Mystery ΨΨΨ
Good performances by Anne Bancroft, Meg Tilly, and Jane Fonda. Fonda plays a court-appointed psychiatrist who must make sense out of pregnancy and infanticide in a local convent. Good examples of *stigmata,* an example of conversion.

Bandits (2001) Comedy ΨΨ
Loosely based on a true story about two criminals who rob banks in a nonviolent way. One of the men (Billy Bob Thornton) is a hypochondriac. In interviews, Thornton stated it was not much of a "stretch to play this role" – he

has acknowledged phobias for both antique furniture and plastic cutlery.

Barbarian Invasions, The (2003) Drama-Comedy ΨΨΨΨ
Friends and family gather to support a stubborn, outspoken man suffering from a terminal illness. The film vacillates from light to heavy, from the somber to the humorous. This Canadian film won an Academy Award for Best Foreign Language Film.

Best Little Girl in the World, The (1981) Drama ΨΨ
Good made-for-TV movie in which a psychiatrist treats a girl who is suffering from anorexia nervosa.

Blue (1993) Drama ΨΨΨΨ
British filmmaker Derek Jarman's last film; he died from AIDS shortly after the movie was completed. Jarman reviews his life and analyzes the ways in which he has been affected by his disease.

Blue Butterfly (2004) Adventure-Drama ΨΨΨ
The mother of a terminally ill boy convinces an entomologist to take her son to the Costa Rican rainforest. The boy's brain cancer disappears and both lives are changed forever. The film is based on a true story.

Bone Collector, The (1999) Suspense-Thriller ΨΨ
Denzel Washington is a crime scene specialist with quadriplegia.

Brief History of Time, A (1992) Biography ΨΨΨ
A documentary about the life of Stephen Hawking, a theoretical physicist coping with amyotrophic lateral sclerosis.

Bubble Boy (2001) Comedy Ψ
Outlandish comedy about a boy born without immunity who must live in a bubble.

Bucket List, The (2008) Comedy ΨΨΨ
Jack Nicholson and Morgan Freeman meet as roommates in a hospital. Both are newly diagnosed with cancer and are given less than 1 year to live. Each makes a list of experiences they want to have before they "kick the bucket." These two very different men spend their last few months together in pursuit of their dreams.

Cactus (1986) Romance ΨΨΨ
Australian film about a woman who loses one eye and considers giving up sight in the other to understand the world of her blind lover more fully.

Center Stage (2000) Drama ΨΨ
A woman fights her way to the top role as a dancer and performs well despite encouragement to drop out. One dancer has bulimia, and the portrayal of the disorder is accurate and well done; however, the film is clichéd and predictable.

Children of a Lesser God (1986) Romance ΨΨΨ
The film examines the complications involved in a love relationship between William Hurt, a teacher in a school for the deaf, and Marlee Matlin, a young deaf woman who works at the school. Much of the conflict in the film revolves around Matlin's refusal to learn to lip-read. Matlin won an Academy Award for Best Supporting Actress for her role in this film.

Chinese Roulette (1976) Drama ΨΨΨ
Fassbinder film about a disabled girl and the ways in which she dominates and manipulates her family.

Chrystal (2004) Drama Ψ
Independent film in which one subplot involves a woman suffering from significant chronic pain caused by a motor vehicle accident.

Cinema Paradiso (1988) Drama ΨΨΨΨΨ
A young boy is mesmerized by a movie theater in a small, post-World War II, Italian town, and befriends a crusty yet warm-hearted projectionist who goes blind after a fire accident. Classic Giuseppe Tornatore film.

Control (2003, Hungary) Crime-Mystery-Comedy ΨΨ
Themes of good versus evil come to life in this farcical film depicting a variety of odd characters interacting in the vast, underground Budapest subway system. One character has narcolepsy.

Common Threads: Stories from the Quilt (1989) Documentary ΨΨΨ
This HBO film examines the lives of five individuals linked by a common illness - AIDS. The movie won the Academy Award for Best Documentary Feature in 1989.

Crash of Silence (1953) Drama ΨΨ
Mother agonizes over whether to keep a hearing-impaired daughter at home or send her to a special school.

Crazy Sexy Cancer (2007) Documentary ΨΨ
Young woman faces the stress of her illness by transforming her lifestyle and attitude.

Cure, The (1995) Drama ΨΨ
Two adolescent boys become best friends. One has AIDS from a blood transfusion, leading the boys to set off in search of a miracle cure.

Dance Me to My Song (1998, Australian) Drama ΨΨΨ
A woman with debilitating cerebral palsy competes with her caretaker for a love interest.

Dancer in the Dark (2000, Denmark) Drama ΨΨΨ
Björk portrays Selma, an immigrant, factory worker and single mother with limited intelligence whose vision is deteriorating. Her impending blindness affects her work, her relationships, and her personal life. Her son Gene will probably suffer the same fate unless she can pay for an operation.

Darius Goes West (2007) Documentary ΨΨΨ
Depiction of a man with Duchenne's muscular dystrophy and his journey with friends to get his wheelchair customized by MTV's "Pimp My Ride."

Deaf Smith and Johnnie Ears (1973) Western ΨΨ
A deaf Anthony Quinn teams up with Franco Nero to cope with the challenges of life in rural Texas.

Diary of a Country Priest (1951, Italy) Drama ΨΨΨΨ
A depressed priest grapples with stomach cancer and his loss of faith.

Diving Bell and the Butterfly, The ΨΨΨΨΨ
(2007, France) Drama-Biography
Jean-Dominique Bauby, editor of *Elle*, emerges completely paralyzed from a 3-week coma following a stroke. He cannot speak or move his body except for his left eye. Bauby responds to his situation with creativity and bravery. Much of the film is presented in the first person to help the viewer identify with his experience.

Doctor, The (1991) Drama ΨΨΨ
William Hurt plays a cold and indifferent physician whose approach to treatment changes dramatically after he is diagnosed with throat cancer.

Dreamland (2006) Drama Ψ
Coming of age story of a young woman in a remote desert trailer park who makes many sacrifices supporting her family and a friend who has multiple sclerosis and chronic pain.

Duet for One (1986) Drama ΨΨ
Julie Andrews plays a world-class violinist who learns to cope with multiple sclerosis. Good illustration of the effect of chronic illness on psychological health. Max von Sydow plays the role of Andrews' therapist.

"Why don't you ask me probing questions about my childhood?"

Stephanie Anderson queries her therapist, in *Duet for One* (1986)

Dummy (1979) Drama ΨΨ
Made-for-TV movie about a hearing impaired and mute teenager who is charged with murder and defended by a deaf attorney.

Deuce Bigalow: Male Gigolo (1999) Comedy Ψ
Rob Schneider takes a job as a male escort - one of his "calls" is for a woman with Tourette's disorder and the other is a woman with narcolepsy. The latter falls asleep in the middle of her bowling stride.

Early Frost, An (1985) Drama ΨΨΨ
Excellent made-for-TV movie (available on video) that explores the pain and anguish involved as a young man explains to his family and friends that he is gay and has AIDS.

Eating (1990) Comedy ΨΨΨ
An extended conversation that examines the relationship among life, love, and food.

Elephant Man, The (1980) Drama ΨΨΨ
David Lynch film about the life of John Merrick, a seriously deformed man who is befriended by a London physician. The film is effective in forcing the viewer to examine prejudices about appearance.

"I am NOT an elephant! I am NOT an animal! I am a human being! I am a man!"

John Merrick in *The Elephant Man* (1980)

Emmanuel's Gift (2005) Documentary ΨΨΨ
Emmanuel was born in Ghana in 1977 with a deformed leg and was destined to become a beggar. However, his mother instilled confidence and hope. This is an inspirational film that challenges negative stereotypes of people with disabilities.

Eye, The (2002) Suspense-Thriller ΨΨΨ
A young, blind woman regains her sight through a cornea transplant. She immediately begins to see ghosts which she identifies as the souls of the dead. Pang brothers' film in the tradition of *The Sixth Sense* and *The Ring*.

Farewell, The (2019) Comedy–Drama ΨΨΨΨ
A charming film that contrasts cultural expectations when the Chinese matriarch of a family develops cancer and her family decides to withhold the diagnosis from her, instead scheduling a wedding that becomes the pretense for a family reunion.

Freud (1962) Biography ΨΨΨ
Montgomery Clift in an interesting account of the early years of Freud's life. The film illustrates paralysis, false blindness, and a false pregnancy, all examples of somatic symptom disorders.

Gaby: A True Story (1987) Biography ΨΨΨ
A true story about a woman with cerebral palsy who goes on to become a respected author. Contrast this story with the life of Christy Brown told in *My Left Foot*.

Godsend (2004) Suspense–Thriller Ψ
Disappointing film starring Robert De Niro as a genetics researcher cloning human beings. He clones a child who begins to experience night terrors, hallucinations, delusions, and murderous behavior.

Hannah and Her Sisters (1986) ΨΨΨ
Comedy–Drama
Mickey (Woody Allen) is a hopeless hypochondriac who was formerly married to Hannah (Mia Farrow). Mickey spends his days worrying - about brain tumors, cancer, and cardiovascular disease.

"A week ago I bought a rifle, I went to the store – I bought a rifle! I was gonna – you know, – if they told me I had a tumor, I was gonna kill myself. The only thing that might have stopped me – MIGHT'VE – is that– my parents – would be devastated. I would have to shoot them also, first. And then I have an aunt and uncle – you know – it would've been a blood bath. "

Mickey contemplates his options if he is found to have a brain tumor, in *Hannah and Her Sisters* (1986)

Heart Is a Lonely Hunter, The (1968) Drama ΨΨ
Alan Arkin stars in this adaptation of Carson McCullers's sad, poignant novel about a simple friendship between two men. One of the men is deaf; the other has an intellectual disability. If you must choose between the film and the novel, read the novel.

Hollywood Ending (2002) Comedy ΨΨΨ
Woody Allen film about a struggling film director (Allen), who develops a conversion disorder (hysterical blindness) and must direct the film blind.

Home of the Brave (1949) Drama–War ΨΨ
An African American soldier develops a conversion disorder following his return from combat.

Honkytonk Man (1982) Drama Ψ
Clint Eastwood produced, directed, and starred in this film about a country and western singer with leukemia who hopes to make it to Nashville before he dies.

Hunchback of Notre Dame, The (1939) ΨΨΨΨΨ
Horror
Charles Laughton plays Quasimodo in this film adaptation of the Victor Hugo novel. The film is a classic in the horror genre, and it explores the relationship between body image and self-concept.

I Sent a Letter to My Love (1981) Drama ΨΨΨ
French film about a sister caring for her paralyzed brother. They each seek romance by writing to a newspaper personals column; without realizing what is happening, each begins corresponding with the other.

Ikiru (*To Live*, 1952, Japan) Drama ΨΨΨΨΨ
A city bureaucrat learns that he is dying of cancer and wants to find some meaning in his life. He becomes assertive in promoting projects for the public good. Until this time, he had lived a very mundane life.

In America (2003) Drama ΨΨΨΨ
Irish family immigrates to the United States to Hell's Kitchen. They befriend a Nigerian painter who is suffering with AIDS.

In for Treatment (1979, Netherlands) Drama ΨΨΨ
Dutch film about the indignities suffered by a cancer patient who must deal with an impersonal health care system.

Inception (2010) Drama ΨΨΨΨΨ
This remarkable movie was made by Christopher Nolan, who directed *Memento* in 2000 and *Oppenheimer* in 2023.. The film stars Leonardo DiCaprio as a thief who has learned to infiltrate the dreams of corporate executives so he can steal their best ideas. The film will teach you little about sleep or sleep disorders per se, but you will leave the theater thinking about the relationship between dreams, sleep, reality, consciousness, and the unconscious. Highly recommended.

Insomnia (2002) Drama–Mystery ΨΨΨΨ
Al Pacino stars as Will Dormer, a cop tracking down a minor writer (Robin Williams) in a murder investigation. Dormer deteriorates with insomnia as he battles guilt,

stress, and an Alaskan environment where the sun doesn't set. Directed by Christopher Nolan.

Italian for Beginners (2002) Comedy-Drama ΨΨΨ
In a hodgepodge of interrelated stories, one character has pancreatic cancer and suffers extraordinary pain.

It's My Party (1996) Drama ΨΨΨΨ
Sensitive film about a man with AIDS who throws one last party before killing himself. Much of the film centers on the issue of voluntary suicide and the ethics of euthanasia.

I Want Someone to Eat Cheese With (2007) Comedy Ψ
Portrayal of binge-eating disorder, the challenges of keeping a diet, and Overeaters Anonymous support group meetings.

Jacquot (1993) Biography ΨΨ
Moving film about the life of French Director Jacques Demy, who died from a brain tumor shortly after the film was released.

Johnnie Belinda (1948) Drama ΨΨ
Jane Wyman (who was Ronald Reagan's wife at the time) earned an Academy Award for her performance as a deaf-mute woman who is stigmatized and raped. The film is dated but still offers insights into the ways in which people who are hearing impaired are perceived.

Kurt Cobain: About a Son (2006) Documentary ΨΨ
Sensitive portrayal of the infamous grunge rock star using only interviewed audio recordings. Documents Cobain's suffering with severe stomach problems and the stress associated with his illness.

La Symphonie Pastorale (1946) Drama ΨΨΨΨ
French adaptation of André Gide novel about a Swiss minister who falls in love with his blind protégée and abandons his wife to be with her. When the blind girl later regains her sight, she is tormented by the decisions he has made because of her.

Leap of Faith (1992) Drama ΨΨ
Steve Martin plays itinerant evangelist Jonas Nightingale, whose faith healing stunts require technological support from backstage assistant Debra Winger. Contrast Martin's role with that of Burt Lancaster in *Elmer Gantry* (1960) and the documentary *Marjoe* (1972).

Life Is Sweet (1990) Drama ΨΨΨ
Mike Leigh film about a dysfunctional British family. One of the twin girls binges and purges on chocolate bars.

Life on a String (1991, China) Drama ΨΨΨ
Lyrical movie about a blind Chinese musician who believes his sight will be restored when he breaks his thousandth banjo string. He grows old and wise while he waits. Directed by Chen Kaige, best known for *Farewell, My Concubine.*

Light That Failed, The (1939) Drama ΨΨ
Adaptation of Kipling novel about a great artist who goes blind because of an injury while in Africa.

Living End, The (1992) Comedy ΨΨ
Two HIV-positive men hit the road and explore what it means to live purposively with their disease.

Longtime Companion (1989) Drama ΨΨΨ
This film explores the ways in which AIDS has affected a group of gay friends and traces the love and loss that is shared between two men as one of them dies from the disease.

"It seems almost inconceivable, doesn't it? That there was ever a time before all this. When we didn't wake up every day, wondering, who's sick now, who else is gone?"

Confronting the reality of AIDS, in *Longtime Companion* (1990)

Lost in Translation (2003) Drama ΨΨΨ
Two Americans (Bill Murray and Scarlett Johansson) stranded in Japan find solace, excitement, and friendship in one another. Both characters suffer with severe insomnia symptoms.

Loverboy (2004) Drama ΨΨ
An overly protective mother illustrates the rare but fascinating phenomenon of factitious disorder by proxy.

Machinist, The (2004, Spain) Mystery-Drama ΨΨΨΨ
Christian Bale lost 80 pounds to play the gaunt Trevor Reznik who suffers from severe insomnia that causes what appear to be symptoms of psychosis (1 year later Bale gained the weight back to play the muscular Batman in *Batman Begins*).

Man Without a Face, The (1993) Drama ΨΨ
Mel Gibson directs and stars in this film about a man whose face becomes terribly disfigured after an automobile accident. He becomes reclusive but finds redemption in his relationship with the 12-year-old boy he tutors.

Marvin's Room (1996) Drama ΨΨΨ
A compelling examination of the way in which chronic illness affects caregivers and families.

Mask (1985) Drama ΨΨΨ
Cher stars in this film about her character's son, Rocky Dennis, a spunky teenager whose life has been dramatically affected by craniodiaphyseal dysplasia, a disorder that distorts the shape of his skull and face. This is a feel-good movie that succeeds. The thwarted love relationship between Rocky and a blind girlfriend underscores our tendency to judge people by their appearance.

Matrix Reloaded, The (2003) Action ΨΨΨ
Keanu Reeves is Neo in this first sequel in a Trilogy by the Wachowski brothers. Neo suffers from insomnia though on a more important level, his insomnia functions as a metaphor for being "awake" and "alive." He also experiences nightmares and frequently worries at night about decisions he needs to make the next day.

Miracle Worker, The (1962) Biography ΨΨΨ
Patty Duke and Anne Bancroft star in this well-known film about the childhood of Helen Keller and the influence of a gifted teacher.

Modify (2005) Documentary ΨΨΨ
An interesting documentary that highlights the many ways in which humans elect to change and improve the bodies with which they were born. In 2020, Americans spent US $16.7 billion on cosmetic surgery.

Motorcycle Diaries (2004, Argentina) Drama ΨΨΨΨ
Based on the true coming of age story of "Che" Guevara. Two men travel the countryside of South America seeing indigenous cultures while logging observations and experiences in a diary. They help in communities and at a hospital in Peru with leprosy patients. One character's struggle with asthma is depicted.

Music Within (2007) Drama–Comedy ΨΨΨ
The true story of Richard Pimentel, a brilliant public speaker, who returned from Vietnam disabled by a severe hearing impairment. He became a passionate advocate for the disabled and is in part responsible for the creation of the 1990 American with Disabilities Act.

My Flesh and Blood (2004) Documentary ΨΨΨ
Moving documentary about Susan Tom, who adopted 11 special needs children and raised them on her own. The children suffer in a variety of ways; their problems include cystic fibrosis, severe burn, developmental disabilities, the absence of legs, and a genetic skin disorder that causes severe pain.

My Life (1993) Drama ΨΨΨ
Michael Keaton learns he is dying from cancer and makes a series of videotapes for his still-unborn son, including one in which he teaches his son how to shave.

My Life Without Me (2003) Drama ΨΨΨ
A 23-year-old woman is diagnosed with ovarian cancer and decides not to tell her family but instead live her life more fully and prepare them for when she is gone. One of her bucket list goals is to have an affair.

My Own Private Idaho (1991) Drama ΨΨ
River Phoenix stars as a young male prostitute who has narcolepsy. He is befriended by Keanu Reeves, and the two leave Portland and travel together. Interesting presentations of dreams that occur during narcoleptic episodes.

Oasis (2002, Korea) Drama ΨΨΨΨ
A quirky young man is released from prison after serving 2.5 years for accidentally killing someone while driving. He becomes curious and interested in the victim's daughter who has cerebral palsy. Both individuals are isolated and outcasts from their families, and they find friendship and comfort in one another.

One Last Thing (2005) Comedy Ψ
A boy with terminal cancer gets a last wish from the Wish Givers Foundation. He gets to spend a week alone with a supermodel.

Open Hearts (*Elsker Dig for Evigt;* 2003, Denmark) Drama ΨΨΨ
Danish film about a random car accident that leaves a man paralyzed from the neck down. He lashes out in anger, unable to accept the reality of his losses. His girlfriend begins an affair with the husband of the woman who caused the accident.

"My whole life disappeared with you that morning."

Grieving, in *Open Hearts* (2003)

Pact of Silence, The (2003, France) Drama ΨΨ
A Jesuit priest tries to make sense out of a nun's psychosomatic fits that turn out to be related to the experiences of the nun's incarcerated twin sister.

Passion Fish (1992) Drama ΨΨΨΨ
The stress of disability and the demands a person with a disability can make on caregivers are nicely chronicled

in this film about a querulous paraplegic actress and her caretaker-companion. The caretaker in the film has been recently hospitalized for cocaine addiction, and the paraplegic actress is an alcoholic.

Patch Adams (1998) Comedy ΨΨ
Robin Williams plays a medical student, nicknamed Patch, who defies the medical institution and crosses boundaries in using humor and holistic medical practices with various patients throughout a hospital. Some humorous and touching scenes occur on the children's cancer ward and with other suffering patients.

Phantom of the Opera, The (1925) Horror ΨΨΨ
A disfigured music lover, played by Lon Chaney, lives in the bowels of the Paris opera house, unable to achieve romantic love because of his hideous face. He is eventually hunted down and killed by an angry mob.

Joe Miller: "What do you love about the law, Andrew?"
Andrew Beckett: "I ... many things ... uh ... uh ... What I love the most about the law?"
Joe Miller: "Yeah."
Andrew Beckett: "It's that every now and again – not often, but occasionally – you get to be a part of justice being done. That really is quite a thrill when that happens."

***Philadelphia* (1993)**

Philadelphia (1993) Drama ΨΨΨ
Tom Hanks won an Academy Award for his portrayal of an AIDS-afflicted attorney who is fired from a prestigious law firm once the partners know of his illness. There is a particularly moving scene in which Hanks plays an opera and explains to Denzel Washington why he loves the music so passionately.

Pieces of April (2003) Drama-Comedy ΨΨΨ
A young woman, estranged from her family, is determined to impress them with a Thanksgiving dinner. She has a particularly tenuous relationship with her cynical mother who is dying of cancer.

Places in the Heart (1984) Drama ΨΨΨ
Sally Field won an Academy Award for Best Actress for her role in this film about a widowed woman struggling to keep her farm and her family in a small Texas town during the Depression. The film links John Malkovich as a blind World War I veteran and Danny Glover as a hapless drifter. The standoff between a blind Malkovich and the local chapter of the Ku Klux Klan is especially memorable.

Promises in the Dark (1979) Drama ΨΨ
Melodrama about a young woman dying from cancer.

Proof (1992, Australian) Drama ΨΨΨ
A blind man takes photographs to document his life and its meaning.

Poison Ivy (1992) Drama Ψ
A newcomer into a pathological family plans to take over the role of wife and mother. The father is an alcoholic and the mother is a hypochondriac.

Primo Amore (2004, Italy) Drama-Romance ΨΨΨ
A goldsmith falls for an art-school model and becomes obsessed with controlling her diet and appearance. This film provides an interesting examination of eating disorders, and it can be viewed as a metaphorical commentary on society's beliefs about the female body.

Queen Margot (1994) Drama ΨΨ
Period film set in 1572 France at a time of heavy religious warfare (Catholic vs. Protestant). The king in the film appears to have a somatoform disorder.

Rails and Ties (2007) Drama ΨΨΨ
Engineer Tom Stark (Kevin Bacon) cannot avoid crashing his train into a parked car occupied by a suicidal mother and her 11-year-old son who escapes the car unscathed. Stark's wife Megan (Marcia Gay Harden) is dying of cancer. The film depicts the relationship between the Starks and the young boy who all help one another cope with life and death.

Rat Race (2001) Comedy Ψ
Several characters travel long distances in a competition for monetary reward. One character, played by Rowan Atkinson, has narcolepsy.

Return to Oz (1985) Adventure-Family Ψ
A follow-up to the classic story, this film depicts Dorothy returning for more adventures in Oz after evading ECT and "dangerous psychiatric treatment." Dorothy struggles with a sleep disorder.

Rory O'Shea Was Here (2005) Comedy-Drama ΨΨΨ
Depicts the quest for independence and friendship between two young men, one coping with muscular dystrophy, the other with cerebral palsy.

Safe (1995) Comedy-Drama ΨΨΨΨ
A rare film almost exclusively focusing on a woman (Julianne Moore) with a somatoform disorder, various treatment approaches, and the effects on her family. This satirical film was cleverly directed by Todd Haynes.

Savage Nights (*Les Nuits Fauves*; 1992, France) Drama-Biography ΨΨΨΨ
This controversial film was directed by French filmmaker Cyril Collard, who died from AIDS 3 days before the film was honored with a Cesar award as the best French film of the year. The movie deals with the existential decisions made by a bisexual antihero who continues to have unprotected sex, even after learning he has AIDS.

Seabiscuit (2003) Drama ΨΨ
Tobey Maguire plays a disc jockey with bulimic symptoms to keep his weight down and compete in horse-racing championships. Bulimic symptoms are common among jockeys, though this is not an emphasis in the film.

Secondhand Lions (2003) Family ΨΨ
A young adolescent (Haley Joel Osment) is forced to live with his two rich uncles (Robert Duvall and Michael Caine), one of whom often sleepwalks.

Secret of Dr. Kildare, The (1939) Drama ΨΨΨ
The good Dr. Kildare works hard to cure a patient's conversion disorder (blindness) in this dated but interesting film.

Send Me No Flowers (1964) Romance-Comedy Ψ
Rock Hudson plays a hypochondriac convinced he will die soon. Hudson sets out to find a suitable replacement so his wife will be able to get along without him.

Shadowlands (1993) Biography ΨΨΨ
Wonderful Richard Attenborough film about the late-life romance of C.S. Lewis (Anthony Hopkins) and Joy Gresham (Debra Winger). Lewis must come to grips with the meaning of pain, suffering, and loss when Joy develops cancer.

Shootist, The (1976) Western ΨΨ
John Wayne's last film, about an aging gunfighter dying from cancer. Also stars Jimmy Stewart, Lauren Bacall, Ron Howard, Harry Morgan, John Carradine, Hugh O'Brian, and Richard Boone. John Wayne, a heavy smoker, died from lung cancer after making this film.

"You aim to do to me what they did with John Wesley Hardin. Lay me out and parade every damn fool in the state past me at a dollar a head, half price for children, and then stuff me in a gunny sack and shovel me under."

John Wayne's character confronts the undertaker, in *The Shootist* (1976)

Shop on Main Street, The (1965, Czech) Drama ΨΨΨΨ
Czechoslovakian film about a man appointed as the "Aryan controller" of a button shop in World War II. He befriends and hides the Jewish owner of the shop, who does not understand the situation because she is deaf. She assumes the new arrival has been sent as her assistant; when he later hides her to avoid deportation to the death camps, she dies. Overcome with remorse, he kills himself. Selected as the Best Foreign Language Film of 1965.

Simple Men (1992) Comedy ΨΨ
Deadpan comedy from auteur director Hal Hartley, that depicts a character suffering with epilepsy.

Smile (2005) Drama ΨΨ
Well-intentioned film depicting the suffering experienced by those with physical deformities such as cleft palates.

Sorry, Wrong Number (1948) Thriller ΨΨ
Barbara Stanwyck and Burt Lancaster star in this murder movie. Stanwyck is a rich heiress who is bedridden with psychosomatic heart disease and paralysis.

Starve (2006) Documentary ΨΨΨ
This film follows the lives of five women with eating disorders.

Storytelling (2001) Comedy-Drama ΨΨ
Two separate stories explore issues of race, sex, and exploitation. In the first story, a teenager allows herself to be exploited by her teacher after getting bored with her boyfriend who has cerebral palsy. In the second story, a shoe-store worker dreams of being a documentary filmmaker and uses a disillusioned teenager and his family as his subjects.

Swallow (2019) Drama ΨΨΨΨΨ
A docile, pregnant housewife finds herself coping with an irresistible urge to swallow inanimate objects like marbles and thumbtacks. Ingesting these items is one of the few ways she can exercise agency and push back against an overbearing husband and his domineering parents. She diagnoses herself with pica, but a diagnosis of obsessive-compulsive disorder would have to be ruled out. The film is in many ways reminiscent of a 1974 film, *The Stepford Wives*.

Tell Me That You Love Me, Junie Moon (1970) Comedy ΨΨ
Otto Preminger film in which three unusual roommates come together as a family. Liza Minnelli is disfigured; another has epilepsy; the third is wheelchair-bound.

Terms of Endearment (1983) Comedy ΨΨΨ
Shirley MacLaine, Debra Winger, and Jack Nicholson star in this poignant but funny movie about relationships, caring, and cancer.

Test of Love, A (1984, Australian) Drama ΨΨ
A film based on a true story of a teacher's successful attempt to reach out to a girl with a disability.

Thin (2006) Documentary ΨΨΨ
Four women with anorexia or bulimia allow their treatment experiences - the struggles, progress, relapse, and symptoms - to be documented on film.

Twelve O'Clock High (1949) War ΨΨΨΨ
Gregory Peck plays the role of General Frank Savage, an effective leader who develops a conversion disorder (psychosomatic paralysis) in response to his role in the death of several of his subordinates. The film is based on a true story.

Unconscious (2004) Drama ΨΨ
A Spanish film that satirizes psychoanalysis; the movie includes examples of hypochondriasis and conversion disorder.

Up in Arms (1944) Musical-Comedy-War Ψ
Danny Kaye plays a hypochondriac in the Army.

Unbreakable (2000) Drama-Suspense ΨΨΨΨ
Samuel L. Jackson plays Elijah, a comic book collector, who was born with a rare genetic bone disease, which makes him highly susceptible to injury. Bruce Willis, on the other hand, plays a security officer who is in a train wreck and is the one survivor who does not have a scratch on him. Second mainstream film by master storyteller, M. Night Shyamalan.

Unfinished Life, An (2005) Drama ΨΨ
A physically abused woman escapes her abuser with her daughter and moves in with her father-in-law (Robert Redford) and a man (Morgan Freeman) he is taking care of. The latter was mauled by a bear, needs daily injections, walks with crutches, and cannot take care of himself.

Vanilla Sky (2001) Drama-Suspense ΨΨΨ
Cameron Crowe film in which Tom Cruise plays a wealthy businessman in NYC who has a car accident and must reestablish his life with a severe facial deformity. This changes his interactions, especially with a woman with whom he is falling in love (Penélope Cruz). He begins to break down further as a dead friend (Cameron Diaz) reappears.

Waking Life (2001) Drama-Animation ΨΨΨ
This unique, creative film follows a character searching for answers to life's most important questions in a world that seems surreal and dream-like. The film is a surrealistic blend of animation and drama with a heavy philosophical and existential bent. The film questions whether we are sleepwalking through our days and our lives, and whether we are more awake when we interact with others or when we dream.

Waterdance, The (1992) Drama ΨΨΨΨ
Realistic film about the way spinal cord injuries have changed the lives of three men who meet in a rehabilitation hospital.

"Got you in a halo, huh. I call that thing a crown of thorns. I thought they was gonna screw it into my brain."

A paralyzed patient describes his rehabilitation, in *The Waterdance* (1992)

Whales of August, The (1987) Drama ΨΨΨ
Vincent Price and Ann Sothern support Lillian Gish and Bette Davis in a remarkable film about what it means to grow old. Davis plays a blind and embittered sister who is still loved by Gish.

Whatever Happened to Baby Jane? (1962) Drama ΨΨΨ
Bette Davis and Joan Crawford portray two elderly sisters. Crawford is wheelchair-bound because of an automobile accident possibly caused by her sister. Davis is obviously demented and terrorizes her younger sister. Watch for the surprise ending.

White Heat (1949) Crime ΨΨΨΨ
James Cagney plays a ruthless gangster who has debilitating migraine headaches that only his mother can cure. The film ties into the psychoanalytic ideas of the day and features a famous ending in which Cagney blows up an oil tank.

"Cody Jarrett. He finally made it to the top of the world. And it blew up in his face."

***White Heat* (1949)**

Wind Will Carry Us, The (1999, France/Iran) Drama ΨΨ
A man and his film crew travel to a remote Iranian village to film the special ceremony that occurs after an old woman dies. Directed by Abbas Kiarostami.

Whose Life Is It Anyway? (1981) Drama ΨΨΨΨ
Richard Dreyfuss plays a sculptor paralyzed from the neck down after a car crash. An unethical physician injects Dreyfuss with Valium, despite his refusal to take the medication. He argues convincingly for the right to die, taking on a hospital staff determined to keep him alive.

Woman's Tale, A (1991, Australian) Drama ΨΨΨΨ
This film chronicles the final days in the life of a 78-year-old woman dying of cancer.

World's Fastest Indian, The (2005, New Zealand) Drama ΨΨΨ
Heart disease threatens the life of New Zealander Burt Munro, who spent years building a 1920 Indian motorcycle. Despite the stress of physical illness, Munro pushes forward to break a land speed record at the Bonneville Salt Flats.

Wrestler, The (2008) Drama ΨΨΨΨ
Randy "the Ram" is a professional wrestler who is forced to retire due to multiple physical problems following use of steroids and body enhancers. He breaks down (vomits and faints) with a heart attack after a challenging match fighting an opponent who uses glass and a staple gun. He attempts a comeback in both his personal life and in wrestling. Directed by Darren Aronofsky.

Yesterday (2004, South Africa) Drama ΨΨΨΨ
A woman named Yesterday focuses largely on the present and future as she takes care of her daughter, her dying husband, and her own HIV.

Sexual Dysfunctions and Gender Dysphoria

Adventures of Priscilla, Queen of the Desert (1994) Comedy ΨΨ
Terence Stamp plays an aging transsexual who joins with two friends to travel from Sidney to Alice Springs in the Australian outback to perform a lip-synching routine. Much of the film revolves around the prejudice and homophobic hostility the three transsexuals encounter.

"Being a man one day and a woman the next isn't an easy thing."

Bernadette complaining about life as a transsexual, in *Adventures of Priscilla, Queen of the Desert* (1994)

AKA (2002) Drama ΨΨΨ
Fascinating artistry where most of the screen is split into three sections, and the viewer is simultaneously shown past and present, different character reactions, different camera angles, and even the internal thoughts and behaviors of a character. The lead character, sexually abused by his father, escapes on a journey exploring his sexual and psychological identity. As with *Memento*, the viewer must pay close attention throughout the film.

All About My Mother (1999, Spain) Drama-Comedy ΨΨ
Pedro Almodóvar film about a nurse who tragically loses her son and, in her grief, meets a transvestite prostitute and a pregnant nun (Penélope Cruz). Winner of an Academy Award for Best Foreign Language Film.

Any Day Now (2012) Drama ΨΨΨ
A drag queen and his attorney lover try to adopt a boy with special needs but come up against societal bias and legal limitations

(A)sexual (2011) Documentary ΨΨ
An examination of the 1% of the population not attracted to either males or females.

Beautiful Boxer (2003, Thailand) Action-Drama ΨΨ
A male-to-female transsexual makes use of her kickboxing skills to pay for a sex change operation.

Birdcage, The (1996) Comedy ΨΨΨ
Mike Nichols and Elaine May's remake of *La Cage aux Folles*. This film is almost as good as the original, thanks to strong performances by Robin Williams and Gene Hackman.

"Al, you old son of a bitch! How ya doin'? How do you feel about that call today? I mean the Dolphins! Fourth-and-three play on their 0-yard line with only 34 seconds to go!"

A gay transvestite trying to act masculine, in *The Birdcage* (1996)

Breakfast on Pluto (2005) Comedy ΨΨΨ
Neil Jordan's film about an Iris Catholic abandoned child who is raised by a parish priest but later becomes a flamboyant transsexual.

Boys Don't Cry (1999) Drama ΨΨΨΨΨ
One of the best films to ever depict the pain and problems that can emerge from gender identity disorder. A brutal, powerful film.

Cowboys (2021) Drama ΨΨΨΨ
A sensitive film about an 11-year-old child who convinces her bipolar father that she is a boy trapped in a girl's body. The child and her father escape to the mountains of Montana, are caught, and the father is jailed. The estranged mother comes to accept her trans child's sexuality, and the family is eventually reunited.

Crying Game, The (1992) Drama ΨΨΨΨ
This Neil Jordan film explores homosexuality, transsexualism, interracial sexuality, and the ability of two human beings to love one another. Too complex to explain simply, the film must be seen to be fully appreciated.

Flawless (1999) Drama-Comedy ΨΨ
Philip Seymour Hoffman plays a drag queen named Rusty who is saving money for a gender modification operation; Robert de Niro plays a homophobic neighbor who takes voice lessons from Rusty following a stroke.

Good Luck to You, Leo Grande (2022)
Comedy-Drama ΨΨΨΨΨ
Emma Thompson is wonderful as Nancy Stokes, a retired religious education teacher and widow, who has never experienced an orgasm or rewarding sex. She hires a male prostitute, Leo Grande, to introduce her to the wonderful world of sexuality.

Gun Hill Road (2011) Drama ΨΨΨ
A man returns from prison to discover that his teenage son is transsexual. He must reevaluate his personal values and beliefs about the trans community to hold his family together.

"I told them my father was a Cultural attaché. What will they think when they find out he lives with a drag queen?"

Renato's son, in *La Cage aux Folles* (1978)

La Cage aux Folles (1978, France/Italy) ΨΨΨ
Comedy
A gay man and his transvestite lover manage a popular St. Tropez nightclub. Much of the humor revolves around sex roles and the folly of trying very hard to be something you're not.

Marie Antoinette (2006) Drama-Biography Ψ
The Queen finds herself in a loveless and asexual relationship with her husband, Louis XVI.

Mrs. Doubtfire (1994) Comedy ΨΨ
Robin Williams cross-dresses as an English nanny to have time with his children.

"Well, I hope you're up for a little competition. She's got a power tool in the bedroom, dear. It's her own personal jackhammer. She could break sidewalks with that thing. She uses it and the lights dim, it's like a prison movie. Amazed she hasn't chipped her teeth."

Daniel Hillard (Robin Williams) tries to discourage Stu, his ex-wife's new lover, in Mrs. *Doubtfire* (1994)

Mystery of Alexina, The (1985) Drama ΨΨ
A story about the psychological sequelae of the decision to raise a male child as a female.

Normal (2003) Drama ΨΨΨ
A man (Tom Wilkinson) after 25 years of marriage tells his wife (Jessica Lange) he is a woman trapped in a man's body, and he wants gender modification surgery.

Oh in Ohio, The (2006) Comedy ΨΨ
A married couple becomes open to new sexual experiences with different partners after a decade of insipid sex. Sexual desire and sexual disorders are depicted.

Princesa (2001) Drama Ψ
Brazilian transvestite moves to Italy and works as a prostitute to earn money for his sex change operation.

Sessions, The (2012) Comedy-Biography ΨΨΨΨ
Helen Hunt plays the role of a sexual surrogate working with Mark, played by John Hawkes, a talented 38-year-old Berkeley student who has spent most of his life in an iron lung.

Soldier's Girl (2003) Drama-Biography ΨΨΨ
Based on the true story of Barry Winchell who entered the military and fell in love with a transsexual dancer at a club. Military peers find out about the secret relationship and the situation ends tragically.

> **"The imagination is the most powerful force known to mankind. And it is my imagined self, the one who is beautiful and loving and worthy of being loved, that has been my guiding force. My inspiration. I can only hope to become the person Barry imagined me to be. I pray for the courage it will take to become a real, live soldier's girl."**
>
> ***Soldier's Girl* (2003)**

Southern Comfort (2001) Documentary ΨΨ
Female-to-male transsexual faces hate and prejudice in this award-winning film.

That's the Way I Like It (1998, Singapore) Drama ΨΨ
A young man who has always tried to please his parents announces that he is in fact a woman who plans to get surgery to make his body conform to his identity. The man attempts suicide but eventually lives and completes his surgery.

Tomboy (2011, France) Drama ΨΨΨΨ
A 10-year-old girl moves into a new neighborhood and is mistaken for a boy. She embraces the mistake and adopts a masculine identify, mystifying her younger sister and upsetting her parents.

Tootsie (1982) Comedy-Romance ΨΨΨΨ
Funny Dustin Hoffman film in which an unsuccessful actor finds success when he impersonates a woman. He learns from the process, and the audience learns some important lessons about gender, sex roles, and human relationships.

> **Director: "I'd like to make her look a little more attractive. How far can you pull back?"**
> **Cameraman: "How do you feel about Cleveland?"**
>
> ***Tootsie* (1982)**

Transamerica (2005) Comedy ΨΨΨΨ
A presurgical male-to-female transsexual takes a cross-country journey with the son she just met for the first time.

Victor/Victoria (1982) Musical-Comedy ΨΨ
Blake Edwards film with Julie Andrews as a down-on-her-luck singer who becomes a sensation when she pretends to be a male-female impersonator.

Wild Tigers I Have Known (2006) Drama ΨΨΨ
A coming of age film about a 13-year-old boy struggling with issues of sexual identity

World According to Garp, The (1982) Comedy-Drama ΨΨ
John Lithgow plays transsexual Roberta Muldoon in a film in which troubled sexuality is commonplace.

Yentl (1983) Musical ΨΨ
Barbra Streisand directed and produced this film, and she has the lead role as a young woman in Eastern Europe who must pass herself off as a man to get an education. Interesting examination of sex roles; terrific performance by Streisand.

Zerophilia (2005) Comedy-Romance Ψ
A young man discovers that he has "zerophilia," which means he can switch sexual identities and experience pleasure as either a man or a woman. The film is a less-than-satisfying exploration of sex roles.

Disruptive, Impulse-Control, and Conduct Disorders

400 Blows, The (1959) Drama ΨΨΨΨΨ
François Truffaut's first feature film based on his own experiences as a young boy. The film depicts ineffectual parenting and inept teachers, and Antoine is portrayed as more rebellious than bad.

> **Psychiatrist: "Your parents say you're always lying."**
> **Antoine Doinel: "Oh, I lie now and then, I suppose. Sometimes I'd tell them the truth, and they still wouldn't believe me, so I prefer to lie."**
>
> **Strange behavior explained, in *The Four Hundred Blows* (1959)**

Afterschool (2008) Drama ΨΨ
A high school boy, addicted to violent online pornography, films the death of two classmates from a drug overdose.

Ali Zaoua: Prince of the Streets (2000) Drama ΨΨΨ
Four young homeless boys, living in poverty on the streets of Morocco, rebel against their gang leader's oppressive rule.

Beautiful Boy (2010) Drama ΨΨΨ
A couple with a strained marriage must cope with additional stress after they learn that their 17-year-old son killed 17 professors and other students at his university before taking his own life.

Beautiful Boy (2018) Biography-Drama ΨΨΨ
Steve Carell plays a father trying to save his 18-year-old son (Nic) who has become addicted to methamphetamine. Based on a memoir written by director David Sheff titled *Beautiful Boy: A Father's Journey Through His Son's Addiction.* Happily, Nic gets treatment and overcomes his addiction.

Beautiful Ohio (2006) Drama Ψ
Independent film about two brothers growing up in the Midwest, one is gifted but also has severe oppositional tendencies.

Behind The Red Door (2001) Drama ΨΨ
Keifer Sutherland plays a man dying of AIDS who exhibits explosive anger.

Carrie (1976) Horror ΨΨ
This Brian De Palma film is based on a Stephen King novel and depicts the cruelty of adolescents and some of the stresses associated with caring for a mentally ill mother. Sissy Spacek's performance is remarkable.

Chorus, The (2004, France) Drama ΨΨΨ
A newly hired boarding schoolteacher tries to transform troubled kids into positive problem solvers through music and positive rewards. The headmaster, who believes in severe punishment, reluctantly agrees to let the new teacher try more positive approaches.

City of God (2003, Brazil) Drama-Foreign ΨΨΨΨ
Painful, sobering, and graphic examination of the violence associated with gang life, drug trafficking, and poverty in Rio de Janeiro. This film depicts young children and adolescents who grow up in an environment in which guns and murder are commonplace.

Dangerous Lives of Altar Boys, The (2002) ΨΨ
Drama-Comedy
High school outcasts express rebellion in a variety of ways, including abuse of an authoritarian nun (played by Jodie Foster).

Don't Come Knocking (2005) Drama ΨΨΨ
A former Western movie star drowns his sorrow in alcohol and self-pity until he discovers he has a son and sets out to find him. The son is oppositional-defiant.

Elephant (2003) Drama ΨΨΨΨΨ
Well-crafted, foreboding, eerie Gus Van Sant film addressing the tragedy of school shootings. Powerful parallels with the Columbine tragedy. Winner of the Palm award at Cannes for Best Picture and Best Director. Sadly, the film is still timely and relevant.

"And most importantly, have fun, man!"

Final words of an adolescent to his co-assassin preparing to enter a school building, in *Elephant* (2003)

Elling (2001) Drama ΨΨΨΨΨ
Norwegian film about two men released from a psychiatric hospital who must prove themselves capable of coping with everyday life. One man suffers from intermittent anger episodes. Oscar nominee for Best Foreign Language Film.

Equus (1977) Drama ΨΨΨ
Richard Burton examines the meaning and purpose of his own life as he attempts to unravel the psychosexual roots that led an adolescent to blind six horses. Wonderful soliloquies by Burton. This Sidney Lumet film is influenced by Freud's case study of Little Hans and the writings of R. D. Laing.

Every Man for Himself and God Against All (1975) Biography ΨΨΨΨΨ
Werner Herzog film based on a true story about a man who spent an isolated childhood virtually devoid of stimulation. This movie should be compared with Truffaut's film *The Wild Child* and the more recent film *Nell.*

Face to Face (1976, Sweden) Drama ΨΨ
Bergman film in which Liv Ullmann plays a suicidal psychiatrist estranged from her husband and 14-year-old daughter. During a coma that results from an overdose of sleeping pills, Ullmann dreams about a childhood experience in which she was punished by being locked in a closet.

Fanny and Alexander (1983, Sweden) ΨΨΨΨΨ
Drama
Bergman film about two young children and the ways in which their lives change when their father dies, and their mother remarries. The film is sensitive, tender, and haunting and shows how the world looks through the eyes of a 10-year-old.

Firestarter (1984) Drama-Suspense-Horror Ψ
A film based on a 1980 novel by Stephen King in which Drew Barrymore portrays a young girl with pyrokinetic, telekinetic, and telepathic powers. Barrymore can set fires simply by staring at whatever she wants to set on fire.

Forbidden Games (1951) War-Drama ΨΨΨΨ
This beautiful French film is about two children who create and share a private fantasy world. The movie juxtaposes the innocence of childhood with the horror of war.

Great New Wonderful, The (2005) Drama ΨΨ
Several stories of New Yorkers converge, including one depicting a child with a serious behavior disorder.

Gummo (1997) Independent ΨΨΨ
This extremely disturbing and unforgettable Harmony Korine film depicts life in a small, rural town after its destruction by a tornado. Despite the lack of a coherent plot, the film gets high marks for its honesty and realism. Various types of psychopathology are presented with an emphasis on conduct disorders.

Happy-Go-Lucky (2008, Britain) Comedy ΨΨΨ
Poppy, an optimistic realist, interacts with a driver education instructor with intermittent explosive disorder in this Mike Leigh film.

Hate (1995, France) ΨΨ
Conduct disorders abound among adolescent gangs in a French suburban ghetto in this film about racism and oppression.

Holes (2002) Family ΨΨΨ
One of the better nonanimated Disney films about troubled youths who are sent to a work camp to dig deep holes in the middle of the desert to help three criminals find a lost treasure. Sigourney Weaver has a memorable role.

Hulk (2003) Action-Drama ΨΨΨ
Director Ang Lee brings the *Incredible Hulk* comic series to film and in doing so creates a wonderful representation of anger and intermittent explosiveness.

Innocents, The (1961) Horror ΨΨΨ
Deborah Kerr plays a governess hired to care for two precocious children. Is she hallucinating or delusional, or are there really ghosts in the house? Interesting sexual tension develops between Kerr and the boy. Based on the Henry James novella *The Turn of the Screw*.

Island on Bird Street (2000) Drama ΨΨΨ
Polish film about an adventurous, high-spirited boy who escapes from Nazi control; inspired by Robinson Crusoe, he creates a hide-out and waits for his father's return.

Kids (1995) Drama ΨΨΨ
Gritty and disturbing film about urban adolescents, sex, drugs, and violence. The main character is a teenager with AIDS who preys on young adolescent girls, taking pride in seducing virgins.

"If you deflower a girl... you're the man. No one can ever do that again. You're the only one. No one, no one, has the power to do that again."

Telly describes his fascination with virgins, in *Kids* (1995)

Klepto (2003) Drama-Comedy ΨΨΨ
Rare film in which the struggles associated with kleptomania are depicted.

Leolo (1992, France/Canada) Comedy ΨΨΨ
Leo, an adolescent boy growing up in an eccentric and very dysfunctional family in Montreal, is unable to accept the reality of his genetic heritage and concocts a fantasy in which he was accidentally conceived by sperm that crossed the Atlantic in a Sicilian tomato. (The film is better than this brief synopsis suggests.)

Life as a House (2001) Drama ΨΨΨ
Touching film about the transformation of the relationship between a rebellious, addicted adolescent (Hayden Christensen) and his terminally ill father (Kevin Kline).

Lilya 4-Ever (2002, Sweden/Denmark) Drama ΨΨΨ
Heartbreaking film about a girl, rejected by her family and society, who seems to meet with tragedy just when it appears she is headed in the right direction. Lilya is physically, emotionally, and sexually abused in the film.

Little Man Tate (1991) Drama ΨΨΨ
Jodie Foster directed this film about a child prodigy and the tensions that arise between his mother and the psychologist to whom the child's education is entrusted. Foster acknowledged that the film is partly autobiographical.

Lord of the Flies (1963) Drama ΨΨ
Film adaptation of William Goldman's novel about a group of schoolchildren who quickly shed the thin veneer of civilization and become savages. Both the film and book raise interesting questions about nature and nurture. Remade in 1990, but the original film is better.

Magdalene Sisters, The (2002) Docudrama ΨΨΨ
Troubled adolescent girls are sent to a dehumanizing boarding home where they are abused, mistreated, and

exploited by the nuns who run the home. One of the abused girls becomes sexually involved with a priest and later becomes psychotic.

Marnie (1964) Thriller-Romance ΨΨ
Hitchcock film about a sexually frigid kleptomaniac who dominates her new husband. As in other Hitchcock films, the protagonist's problems are found to be rooted in childhood trauma, and she overcomes them once she experiences catharsis. Watch for the use of a word association test administered by her husband, a young Sean Connery. Bruce Dern has a minor role as a drunken sailor who rapes Marnie's mother. (Also see *Spellbound*.)

Monsieur Ibrahim (2003) Drama ΨΨΨ
Heart-warming French film about an adolescent boy raised by a critical, neglecting father; he develops a meaningful friendship with a local store owner.

Mortal Transfer (2001) Mystery-Drama ΨΨΨ
French film depicting a patient undergoing psychoanalysis and struggling with kleptomania and sexual sadomasochism. Her therapist falls asleep; when he wakes up, his patient is dead.

My First Mister (2001) Drama ΨΨ
Adolescent girl struggles with severe isolation, depression, self-injurious behavior, and other acting out behaviors until she befriends a 49-year-old man. The teen has a host of behavioral problems including "huffing," autoerotic asphyxiation, isolation from her family, and prostitution.

My Flesh and Blood (2004) Documentary ΨΨΨ
Moving story of Susan Tom, who adopted 11 special needs children and raised them on her own. One has cystic fibrosis and severe anger and oppositional behavior.

Nell (1994) Drama ΨΨΨ
Jodie Foster plays a feral child raised in isolation in the North Carolina woods. She is terrified of the doctor who discovers her, and she eventually develops her own odd language. The doctor consults an expert on child psychology. Interesting examination of Rousseau's concept of the "noble savage."

Noise (2007) Comedy ΨΨ
Street noise is a stressor for David Owen (Tim Robbins) who becomes the Rectifier, a vigilante who takes noise personally. He damages noisy cars and destroys car alarms. He also seriously damages his relationships and loses his job and family.

Noi the Albino (*Nói Albinói;* 2003, Iceland) ΨΨΨ
Drama
A film about a troubled but gifted teen who struggles with conduct problems in Iceland. The movie provides a realistic evaluation of a gifted adolescent who is out of place in both school and life.

Pelle the Conqueror (1986) Drama ΨΨΨΨ
Moving film about lust, passion, dreams, aging, hope, pragmatic romance, and, most of all, the love between a father and his son. The film won the Grand Prix at the Cannes Film Festival and an Academy Award for Best Foreign Language Film.

Pieces of April (2003) Comedy ΨΨΨ
Previously troubled adolescent estranged from her family tries to create a pleasant, memorable experience for her dysfunctional family's Thanksgiving dinner. Well-acted by Katie Holmes and Patricia Clarkson.

Pixote (1981) Drama ΨΨΨΨΨ
A powerful film about the squalid, depressing lives of street children in Sao Paulo. In the film, a homeless child, Pixote, commits his first murder at the age of 10. Tragically, the film's child star was shot and killed by the police 5 years after the film was released.

Popeye (1980) Drama ΨΨ
The archetypal Bluto, a character with an intermittent explosive disorder, is foiled by the heroic Popeye, played by Robin Williams.

Punch Drunk Love (2002) Drama-Comedy ΨΨΨ
Adam Sandler in a serious role about a man who alternates from an awkward passivity to explosive anger. Falling in love changes him. Quirky cinematic elements are added by director Paul Thomas Anderson.

Ratcatcher, The (1999) Drama ΨΨΨ
Young adolescent living in Glasgow must cope with trash-covered streets, lice, and dead rats. He acts out as he tries to cope with poverty.

Rebel Without a Cause (1955) Drama ΨΨΨ
Dated but still interesting examination of teenage alienation, violence, and family pathology. James Dean is the rebellious protagonist. All three stars (Dean, Natalie Wood, and Sal Mineo) met violent deaths in real life (a car wreck, a drowning, and a murder, respectively).

"Boy, if, if I had one day when I didn't have to be all confused and didn't have to feel that I was ashamed of everything"

***Rebel Without a Cause* (1955)**

Salaam Bombay! (1988) Drama ΨΨΨ
Remarkable story about the way indigent children manage to survive to adulthood on the mean streets of Bombay.

Splendor in the Grass (1961) Drama ΨΨ
A teenage girl unable to come to grips with adolescent sexuality winds up in a psychiatric hospital.

Squid and the Whale, The (2005) Drama ΨΨΨΨ
This excellent film depicts the trauma involved when the parents in a family of four go through a divorce. The film stars Jeff Daniels and Laura Linney. The two children act out in significant ways.

Thirteen (2003) Drama ΨΨΨΨ
Important film about the rise and fall of teen friendships, sexual promiscuity, self-hate, rebellion, and the intense need for adolescents to fit in and be accepted. Holly Hunter plays the recovered alcoholic mother struggling with the delicate balance between giving her daughter appropriate levels of freedom and setting limits.

Tin Drum, The (1979) Drama–War ΨΨΨΨ
Political allegory about a child who decides to stop growing. Based on a Gunter Grass novel, the film won an Academy Award for Best Foreign Language Film. The film received considerable attention because a scene in which the child has oral sex with an adult was judged to be obscene under Oklahoma law. The ACLU defended the film.

To Kill a Mockingbird (1962) Drama ΨΨ
Robert Duvall makes his film debut as Boo Radley, a man with an intellectual disability who kills another man to protect two children. This is a classic film that I love; it just doesn't teach us much about psychopathology.

"She did something that in our society is unspeakable. She kissed a black man. Not an old uncle, but a strong, young Negro man. No code mattered to her before she broke it, but it came crashing down on her afterwards."

To Kill a Mockingbird **(1962)**

United States of Leland, The (2004) Drama ΨΨ
Interesting story about Leland P. Fitzgerald (Ryan Gosling), an adolescent who kills a boy with autism but can't explain why. His emotions are blunted, his social behavior is quirky, yet his thoughts are often insightful and perceptive. Kevin Spacey co-stars.

Weather Man, The (2005) Drama ΨΨ
A meteorologist struggles in his personal life, which includes supporting his depressed daughter.

Welcome to the Dollhouse (1995) Comedy ΨΨΨ
Interesting examination of families, emerging sexuality, and the cruelty of adolescents.

Wild Child, The (*L'enfant Sauvage;* 1969, France) Drama ΨΨΨΨΨ
François Truffaut's engaging black-and-white, subtitled film about the life of a feral child, the "Wild Boy of Aveyron." Based on a true story and the journal of Jean Itard, the doctor who set out to educate the child. Truffaut plays the role of doctor Itard.

Willy Wonka and the Chocolate Factory (1971) Family ΨΨ
Five lucky children win a free tour of a wonderful chocolate factory. Four of the five children (excluding the hero, Charlie) are either oppositional, obsessed, or enormously selfish. Gene Wilder stars as Willy Wonka.

Wish You Were Here (1987) Drama ΨΨ
A teenage girl coming of age in Great Britain in the early 1940s must come to grips with her emerging sexuality.

The Young and the Damned (*Los Olvidados;* 1950, Mexico) Drama ΨΨΨ
Luis Buñuel film about juvenile delinquency in the squalid slums of Mexico City. Highly recommended.

Substance-Related and Addictive Disorders

Alcoholism

16 Blocks (2006) Drama ΨΨΨ
A corrupt, burnt out, alcoholic cop risks his job and life by confronting authority to save a criminal from being killed. He drinks on the job, is unshaven, overly fatigued, has poor stamina, and lethargy, and colleagues repeatedly comment about his alcohol abuse.

16 Years of Alcohol (2003, UK) Drama ΨΨ
The impact of parental alcoholism on a boy who eventually becomes an alcoholic himself. A transformation occurs when he becomes a member of AA and works at letting go of his anger and violent patterns.

28 Days (2000) Drama ΨΨΨ
A writer (Sandra Bullock) is court-ordered into a drug/alcohol rehabilitation center after a drinking and driving accident. The film depicts symptoms of alcoholism and its impact on a family.

Another Round (2020, Danish) Comedy-Drama ΨΨ
Four middle-aged men deal with their midlife crisis by resolving to be a little drunk each day while at work, but eschewing alcohol evenings and weekends. They monitor their breath to ensure blood alcohol levels of 0.05%. You must be comfortable with subtitles to enjoy the film.

Arthur (1981) Comedy Ψ
Dudley Moore as a drunken millionaire who falls in love with Liza Minnelli. A genuinely funny film but upsetting in its cavalier approach to alcoholism and drunk driving.

Susan: "A real woman could stop you from drinking."
Arthur: "It'd have to be a real BIG woman."

***Arthur* (1981)**

Bad News Bears (2005) Comedy Ψ
Richard Linklater remake portraying a despicable alcoholic (Billy Bob Thornton) who attempts to coach a little league baseball team that has limited potential.

Barfly (1987) Comedy-Romance-Drama ΨΨΨΨ
Faye Dunaway and Mickey Rourke play two alcoholics whose lives briefly touch. Good examination of skid row alcoholism; the film is based on a story by cult poet Charles Bukowski.

Basketball Diaries, The (1995) Drama ΨΨΨ
Adolescent basketball stars succumb to drug abuse in this film that stars Leonardo DiCaprio and Mark Wahlberg. Adapted from a Jim Carroll novel.

Be Here to Love Me: A Film About Townes Van Zandt (2004) Documentary Biography ΨΨΨΨ
An examination of the all-too-short life of Townes Van Zandt and the ways in which his life was affected by abuse of both alcohol and drugs. In one scene, Van Zandt describes passing out in military school as a young man after sniffing glue.

Being Flynn (2012) Drama ΨΨ
Robert De Niro plays the role of Flynn, an aging and homeless poet, conman, and alcoholic.

Beloved Infidel (1959) Biography ΨΨ
Gregory Peck plays F. Scott Fitzgerald and Deborah Kerr is columnist Sheila Graham, who tries to save Fitzgerald from his alcoholism.

Bob and the Monster (2011) Documentary ΨΨΨΨ
This film traces the life of indie-rock musician, Bob Forrest, documenting his struggles with drugs and alcohol and his eventual recovery. Today Forrest is a drug and alcohol counselor working with some of Hollywood's biggest names.

Born on the Fourth of July (1989) ΨΨΨΨ
Drama-War-Biography
Tom Cruise plays paralyzed and alcoholic Vietnam veteran Ron Kovic in Oliver Stone's film. Stone won an Oscar as Best Director for this film.

"You're a T6 – paralyzed from the mid-chest down ... you'll be in a wheelchair for the rest of your life."

Ron Kovic's grim prognosis, in *Born on the Fourth of July* (1989)

Capote (2005) Drama-Biography ΨΨΨ
Philip Seymour Hoffman portrays the writer Truman Capote, and a segment of his life in which Capote gets material from a man who killed a family of four in Kansas for his book *In Cold Blood*. Capote becomes depressed when he is unable to prevent the man from being hanged. He abuses alcohol and loses his will to write.

Cat Ballou (1965) Comedy-Western Ψ
Light-hearted film, with Jane Fonda playing a schoolteacher turned outlaw. Lee Marvin got an Oscar for his role as an alcoholic gunman. The film perpetuates the myth of the down-and-out drunk whose shooting skills return after he has had a few drinks. Marvin won an Oscar as Best Actor for his role in this film.

Cat on a Hot Tin Roof (1958) Drama ΨΨΨ
Paul Newman, Elizabeth Taylor, and Burl Ives in a subdued adaptation of Tennessee Williams' play about "mendacity." Alcohol plays a prominent role in the life of almost all the characters' lives.

"Big Daddy! Now what makes him so big? His big heart? His big belly? Or his big money?"

***Cat on a Hot Tin Roof* (1958)**

Changing Lanes (2002) Drama ΨΨ
A successful lawyer from a corrupt firm collides with an alcoholic insurance salesman who is on his way to court for a custody hearing and misses the court appearance. The role of Alcoholics Anonymous and the ongoing struggle associated with recovery are depicted.

Charlie Wilson's War (2007) Drama–Biography ΨΨ
Mike Nichols film about a legendary congressman who is also an alcoholic.

Children of Men (2006) Thriller–Drama Ψ
Alcohol abuse and marijuana abuse are depicted in this film about saving the human race.

Come Back, Little Sheba (1952) Drama ΨΨΨ
Burt Lancaster and Shirley Booth in a film about alcoholism and marriage. Booth won an Academy Award for Best Actress for her role.

Come Fill the Cup (1951) Drama ΨΨ
James Cagney and Jackie Gleason star in this serious examination of the problems of alcoholism in an ex-newspaperman.

Crazy Heart (2009) Drama ΨΨΨΨΨ
Academy Award–winner Jeff Bridges, plays Bad Blake, a 57-year-old, four-time divorced, small-time musician. Blake is an alcoholic who travels around the southwest for small-time gigs, spending his days and nights drinking and womanizing, ending each night isolated and poor. He develops a meaningful relationship with a young woman and her son, but his alcohol dependence seriously affects his relationship with both. It is interesting to compare this film with other musician–addiction films, such as *Ray, Walk the Line*, and especially *Tender Mercies*.

Crazy Wisdom: The Life & Times of Chogyam Trungpa Rinpoche (2011) Documentary Ψ
This documentary explores the complicated life of Chogyam Trungpa Rinpoche, someone known as the "bad boy of Buddhism." Rinpoche smoked, abused alcohol, and slept with his female followers – and sometimes the wives of his followers.

Dark Obsession (1989) Drama–Mystery ΨΨ
Five drunken British military officers are involved in a hit-and-run accident in which the victim dies. The five men take a vow of silence; one is troubled by the decision. Interesting analysis of responsibility for one's behavior while intoxicated.

Days of Wine and Roses (1962) Drama ΨΨΨΨ
Blake Edwards film starring Jack Lemmon and Lee Remick. Lemmon teaches Remick how to drink. Lemmon is saved by AA; Remick is unable to stop drinking, despite the consequences. This is a classic film.

"You see, the world looks so dirty to me when I'm not drinking. Joe, remember Fisherman's Wharf? The water when you looked too close? That's the way the world looks to me when I'm not drinking."

Kristen describes why she continues to drink, in *Days of Wine and Roses* (1962)

Drunks (1995) Drama ΨΨΨΨ
This film is the best available introduction to Alcoholics Anonymous. It is highly recommended for any student who will be working with substance abuse issues.

Educating Rita (1983) Drama ΨΨ
Michael Caine as an alcoholic college professor who takes on the task of educating a working-class woman.

Everything Must Go (2011) Comedy–Drama ΨΨΨ
Will Ferrell's character Nick loses his wife and his job and copes by setting up a yard sale on his front lawn. He spends each day drinking beer from morning to night, but eventually makes contacts who help him put his life back together again.

Factotum (2005) Comedy ΨΨ
A struggling writer works multiple odd jobs and sleeps with multiple partners. He consistently drinks on the job and while writing. He loses several jobs but is unable to stop drinking. The film accurately portrays alcohol dependence.

Fire Within, The (*Le Feu Follet;* 1963, France) Drama ΨΨΨΨΨ
French filmmaker Louis Malle's remarkable black-and-white account of alcoholism, suicide, and the existential choices that confront us all. Roger Ebert wrote, "the film is a triumph of style ... inspired by Scott Fitzgerald's *Babylon Revisited.*"

Flight (2012) Drama ΨΨΨΨ
Denzel Washington plays Whip Whitaker, a handsome and talented airline pilot who abuses alcohol, cocaine, and other drugs. His skill as a pilot allows him to land a damaged plane in a field, saving the lives of almost all of the passengers and crew. The film is misleading in its premise that someone can be very intoxicated and still perform well-rehearsed skills at a very high level.

For One More Day (2007) Drama ΨΨ
A child of divorced parents grows up feeling guilty about his mother's death. As an adult, he becomes depressed and an alcoholic. His suicide attempt is interrupted by his deceased mother who gives him one last day to spend with her. Based on Mitch Album's novel.

Genius (2016) Historical-Biography ΨΨ
The film focuses on the relationship between Scribner editor Max Perkins and authors Thomas Wolfe, Ernest Hemingway, and F. Scott Fitzgerald. All three authors were alcoholic, Hemingway was depressed, and Wolfe was probably bipolar - which may have resulted in a prodigious achievement, *Look Homeward Angel.*

Gervaise (1956, France) Drama ΨΨΨΨΨ
French film based on Emile Zola's novel *L'Assomoir,* depicting the fatal degeneration of a family, mainly because of alcoholism.

Graduate, The (1967) Drama-Comedy ΨΨΨ
A telling indictment of the shallow values of the time (e.g., plastics). Mrs. Robinson's alcoholism impairs her judgment and ruins her life.

"Mrs. Robinson, you're trying to seduce me. Aren't you?"

***The Graduate* (1967)**

Great Man Votes, The (1939) Drama ΨΨ
John Barrymore plays an alcoholic college professor fighting to maintain custody of his children.

Harvey (1950) Comedy-Drama ΨΨΨΨ
Elwood P. Dowd's (Jimmy Stewart) imaginary friend is a 6-foot white rabbit named Harvey with whom he has a good relationship. Dowd drinks daily, goes to taverns, and has hidden bottles behind books. He always gets two drinks, one for himself and one for Harvey, and therefore has two drinks at a time.

Henry Fool (1997) Comedy-Drama ΨΨ
Hal Hartley film about a taciturn garbage man who befriends a roguish alcoholic.

Iceman Cometh, The (1973) Drama ΨΨ
Lee Marvin in an adaptation of Eugene O'Neill's play about alcoholism and the pathos of dreams unfulfilled.

I'll Cry Tomorrow (1955) Biography ΨΨΨ
Singer Lillian Roth (Susan Hayward) attempts suicide as a way of coping with her alcoholism before AA support helps her find her way.

Ironweed (1987) Drama ΨΨΨΨ
Jack Nicholson and Meryl Streep in compelling roles as homeless alcoholics. The film, a very realistic portrayal of life on skid row, should be compared with another excellent film made the same year, *Barfly.*

Julia (2008) Drama ΨΨΨ
Tilda Swinton stars as Julia, a manipulative but charismatic woman with a long history of alcoholism. When drunk, she makes a series of terribly bad decisions, including a plan to kidnap a child. It doesn't go well.

Key Largo (1948) Crime ΨΨΨ
Claire Trevor won an Academy Award for Best Supporting Actress for her role as an alcoholic singer forced to beg gangster Edward G. Robinson for a drink during a hurricane in Key West.

Krisha (2015) Drama ΨΨΨΨΨ
A remarkable first film by director Trey Shults. The movie powerfully portrays the ways in which a happy family is affected by reunion with a long-estranged relative whose addiction to alcohol and drugs winds up ruining their Thanksgiving dinner.

Last Night at the Alamo (1983) Drama ΨΨΨ
Fascinating examination of bar culture in a small Texas town. Unforgettable characters, most of whom are coping with alcoholism and adultery.

Leaving Las Vegas (1995) Drama ΨΨΨΨΨ
Nicholas Cage delivers a stunning performance as an alcoholic who has no interest in quitting. He develops a relationship with a prostitute (Elisabeth Shue) who is the first to truly understand him. Gripping alcohol dependence portrayal and a painful depiction of delirium tremens.

Ben Sanderson: "Don't you think you'll get a little bored, living with a drunk?"
Sera: "Well, that's what I want."
Ben Sanderson: "You haven't seen the worst of it. These last few days, I've been very controlled. But I knock things over and throw up all the time. But, right now, I feel really good. You're like some sort of antidote that mixes with the liquor and keeps me in balance. But that won't last forever."

Ben warns Sera about what to expect from his drinking, in *Leaving Las Vegas* (1995)

Legend of Bagger Vance, The (2000) ΨΨΨ
Drama-Inspiration
Matt Damon plays Rannulph Junuh, a talented golfer whose game has deteriorated because of his war

experiences. He isolates himself, drinks heavily, and plays cards all night. He returns to golf in a promotional event with the help of an inspirational caddy and mentor, Bagger Vance (Will Smith).

Libertine, The (2004) Drama ΨΨ
John Wilmot, the second Earl of Rochester in the 17th century, a poet and author and close friend of Charles II (John Malkovich), desperately uses alcohol to cope with banishment. He drinks constantly for 5 years, and the long-term consequences of alcohol use are illustrated.

Lonely Passion of Judith Hearne, The (1987) Romance ΨΨ
Maggie Smith plays a lonely alcoholic who mistakenly believes she has a last chance to find love and meaning in her life.

Long Day's Journey Into Night (1962) Drama ΨΨΨΨΨ
Alcohol is a part of daily life for this deeply troubled family. Numerous examples of family pathology, conflict between father and sons, and denial.

> **"It shrinks my liver, doesn't it, Nat? It pickles my kidneys, yeah. But what it does to the mind? It tosses the sandbags overboard so the balloon can soar. Suddenly I'm above the ordinary. I'm competent. I'm walking a tightrope over Niagara Falls. I'm one of the great ones."**
>
> **Don Birnam talking to his bartender about what it feels like to be drunk, in *The Lost Weekend* (1945)**

Lost Weekend, The (1945) Drama ΨΨΨΨΨ
Billy Wilder classic starring Ray Milland as a writer struggling to overcome his alcoholism. Some scenes were filmed at Bellevue Hospital in New York City, and the portrayals of delirium tremens are convincing. Polanski borrowed scenes from *The Lost Weekend* as models for his film *Repulsion*. I have used excerpts from this film in classes for years.

Love Song for Bobby Long, A (2004) Drama ΨΨ
A young woman returns to her hometown, New Orleans, for a funeral and finds two drunken dwellers living in her deceased mother's home. Bobby Long(John Travolta), an English professor, and his former assistant have no intentions of moving.

Love Streams (1984) Drama ΨΨΨΨ
John Cassavetes film in which Cassavetes plays a writer addicted to alcohol and gambling, and Gena Rowlands plays his sister. Cassavetes' character has an 8-year-old son he has never seen; when he is forced to care for the child, he takes his son gambling and teaches the 8-year-old how to drink. In real life, Cassavetes and Rowlands were married until his death in 1989.

Misfortunates, The (2009, Belgium) Drama ΨΨΨ
A 13-year-old boy grows up with an alcoholic father and several alcoholic uncles.

My Beautiful Laundrette (1985) Drama ΨΨ
The two lead characters are gay, although this fact is almost incidental to the story about alcoholism, street gangs, race relations, and social class.

My Favorite Year (1982) Comedy ΨΨΨ
A great actor (modeled after John Barrymore and Errol Flynn) who has become a pathetic drunk must confront one of the greatest challenges of his career – a live television performance.

My Name Is Bill W. (1989) ΨΨΨ
Made-for-TV movie about the founding of Alcoholics Anonymous.

My Name Is Joe (1998, Britain) Drama ΨΨ
A film about an unemployed alcoholic and a health care worker. The title comes from the characteristic opening of Alcoholics Anonymous meetings. There is a dramatic and surprising ending to the film.

My Name Was Bette: The Life and Death of an Alcoholic (2012) Documentary ΨΨΨΨ
This film is a sensitive examination of the life and death of Bette VanderAkker, a nurse and mother who died from alcoholism. The film was made by Bette's daughter, and it provides considerable insight into the problem of alcoholism in women.

National Lampoon's Animal House (1978) Comedy ΨΨ
One of the best of a hundred or so college films that portray fraternity life as a series of beer busts interspersed with an occasional class. At one point, the character played by John Belushi, not the brightest of the fraternity brothers, chugs a fifth of Jack Daniels.

Night of the Iguana, The (1964) Drama ΨΨ
Richard Burton and Ava Gardner star in John Huston's adaptation of Tennessee Williams' play. Burton plays a very convincing alcoholic and erstwhile clergyman.

No Such Thing (2001, Iceland/US) Ψ
Hal Hartley film about a belligerent, foul-mouthed, mythical monster who is also an alcoholic.

Pay It Forward (2000) Drama-Inspiration ΨΨ
Haley Joel Osment plays a seventh grader implementing a class assignment that has profound effects on the people around him. His mother (Helen Hunt) is a struggling alcoholic.

> **"Think of an idea to change our world ... and put it into action."**
>
> **A student assignment, in *Pay It Forward* (2000)**

Prize Winner of Defiance, Ohio, The ΨΨΨΨΨ
(2005) Drama
A stay-at-home mother (Julianne Moore) in the 1950–60s, confronts her alcoholic and dependent husband (Woody Harrelson) with unswerving optimism. The film illustrates the social expectations of women who stay in relationships with abusive husbands.

Proud and the Beautiful, The (1953) Romance ΨΨ
A film about a woman who helps an alcoholic physician overcome his problems and regain some sense of dignity. Filmed in France and Mexico.

Sideways (2004) Comedy ΨΨΨΨ
Two men tour California's wine country. One is a depressed alcoholic craving a relationship; the other is going to be married later that week, but he begins an affair with a woman he meets on the trip.

> **Jack: "If they want to drink Merlot, we're drinking Merlot."**
> **Miles Raymond: "No, if anyone orders Merlot, I'm leaving. I am NOT drinking any fucking Merlot!"**
>
> **Merlot sales plummeted and pinot noir sales soared after *Sideways* was released**

Skin Deep (1989) Comedy ΨΨ
A funny Blake Edwards film about an alcoholic writer who continues to deny his alcoholism long after it has become apparent to everyone else.

Smashed (2012) Drama ΨΨΨ
A couple finds their entire married life revolves around alcohol. The wife realizes her life is out of control when she urinates on the floor of a convenience store and steals a bottle of wine. A good introduction to Alcoholics Anonymous.

Smash-Up, the Story of a Woman (1947) Drama ΨΨ
Melodramatic Susan Hayward film about a movie star who must come to grips with her alcoholism.

Some Like It Hot (1959) Crime-Comedy ΨΨ
Marilyn Monroe portrays a performer constantly sneaking drinks; she is nearly fired for alcohol abuse.

Spectacular Now, The (2013) Comedy-Drama ΨΨΨ
A coming-of-age story that features a boy who passes out on the lawn of a girl he eventually winds up dating. The film involves lots of teenage drinking.

Streamers (1983) Drama ΨΨΨ
Robert Altman film about three soldiers waiting to go to Vietnam. The film deals with themes of homosexuality, violence, and racism, but also illustrates the alcohol abuse that is so pervasive in military life.

Sweet Bird of Youth (1962) Drama ΨΨ
Paul Newman in an adaptation of Tennessee Williams' play about a has-been actress (played by Geraldine Page) addicted to alcohol and drugs who takes up with a young, vital Newman.

Taxi Blues (1990, Soviet Union) Drama ΨΨΨ
An alcoholic jazz musician becomes friends with an anti-Semitic taxi driver. This Russian film won the prize for Best Director at Cannes. Fascinating examination of the role of alcohol in the daily lives of the Moscow protagonists.

Tender Mercies (1983) Drama ΨΨΨΨΨ
Sensitive and optimistic film in which Robert Duvall plays a successfully recovering alcoholic songwriter. Duvall won an Oscar for this almost perfect performance. Contrast with *Crazy Heart*.

Tree Grows in Brooklyn, A (1945) Drama ΨΨΨ
Elia Kazan film about a poor Irish family living in Brooklyn at the turn of the century. The family's problems are complicated by the father's alcoholism.

Trees Lounge (1996) Comedy ΨΨΨΨ
Steve Buscemi wrote and directed this compelling film, and he plays the lead character, a 31-year-old unemployed auto mechanic. Few contemporary films present a more vivid picture of the problems associated with alcoholism.

Under Capricorn (1949) Drama Ψ
A little-known Hitchcock film starring Joseph Cotton and Ingrid Bergman. Bergman is a wealthy socialite whose life is ruined by her alcoholism.

Under the Volcano (1984) Drama ΨΨΨΨ
John Huston directing Albert Finney; the film is an excellent portrayal of chronic alcoholism.

Verdict, The (1982) Drama ΨΨΨΨ
Paul Newman in a wonderful role as a disillusioned alcoholic lawyer who becomes genuinely involved with a brain-injured client who is the victim of medical malpractice. He wins the case but continues to drink. Interesting analysis of codependency.

Edward J. Concannon: "Why wasn't she getting oxygen...?"
Dr. Robert Towler: "Well, many reasons, actually ..."
Edward J. Concannon: "Tell me one?"
Dr. Robert Towler: "She'd aspirated vomitus into her mask..."
Edward J. Concannon: "She threw up in her mask. Let's cut the bullshit. Say it: She threw up in her mask."

***The Verdict* (1982)**

Vital Signs (1986) Drama ΨΨ
Ed Asner in a surpassingly good made-for-TV movie about a father and son, both surgeons, fighting the twin problems of alcoholism and drug abuse.

Vodka Lemon (2003, France/Armenia) Comedy ΨΨΨ
Minimalist film about grieving widows who befriend one another in a culture where everyone seems to drink vodka.

Way Back, The (2020) Drama ΨΨΨΨ
Ben Affleck spends every evening at a local bar. He was a high school basketball player who turned his back on a college scholarship to take a construction job. He is given a shot at redemption when he is asked to substitute as a basketball coach at his former high school.

What Price Hollywood? (1932) Drama ΨΨ
An alcoholic director helps a Hollywood waitress become a star. The figure of the alcoholic director may have been modeled after John Barrymore.

When a Man Loves a Woman (1994) Drama ΨΨ
Meg Ryan as a middle-class alcoholic. This is a melodramatic and somewhat predictable film, but an interesting introduction to AA and Al-Anon. The film explores the role of codependency and a husband's role in his wife's alcoholism.

Drug Abuse

21 Grams (2003) Drama-Mystery ΨΨΨΨ
Complicated, well-integrated stories of an ex-con and recovering alcoholic (Benicio Del Toro), a cocaine addict (Naomi Watts), and a terminal man awaiting a transplant (Sean Penn), all brought together by an accidental death.

"They say we all lose 21 grams at the exact moment of death ... everyone. The weight of a stack of nickels. The weight of a chocolate bar. The weight of a hummingbird."

***21 Grams* (2003)**

Answer Man, The (2009) Drama ΨΨ
The author of the hit self-help book *Me and God* helps a single mother and a young man who has just been released from a drug rehabilitation facility find meaning in their lives.

Awakening of the Beast (1969) Drama Ψ
Cult film involving four subjects who take LSD as an experiment to provide data for a book a psychiatrist is writing about the effects of drugs.

Bad Lieutenant (1992) Drama ΨΨΨ
Harvey Keitel stars in one of his most powerful roles, as a police lieutenant addicted to cocaine, alcohol, and prostitutes. The film illustrates stark abuse of power and the deterioration of family life that accompanies addiction. Keitel's character has a hallucination in which Jesus Christ comes to him.

Big Lebowski, The (1998) Comedy ΨΨ
Coen brothers film portraying "the Dude" (Jeff Bridges), a cannabis-smoking, unemployed drifter in an entertaining, film noir comedy.

Bird (1988) Biography ΨΨ
Clint Eastwood directed this biographical film of the life of jazz great and drug addict Charlie "Bird" Parker. Parker was an addict for all his adult life, and his addiction killed him at the age of 34.

Blow (2001) Drama ΨΨΨ
Johnny Depp stars as George Jung, a man who claimed to have imported about 85% of all cocaine in America in the late 1970s.

Candy (2006, Australia) Drama ΨΨΨ
Candy is both the name of the female lead in the film (Abbie Cornish) and a slang term for heroin. The film accurately portrays heroin addiction and withdrawal.

Geoffrey Rush is very convincing as a chemistry professor who supports the habits of his young friends and who eventually dies from an overdose.

Chappaqua (1966) Drama Ψ
Heroin addict checks in for treatment. The film is most notable for short roles by William Burroughs, Ravi Shankar, and Allen Ginsburg.

Christiane F. (1981) Drama ΨΨΨΨ
Powerful and frightening examination of the life of a teenage drug addict in West Berlin. Based on a true story, the film is still gripping 4 decades after it was made.

Clean and Sober (1988) Drama ΨΨΨΨ
Good portrayal of AA, cocaine addiction, and alcoholism.

> **"I woke up one morning, and when I looked in the mirror, I noticed my nose was bent over entirely onto one side of my face. So, I got a hammer, and started banging my nose back to a right angle with my face. Suddenly, I looked at myself in the mirror, hammer in hand, blood streaming down my chin, and I realized my life was no longer manageable."**
>
> ***Clean and Sober* (1988)**

Cocaine Fiends, The (1936) Drama Ψ
Another "word of warning" film that portrays the dangers of cocaine. Made in the same year as *Reefer Madness.* The message in this film is exaggerated and histrionic but somewhat more realistic then *Reefer Madness* in its estimate of the dangers of the drug.

Coffee and Cigarettes (2003) Comedy ΨΨΨ
Various conversational skits (starring a variety of talented individuals, including Bill Murray, Roberto Benigni, Cate Blanchett, Iggy Pop, and Steve Buscemi) linked through the characters' consumption of coffee and tea and smoking. Portrayals of compulsive use of each drug, side effects, and the desire to quit or avoid the substance.

Connection, The (1961) Drama ΨΨΨ
Heroin addicts in New York wait for their pusher.

Dead Ringers (1988) Drama ΨΨΨ
A David Cronenberg film about two twin brothers who are renowned gynecologists. They are also addicted to amphetamines and barbiturates. Based on a true story about two twin physicians who died from barbiturate withdrawal.

Dopamine (2003) Drama-Comedy ΨΨ
Independent film explores the chemistry behind male-female relationships. One character uses amphetamine pills and large quantities of caffeine. Interesting debate on how physical attraction emerges.

Drugstore Cowboy (1989) Drama ΨΨΨΨ
Matt Dillon leads a group of junkies who rob pharmacies to support their habit. William Burroughs plays a junkie priest.

> **"Most people don't know how they're gonna feel from one moment to the next. But a dope fiend has a pretty good idea. All you gotta do is look at the labels on the little bottles."**
>
> **Addict reflecting on the pleasures of drugs, in *Drugstore Cowboy* (1989)**

Easy Rider (1969) Drama ΨΨΨ
Classic film of the late 1960s with Jack Nicholson as an alcoholic lawyer and Peter Fonda and Dennis Hopper as marijuana-smoking, LSD-using free spirits. The film is dated but still worth seeing.

> **"The governor of Louisiana gave me this. Madame Tinkertoy's House of Blue Lights, corner of Bourbon and Toulouse, New Orleans, Louisiana. Now, this is supposed to be the finest whorehouse in the south. These ain't no pork chops! These are U.S. Prime!"**
>
> **Jack Nicholson plans for his trip to New Orleans, in *Easy Rider* (1969)**

Fear and Loathing in Las Vegas (1998) ΨΨ
Drama-Fantasy
Terry Gilliam's adaptation of Hunter S. Thompson's gonzo journalism classic. The book is better than the film; although the movie does not glorify drug use, it clearly models the behavior and tacitly condones the practice of driving while intoxicated.

Half Baked (1998) Comedy Ψ
Exaggerated comedy about smoking "weed." Interesting for its classification of different types of marijuana smokers: the "you should have been there smoker," the "scavenger," the "enhancer," the "medicinal," the "after school special," the "father, I'm 40 and still cool," the "MacGyver smoker," the "straight-up potheads," and the "I'm only creative if I smoke" users.

Half Nelson (2006) Drama ΨΨΨ
A drug-addicted teacher-coach (Ryan Gosling) at an inner-city school uses cocaine regularly and smokes crack in the girls' locker room after a game. He has a history of failed rehabilitation, and tries to rebuild relationships, but he struggles with anger and is disengaged from his family.

Hatful of Rain, A (1957) Drama ΨΨ
Melodramatic film about the life and problems of a drug addict. This was one of the earliest films to honestly examine the problem of drug addiction.

High Art (1998) Drama-Comedy ΨΨ
Realistic, well-acted independent film about several people whose lives intersect for drugs, support, and conversation in a New York City apartment.

Honey Boy (2019) ΨΨΨΨ
Shia LeBeouf wrote the screenplay and stars in this engaging film. Watching the movie will help you better understand drug rehabilitation and Alcoholics Anonymous, and it will likely give you some ideas about how bad parenting can affect child development (e.g., in one scene, LeBeouf's father ridicules the size of his son's penis). The film illustrates alcoholism and drug abuse, but focuses on the deleterious effects of bad parenting.

Hustle and Flow (2005) Drama ΨΨΨΨ
In this Sundance Audience Choice Award film, an aspiring Memphis disc jockey works to get his first record made as he approaches mid-life. He is a pimp, drug user, and dealer who questions his life's purpose and the decisions he has made along the way.

I Don't Buy Kisses Anymore (1992) ΨΨ
Comedy-Romance
Lightweight but entertaining film about an obese male who falls in love with a woman using him as a subject for her master's thesis.

I'm Dancing as Fast as I Can (1982) Drama ΨΨ
Jill Clayburgh plays the role of a high-powered documentary filmmaker who becomes addicted to Valium and requires hospitalization in a special program for addicts. Based on a true story.

I'm Still Here (2010) Drama-Documentary ΨΨ
Casey Affleck film that is a mockumentary about Joaquin Phoenix, his drug use, and his announced (but fake) retirement from films to concentrate on making rap/hip-hop music.

Jungle Fever (1991) Drama-Romance ΨΨΨ
Interesting film about race relations and sexual stereotypes, with a subplot involving Gator, the crackhead brother of the protagonist, who is destroying his middle-class family.

Kurt Cobain: About a Son (2006) Documentary ΨΨ
Cobain discusses his chronic pain and irritable bowel syndrome, as well as his suicidal ideation and heroin addiction.

La Femme Nikita (1990) Action-Drama ΨΨ
A sociopathic and drug-addicted woman is sentenced to die for murder and then is transformed into a government agent. Most memorable for the drugstore robbery that opens the film.

Lady Sings the Blues (1972) Biography-Musical ΨΨ
Diana Ross plays heroin addict Billie Holiday.

Long Day's Journey Into Night (1962) ΨΨΨΨΨ
Drama
Katharine Hepburn plays a morphine-addicted, histrionic mother with an alcoholic son (Jason Robards) and husband. One of O'Neill's greatest plays; one of Hepburn's greatest roles. Hepburn's character is a good illustration of a histrionic personality disorder. This film is better than any of the subsequent remakes.

Love and Diane (2002) Documentary ΨΨ
A mother recovers from an addiction to crack as she attempts to start a new life and connect with the children she had abandoned.

Love Liza (2002) Drama-Comedy ΨΨΨΨ
Philip Seymour Hoffman skillfully plays a man who huffs gasoline in response to his wife's suicide. A rare and illuminating depiction of inhalant abuse and intoxication.

Luna (1979) Drama Ψ
Disappointing Bernardo Bertolucci film, with Jill Clayburgh playing the mother of a drug addict son. The film depicts an incestuous relationship between mother and son.

"What the fuck do I need to be sober for so I can see how fucked up shit really is, please. High is how I am gonna be. I'm high till I die."

A crack addict, in *MacArthur Park* (2001)

MacArthur Park (2001) Drama ΨΨΨΨ
A crack addict struggles to overcome drug dependence and leave his home in the park to live with his estranged son. A quality independent film.

Man With the Golden Arm, The (1955) Drama ΨΨ
Frank Sinatra and Kim Novak in a dated but interesting portrayal of drug addiction. Good example of the challenge of "cold turkey" withdrawal.

Maria, Full of Grace (2004) Drama ΨΨΨ
Fascinating, independent film depicting the realities and dangers young girls from Colombia face as they take jobs as "mules," smuggling drugs into the United States by swallowing them in large latex packages. While this film is not directly about substance abuse, it depicts the drug trade and problems related to ingesting drugs for illegal purposes.

Mask (1985) Biography ΨΨΨ
Bogdanovich film with Cher as the mother of deformed but spunky teenager Rocky Dennis. Sympathetic portrayal of motorcycle gangs. Cher struggles with her angry father and her compulsive use of alcohol and drugs as she works hard to be a good mother.

Mighty Wind, A (2003) Comedy ΨΨ
Hilarious Christopher Guest parody of folk music. One character displays significant remnants of years of drug abuse.

Molly's Game (2017) Drama ΨΨΨ
An engaging movie based on a true story about a world-class skier who has a disastrous accident and winds up running a high-stakes poker game. The game eventually falls apart, and she is arrested by the FBI; her failure in part results from her addiction to alcohol and drugs.

Father: "What did everyone learn in school today?"
Molly: "I learned that Sigmund Freud was both a misogynist and an idiot, and that anyone who relies on his theories of human psychology is a quack. ... he believed that a woman's life is about her reproductive function."
Father: "I'm a professional psychologist, not a quack."

Molly Bloom baits her psychotherapist father, in *Molly's Game* (2017)

Naked Lunch (1991) ΨΨ
Drama–Science Fiction–Fantasy
This film is based on the novel by William Burroughs and deals with drug abuse, paranoia, and homicide. Burroughs killed his second wife in 1951 in Mexico City while drunk and attempting a "William Tell stunt."

New Jack City (1991) Action–Crime ΨΨ
Wesley Snipes and Ice-T in a realistic movie about the business of drugs. Good introduction to cocaine addiction and Narcotics Anonymous.

Pain and Glory (2019, Spain) Drama ΨΨΨΨΨ
This is a superb semiautobiographical film, directed by Pedro Almodóvar, that stars Antonio Banderas and Penélope Cruz. The film portrays a washed-up director who grieves over his loss of creativity and productivity. His life is limited by chronic pain, and he turns to smoking heroin to cope with his numerous infirmities. The film includes numerous flashbacks to the protagonist's childhood and his earliest sexual experiences.

"If the First Amendment will protect a scumbag like me, it will protect all of you."

Larry Flint on free speech, in *The People vs. Larry Flynt* (1996)

People vs. Larry Flynt, The (1996) ΨΨΨ
Biography–Drama
A good movie about a controversial figure, the film forces the viewer to examine their views on pornography and free speech. The film is included in this section because of the effects of drugs on the lives of Flynt and his wife, Althea (Courtney Love), after he is shot and becomes addicted to narcotics.

Pineapple Express (2008) Drama Ψ
Enthusiastic marijuana users quickly find themselves embroiled in the complex world of drug dealing.

Platoon (1986) War ΨΨΨΨ
Vietnam veteran Oliver Stone directed *Platoon*, one of the most realistic of dozens of war movies. There is an interesting juxtaposition of "boozers" (those who use alcohol to escape) and "heads" (those who take refuge in marijuana and other illegal drugs).

Postcards from the Edge (1990) ΨΨΨ
Comedy–Drama
Mike Nichols' adaptation of a Carrie Fisher story about life as the daughter of a famous actress. The mother is alcoholic; the daughter abuses multiple drugs, including cocaine and sedatives. There are brief scenes of psychotherapy and a terrific cast.

Pulp Fiction (1994) Drama ΨΨΨΨΨ
Quentin Tarantino film about drugs, crime, depravity, the underworld, and life in urban America. One especially memorable scene involves Vincent Vega (John Travolta) smashing an adrenaline-filled needle into Mia Wallace's (Uma Thurman) chest to revive her after she inadvertently overdoses on heroin (see Figure 36).

"What now? Let me tell you what now. I'm calling a couple of hard, pipe-hittin' niggers, who'll go to work on this soon-to-be-dead hillbilly rapist here with a pair of pliers and a blow torch. You hear me talkin', hillbilly boy? I ain't through with you by a damn sight. I'm a gonna get medieval on your ass."

Marsellus Wallace planning revenge in *Pulp Fiction* (1994)

Quitting (2001) Drama ΨΨΨΨ
Slow-moving but interesting Chinese film about a onetime famous actor who deteriorates due to a heroin addiction. The emotional and psychological withdrawals depicted are memorable. This is an important film on addiction and withdrawal.

Ray (2004) Drama ΨΨΨΨΨ
This award-winning film depicts 20 years in the life of Ray Charles when he was addicted to heroin. Physical disability (blindness) and childhood psychological traumas shape the personal life of this renowned artist.

Reefer Madness (1936) Drama Ψ
Campy film depicting the dangers of marijuana. Ironically, thousands of college students have gone to see this film high on the very drug the film condemns.

Requiem for a Dream (2000) Drama ΨΨΨΨ
Disturbing film about four drug addicts whose lives deteriorate. Unforgettable performances and critically acclaimed. Excellent direction by Darren Aronofsky.

Harry Goldfarb: [Harry has just found out that Sara is on diet pills] "Does he give you pills?"
Sara Goldfarb: "Of course he gives me pills. He's a doctor!"
Harry Goldfarb: "What kind of pills?"
Sara Goldfarb: "Uh, uh, a blue one, a purple one, an orange one..."
Harry Goldfarb: "I mean, like, what's in 'em."

***Requiem for a Dream* (2000)**

Rose, The (1979) Musical-Biography-Drama ΨΨ
Bette Midler portrays Janis Joplin and her problems with Southern Comfort and drugs.

Rush (1991) Crime-Drama ΨΨΨ
Two undercover narcotics agents find addiction to be an occupational hazard.

Scarface (1983) Crime ΨΨΨ
Brian De Palma movie starring Al Pacino as a Cuban immigrant mobster who becomes addicted to the cocaine he is marketing. This long film, which tends to be loved or hated, is based on a 1932 Howard Hawks classic film with the same name.

Seven Percent Solution, The (1976) Mystery ΨΨ
Sigmund Freud treats Sherlock Holmes' cocaine addiction. The film is historically accurate in documenting Freud's early enthusiasm for cocaine.

Shadow Hours (2000) Drama Ψ
A wealthy man manipulates a young gas station attendant into drug relapse and fraternizing with three types of "night owls": (1) those who find their prince charming or princess before midnight, (2) vampires - prostitutes, drug dealers, and (3) Mr. Hydes - those who can't sleep.

Sherrybaby (2006) Drama ΨΨΨ
Maggie Gyllenhaal's character leaves prison after a 3-year conviction for heroin use. She tries to reunite with her daughter, but finds it more difficult than she had anticipated.

Sid and Nancy (1986) Biography ΨΨΨΨ
Compelling biography of Sid Vicious of the Sex Pistols; the film offers insight into the worlds of drugs and rock and roll.

Side Effects (2013) Drama ΨΨΨ
A severely depressed woman who has made several suicide attempts is prescribed a new medication; she subsequently murders her husband, apparently because of the medication. She is sent to a psychiatric hospital, and the doctor who originally prescribed the drug sees his practice ruined. However, things turn out to be much more complicated than the viewer first believes.

Spun (2002) Drama-Comedy ΨΨΨ
A well-done, intense film about methamphetamine addiction.

"Dog had a litter of about 8, and my mother was bending over killing each one of these little puppies in the bathtub. I remember I said 'why?'... She said, 'I'm just killing what I can't take care of.' Then my momma said to me, she looked at me and she said, 'I wish I could do that to you.'"

A recollection by the cook in *Spun* (2002)

Stardust (1975) Drama Ψ
British film about a rock star whose success is tarnished by drug addiction and mental illness.

Sweet Nothing (1996) Drama ΨΨΨ
An effective examination of the futility, desperation, and violence associated with crack addiction. This is a true story based on diaries found in a Bronx apartment in March of 1991.

Synanon (1965) Drama ΨΨ
Interesting only insofar as the film documents the treatment methods practiced in this highly praised treatment program.

This Wretched Life (2010) ΨΨ
An addict, Chris, wakes up after a near fatal overdose and discovers he has a second chance. The film illustrates a 12-step program, and shows interaction between Chris and his psychiatrist, someone he is mandated to see.

Tideland (2005) Drama-Fantasy Ψ
A disappointing Terry Gilliam film about a young girl with drug-addicted parents; the mother dies from a drug overdose and the father takes his daughter to hide in the country at his mother's home.

Traffic (2000) Drama ΨΨΨΨΨ
This Steven Soderbergh film thematically intersects the lives of a newly hired government drug czar (Michael Douglas), his daughter who experiments with crack, police officers struggling with drug cartels, and a suburban wife of a drug lord.

"I've been known to sniff it, smoke it, swallow it, stick it up my arse and inject it into my veins. I've been trying to combat this addiction, but unless you count social security scams and shoplifting, I haven't had a regular job in years."

***Trainspotting* (1996)**

Trainspotting (1996) Drama-Comedy ΨΨΨ
A realistic and disturbing film about the heroin scene in Edinburgh. The film presents accurate depictions of cold turkey withdrawal. There is one memorable scene in which a young mother's baby dies while she is high, and she immediately needs a fix to cope with her grief. Several scatological scenes seem gratuitous and unnecessary.

Veronika Voss (1982) Drama ΨΨ
Rainer Werner Fassbinder film about a German movie star who becomes addicted to morphine. Fassbinder himself died from an overdose of cocaine and barbiturates.

Wasted (2002) Drama ΨΨ
Teens, covering up inner pain, fear, and loneliness, battle their heroin addiction.

What's Love Got to Do with It? (1993)
Musical-Biography ΨΨ
Excellent film biography of singer Tina Turner; it includes some memorable scenes of husband Ike strung out on cocaine.

Who'll Stop the Rain? (1978) Crime-Drama ΨΨ
Also known as *Dog Soldiers,* this film explores the world of drug smuggling and addiction.

Megan: "What are we ever gonna do with you, baby girl?"
Ree: "Kill me I guess."
Megan: "That idea's been said already. Got any others?"
Ree: "Help me. Nobody's said that idea yet, have they?"

Ree Dolly (Jennifer Lawrence) uses her social intelligence to get out of a difficult situation, in *Winter's Bone* (2010).

Winter's Bone (2010) Drama ΨΨΨΨ
Jennifer Lawrence is wonderful as the 17-year-old Ree Dolly, a character who struggles to find her methamphetamine-addicted father and keep her Ozark family together.

Gambling and Other Nonsubstance-Related Addictions

21 (2008) Drama ΨΨ
A young man is accepted into Harvard medical school but to afford the tuition, he joins a group of card counters led by their professor. Kevin Spacey plays the ringleader.

2046 (2004, China/Hong Kong) Fantasy-Drama ΨΨ
One character has a compulsive gambling problem in this film that blends present and future; the movie is directed by War Kar Wai, who films without a script. "Love is all a matter of timing – it's no good meeting the right person too soon or too late."

Basic Instinct (1992) Suspense-Thriller ΨΨ
Psychological thriller about a novelist (Sharon Stone) who is a sex addict who entangles an investigator (Michael Douglas) in a complex mystery of murder, sex, and fascination. The scene in which Sharon Stone uncrosses her legs while being interrogated has become iconic.

Psychologist: "Nick, when you recollect your childhood, are your recollections pleasing to you?"
Nick: "Number 1, I don't remember how often I used to jerk off, but it was a lot. Number 2, I wasn't pissed off at my dad, even when I was old enough to know what he and mom were doing in the bedroom. Number 3, I don't look in the toilet before I flush it. Number 4, I haven't wet my bed for a long time. Number 5, why don't the two of you go fuck yourselves; I'm outta here."

Nick feels threatened by a psychological interview, in *Basic Instinct* (1992)

Belle de Jour (1967) Drama ΨΨΨΨΨ
Luis Buñuel film with Catherine Deneuve playing a bored housewife who amuses herself by working in a brothel from two until five every afternoon, at least until her sexual obsessions begin to complicate her life. Buñuel may be filming what is just an erotic dream.

Bookies (2003) Drama ΨΨ
Three college roommates, obsessed with gambling, secretly launch a "bookie" operation.

Burn After Reading (2008) Comedy ΨΨ
Clever, dark comedy by the Coen brothers in which George Clooney's character has a sexual addiction.

California Split (1974) Comedy ΨΨ
Robert Altman movie starring George Segal and Elliott Gould as two compulsive gamblers. Not as strong a film as *The Gambler*.

Carnal Knowledge (1971) Drama ΨΨ
This Mike Nichols film traces the sexual lives of two college roommates, played by Jack Nicholson and Art Garfunkel, as they age and become increasingly disenchanted with sex, love, and the possibilities inherent in relationships.

Casino (1995) Drama ΨΨ
Martin Scorsese film explores the mafia's relationship to Las Vegas and gives an inside look at casinos and gambling addictions. A strong cast includes Robert De Niro, Joe Pesci, Sharon Stone, and James Woods.

Choke (2008) Drama ΨΨ
A sex addict and medical school dropout feigns choking to raise money for care of his mother with Alzheimer's disease.

Closer (2004) Comedy-Drama ΨΨΨ
A quality film with good dialogue and superb acting by Jude Law, Natalie Portman, Julia Roberts, and Clive Owen. Important issues related to sexuality are portrayed, including deceit, infidelity, the failure to self-disclose, dependency, the impact of guilt and shame, and relationship testing. One scene depicts an amusing online conversation between two men sending erotic instant messages.

Comfort of Strangers, The (1990) Drama ΨΨ
Sexual conflict and disorders abound as two couples find themselves entangled with one another in Venice.

Cooler, The (2003) Drama ΨΨΨ
An unlucky, depressed man (William H. Macy) walks around the casino as "the cooler," someone paid to bring bad luck to successful gamers by appearing near their gambling tables. He is paying off enormous gambling debts owed to the casino owner, played by Alec Baldwin.

Crime of Father Amaro, The (2002, Mexico) ΨΨΨ
Drama
A young priest, newly ordained, goes to a small, Mexican town to serve a parish. He witnesses his superior having sex with women, and he becomes involved with a woman whom he secretively uses for sex until she becomes pregnant.

Damage (1992) Drama ΨΨΨ
A Louis Malle film starring Jeremy Irons as a man who develops a sexual obsession for his son's fiancée. Both the father and the son's girlfriend seem powerless to control their erotic attachment despite its inevitable consequences.

De-Lovely (2004) Musical-Comedy-Biography ΨΨ
The story of the life of Cole Porter and his sexual addiction. An earlier film, *Night and Day* (1946) starred Cary Grant and ignored the fact that the composer was gay.

Diary of a Nymphomaniac (2009, Spain) Drama ΨΨ
A 28-year-old woman has an insatiable appetite for sex and eventually ends up in a brothel. Lar von Trier's two films *Nymphomaniac: Vol. 1* and *Nymphomaniac: Vol. 2* are much more powerful and illustrative of sexual addiction.

Diary of a Sex Addict, The (2001) Drama ΨΨ
Depiction of a classic sex addict who denies, rationalizes, and continues a series of affairs until he finally can deceive no longer. He continues his compulsive behavior, even after the consequences of this behavior are almost fatal. The film offers a realistic portrayal of a sex addict.

Therapist: "Which one is really you? The family man or the other guy?"
Patient: "Both"

***The Diary of a Sex Addict* (2001)**

Dinner Rush (2001) Drama-Comedy ΨΨ
A New York City restaurant is frequented by highbrow customers, self-centered art critics, hoodlums from Queens, and casual customers. One of the cooks has a gambling problem.

Dirty Shame, A (2004) Comedy Ψ
A woman becomes promiscuous after a head injury.

Don Jon (2013) Drama ΨΨ
A young, unmarried man finds that his addiction to online pornography gets in the way of meaningful sexual interactions; each week he confesses the same sins (masturbating to pornography and sex outside of marriage) to his priest.

Far From Heaven (2002) Drama ΨΨΨ
Julianne Moore, living in a conservative area in a conservative time, finds out her husband is a homosexual. This is an interesting film that explores racism, stereotypes, and secrets.

Felicia's Journey (1999, Canada, UK) Drama ΨΨ
A pregnant young woman leaves Ireland for England to find her boyfriend; upon arrival, she is befriended by a middle-aged caterer who has a history of exploiting women in similar situations.

Gambler, The (1974) Drama ΨΨΨΨ
James Caan plays a university professor of literature who can't control his compulsive gambling. This is one of the best film portrayals of pathological gambling.

Good Thief, The (2002) Drama ΨΨ
Nick Nolte plays an aging junkie gambler who attempts to rob a casino.

Harold and Maude (1972) Comedy ΨΨΨ
A cult film that examines sexual and romantic attraction across generations; this movie will force you to reexamine your feelings about age and death.

House of Games (1987) Crime ΨΨ
A David Mamet film about a psychiatrist specializing in the treatment of gambling addiction. Fascinating introduction to the world of the con.

Hysteria (2011) Romantic Comedy ΨΨ
Maggie Gyllenhaal and Hugh Dancy star in this amusing story about two gynecologists who very properly masturbate their Victorian clients, initially using digital stimulation and later using a mechanical vibrator they invent. (The word "hysteria" comes from the Greek term for "wandering uterus," and it was once believed only women could develop hysteria. The term is not found in the DSM-5.)

I Am a Sex Addict (2005) Biography-Comedy Ψ
A recovering sex addict describes how his life and marriages have been changed by his addiction to prostitutes.

Kiss of the Spider Woman (1985) Prison ΨΨΨΨ
A homosexual and a political activist share a prison cell and grow to understand and appreciate each other. William Hurt won an Academy Award for his performance.

Last Tango in Paris (1973) Drama ΨΨΨΨ
Marlon Brando stars in a classic Bernardo Bertolucci film about a man who begins a casual sexual liaison on the day his wife commits suicide. The two lovers never exchange names. The film includes themes of depression, sexuality, loneliness, and cynicism.

Lianna (1983) Drama ΨΨΨ
Sensitive film portraying the emotional life of a woman who leaves her husband and two children after she

becomes romantically involved with a lesbian professor teaching a night course in child psychology.

Magenta (1996) Drama Ψ
A happily married physician crosses boundaries sexually with his sister-in-law, creating havoc in his family.

Maverick (1994) Western Drama ΨΨ
Mel Gibson and Jodie Foster star as charming gamblers and cons in a game of high stakes poker.

Maxed Out (2006) Documentary ΨΨ
Interesting statistics and depiction of the struggles and realities of American credit card debt. The film depicts the consequences of spending addictions and impulse control disorders.

Midnight Cowboy (1969) Drama ΨΨΨΨΨ
Jon Voight leaves Texas to make his fortune in New York City working as a stud; instead, he winds up hanging out with Ratso Rizzo who dies before the two men can escape to Florida. This film is a fascinating and complex character study.

> **"Well, I'll tell you the truth now. I ain't a real cowboy, but I am one helluva stud."**
>
> **Joe Buck in *Midnight Cowboy* (1969)**

Oscar and Lucinda (1997) Drama-Romance ΨΨΨΨ
Pathological gambling and concomitant anxiety disorders are clearly depicted in this film set in mid-1800s England, starring Ralph Fiennes and Cate Blanchett.

Owning Mahowny (2003) Drama ΨΨΨΨ
Philip Seymour Hoffman, one of today's finest character actors, plays a pathological gambler. Accurate portrayal of the addictive cycle and elements of denial, deterioration, and self-destruction. The film is based on a true story.

Personal Best (1982) Sports ΨΨΨ
Fascinating film that explores the sexual relationship that develops between two women competing for a position on an Olympic team.

Reflections in a Golden Eye (1967) Drama ΨΨ
A John Huston film in which Richard Burton plays the role of a repressed homosexual Army major serving on a small Georgia military base. Elizabeth Taylor is his sadistic and sexually liberated wife who has an affair with an enlisted man. The film was banned by the Catholic Film Board.

Romance (1999, France) Drama Ψ
A young schoolteacher is ignored sexually by her boyfriend, so she engages in a desperate search for love and sexual fulfillment.

Rounders (1998) Drama ΨΨ
Matt Damon stars as a poker player who has gambled away his life savings to a Russian mobster, gives up gambling, and is lured back into the game by his friend played by Edward Norton.

Sailor Who Fell from Grace with the Sea, The (1976) Drama ΨΨΨΨ
After his father dies, a young boy plots to take revenge on his mother's new lover. Interesting story of adult romance and child psychopathology; based on a novel by Yukio Mishima.

Shame (2011) Drama ΨΨΨΨ
This Steve McQueen film stars Michael Fassbender as Brandon, a man with a seemingly unquenchable need to have sex with multiple women (and occasionally men). Although not an official diagnosis in the DSM-5, many clinicians believe sexual addiction is a bona fide psychological disorder.

Swept Away (1975) Drama-Comedy ΨΨΨ
Lina Wertmuller's examination of sex roles. A rich woman and a poor deckhand are marooned on an island and find sexual excitement and satisfaction in the new roles each assumes.

That Obscure Object of Desire (1977) Drama ΨΨΨΨΨ
Surrealistic film by Luis Buñuel about violence, love, and sexual obsession in a middle-aged man. The film is complex, intriguing, and full of symbolism, including two actresses playing the same character. This was the last film Buñuel ever directed.

This Girl's Life (2003) Drama Ψ
A female porn star starts a business by getting women concerned about their husbands' fidelity to pay her to attempt to seduce them.

To Live (1994) Drama ΨΨΨΨΨ
This epic film by Zhang Yimou follows a Chinese family through tragic and wonderful times. One of the early struggles of the lead character, Fugui, is gambling; he loses his family home and his fortune gambling with dice.

To Our Loves (*A Nos Amours;* 1983, France) ΨΨΨ
Drama
A French film exploring the sexuality of a 15-year-old girl and the way it affects her family.

Two for the Money (2005) Drama ΨΨΨ
A young, savvy, football game expert (Matthew McConaughey) gets hired by a pathological gambler (Al Pacino) to work in a fast-paced business as an advisor to gamblers betting on football games. Based on a true story.

Unbearable Lightness of Being, The (1988) ΨΨΨ
Romance
A highly sensual film about a Prague neurosurgeon and his inability to separate sex and love. The film is based on the novel of the same name by Milan Kundera.

We Don't Live Here Anymore (2004) Drama ΨΨΨ
Two couples (played by Peter Krause, Naomi Watts, Mark Ruffalo, and Laura Dern) find both their marriages failing, in part due to adultery. The movie includes themes of deceit, manipulation, lack of integrity, and the excitement of secrecy. Each couple battles against boredom and idleness, using sex to escape the emptiness of their lives.

Young Adam (2003) Drama ΨΨ
Ewan Macgregor as a sexual addict who becomes intimately involved with his boss's wife, her sister, and a woman he meets at a ship's port.

Neurocognitive Disorders

50 First Dates (2004) Comedy Ψ
Adam Sandler plays a veterinarian and womanizer who falls in love with a woman (Drew Barrymore) who has lost the ability to consolidate memories. She awakens each morning forgetting everything from the day before (so she repeats the same activities each day, enabled by her family). A flawed *Memento.*

Accidental Hero, The (2002, France) Drama ΨΨ
A boy comes to appreciate his mother more fully after she is involved in a serious car accident and experiences a profound retrograde amnesia.

Alzheimer's Project, The (The Memory Loss Tapes) (2009) Documentary ΨΨΨΨ
Poignant and important HBO series integrated into a deeply meaningful film revealing seven vignettes of individuals at various stages of Alzheimer's disease and their families. The film addresses both the suffering caused by the disease and the challenges of the caregiver, such as themes of the adult-child role reversal, wandering, loss of independence, and the emotional grieving process.

Amour (2012, France) Drama ΨΨΨΨΨ
Georges and Anne are two retired music teachers living in Paris. When Anne has a stroke, Georges promises to keep her out of the hospital and out of a nursing home. She becomes increasingly debilitated, and this forces Georges to make difficult decisions about their relationship and future. This film can be a wonderful springboard for class discussions about aging, long-lasting love, the impact of neurocognitive disorders, and euthanasia.

Assisted Living (2003) Comedy-Drama ΨΨ
This movie was filmed in an actual nursing home. A pot-smoking janitor interacts with the residents and slowly learns to care about the patients in the home.

Awakenings (1990) Drama ΨΨΨ
Robin Williams as neurologist Oliver Sacks treats patient Robert De Niro in a Bronx hospital. The film documents the use of L-Dopa in the treatment of patients with advanced Parkinson's disease. Good portrayal of the daily life of a mental hospital.

Away From Her (2006, Canada) Drama ΨΨΨΨΨ
Sarah Polley's directorial debut about a woman (Julie Christie) who realizes she has Alzheimer's disease and convinces her husband (Gordon Pinsent) to take her to a care facility. He visits her regularly, despite discovering that she has fallen in love with another man. Sexual relations in which one partner is losing the cognitive ability to give consent presents a challenging ethical dilemma.

Fiona: "I'd like to make love, and then I'd like you to go. Because I need to stay here and if you make it hard for me, I may cry so hard I'll never stop."

Fiona checks into the memory care unit of a nursing home, in *Away From Her*

Ballad of Narayama, The (1958, Japan) Drama ΨΨΨ
This Japanese film tells the story of a small village in which, by tradition, all old people are taken up to the top of a mountain and left to die so they won't be a financial burden for their children and village. This was the final

film added to Roger Ebert's list of great movies before he died in 2013. Remade in 1983 with the same title.

Barney's Version (2010) Drama ΨΨΨ
Paul Giamatti portrays a small-time television producer who struggles with intimacy, alcohol dependence, and an early onset memory disorder.

Business of Amateurs (2016) Documentary ΨΨΨ
An expose examining the NCAA and their exploitation of student athletes. The film addresses the consequences of chronic traumatic encephalopathy (CTE), a progressive brain disorder caused by repeated blows to the head.

City of No Limits, The (2002) Drama ΨΨ
A family patriarch becomes paranoid and delusional because of a brain tumor; as a result, he shares long hidden family secrets.

Dark Victory (1939) Drama ΨΨΨ
Bette Davis, George Brent, and Humphrey Bogart star, but also watch for Ronald Reagan. Davis's character has a fatal brain tumor, and she spends what little time she has left with her brain surgeon husband. The "dark victory" refers to living life well, even when facing death. Remade (not very effectively) with Susan Hayward, as *Stolen Hours* (1963).

Death Be Not Proud (1975) Biography ΨΨ
A made-for-TV film based on John Gunther's moving account of his son's struggle with a brain tumor, which killed the boy when he was only 17 years old. The book itself provides considerable insight into the neurology of brain lesions.

Do You Remember Love? (1985) Drama ΨΨ
Joanne Woodward won an Emmy for her portrayal of a middle-aged college professor who develops Alzheimer's disease.

Father, The (2020) Drama ΨΨΨΨΨ
A remarkable film starring Anthony Hopkins as an octogenarian with dementia, supported by Olivia Colman playing his daughter. Few films are as powerful in portraying the confusion, paranoia and memory loss associated with dementia. Both lead actors are magnificent.

Harder They Fall, The (1956) Sports ΨΨΨΨ
Humphrey Bogart in his last film, made the year before his death. The movie is very critical of the sport of boxing and the exploitation of fighters by promoters. A slow-witted boxer has a brain clot and is almost killed in his last fight. Both prize fighters and football players often experience chronic traumatic encephalopathy (CTE).

Iris (2001) Drama-Biography ΨΨΨΨ
Based on the life of the famous British novelist and philosophical writer, Iris Murdoch (played by Judi Dench), who deteriorates because of Alzheimer's disease. Oscar-winner, Jim Broadbent plays John Bayley, Murdoch's loving husband. A powerfully realistic and emotional film.

Jacket, The (2005) Drama-Thriller ΨΨ
Adrien Brody portrays a man with retrograde amnesia who is mistreated in a psychiatric hospital in this avant-garde film.

Last Days of Ptolemy Grey, The (2022) Drama ΨΨΨΨ
Although a TV miniseries, I found this show interesting and accurate in its depiction of a man in the early stages of dementia. As always, Samuel L. Jackson is magnificent.

Lookout, The (2007) Drama ΨΨΨ
A high school student suffers a brain injury, and his life is changed forever. The film is a good introduction to many of the symptoms experienced by someone with a traumatic brain injury.

Lorenzo's Oil (1992) Drama ΨΨΨ
Nick Nolte and Susan Sarandon star in the true story of the Odone family and their desperate struggle to save their son's life. The boy has a rare neurological disease that they are told is ultimately fatal. Good illustration of the effects of chronic illness on family functioning.

Majestic, The (2001) Drama ΨΨ
Jim Carrey plays a disenfranchised screenwriter who develops amnesia after his car topples over a bridge. He washes on the shore of a small town whose citizens take him in as a lost war hero.

Man Without a Past, The (2002) Drama ΨΨΨ
A man is severely beaten while sleeping outside and is proclaimed dead. He awakens with amnesia and begins to create a new life for himself before eventually discovering parts of his old life.

Memento (2001) Suspense-Mystery ΨΨΨΨΨ
Christopher Nolan directs this one-of-a-kind, exquisitely crafted film about a man suffering from anterograde amnesia. The film demands the viewer have very good short-term memory as the major plot progresses backwards scene by scene while juxtaposing past events (going forward) in black and white. This is a film not to be missed.

Natalie: "But even if you get revenge, you're not going to remember it. You're not even going to know that it happened."
Leonard Shelby: "My wife deserves vengeance. Doesn't make a difference whether I know about it. Just because there are things I don't remember doesn't make my actions meaningless."

Leonard contemplates his need to avenge his wife's murder, in *Memento* (2001)

Memories of Me (1988) Comedy ΨΨ
Henry Winkler directs Billy Crystal in the role of a high-powered surgeon who has just had a heart attack, and Alan King, his actor father who may have Alzheimer's. It turns out that an aneurysm is present, and father and son eventually learn to care for one another.

Memory of a Killer, The (2003) Drama ΨΨ
A hit man in the early stages of dementia attempts to do one last job before retiring.

Mercy or Murder? (1987) Drama ΨΨ
Made-for-TV movie about a Florida man who went to prison after killing his wife because she had advanced Alzheimer's disease. The film raises interesting questions that society will increasingly be forced to confront (especially since it appears that COVID-19 dramatically increases the risk of Alzheimer's).

Million Dollar Baby (2004) Drama ΨΨΨΨ
A female prize fighter (Hilary Swank) is paralyzed from the neck down after being hit from behind with a chair by an angry opponent; she pleads with her trainer (Clint Eastwood) to end her life before she loses the memory of the crowd's applause.

Mulholland Drive (2001) Mystery-Drama-Suspense ΨΨΨΨ
David Lynch film about a woman who experiences a head injury from a car accident, becomes amnestic, and finds refuge in an aspiring Hollywood actress's condominium. This is characteristic Lynch in its nonlinearity with themes of reality versus illusion, identity confusion, and nightmarish dream sequences.

My Girl (1991) Drama-Comedy ΨΨ
An 11-year-old girl is a hypochondriac with a mortician for a father and a grandmother who has Alzheimer's disease.

No Home Movie (2015) Documentary ΨΨΨΨ
Director Chantal Akerman documents the life and decline of her mother, a Polish woman who survived Auschwitz. The film pays homage to motherhood, memory and loss. Akerman committed suicide shortly after the film was released.

Notebook, The (2004) Drama ΨΨΨ
Gena Rowlands and James Garner play a couple coping with her ever worsening Alzheimer's disease. Based on the best-selling novel by Nicholas Sparks.

On Golden Pond (1981) Drama ΨΨΨΨ
Sensitive portrayal of an aging couple (Henry Fonda and Katharine Hepburn) cherishing their time together and struggling with his increasingly apparent dementia.

On the Waterfront (1954) Drama ΨΨΨΨΨ
Classic Elia Kazan film starring Marlon Brando as Terry Malloy, a prizefighter with limited intelligence who is exploited by almost everyone around him. Brando won an Oscar as Best Actor for his performance depicting a fighter who took a dive and spent the rest of his life regretting it.

"You was my brother, Charley, you should've looked out for me just a little bit so I wouldn't have to take them dives for the short-end money."

***On the Waterfront* (1954)**

Pride of the Yankees, The (1942) Biography ΨΨΨ
Gary Cooper stars in this Samuel Goldwyn film about legendary Yankees' first baseman Lou Gehrig, who had to give up baseball due to amyotrophic lateral sclerosis, which came to be widely known by the eponym "Lou Gehrig's disease."

"Some people say I've had a bad break, but I consider myself to be the luckiest man on the face of the earth."

Lou Gehrig giving up baseball, in *The Pride of the Yankees* (1942)

Private Matter, A (1992) Biography ΨΨ
Provocative made-for-TV movie starring Sissy Spacek as a TV personality who gets national attention after her decision to abort a child likely to be affected by the drug thalidomide. The film seems more timely after the Supreme Court's 2022 Dobbs decision overturning Roe v. Wade and a half-century of established law.

Random Harvest (1942) Drama ΨΨΨΨ
A shell-shocked, amnestic soldier (Ronald Coleman) is hospitalized in an asylum after World War I. He wanders away and becomes romantically involved with a cabaret singer (Greer Garson), eventually marrying her, and establishing a new career as a writer. Three years later he is hit by a car – he can then remember all the details of his privileged life prior to World War I, but nothing of his new life with Greer Garson's character. She eventually tracks him down but doesn't reveal her identity upon the advice of a psychiatrist who cautions her that the shock would be too much for him. She becomes his personal secretary, and – not surprisingly – he falls in love with her all over again.

Raging Bull (1980) Biography–Sports ΨΨΨΨΨ
Powerful film depicting the psychological, moral, and mental decline of a prizefighter. Robert De Niro won an Oscar for his portrayal of Jake LaMotta.

Regarding Henry (1993) Drama ΨΨ
An attorney has his life permanently altered following a head injury; his values change as well as his personality.

Safe House (1998) Thriller ΨΨ
An ex-intelligence operative begins to develop Alzheimer's disease.

Savages, The (2007) Drama ΨΨΨ
A brother and sister (Philip Seymour Hoffman and Laura Linney) find themselves becoming closer as they attempt to cope with the challenges associated with caring for their father, who is suffering from Alzheimer's disease.

Sea Inside, The (*Mar Adentro;* 2004, Spain) ΨΨΨΨ
Biography–Drama
Javier Bardem stars in this sensitive and moving story about a Spanish citizen's quest to end his life.

Separation, A (2001, Iran) Drama ΨΨΨΨ
The wife wants to move to America; the husband insists on staying in Iran so they can take care of his father, a man coping with Alzheimer's disease.

Shattered (1991) Mystery–Suspense ΨΨ
A man in a near-fatal car accident experiences amnesia and undergoes reconstructive facial surgery. He begins to find inconsistencies in stories from loved ones about his past and his own memories, only to face a shocking truth.

Song for Martin, A (*En Sång för Martin;* 2002, Sweden) Drama ΨΨΨ
An interesting portrayal of the ways in which a married couple deeply in love are affected by his Alzheimer's disease.

Son of the Bride (*El Hijo de la Novia;* 2001, Argentina) Drama–Comedy–Romance ΨΨΨΨ
Moving drama with many inspirational and comic moments about a man too busy for his family until he reevaluates his life following a heart attack. A major substory is the man's aging father, who steadfastly expresses unconditional love to his wife who is deteriorating with Alzheimer's disease.

Still Alice (2014) Drama ΨΨΨΨΨ
Julianne Moore as a brilliant Columbia professor who is diagnosed with early-onset Alzheimer's. The film is shown from her point of view, and her sadness and frustration is palpable as we watch the insidious progression of the disease.

"Who can take us seriously when we are so far from who we once were? Our strange behavior and fumbled sentences change other's perception of us and our perception of ourselves. We become ridiculous, incapable, comic. But this is not who we are, this is our disease."

Dr. Alice Howland, a linguistics professor, noting the difference between herself and her disease, in *Still Alice* (2014).

Tell Me Who I Am (2019, UK) Documentary ΨΨΨΨΨ
Ed Perkins directed the remarkable documentary about twin brothers Marcus and Alex Lewis. Alex was involved in a near-fatal motorcycle accident at age 18, and had profound retrograde amnesia after the accident. He retained a memory of this twin, but not his parents, girlfriend, or any of his other friends. Marcus helps Alex reconstruct the past, but he leaves out significant events, only becoming totally honest about their past at age 54. The film is highly recommended.

Tuesdays with Morrie (1999) Drama–Inspiration ΨΨ
Made-for-TV movie based on the best-selling Mitch Albom book about a journalist who befriends and finds inspiration from a man dying of amyotrophic lateral sclerosis (ALS; also known as Lou Gehrig's disease).

Vow, The (2012) Drama ΨΨ
A recently married couple are in an automobile accident, and the wife sustains a serious head injury. She awakes from her coma profoundly amnestic with no memories of her marriage or husband. She returns home to live with her parents where she resumes a relationship with a former boyfriend.

Waltz With Bashir (2008, Israel) ΨΨΨΨ
Animation–Biography
An exploration of the construction and shifting nature of memory. Ari Folman served in the Israeli army during the Lebanon War of 1982 but has no recollection of these events, and he attempts to reconstruct them in this film. The opening animation and the closing, unanimated, scene are especially vivid. Watching this film will help you understand PTSD and how trauma can cause amnesia.

Personality Disorders

25th Hour (2002) Drama ΨΨΨΨ
A Spike Lee film about a young man (Edward Norton) about to go away to prison for 7 years for marijuana trafficking. In making the most of his final hours, he meets with his recovering alcoholic father, girlfriend, friends, and an underground boss and his henchmen. Look for tributes to 9/11 throughout the film (this was the first film to use Ground Zero in a film scene).

Accidental Tourist, The (1988) Comedy ΨΨΨ
William Hurt plays a withdrawn, unemotional writer whose isolation is compounded when his 12-year-son is senselessly murdered in a fast-food restaurant.

Alfie (2004) Comedy ΨΨΨ
Jude Law stars as a man with a narcissistic personality who prides himself in being a womanizer and not committing to relationships. Law's asides to the audience provide insight into his narcissistic thinking. By the end of the film, Alfie begins to face the impact of his behavior on others.

Amélie (2001, France) Comedy–Romance ΨΨΨΨΨ
Audrey Tautou stars as Amélie, an avoidant woman who wants an intimate relationship with others but is unable to be direct. Upon deciding to change her life by making a difference in others' lives, she adopts extreme and creative measures to bring joy to others and make connections. Brilliantly directed by Jean Pierre-Jeunet.

American Beauty (1999) Comedy–Drama ΨΨΨΨΨ
Kevin Spacey has the lead role in this remarkable film about a very dysfunctional family and the ennui that accompanies life in suburbia. Annette Bening plays a woman with a classic histrionic personality disorder. Almost every character exhibits some degree of psychopathology. The film is a compelling examination of the psychopathology of everyday life.

American Gangster (2007) Crime–Drama ΨΨΨ
An honest detective (Russell Crowe) tries to bring down a heroin kingpin (Denzel Washington) in this Ridley Scott film.

American History X (1998) Drama–Suspense ΨΨΨ
Edward Norton plays an antisocial, White supremacist who decides to change his life when he sees his younger brother is following his example.

Anatomy of a Murder (1959) Drama ΨΨΨΨ
Jimmy Stewart as an attorney defending a man accused of murder. His case rests on the contention that the defendant could not help behaving as he did, because the man he murdered had raped the defendant's wife. The film raises interesting questions about the irresistible impulse defense.

Anchorman: The Legend of Ron Burgundy (2004) Ψ and **Anchorman 2: The Legend Continues** (2013) Comedy
A narcissistic anchorman (Will Ferrell) competes with an ambitious female journalist as well as rival newscasters.

Animal Kingdom (2010, Australia) Drama ΨΨΨΨ
A 17-year-old boy is sitting on a couch with his mother and watches as she overdoses on heroin and dies. He goes to live with his extended family, a group of criminals and drug addicts.

Anything Else (2003) Comedy ΨΨ
Woody Allen film about a young man with a dependent personality disorder who falls for an erratic young woman (Christina Ricci).

Apostle, The (1997) Drama ΨΨΨΨ
Robert Duvall directs, writes, and stars as a philandering but dedicated minister who flees his hometown after committing a violent act. His redemptive journey takes him to a small town where he builds a ministry until his past catches up with him.

> **"All I can say is that whenever you've been on the radio, most all the white people think you're black. Now, most all the colored people know you ain't black; but they sure do like your style of preaching."**
>
> ***The Apostle* (1997)**

Apt Pupil (1998) Drama–Suspense ΨΨΨ
A high school student becomes fascinated with his discovery of a man (Ian McKellen) who was formerly a Nazi

henchman. Kurt Dussander is living (and hiding out) in a local town. The student manipulates him to tell him detailed stories about his previous life.

Arsenic and Old Lace (1944) Comedy ΨΨ
Frank Capra film about Cary Grant's two aunts who practice mercy killing by giving their gentlemen guests poisoned elderberry wine. Grant worries about the fact that mental illness not only runs in his family, it gallops!

Assassination of Jesse James by the Coward Robert Ford, The (2007) Crime ΨΨΨ
The humanization and glorification of infamous outlaw, Jesse James (Brad Pitt) is depicted, along with the young, timid Robert Ford who shot him. James was an antisocial personality who was (understandably) paranoid.

Bad Santa (2003) Comedy Ψ
This Terry Zwigoff film stars Billy Bob Thornton as a rule-breaking, crass alcoholic who works as Santa Claus at a department store. The female costar has a "Santa fetish."

Bad Seed, The (1956) Drama Ψ
Interesting examination of whether evil is congenital; a sociopathic, adopted child turns out to be the daughter of a serial killer. Contrast this film with *We Need To Talk About Kevin* (2011).

Bartleby (1970) Comedy ΨΨΨ
Original black-and-white version of the Herman Melville short story, "Bartleby the Scrivener." More slow, dark, and dreary than its recent counterpart, yet still an excellent depiction of schizoid personality.

Bartleby (2001) Comedy ΨΨΨ
This dark comedy brilliantly casts Crispin Glover as the aloof, quirky clerk, Bartleby, who repeats the same phrase, "I would prefer not to," when asked to work. Ironically colorful set design and a hodgepodge of quirky personalities as supporting cast. This is clearly a "love it or hate it" film, based on a short story by Herman Melville. Bartleby's character is a classic depiction of a person with a schizoid personality.

Basic Instinct (1992, 2006) Thriller-Drama Ψ
Sharon Stone as Catherine Tramell, a seductive and manipulative woman with numerous borderline traits. He manipulation of detectives during an interrogation is a classic scene.

Before the Devil Knows You're Dead (2007) Drama-Crime ΨΨΨ
Sidney Lumet directs Philip Seymour Hoffman, Ethan Hawke, Marisa Tomei, and Albert Finney in a film about a heist (of one's own family) gone terribly wrong.

Being Julia (2004) Drama-Comedy ΨΨΨ
Annette Bening portrays an actress with features of each of the Cluster B personality disorder traits, in addition to a work addiction.

Believer, The (2001) Biography-Drama ΨΨΨ
Fascinating character study of Danny Burrows who is living his life in an impossible contradiction as a Jewish Nazi. As he faces his true self, his ruthless antisocial characteristics begin to crumble. Based on a true story of events that occurred in Burrows' life in the fall of 1965.

Bitter Moon (1992) Drama ΨΨΨΨ
Roman Polanski film in which a couple becomes entangled with a woman who meets several criteria for borderline personality.

Black Snake Moan (2006) Drama ΨΨΨ
Samuel L. Jackson plays a broken man who rescues a promiscuous, erratic woman (Christina Ricci) left for dead on the road. Both characters face and share their dark sides.

Blue Jasmine (2013) Comedy-Drama ΨΨΨΨΨ
Woody Allen pays homage to the film version of a *Streetcar Named Desire* (1951) in this intriguing film. It is one of the best examples of a histrionic personality disorder, and I use clips in lectures to medical students about personality disorders.

"Anxiety, nightmares and a nervous breakdown, there's only so many traumas a person can withstand until they take to the streets and start screaming."

A histrionic Jasmine – who had just flown first class – contemplates life's challenges, in *Blue Jasmine* (2013)

Box of Moonlight (1996) Drama ΨΨΨ
A rigid, orderly, rule-obsessed man, played by John Turturro, takes extra time off from his job and family to rediscover his lost adolescence. The title becomes a beautiful, transformational metaphor in the film.

Breach (2007) Biography-Thriller-Drama ΨΨΨ
A pathological, manipulative CIA official (Chris Cooper) leads a double life in this intriguing thriller. Based on the true story of the worst FBI spy in US history, someone who eventually cost the US government billions of dollars.

Breathless (*A Bout De Souffle;* 1960, France) ΨΨΨΨΨ
Drama-Crime
Classic antisocial hoodlum in a classic film by French New Wave director, Jean-Luc Godard. The protagonist impulsively murders a motorcycle policeman but feels no guilt. The pacing of the film justifies the title, as does the lead performance of the antihero.

Bruce Almighty (2002) Comedy Ψ
Whimsical comedy about a man (Jim Carrey) given the opportunity to "be God" for a day.

Butley (1974) Drama ΨΨΨΨ
Alan Bates in a Harold Pinter film adaptation of a London play about the life of a British university professor. Bates's wife and lover are both leaving him, and his colleagues are estranged. Bates seems to fail in every interpersonal encounter.

Caine Mutiny, The (1954) Drama ΨΨΨ
Humphrey Bogart is the ship's paranoid captain, who decompensates under the pressure of testimony when he is called to the witness stand. Bogart is magnificent in the role of Captain Queeg.

Catch Me If You Can (2002) Biography-Drama ΨΨΨ
Steven Spielberg directs Leonardo DiCaprio in the role of a manipulative con man with an antisocial personality. He repeatedly changes his identity while defrauding banks and keeping an FBI agent (Tom Hanks) one step behind him. Based on the true story of Frank Abagnale Jr.

Character (*Karakter;* 1997, The Netherlands)
Drama ΨΨΨ
Winner of an Academy Award for Best Foreign Language Film, about a young man's personal and financial struggle to be free of his antisocial father. His mother appears to have a schizoid personality disorder.

> **"That boy, I'll strangle him for nine tenths and the last tenth will make him strong."**
>
> **Dreverhaven describing his son, in *Character* (1997)**

Charlie and the Chocolate Factory (2005) ΨΨΨΨ
Drama-Comedy
Tim Burton remake of the classic story is well-casted, with beautiful set designs. Johnny Depp's portrayal of an eccentric, isolated, and perceptually disturbed Willy Wonka is one of the best depictions of schizotypal personality captured on film.

Child, The (*L'enfant;* 2005, France) ΨΨΨ
Drama-Crime
Bruno, who leads a gang of petty thieves, decides to sell his newborn for money.

Citizen Kane (1941) Drama ΨΨΨΨΨ
Orson Wells and Joseph Cotton star in this classic film that is a staple in film history courses. For our purposes, the film offers a dramatic illustration of narcissistic personality disorder.

Come Back to the 5 & Dime, Jimmy Dean, Jimmy Dean (1982) Drama ΨΨ
A Robert Altman film in which Sandy Dennis plays a local woman in a small Texas town who is convinced she bore a son by James Dean, impregnated when he was in town filming *Giant*.

Compulsion (1959) Drama-Crime ΨΨΨ
Two young fraternity brothers believe their perfect crime of murder is "the true test of a superior intellect." Their defense attorney (Orson Welles) gives a memorable speech to save their lives.

Conspiracy Theory (1997) Drama ΨΨ
Mel Gibson plays a cab driver with virtually no personal life, who is obsessed with a woman, and who writes a newsletter on conspiracies. His paranoia takes him to every possible place and situation, including one conspiracy that turns out to be true.

Conversation, The (1974) Drama ΨΨΨ
A Francis Ford Coppola film in which Gene Hackman plays a surveillance expert with a paranoid personality.

Corporation, The (2004) Documentary ΨΨ
Interesting, albeit one-sided, review of corporations that documents the similarities between them and the characteristics of a psychopathic personality disorder.

Criminal (2004) Drama-Crime Ψ
John C. Reilly portrays an antisocial con artist who tries to sell a fake copy of a rare bill to a collector. The film suffers from a contrived ending, standard fare for con films.

Crush, The (1993) Drama-Suspense Ψ
Alicia Silverstone plays a 14-year-old temptress who is obsessed with a 28-year-old man who spurns her sexual overtures. This is an engaging portrayal of a character who is likely to qualify for a diagnosis of antisocial personality disorder as soon as she turns 18.

Dark Knight, The (2008) Action-Crime ΨΨΨΨ
Christopher Nolan's follow-up to *Batman Begins* stars Heath Ledger in incredible form as "the Joker," a clever and fearless psychopath who battles Batman (Christian Bale).

Decalogue, The (1989, Poland) Drama ΨΨΨΨΨ
Ten, 1-hr films loosely based on the 10 Commandments, originally made for Polish television by director Krzysztof Kieslowski. This set of films was hailed as one of the most significant productions in recent history, and the late Stanley Kubrick once said it is the only film masterpiece he knows. Multiple psychological disorders are portrayed in various characters living in an apartment complex.

Dementia 13 (1963) Horror Ψ
Third-rate film about an axe murderer; interesting primarily because it is Francis Ford Coppola's first serious film.

Henry Barthes: "You know it's funny, I spend a lot of time trying to not have to deal ... to not really commit. I'm a substitute teacher, there's no real responsibility to teach. Your responsibility is to maintain order, make sure nobody kills anybody in your classroom and then they get them to their next period."

Henry Barthes explains his passivity, in *Detachment* (2012)

Detachment (2012) Drama ΨΨΨ
Adrien Brody stars as Henry Barthes, a substitute teacher who drifts from job to job, avoiding meaningful attachments with his students or other teachers. Students may want to debate the merits of a diagnosis of either schizoid personality disorder or avoidant personality disorder.

Divine Secrets of the Ya-Ya Sisterhood (2002) ΨΨ
Drama-Comedy
A group of friends teach a young woman (Sandra Bullock) about her troubled mother. Ashley Judd and Ellen Burstyn plays the (young and old) erratic, labile, and abusive mother.

Dogville (2003, Denmark) Drama ΨΨΨ
A Lars von Trier film in which Nicole Kidman stars as a woman on the run who finds refuge in a small, isolated town. If a town could be diagnosed, this one would clearly be "antisocial," as group contagion results in manipulation, deceit, and abuse. Unique set design of a town without any houses or doors, and the film is staged as if we are watching an actual play.

Dot the I (2003, UK/Spain/US) Drama-Romance Ψ
A love triangle set in London with various twists of deceit and sabotage that leave the viewer wondering who is manipulating whom.

Dream Lover (1994) Drama Ψ
A sociopathic woman plots to marry a man and then have him committed to an insane asylum.

Employee of the Month (2004) Comedy-Drama Ψ
Dark comedy with Matt Dillon experiencing a day when everything in his perfect life goes wrong. Watch for numerous Buddhist references to the fact that "everything is an illusion."

End of Violence, The (1997) Drama ΨΨΨ
Wim Wenders film about a paranoid personality played by Bill Pullman.

Enron: The Smartest Guys in the Room (2005) ΨΨ
Documentary
Depicts the antisocial personalities of the Enron corporation leaders and the backstory of their rise to power and eventual downfall.

Equilibrium (2002) Action ΨΨ
This film depicts a futuristic society in which everyone must take a drug to block the disease called "human emotion."

Eraserhead (1976) Drama ΨΨΨ
This early David Lynch film has become a cult classic. It depicts Henry Spencer as someone with a schizoid personality: He is an awkward loner who doesn't know how to interact with others; he has flat and frequently inappropriate affect; he has few friends; and he is seemingly indifferent to criticism or praise.

Evita (1997) Drama-Musical ΨΨ
Madonna portrays Argentina's first lady, Eva Peron, and depicts her rise from poverty and scandal to fame, fortune, and the adulation of a nation. Eva (Evita) does what it takes to climb the ladder of success, eventually marrying military leader Juan Peron. She speaks out on his behalf, mobilizes the people of Argentina, frees him from jail, and helps him get elected. Antonio Banderas plays her alter ego with running commentary, warnings, criticism, and song.

Family Man, The (2000) Family-Comedy ΨΨ
A corporate executive (Nicholas Cage) who is obsessed with money, fame, and power gets an opportunity to see

how his life would have turned out if he had married his college sweetheart. The film includes obvious parallels with *It's a Wonderful Life*.

Fatal Attraction (1987) Thriller-Romance ΨΨΨΨ
Glenn Close displays classic characteristics of borderline personality disorder, including fears of abandonment, unstable interpersonal relationships, impulsivity, suicidal gestures, inappropriate and intense anger, and affective instability. This remarkable film is flawed by a contrived and artificial ending, but it is an excellent teaching tool.

Fargo (1996) Comedy ΨΨΨΨΨ
Dark comedy from the Coen brothers about a car salesman (William H. Macy) whose plot to kidnap his wife has gone horribly awry. Frances McDormand has a memorable role as police chief Marge Gunderson.

Finding Forrester (2000) Drama ΨΨ
A high school student befriends an aloof, retired professor and writer who has avoided people for years. Their relationship gets off to a shaky start and takes many turns, yet each has a profound impact on the other.

Five Easy Pieces (1970) Drama ΨΨΨ
Jack Nicholson, raised in an upper class and gifted family, is a talented pianist who left his affluent life to work in the oil fields. The plot is thin, but the character Nicholson plays is complex and fascinating.

Fracture (2007) Thriller-Drama Ψ
Anthony Hopkins and Ryan Gosling star in this courtroom suspense film in which Hopkins kills his wife and gets away with it.

Freaks (1932) Horror ΨΨΨΨ
Fascinating film about a normal trapeze artist who marries a midget for his inheritance, and then tries to poison him. When his friends find out, they kill her strong-man lover and turn her into one of them.

From Dusk Till Dawn (1995) Horror Ψ
Quentin Tarantino and George Clooney portray psychopaths who rendezvous at a biker bar that turns out to be run by vampires. The film presents as two very different movies combined – the first is Tarantino-like in character interaction and dialogue, and the second half is a horror show. Robert Rodriguez directs the film.

From the Life of the Marionettes ΨΨΨ
(*Aus dem Leben der Marionetten;* 1980, Germany) Drama
Bergman film in which an executive rapes and kills a prostitute. This is Bergman's only film shot in the German language; he had moved to Germany to avoid paying taxes in Sweden.

Ghost Dog: The Way of the Samurai (1999) ΨΨΨ
Crime-Drama
Jim Jarmusch film about a reclusive man who lives with pigeons and believes he is indebted to a mob boss who once saved his life.

Heart in Winter, A (*Un Coeur en Hiver;* 1992, France) Drama ΨΨΨ
This film depicts a complicated love triangle which includes an emotionally distant violin restorer who is already married. The married man is cold and indifferent, and he meets DSM-5 criteria for schizoid personality disorder.

Susanna: [reading from a book] "'Borderline Personality Disorder. An instability of self-image, relationships and mood... uncertain about goals, impulsive in activities that are self-damaging, such as casual sex.'"
Lisa: "I like that."
Susanna: "'Social contrariness and a generally pessimistic attitude are often observed.' Well, that's me."

***Girl, Interrupted* (1999)**

Girl, Interrupted (1999) Drama ΨΨΨ
A depressed, young woman, Susanna (Winona Ryder), is sent to a psychiatric hospital and labeled with borderline personality disorder. She soon encounters a dangerous patient, Lisa (Angelina Jolie), with an antisocial personality disorder.

Godfather, The (1972, 1974, 1990) ΨΨΨΨΨ
Crime-Drama
A classic trilogy directed by Francis Ford Coppola about a New York Mafia family that is kind and generous to those who support the family and ruthless to those who oppose it.

God Is Great and I Am Not (*Dieu Est Grand, Je Suis Toute Petite;* 2003, France) Comedy ΨΨ
Audrey Tautou plays a dependent woman who obsessively conforms to the religion of any man she is dating.

Gone With the Wind (1939)
Romance-Drama ΨΨΨΨΨ
In the classic love story, Scarlett O'Hara meets full criteria for histrionic personality disorder; however, some have argued that these surface features are the result of

the social forces of her culture and time and that her deeper character structure would not be considered histrionic.

Good Nurse, The (2022) ΨΨΨ
Biography-Crime-Drama
A male nurse is responsible for multiple patient deaths at each of the hospitals in which he works, and he continues moving from hospital to hospital until a good nurse agrees to work with detectives to get him to confess.

Greenberg (2010) Drama-Comedy-Romance ΨΨ
A neurotic and self-centered man (Ben Stiller) discharged from a psychiatric hospital goes to house sit for his brother. Greenberg is obsessed with imperfections, and he meets almost of the DSM-5 criteria for obsessive-compulsive personality disorder.

Grey Gardens (2009) Drama-Biography ΨΨΨ
Drew Barrymore and Jessica Lange portray the infamous mother and daughter, Edie and Edith Beales. Lange's character was a first cousin to Jackie Onassis-Kennedy; she displays a dependent personality disorder and extreme symptoms of what might be agoraphobia. The extreme avoidance and pathology of the characters results in their mansion deteriorating into a cesspool of filth and cat urine.

Grifters, The (1990) Crime ΨΨΨΨ
Anjelica Huston stars in this fascinating introduction to the world of the con. Contrast this film with a movie almost as good, David Mamet's *House of Games*.

Guy (1997) Drama ΨΨ
Fascinating story about a documentary filmmaker (Hope Davis) who chooses one person (Vincent D'Onofrio) at random and relentlessly follows him, filming his daily life for several days despite the victim's resistance and threats. Her obsession of filming him becomes his obsession with being filmed. The movie addresses narcissism and suggests that obsessions are a core part of human nature.

Heavy (1995) Drama ΨΨΨ
An obese, schizoid man loses his mother (with whom he lived) and becomes even more withdrawn as he grieves.

I, Robot (2004) Action-Suspense ΨΨ
Surprisingly high-quality action film about an agent who battles robots threatening to take over the world. Will Smith's role illustrates paranoid personality traits.

In the Company of Men (1997) Comedy ΨΨΨ
Misogynistic satire of two men (with varying levels of narcissism) who deliberately seduce the same vulnerable girl, lead her on, and then abandon her. Directed by Neil LaBute.

Iron Man (2008) Drama ΨΨΨ
In this film and its sequel (2010), Robert Downey Jr. plays a grandiose, egotistical man who meets criteria for a diagnosis of narcissistic personality disorder.

Jobs (2013) Biography Ψ
Ashton Kutcher plays Steve Jobs in a disappointing film; however, it is a useful pedagogical exercise to watch the film and to see if Jobs meets the DSM-5 diagnostic criteria for narcissistic personality disorder.

Jonestown: The Life and Death of Peoples Temple (2006) Documentary-Biography ΨΨ
Discussion and explanation of the events that led up to the largest mass suicide in modern history, brought about by the manipulative tactics of the antisocial preacher Jim Jones.

Kalifornia (1993) Thriller ΨΨ
Early Brad Pitt performance as a quirky, ruthless, psychopathic killer who teams up with his naïve sweetheart (Juliette Lewis), a woman with a borderline IQ. There is not a hint of remorse or empathy in Pitt's character.

Knife in the Water (1962) Drama ΨΨΨΨ
One of Roman Polanski's earliest films. A man and his wife on a sailing holiday pick up a hitchhiker. There is mounting sexual tension between the older man and his younger rival. The younger man eventually makes love to the wife after a complex turn of events that occur when the couple becomes convinced the young man has drowned.

La Cage aux Folles (1978) Comedy ΨΨΨ
Zaza (Albin), a transvestite nightclub performer, is a wonderful example of a histrionic personality. He is dramatic and flamboyant and threatens suicide when things do not go his way.

Ladies Man, The (2000) Comedy Ψ
Tim Meadows plays a narcissistic talk-show host and "player." Spin-off of a successful Saturday Night Live skit.

Ladykillers, The (2004) Comedy ΨΨ
Tom Hanks leads a group of thieves in a caper to steal money from a casino by digging underground from the home of an oblivious, good-hearted, elderly woman.

Good portrayal of how people with antisocial personalities can use language to manipulate their victims. Directed by the Coen brothers.

Lakeview Terrace (2009) Drama–Thriller ΨΨΨ
Samuel L. Jackson portrays a police officer who terrorizes his next-door neighbors because they are an interracial couple. His character would meet criteria for a paranoid personality.

Land of Plenty (2004, US/Germany) Drama ΨΨΨΨ
Wim Wenders film about misguided patriotism and paranoia in post-9/11 times in America; the protagonist is a classic paranoid personality disorder; this condition has rarely been portrayed so well.

Last King of Scotland, The (2006)
Drama–Biography ΨΨΨ
Forest Whitaker in an unforgettable, terrifying role as Idi Amin, the charming, charismatic, and paranoid ruler of Uganda who killed over 300,000 people during his reign.

Last Station, The (2009)
Drama–Biography–Romance ΨΨΨ
A film about the last year in the life of novelist Leo Tolstoy. Tolstoy's wife, Countess Sofya Andreevna Tolstoy, is upset because her husband's new will leaves all his writings – and all his royalties – to the Russian people rather than to her and her children. She meets all the DSM-5 criteria for the diagnosis of histrionic personality disorder.

Last Supper, The (1996) Comedy Ψ
Dark comedy of five liberal graduate students seeking revenge against reactionary and conservative dinner guests. The film depicts elements of antisocial and compulsive behavior.

Leave Her to Heaven (1945) Romance–Crime ΨΨ
Protagonist commits multiple murders, watches her brother-in-law drown, and terminates her pregnancy by throwing herself down a flight of stairs with no sense of shame or remorse. Dated but interesting portrayal of an antisocial personality.

Le Boucher (1970, France) Thriller ΨΨΨ
Claude Chabrol film in which a butcher who is also a murderer commits suicide when the woman he loves realizes he is a criminal.

Levity (2003) Drama ΨΨΨ
Billy Bob Thornton plays a "recovered antisocial," who, after his release from prison, seeks to achieve redemption by making amends with a family member (Holly Hunter) of a boy he killed decades ago. Morgan Freeman plays an antisocial preacher.

Lord of War (2005) Action–Drama Ψ
Nicholas Cage portrays Uri Orlov, an antisocial man who sells illegal arms to various countries. Based on actual events.

Love Exposure (2008, Japan) Drama ΨΨΨ
The character Kaori has a borderline personality disorder. She falls hopelessly in love with a priest and attempts to seduce him in a confessional booth, claiming "Father, listen to my confession! If you turn away from me, I'll kill myself. Please listen to me." The two eventually become lovers. The priest is a widower with a son who takes surreptitious photos of women's panties so he will have sufficient sins to confess to his demanding father.

Lovelife (1997) Comedy ΨΨ
Film about a group of friends and their struggles in relationships, many with symptoms of disorders that prevent them from connecting – the depressed intellectual, the dependent woman, and the neurotic voyeur – but the standout is the narcissist professor.

Mad Love (*Juana la Loca;* 2002, Spain) ΨΨ
Spanish film about a princess who marries and later becomes queen and is nicknamed "Joan the Mad" because of her worries about her philandering husband.

Man from Elysian Fields, The (2001) Drama ΨΨ
A married man (Andy Garcia) becomes an escort, and his life falls apart because of this decision.

Man Who Cried, The (2000) Drama ΨΨ
Slow-moving film of a young woman (Christina Ricci) who left a very poor Russian family years ago to make it as a dancer in the theater. This is a disappointing film despite an all-star cast including Johnny Depp, Cate Blanchett, and John Turturro.

Man Who Wasn't There, The (2001) Drama ΨΨΨΨ
This Coen brothers film noir is a fascinating character analysis of Ed Crane (Billy Bob Thornton) who is an aloof, taciturn, and unemotional barber struggling to find purpose. An excellent illustration of schizoid personality disorder, a Cluster A disorder.

Margot at the Wedding (2007) ΨΨΨ
Comedy–Drama
Nicole Kidman portrays Margot, a woman with a borderline personality disorder who displays loose boundaries, lability, anger, impulsivity, inappropriate affect, and fears of abandonment during a short visit to her sister's house.

Marriage of Maria Braun, The (1978) Drama–War ΨΨΨ
This Fassbinder film, an allegory about postwar Germany, portrays the dehumanizing effects of war and its aftermath, as we watch the commercial success and personal failures of Maria Braun. There is an explosive finale.

Master, The (2012) Drama ΨΨΨ
A Navy veteran coping with alcoholism and PTSD is drawn into the inner circle of a charismatic cult leader played by Philip Seymour Hoffman, but begins to doubt the sincerity of the leader. Several of the cult followers meet criteria for dependent personality disorder. The film was inspired by the life of Scientology founder L. Ron Hubbard.

Match Point (2005) Drama–Crime ΨΨΨΨ
Very dark but engaging Woody Allen film about a young man who inadvertently murders someone and then demonstrates significant antisocial traits that keep him from getting caught.

Me and You and Everyone We Know (2005) Comedy Ψ
Several odd and quirky characters exhibit subclinical syndromes and features of personality disorders.

Minus Man (1999) Drama ΨΨ
Owen Wilson stars as a charming, kind, drifting serial killer. The film does not explain his behavior, which he claims is spontaneous.

Mommie Dearest (1981) Drama–Biography ΨΨΨΨΨ
Biographical film based on a book by Joan Crawford's adopted daughter. Faye Dunaway plays Crawford. The film suggests the great star was tyrannical, narcissistic, alcoholic, and probably bipolar. Other potential diagnoses include borderline personality disorder and obsessive-compulsive personality disorder.

> **"What are wire hangers doing in this closet? Answer me! I buy you beautiful dresses, and you treat them like they were some dishrag. You do! Three-hundred-dollar dress on a wire hanger!"**
>
> **Joan Crawford in a manic state berates her daughter, in *Mommie Dearest* (1981)**

Monster (2004) Docudrama ΨΨΨΨ
Graphic, disturbing film based on the life of Aileen Wuornos, a prostitute and drifter turned serial killer. Charlize Theron won an Oscar for her powerful performance as Wuornos.

My Summer of Love (2004) Drama–Romance Ψ
Coming-of-age tale of a girl who falls in love with another girl her age who turns out to be suffering from a burgeoning case of antisocial personality disorder (compare this film with Neil Labute's *The Shape of Things*).

My Super Ex-Girlfriend (2006) Comedy–Romance Ψ
Uma Thurman portrays G-Girl, a superheroine with great powers but one who also exhibits borderline traits, fear of abandonment, hostility, all-or-none thinking, and revengeful behavior.

My Week With Marilyn (2011) Biography Drama ΨΨ
Marilyn Monroe, as depicted in this film, meets many of the criteria for borderline personality disorder, including an extreme fear of abandonment, impulsivity, insecurity, an unstable self-image, and intense but labile interpersonal relationships.

Naked (1993) Drama ΨΨΨΨΨ
Fascinating story about an "existential antisocial," Johnny, wandering the streets of London exchanging philosophical observations with other quirky characters. Comedy, love, drama, and violence flow throughout this film. Written and directed by renowned British director Mike Leigh.

No Country For Old Men (2007) Drama–Crime ΨΨΨΨΨ
Javier Bardem gives one of the most chilling portrayals of psychopathology in cinema history in the role of Anton Chigurh, an evil man who plays with the destiny of everyone he encounters.

Notes on a Scandal (2006) Drama ΨΨΨΨ
Judi Dench and Cate Blanchett engage in a battle of manipulation and deceit in a movie that depicts ephebophilia, emptiness, objectification, obsession, and borderline traits.

Odd Couple, The (1968) Comedy ΨΨΨΨ
Jack Lemmon is magnificent as the obsessive-compulsive Felix Unger, who uses air freshener and leaves notes on the pillow of his housemate (Walter Matthau).

One Hour Photo (2002) ΨΨΨ
Robin Williams in a quirky, dramatic, and disturbing role as the personality disordered Sy, the Photo Guy. Sy collects photographs from a customer's family and finds meaning through their lives until he discovers they are not the perfect family.

Orphan (2009) Drama–Horror ΨΨ
A young couple decides to adopt a 9-year-old Russian girl after the mother miscarries; however, the child does not measure up to the fantasies of the parents.

Overnight (2003) Documentary-Drama ΨΨ
A rags to riches to rags story about a narcissistic bartender, Troy Duffy, who is offered an attractive deal by Miramax for his screenplay only to have his pathology eventually sabotage this opportunity.

Pacific Heights (1990) Drama-Suspense ΨΨΨ
Michael Keaton plays a classic antisocial personality who becomes a tenant of a Victorian home and refuses to leave or pay rent, reaping significant havoc.

Paper Moon (1973) Comedy-Drama ΨΨ
Fun Peter Bogdanovich film, with Ryan O'Neal and daughter Tatum working together as a pair of con artists in the early 1930s.

Pawn Sacrifice (2014) History-Drama ΨΨΨΨ
Tobey Maguire plays the role of troubled chess genius Bobby Fischer, and Fischer's character is an excellent illustration of paranoid personality disorder.

Perfume: The Story of a Murderer (2006, Germany) Drama-Crime ΨΨΨΨ
A young man with a phenomenal sense of smell becomes obsessed with capturing the perfect scent, but he takes his obsession too far. Directed by Tom Tykwer.

Phone Booth (2003) Action-Suspense Ψ
A one-dimensional, narcissistic New Yorker begins to unravel as he is manipulated and forced to stay on the phone on the busy streets of Manhattan with a serial killer (Kiefer Sutherland). Worth seeing for the ending that cinematically shows the deep wounds underlying many narcissistic personality disorders.

Plumber, The (1979, Australia) Mystery-Drama ΨΨ
In this early Peter Weir film, a strange and mysterious plumber seems to be manipulating a woman as he repeatedly returns to her house to check pipes and fix the plumbing. The film raises important questions about trust and class.

Pumpkin Eater, The (1964) Drama ΨΨ
Most memorable for the scene in which Anne Bancroft, responding to the stress of eight children and an unfaithful husband, breaks down in Harrods.

Rampage (1992) Drama-Thriller ΨΨΨ
A film that explores the insanity defense, sociopathy, and mass murder. Directed by William Friedkin, who was also the director for *The Exorcist*.

Reign Over Me (2007) Drama ΨΨΨΨ
Adam Sandler portrays Charlie Fineman, a man with a schizotypal personality who is lost in pathological grief. An old friend (Don Cheadle) works hard to reorient him back to the world around him. Winner of a Voice Award.

"Charlie, before you go, I'd like to say something. Look, the fact is you had a family and you suffered a great loss, and until you discuss that, and we can really talk about that, this is all just an exercise. I can be patient, Charlie, but you need to tell someone your story. It doesn't have to be me, but someone."

Psychologist Angela Oakhurst works with Charlie Fineman, in *Reign Over Me* (2007)

Remains of the Day (1994) Romance-Drama ΨΨΨΨ
Anthony Hopkins plays a butler whose rigid personality will not allow him to experience intimacy or genuine love. Few films have been more effective in presenting this reserved, over-controlled, and limiting personality type.

Rick (2003) Comedy-Drama ΨΨΨ
Satirical comedy starring Bill Pullman as Rick, a narcissistic corporate executive who is self-serving, misanthropic, and cruel.

Robber, The (2010, Germany) Biography ΨΨΨ
This film is based on the true story of Johann Rettenberger, a world-class marathon runner who robbed banks in his spare time.

Roger Dodger (2002) Comedy ΨΨΨ
Manhattan executive teaches his 16-year-old nephew about women in one night by taking him to the streets of New York. Great portrayal of narcissism.

Royal Tenenbaums, The (2001) Comedy ΨΨΨΨ
Dark comedy classic about the highly dysfunctional Tenenbaum family. The parents (Gene Hackman and Angelica Huston) raise three genius children (Ben Stiller, Gwyneth Paltrow, and Luke Wilson) who must cope with significant problems including paranoia, depression, incest, and suicidal thoughts. The family is reunited when the narcissistic father returns home claiming he is dying of stomach cancer. We are left to see the dysfunctional dynamics of the family take place in comical form. A schizotypal personality is also portrayed (Owen Wilson) – a cinematic rarity.

Saw (2004) Horror Ψ
Jigsaw, a serial killer and torturer, manipulates people whom he believes are ungrateful, to test how far they will go to save themselves, such as cutting off one's own foot with a rickety saw to set oneself free. There are numerous sequels to the original *Saw*, but few are worth seeing unless one truly loves the genre.

Séance on a Wet Afternoon (1964, Britain) ΨΨΨΨ
Crime
A British film in which Kim Stanley plays a medium who persuades her husband (Richard Attenborough) to kidnap a child so they can then use her power of clairvoyance to "find" the missing child.

Series of Unfortunate Events, A (2004) ΨΨΨ
Comedy–Drama
Jim Carrey plays a comical psychopath who adopts multiple disguises to inherit a family fortune that rightfully belongs to three orphans whose parents have died in a fire.

Servant, The (1963) Drama ΨΨΨ
Joseph Losey film in which a wealthy British gentleman and his manservant wind up switching roles. There are strong homosexual overtones in the relationship between the two men, and a complex relationship develops with two women. The film is an interesting examination of dominance and submission.

Sexy Beast (2001) Drama ΨΨΨ
Ben Kingsley portrays a brutal antisocial personality who is anything but sexy.

Shadow of Fear (2004) Drama–Suspense Ψ
Disappointing film about a young businessman who is blackmailed after he accidentally kills a man with his car and tries to cover it up. James Spader's character displays strong antisocial characteristics.

Shape of Things, The (2003) Comedy ΨΨΨ
Disturbing comedy of a woman who helps transform an anxious, insecure man through physical alteration and love only to later reveal it was all a manipulative, self-serving project. Another film by director Neil LaBute who has been appropriately nicknamed by some film critics as Neil La-Brute because of his brutal character portrayal of people and society.

Shattered Glass (2003) Drama ΨΨΨ
Based on a true story of a young journalist for the popular *New Republic* magazine, Stephen Glass (well-acted by Hayden Christensen), who in 1998 made up several of his published stories. He was fraudulent with people, places, and events, making up fake business cards, notes, websites, phone numbers, and voice mails. The film depicts "the antisocial in trouble," a situation in which the person becomes neurotic and remorseful. The real-life Glass, a self-proclaimed pathological liar, admitted that 27 of his 41 published magazine stories were partially or completely made up.

Silence of the Lambs, The (1991) ΨΨΨΨΨ
Drama–Suspense
Anthony Hopkins plays one of film history's greatest antisocial personalities, psychiatrist and cannibal Hannibal Lector. Jodie Foster is the FBI agent.

"A census taker once tried to test me. I ate his liver with some fava beans and a nice Chianti."

The Silence of the Lambs **(1991)**

Sleeping With the Enemy (1991) Suspense ΨΨ
Julia Roberts plays the battered wife of a possessive and sadistic husband played by Patrick Bergin. Roberts fakes her death and assumes a new identity in a desperate attempt to escape.

Small Time Crooks (2000) Comedy Ψ
Woody Allen plays a "foolish antisocial" who devises a plan to rob a bank with his not-so-bright pals. Hugh Grant plays a manipulative, charming, self-serving narcissist.

Sneakers (1992) Drama–Comedy ΨΨ
This film has a star cast that includes Dan Akroyd, who plays an ex-convict with paranoid traits who sees conspiracy in almost every situation.

Solitary Man (2009) Drama ΨΨΨ
Michael Douglas plays the role of Ben Kalmen, a man with a narcissistic personality disorder who has failed as a salesman, father, grandfather, husband, lover, and friend.

Speed (1994) Drama ΨΨ
Dennis Hopper plays a deranged sociopath who programs a bomb to explode if a city bus slows to less than 50 miles per hour.

Stagecoach (1939) Western ΨΨΨ
Classic John Ford movie, with Thomas Mitchell playing a drunken physician. Mitchell won an Academy Award for Best Supporting Actor for his role.

Strangers on a Train (1951) Thriller ΨΨΨΨΨ
Classic Hitchcock film in which Farley Granger is unable to extricate himself from his involvement with sociopath Robert Walker.

Streetcar Named Desire, A (1951) Drama ΨΨΨΨΨ
Elia Kazan film starring Marlon Brando and Vivian Leigh. Blanche DuBois offers a striking example of a histrionic personality. Brando is unforgettable in the role of Stanley Kowalski. (Compare this film with Woody Allen's *Blue Jasmine*.)

Sunset Blvd. (1950) Drama ΨΨΨΨ
Billy Wilder film in which a narcissistic, histrionic, and delusional Gloria Swanson clings to the memories of her former greatness as a silent screen star. William Holden plays a young man who exchanges attention and sexual favors for security.

"They're dead, they're finished! There was a time in this business when they had the eyes of the whole wide world. But that wasn't good enough for them. Oh, no. They had to have the ears of the world, too. So they opened their big mouths, and out came talk. Talk! Talk!"

Gloria Swanson as Norma Desmond, in *Sunset Blvd.* (1950)

Suspect Zero (2004) Thriller-Crime ΨΨ
Ben Kingsley plays a serial killer who tries to catch a serial killer by attempting to tune into the killer's thoughts, intentions, and feelings.

Swimfan (2002) Drama-Suspense Ψ
A high school senior's one-night-stand with a fellow classmate shifts from infatuation to the conviction. "If I can't have you, no one will."

Swimming Pool (2002) Drama-Mystery ΨΨΨΨ
A mystery writer leaves London to find peace, quiet, and inspiration at her publisher's secluded home in a French village. She overcomes her writer's block by writing about the adventures of a seductive, provocative young woman, the publisher's daughter, who has spontaneously moved in.

Swimming With Sharks (1994) Comedy ΨΨ
Dark comedy with Kevin Spacey as a nasty, heartless, business executive who is held hostage and tortured by an employee he has verbally abused over the years.

Talented Mr. Ripley, The (1999) Drama ΨΨΨΨΨ
Matt Damon is the deceitful, charming, clever impersonator, Tom Ripley, who manipulates anyone in his path until he can no longer get away with his deceit. Breakthrough film for supporting actor Jude Law.

"I always thought it would be better to be a fake somebody than a real nobody."

Tom Ripley describing his secretive double life, in *The Talented Mr. Ripley* (1999)

Tao of Steve, The (2000) Comedy Ψ
Self-serving, amateur philosopher uses some ideas from Buddhist philosophy to pursue and sleep with women.

Tape (2001) Drama ΨΨΨΨ
Creative, engaging, and honest story of how people manipulate one another to meet their own desires and how they react when their secrets are exposed. It also shows what can happen when someone has unresolved psychological issues. The entire film takes place in one motel room with only three characters – all young veterans – Ethan Hawke, Robert Sean Leonard, and Uma Thurman.

Taxi Driver (1976) Drama ΨΨΨΨΨ
The premorbid personality of Travis Bickle illustrates delusional paranoid thinking. Bickle would probably meet the criteria for a diagnosis of schizotypal personality disorder.

"You talkin' to me? [slower] You talking to me? You talking to me? Well, then, who the hell else are you talking – you talking to me? Well, I'm the only one here."

Travis Bickle rehearsing, in *Taxi Driver* (1976)

There Will Be Blood (2007) Drama-Thriller ΨΨΨΨ
Daniel Day-Lewis portrays Daniel Plainview, a charismatic, ruthless oil prospector in this story of greed, religion, and family. Plainview is a good illustration of an antisocial personality disorder.

Thin Blue Line, The (1988) Documentary ΨΨΨ
Gripping documentary examining the unjust incarceration of a man accused of the murder of a Texas policeman.

To Die For (1995) Drama ΨΨ
Nicole Kidman plays the role of a newswoman who will do anything to advance her career, including having her husband killed.

Toto the Hero (*Toto le Heros;* 1991, France) ΨΨΨΨ
Drama-Comedy
An old man in a nursing home reviews his life and his lifelong hatred for his next-door neighbor, who appeared to have every advantage. Wonderful example of a paranoid personality disorder.

Town, The (2010) Drama ΨΨΨ
A bank robber seduces the teller he and his partners had earlier taken hostage; he falls in love with her but finds it hard to leave his criminal past behind him. Ben Affleck's character meets many of the criteria for antisocial personality disorder.

Treasure of the Sierra Madre, The (1948) ΨΨΨΨ
Drama
This is a wonderful John Huston film starring Humphrey Bogart. The movie explores obsessive greed, the folly of avarice, and the ways in which love of money can come to be the dominant force in one's life. Bogart's character is an example of a paranoid personality disorder.

"Badges? We ain't got no badges! We don't need no badges. I don't have to show you any stinkin' badges!"

***The Treasure of the Sierra Madre* (1948)**

Trucker (2008) Drama ΨΨ
A self-reliant woman finds her isolated life is turned upside down when her long-abandoned 11-year-old son turns up. It is useful for students to speculate about whether Michelle Monaghan's character meets DSM-5 criteria for a personality disorder.

Tsotsi (2005, South Africa/UK) Crime-Drama ΨΨΨΨ
An African gangster accidentally kidnaps an infant and in learning to care for the child makes some changes in himself.

Unfaithful (2002) Drama-Suspense ΨΨ
A married man (Richard Gere) finds out his wife (Diane Lane) is having an affair, and he seeks revenge.

Very Bad Things (1999) Comedy Ψ
Dark comedy about a bachelor party gone horribly wrong. As the five men try to cover up an accidental murder, more problems arise.

Vicky Cristina Barcelona (2008) Drama ΨΨΨ
Woody Allen film about two young women touring Barcelona for the summer who encounter a handsome man and his erratic, labile ex-wife (Penélope Cruz).

Violette Noziere (1978) Biography-Crime ΨΨ
Claude Chabrol film based on a true story about a teenage girl who poisoned her parents, eventually killing her father, whom she claimed had raped and abused her.

Wall Street (1987) Drama ΨΨΨΨ
Michael Douglas is memorable as Gordon Gekko, a man who clearly meets criteria for a diagnosis of antisocial personality disorder.

"The richest one percent of this country owns half our country's wealth, five trillion dollars. One third of that comes from hard work, two thirds comes from inheritance, interest on interest accumulating to widows and idiot sons and what I do, stock and real estate speculation. It's bullshit. You got ninety percent of the American public out there with little or no net worth. I create nothing. I own. We make the rules, pal."

Gordon Gekko explains capitalism to Bud Fox, in *Wall Street* (1987)

Wall Street: Money Never Sleeps (2010)
Drama ΨΨΨ
Gordon Gekko returns to Wall Street after serving an 8-year sentence for securities fraud.

Wannsee Conference, The (1984)
Historical-War ΨΨΨ
Recreation of the Berlin meeting in which Nazi officers first outlined the "final solution" for dealing with the Jewish problem.

Welcome to Me (2014) Comedy-Drama ΨΨΨ
A woman being treated for borderline personality disorder wins the lottery, stops taking her medications, and buys her own talk show because she "wants to be like Oprah."

Whisperers, The (1966) Drama Ψ
Dame Edith Evans stars as a lonely old woman, divorced from her husband and estranged from her son, who devotes her days to worry and paranoid ramblings.

White Oleander (2002) Drama ΨΨΨΨ
A young girl is moved from home to home when her mother is incarcerated. The mother figures include characters played by Michelle Pfeiffer (antisocial), Renée Zellweger (dependent), and Robin Wright-Penn (histrionic). Fascinating dynamics of a young girl's resilience with each personality disordered mother figure.

Who Loves the Sun (2006) Drama ΨΨ
Will discovers that his wife is having an affair with Daniel, the best man from their wedding, and he copes by

dropping out of sight for 5 years. Daniel's character illustrates narcissistic personality disorder.

Wild at Heart (1990) Comedy–Drama–Romance ΨΨΨ
David Lynch film starring ex-con Nicolas Cage and his lover, Laura Dern, as two antisocial personalities (despite their apparent commitment to each other). This film won the Palme d'Or at Cannes, but not all critics were impressed – too violent for some tastes.

Willard (2003) Drama Ψ
Crispin Glover plays a schizoid man whose only contact is his critical mother and numerous rats living in his basement. He uses the rats for revenge until they turn on him.

Wise Blood (1979) Drama ΨΨΨ
John Huston's adaptation of Flannery O'Connor's gothic Southern novel about an obsessed preacher.

Zoolander (2001) Comedy Ψ
Absurd, over-the-top depiction of a narcissistic model who is brainwashed to become an assassin. Ben Stiller directed, cowrote, and starred in this film.

Paraphilic Disorders

8MM (1999) Mystery–Thriller ΨΨ
Joel Schumacher film about the underground world of "snuff" films. Stars Nicolas Cage, Joaquin Phoenix, and James Gandolfini, and depicts the worst kind of sadism.

Adjuster, The (1991) Drama ΨΨΨ
This interesting Canadian film explores voyeurism and exhibitionism.

Aleksandr's Price (2013) Drama ΨΨ
A Russian immigrant loses his mother, becomes involved with drugs, and then is drawn into the gay underworld as a male prostitute.

Angels and Insects (1995) Drama ΨΨΨ
Complex drama about social class, passion, incest, and hidden sexual secrets in a wealthy Victorian household.

Another Time, Another Place (1983) Drama ΨΨΨ
Sensitive film in which a Scottish woman in an unhappy marriage has a brief affair with an Italian prisoner of war working as a laborer on the farm. The man is accused of a rape he did not commit; his lover can save him, but only at the cost of revealing her adultery.

Antichrist (2009) Drama–Horror ΨΨΨ
A controversial Lars von Trier film about a grieving couple who lost their infant son when the child fell from a window while the man and his wife were making love. They retreat to a country cabin where the woman quickly decompensates and becomes psychotic, and the couple engage in sadomasochistic behavior. The film has four chapters, titled "Grief," "Pain (Chaos Reigns)," "Despair (Gynocide)," and "The Three Beggars." The film, dedicated to the Russian director Andrei Tarkovsky, stars Willem Dafoe as the therapist husband and Charlotte Gainsbourg as the grieving wife.

Bad Timing: A Sensual Obsession (1980) Drama ΨΨ
Art Garfunkel (playing a psychology professor), Harvey Keitel, and Theresa Russell star in a provocative and explicit film about a psychiatrist who becomes sexually obsessed with a young woman after she makes a suicide attempt.

Beginner's Luck (1983) Comedy ΨΨ
Lightweight comedy about a law student who becomes involved in a ménage à trois.

Blame It on Rio (1984) Comedy ΨΨ
Two men take their teenage daughters to Rio's topless beaches, and one of the men, 43 years old, has an affair with the 15-year-old daughter of the other. The film has a vaguely incestuous theme and is modeled after the French film *One Wild Moment*. Also see the 2013 film *Adore* in which two mothers commit boundary violations, each with the other's son.

Bliss (1997) Drama ΨΨ
A very fragile woman with a borderline personality disorder goes to a charming sex therapist (Spalding Gray) who sleeps with his patients. After confronting the therapist, the husband converts and becomes his disciple. The film illustrates numerous ethical violations, and it demeans sacred Hindu tantric practices. (Note that there are about a dozen films titled *Bliss*. The 2021 German version is the best.)

Bliss (*Glück;* 2021, Germany) Drama ΨΨΨ
Two sex workers in a Berlin brothel fall in love; one is satisfied with her life, while the other one longs for more. Dialogue is in both German and English, but English subtitles are provided when German is spoken.

Blue Angel, The (1930) Drama ΨΨΨΨΨ
Classic film about a phlegmatic professor who loses everything because of his obsession with a cabaret singer.

Blue Car (2002) Drama ΨΨΨ
Independent film about an adolescent girl who is seduced by her teacher. Good depiction of the disturbing, subtle aspects of seduction and sexual exploitation.

Blue Velvet (1986) Mystery ΨΨΨΨ
A powerful and engrossing David Lynch film about drugs, sexual violence, and sadomasochism. Dennis Hopper portrays Frank Booth, one of the most sociopathic and sadistic villains in film history.

Bound (1996) Suspense-Drama ΨΨ
A tough female ex-con and her new female lover concoct a scheme to steal mob money. This film noir is the Wachowski brothers' directorial debut.

Breaking the Waves (1996, Denmark) Drama ΨΨΨ
A Danish film set in Scotland in which a devout Catholic wife submits to sexual degradation to satisfy the voyeuristic demands of her paralyzed husband. Directed by Lars von Trier.

Dr. Richardson: "Look for Christ's sake, he's... he's forcing you to get screwed by every Tom, Dick and Harry... it's just not you."
Bess McNeill: "I don't make love with them. I make love with Jan, and I save him from dying."
Dr. Richardson: [exhales] "Well I'm sorry, but, you know, to me seems more like a dirty old man who wants to play the Peeping Tom."

Bess tries to explain her behavior, in *Breaking the Waves* (1996)

Cabaret (1972) Musical-Drama-Dance ΨΨΨΨ
Liza Minnelli in a film about sadomasochism, bisexuality, and the relationship between sex and power. *Cabaret* won Oscars for Best Actor, Best Actress, and Best Director. One scene in the film is as unforgettable as the classic confession of incest in *Chinatown*.

Caesar and Rosalie (1972) Comedy-Romance ΨΨ
Lighthearted and amusing examination of a ménage à trois.

Capturing the Friedmans (2003) ΨΨΨΨ
Documentary
Extraordinarily disturbing and emotional documentary about a father and son accused of pedophilia. Important film to see regarding sex addiction, pedophilia, and the importance of not casting judgment too quickly.

"Don't worry, you've got everything under control."

A therapist's comments to a pedophile who was worried he might molest his own children; he later molests numerous children in a class he teaches out of his home, in *Capturing the Friedmans* (2003)

Chinatown (1974) Mystery ΨΨΨΨ
A film about power, incest, and the complexity of human relationships. Actors includes Jack Nicholson, Faye Dunaway, and John Huston.

"You see, Mr. Gettes, most people never have to face the fact that, at the right time and in the right place, they are capable of anything."

***Chinatown* (1974)**

Claire's Knee (1971, France) Drama ΨΨΨ
An intelligent film in which a middle-aged man becomes obsessed with a young girl's knee.

Close My Eyes (1991) Drama ΨΨ
A British film about brother-sister incest.

Collector, The (1965) Drama ΨΨΨ
Terence Stamp stars as a young man who collects butterflies. He becomes obsessed with Samantha Eggar, kidnaps her, and winds up inadvertently killing her.

Crash (1996) Drama ΨΨΨ
A David Cronenberg film about people who become sexually aroused by automobile accidents. The film presents a plausible hypothesis: People have developed fetishes for stranger things, and there are erotic overtones to both cars and speed.

"You couldn't wait for me? You did the Jane Mansfield crash without me!"

One of many strange interactions in *David Cronenberg's Crash* (1996)

Cruising (1980) Crime Ψ
Controversial William Friedkin film starring Al Pacino as an undercover police officer who infiltrates gay bars and bathhouses. Gay activists condemned the film because it perpetuates stigma and stereotypes.

Dahmer (2002) Biography-Drama ΨΨ
A docudrama about the life of serial killer and cannibal Jeffrey Dahmer who served 2 years of a life sentence before being killed by another inmate on November 28, 1994. Dahmer was 34 years old when he died.

Day in the Country, A (1936) Romance ΨΨΨΨ
Jean Renoir's adaptation of a short story by Guy de Maupassant that describes the seductions of a man's wife and daughter.

Dark Tourist (2013) Drama ΨΨ
Michael is a "dark tourist" – he travels to places where atrocities have been committed such as mass murders. While visiting an arson site in California, Michael becomes involved with a waitress played by Melanie Griffith.

Desert Flower (2009) Biography ΨΨΨ
This autobiographical film details the life of a Somalian nomad who was subjected to female genital mutilation (FGM) as a child to ensure she would not be able to experience sexual pleasure as an adult. She was forced to marry a much older man when she was 13 but escaped and moved to London where she eventually became a celebrated model – and an outspoken opponent of FGM.

Disconnect (2013) Drama ΨΨΨ
This film presents three stories, all of which relate to social media and online communications. One story involves a teenage male prostitute who engages in online chat room sex; one involves identity theft of a couple, both of whom are involved with illicit online activities; and one story is about two high school boys who impersonate a girl and persuade a shy boy to send them a nude photo of himself. The photo is sent to everyone in his high school class, and he subsequently attempts suicide, ending up in a coma.

Door in the Floor, The (2003) Drama ΨΨ
A couple separates after the deaths of their twin sons. The catalyst for the breakup is Eddie, a 16-year-old who takes a job as Jeff Bridges' assistant. Eddie is infatuated by Kim Bassinger's character and masturbates using her photos and undergarments to become aroused. Bassinger eventually seduces Eddie, who reminds her of her dead sons. Based on a novel by John Irving.

Dreamers, The (2003) Drama ΨΨΨ
Fraternal twins take in a roommate in this Bernardo Bertolucci exploration of politics, cinema, and sexuality. The dynamics become complicated when the new roommate falls in love with the female twin, taking her virginity and challenging her enmeshment with her brother.

"A filmmaker is like a peeping Tom, a voyeur. It's as if the camera is the key to your parent's bedroom and you spy on them, and you're disgusted, and you feel guilty, but you can't ... you can't look away."

***The Dreamers* (2003)**

Eros (2004) Drama ΨΨΨ
Three noted directors (Michelangelo Antonioni, Steven Soderbergh, and Wong Kar Wai) each contribute a short film dealing with some aspect of sexuality (e.g., a ménage à trois, voyeurism, and prostitution).

Everything You Always Wanted to Know About Sex * But Were Afraid to Ask (1972) Comedy ΨΨ
Woody Allen classic includes vignettes on crossing dressing, bestiality, sex in public, and the inner workings of the brain during sexual excitement.

Evil Alien Conquerors (2002) Comedy Ψ
Painfully bad film in which former Saturday Night Live star, Chris Parnell, has a foot fetish.

Eyes Wide Shut (1999) Drama ΨΨΨΨΨ
The final Stanley Kubrick film about a man (Tom Cruise) who discovers a sexual underworld after his wife (Nicole Kidman) tells him of her fantasies and previous sexual encounters. Depiction of ephebophilia (sexual attraction of adults to adolescents), orgies, sexual rituals, exhibitionism, prostitution, infidelity, sexual fantasy, seduction, and betrayal. Mythological and Jungian psychology themes are omnipresent.

Feed (2005) Mystery Ψ
A sociopath with a fat fetish houses, feeds and videotapes morbidly obese women, putting the tapes he makes on a pornographic website and taking bets on how long each woman will live.

Fellini Satyricon (1970) Historical ΨΨΨΨ
Controversial Fellini film about the decadence of ancient Rome. The film is visually stunning and explores human vices ranging from pedophilia to cannibalism. The film can be a springboard for a discussion of hedonism.

Female Perversions (1996) Drama ΨΨΨ
Confused and often confusing examination of the relationship between women, power, sexuality, and psychopathology. Based on a scholarly book with the same title by psychoanalyst Louise J. Kaplan.

Fetishes (1996) Documentary ΨΨΨ
True examination of the clients of Pandora's Box, an elite club catering to the sexual fetishes in New York City.

Fist in His Pocket (1966) Drama ΨΨΨ
Italian film about a dysfunctional family with multiple examples of psychopathology including epilepsy, murder, and incest.

Girl 6 (1996) Drama-Comedy Ψ
Spike Lee film about a woman who takes a job as a phone sex operator for the money.

God's Little Acre (1958) Drama Ψ
Buddy Hackett and Michael Landon star in this adaptation of Erskine Caldwell's tale of depravity and Georgia farm life.

Good Mother, The (1988) Drama ΨΨΨ
A provocative film in which Diane Keaton plays the divorced mother of a 6-year-old daughter. Keaton falls in love with an iconoclastic artist, who allows the daughter to touch his penis when she sees him in the shower and expresses normal childhood curiosity. Keaton is eventually forced to denounce her new lover to maintain a relationship with her daughter.

Happiness (1998) Comedy-Drama ΨΨΨ
Disturbing dark comedy portraying a variety of quirky characters. The most striking are the pedophiliac psychiatrist who drugs and rapes his son's best friend, and Philip Seymour Hoffman as a man who is obsessed with telephone scatologia. Director Todd Solondz has a cameo as a doorman.

Joe: "What do you think would happen if I got him a professional ... you know ..."
Bill: "A professional?"
Joe: "Hooker. You know, the kind that can teach things ... first-timers, you know ... break him in."
Bill: "But Joe, he's 11."
Joe: "You're right, you're right. It's too late."

Cultures clash in *Happiness* (1998)

Hard Candy (2005) Drama ΨΨ
A pedophile arranges to meet a 14-year-old girl who turns things around and winds up being the aggressor.

Henry & June (1990) Drama ΨΨ
Adaptation of Anais Nin diary detailing her ménage à trois with novelist Henry Miller and his wife June.

Holy Smoke (1999) Drama ΨΨΨ
Jane Campion film about a family who believes their daughter (Kate Winslet) is under the power of a cult leader. They hire a renowned "cult exiter" (Harvey Keitel) whose role is to isolate the subject, provoke them, and then reintegrate them into the family. After an interesting role reversal, he finds himself developing a sexual obsession.

Human Nature (2001) Comedy ΨΨ
Fascinating study on instinct and desire, about a man raised in the wild and the scientists he encounters.

Hunt, The (2013, Denmark) Drama ΨΨΨ
A schoolteacher loses his job and is going through a divorce; however, his life seems to be improving until he is unfairly accused of pedophilia.

In the Realm of the Senses (1977, Japan) Drama ΨΨΨ
A sadomasochistic relationship intensifies into highly graphic and unforgettable scenes of autoerotic asphyxiation and the severing of a penis.

Intimacy (2000) Drama ΨΨ
A depressed man and woman meet for anonymous sex in a dilapidated apartment once a week. The man becomes curious about the woman and follows her to learn more about her. Slow, dark film that depicts the double life of the addict.

Ju Dou (1990, China) Drama-Historical-Romance ΨΨΨΨ
Wonderful, visually stunning film examining the complex links that bind a husband, his wife, her lover, and the son of the illicit union. Good illustrations of sexual passion and sexual torment.

Jules and Jim (1962, France) Drama ΨΨΨΨΨ
Beautiful and engaging Truffaut film about a complex ménage à trois and an ultimate suicide. The film deals with far more than sexuality; it explores fundamental dimensions of human relationships and the boundaries of friendship and love.

"Love is the answer, isn't it? But sex raises a lot of very interesting questions."

***Kinsey* (2004)**

Kinsey (2004) Drama-Biography ΨΨΨΨ
Examination of the life of Alfred Kinsey, a sex researcher who revolutionized the way Americans viewed sexuality. The film depicts Kinsey's obsessive-compulsive

personality, his inability to connect in a deep way, and the failure to set boundaries for his own (and his research team's) sexual practices.

Kissed (1996) Drama ΨΨΨ
A controversial but sensitive film dealing seriously with necrophilia. Molly Parker is the protagonist, a young woman obsessed from childhood with death. She gets a job in a mortuary and has ritualistic sex ("crossing over") with the bodies she embalms. Her boyfriend commits suicide when he realizes this is the only way to fully earn her affection and attention.

Last Exit to Brooklyn (1989) Drama ΨΨ
A film based on a controversial book about life in a sordid Brooklyn neighborhood. The film deals with rape, prostitution, homosexuality, and transvestism, but mostly with the sad and bleak reality of the lives of its characters.

Leap Year (2011, Mexico) Drama ΨΨΨΨ
Laura, a 25-year-old journalist, has numerous one-night stands until she meets Arturo who introduces her to the world of sadomasochistic sex. She embraces and expands this new sexual role as her lover beats her, urinates on her, chokes her, burns her, and rubs a knife over her naked body.

Leaving Neverland (2019, Britain) Documentary ΨΨΨ
This controversial film involves interviews with two grown men who alleged that they were sexually abused by Michael Jackson when they visited his Neverland Ranch as children.

Little Children (2007) Drama ΨΨΨΨ
This film portrays several sexually troubled characters but is especially memorable for the roles of Jackie Earle Haley playing a pedophile, and Kate Winslet playing the role of a parent who overcomes her repugnance to befriend him.

Lolita (1962) Drama ΨΨΨΨ
James Mason and Sue Lyons star in a loose adaptation of Vladimir Nabokov's novel about pedophilia and murder. Laurence Olivier turned down the role of Humbert Humbert. Directed by Stanley Kubrick; watch for Peter Sellers as Dr. Zempf, the Beardsley High School psychologist.

> **"What drives me insane is the twofold nature of this nymphet ... this mixture in my Lolita of tender, dreamy childishness and a kind of eerie vulgarity."**
>
> **Humbert Humbert in *Lolita* (1962)**

Luna (1979) Drama ΨΨ
A Bertolucci film that explores mother-son incest and addiction; a recently widowed mother begins a sexual relationship with her 15-year-old son to help him overcome his heroin addiction. The film is not Bertolucci's best effort.

Lust, Caution (2007) Drama ΨΨΨ
An Ang Lee film about a young Chinese woman who seduces a sadistic Japanese leader.

M (1931, Germany) Crime-Drama-Thriller ΨΨΨΨ
A Fritz Lang film about a psychopathic Berlin pedophile who is murdering young children.

Manhattan (1979) Comedy-Romance ΨΨΨΨ
Classic Woody Allen film in which a character's former wife, played by Meryl Streep, has taken a lover, found happiness, and written a book to tell the world about her former husband's kinky habits. The protagonist (in an example of art imitating life) is consumed with guilt over the fact that he is living with a 17-year-old high school girl.

Mark, The (1961) Drama ΨΨΨΨ
A British film about a pedophile who serves his sentence and is released, supposedly cured. However, a journalist who reveals the man's past hampers his rehabilitation. Interesting film considering recent court decisions about sex offenders.

Matador (1986) Comedy-Drama ΨΨ
Almodóvar film about a bullfighter who acts in snuff films.

Menage (1986, France) Comedy ΨΨ
A French film that examines sex roles, sexual stereotypes, and the need for novelty and excitement in sexual relationships.

Midsummer Night's Sex Comedy, A (1982) ΨΨ
Excellent Woody Allen film about friends and acquaintances who gather at a country house in the woods at the turn of the century. Sexual boundaries blur in this homage to Shakespeare, Renoir, and others.

Mona Lisa (1986) Crime ΨΨΨ
Interesting Neil Jordan film about prostitution, exploitation, drug addiction, and love. Filmed in Soho, the film gives some insight into the two different worlds of prostitution: that of the call girl and that of the streetwalker.

Murmur of the Heart (*Le Souffle Au Coeur;* 1971, France) Comedy–Drama ΨΨ
A sensitive, intelligent, and funny French film about an incestuous relationship between a young mother and her adolescent son.

My Favorite Season (*Ma Saison Préférée;* 1993, France) Drama ΨΨΨ
A French film dealing with adolescent sexuality, family dynamics, and love between a brother and sister. Catherine Deneuve stars in the film.

My Life to Live (1962, France) ΨΨΨ
Jean-Luc Godard's 12-part examination of the life of a prostitute, starring Anna Karina.

My Own Private Idaho (1991) Drama ΨΨ
River Phoenix, who subsequently died of a drug overdose, plays a homosexual prostitute.

Nine ½ Weeks (1986) Drama–Suspense ΨΨ
Excellent character portrayals by Mickey Rourke and Kim Bassinger who meet at a grocery store and later engage in sensual sexual exploration and mild sadomasochism.

Of Human Bondage (1934) Drama ΨΨ
Bette Davis stars in this film about the sexual obsession of a club-footed physician for a cruel, vulgar, and manipulative waitress. Based on a novel by Somerset Maugham. This film is far superior to the two adaptations that followed it, and none of the films are quite as good as the novel.

"You dirty swine! I never cared for you ... It made me sick when you kissed me. I only did it because you drove me crazy. And after you kissed me, I always used to wipe my mouth – wipe my mouth!"

***Of Human Bondage* (1934)**

Oldboy (2003) Drama ΨΨΨΨ
This is an unforgettable Korean film directed by Chan-Wook Park about a man kidnapped and imprisoned for 15 years who becomes involved in an unwitting incestuous relationship with the daughter he had not seen for 15 years.

On Line (2002) Drama ΨΨΨ
A film about Internet addiction. The emphasis is on the lack of connection and relational intimacy of the addict. Depicts an obsession with fantasy that becomes confused with reality.

Oscar Wilde (1960) Biography Ψ
Robert Morley plays Oscar Wilde, a playwright who was convicted of sodomy in 1895.

Peeping Tom (1960) Thriller ΨΨΨ
Controversial film about a sexual psychopath who photographs his victims as they are dying. Look for the full-length version of the film, which was released in 1979. The protagonist's father is a psychologist.

Pervert Park (2014) Documentary ΨΨΨΨ
Frida and Lasse Barkfors interview the residents of a trailer park in St. Petersburg, Florida set aside for 120 registered sex offenders. The residents tell their stories, and you may find yourself feeling empathetic and supportive of the efforts of these men to turn their lives around.

Piano Teacher, The (*La Pianiste;* 2001, France) Drama ΨΨΨΨ
This is a powerful film about a prominent, masochistic piano teacher who becomes sexually involved with one of her pupils. The film makes sexual obsession understandable and plausible.

"It's being aware of what it means to lose oneself before being completely abandoned."

***The Piano Teacher* (2001)**

Pillow Book (1997) Drama ΨΨΨΨ
Complex Peter Greenaway film about a woman who becomes sexually obsessed with calligraphy. This film is a meditation on love, art and imagination, eroticism, order, and decay.

Pretty Baby (1978) Drama ΨΨ
This Louis Malle film about pedophilia introduces Brooke Shields as a 12-year-old New Orleans prostitute.

Pretty When You Cry (2001) Drama–Suspense Ψ
Mostly flashbacks as detectives follow up a murder investigation with a young man who tells the story of his infatuation and love for a beautiful woman who was in an abusive relationship. The masochistic-sadistic relationship is portrayed, as well as physical, verbal, and emotional abuse.

Priest (1994) Drama ΨΨ
A priest struggles to deal with the sanctity of confession after a young girl tells him she is being molested by her father.

Private Lessons (1981) Drama Ψ
A French maid seduces a 15-year-old boy and betrays his trust.

Private Parts (1997) Comedy Ψ
Inside look at radio personality Howard Stern and his obsession with sex and outlandish comedy

Psychopathia Sexualis (2006) Drama Ψ
Based directly on the classic Krafft-Ebing text, the film depicts a variety of fetishes and other paraphilias.

Pulp Fiction (1994) Drama ΨΨΨΨΨ
This Quentin Tarantino film depicts an underworld sadomasochistic den of iniquity run by two sexual sadists in the basement of an Army surplus store. A masochistic slave dressed totally in leather lives in a box in the back of the room.

> **"Look, maybe your method of massage differs from mine, but touchin' his lady's feet, and stickin' your tongue in her holiest of holies, ain't the same ballpark, ain't the same league, ain't even the same fuckin' sport. Foot massages don't mean shit."**
>
> **A discussion of foot massage, in *Pulp Fiction* (1994)**

Quills (2000) Drama ΨΨΨ
Depiction of the last years of the Marquis de Sade (well played by Geoffrey Rush) who was sent to the Charenton Insane Asylum as punishment for his erotic writings. Interesting portrayal of various paraphilias.

Reader, The (2008) Drama ΨΨΨΨ
Kate Winslet plays Hanna Schmitz, a Nazi concentration camp guard who seduces a young boy who later grows up and becomes a prominent attorney.

Rita, Sue and Bob Too (1986) Comedy ΨΨΨ
British film about a married man who winds up in a sexual relationship with the two working-class teenage girls who babysit for his children. Interesting examination of the appropriate age for consent and issues of sexual exploitation.

Rocky Horror Picture Show, The (1975)
Comedy-Horror-Musical-Dance Ψ
A fun film about a Transylvanian transsexual. From a psychological perspective, the film is not nearly as interesting as the fans are who have turned it into a cult classic.

Salò, or the 120 Days of Sodom (1975, Italy) Drama Ψ
Based on the writings of the Marquis de Sade, and arguably an allegory denouncing the excesses of fascism. Some reviewers consider this controversial last film of Italian director Pier Paolo Pasolini a classic. I disagree and believe the coprophagia and extreme sexual violence are largely gratuitous.

Secretary (2002) Drama ΨΨΨ
A self-injurious, depressed woman is hired as a secretary after leaving a mental hospital; she takes a new job and begins to enjoy the criticism and punishment inflicted by her boss. They develop a sadomasochistic relationship in the work setting and eventually fall in love and marry.

> **"In one way or another I've always suffered. I didn't know why exactly. But I do know that I'm not so scared of suffering now. I feel more than I've ever felt, and I've found someone to feel with. To play with. To love in a way that feels right for me."**
>
> **Reflections on masochism, in *Secretary* (2002)**

Sergeant, The (1968) Drama ΨΨ
Rod Steiger plays an Army sergeant sexually obsessed with a young private in his outfit. The film underscores the difficulties associated with being gay in the military.

Sex and Zen (1993) Comedy Ψ
Second-rate film about a Buddhist who leaves his master and new wife to seek out a life of debauchery and erotic pleasures.

Sex Is Zero (2002) Comedy Ψ
A Korean *Animal House*, but not as clever. The film involves lots of teens sexually acting out in a variety of ways.

Sex, Lies and Videotape (1989) Drama ΨΨΨ
A Steven Soderbergh film about an impotent man who can achieve orgasm only when masturbating while watching videotapes of women whom he has persuaded to share the most intimate details of their sexual lives. This film won the top award at the Cannes Film Festival.

Sexting in Suburbia *(*2012) Drama ΨΨ
A teenage girl commits suicide in response to the cyberbullying that resulted after her boyfriend shared nude photos of her with her classmates. Also known under the title *Shattered Silence*.

Short Cuts (1993) Drama ΨΨ
Most memorable for a scene in which a bored woman talks dirty on the phone to earn a few dollars while she changes her baby's diapers. Her husband wonders why she never talks to *him* like that.

Short Eyes (1977) Prison ΨΨΨΨ
A powerful film about life in The Tombs, New York City's Men's House of Detention. Short Eyes is prison slang for a child molester.

Short Film About Love, A (1988, Poland) Drama ΨΨ
This Krzysztof Kieslowski film deals with themes of voyeurism, exhibitionism, humiliation, and suicide.

Skin I Live In, The (*La Piel Que Habito;* 2011, Spain) Thriller ΨΨΨΨ
Pedro Almodóvar film starring Antonio Banderas as Dr. Robert Ledgard, a gifted but troubled plastic surgeon. This film is too good to spoil with a plot summary, but it is highly recommended.

Sliver (1993) Drama Ψ
William Baldwin plays a voyeur who is the landlord of an apartment complex with high tech cameras set up in the tenants' rooms.

Something About Amelia (1984) Drama ΨΨ
Popular made-for-TV movie about father-daughter incest. The film illustrates the family dynamics involved when a daughter accuses her father of sexual abuse.

Strange One, The (1957) Drama ΨΨ
Ben Gazzara stars in this film about homosexuality and sadism in a Southern military academy.

Tale, The (2018) Drama ΨΨΨΨΨ
A documentary filmmaker (Laura Dern) who has repressed childhood memories of grooming and abuse eventually confronts the running coach and riding instructor who had abused her. The film raises interesting questions about how salient events (like rape) can be repressed or ignored, and sometimes entirely forgotten.

This World, Then the Fireworks (1997) Drama ΨΨ
This film traces the development of incestuous twins who eventually become con artists.

Three (2010, Germany) Drama ΨΨ
In this Tom Tykwer film, a long-time couple wind up independently having an affair with the same man who is both a stem cell scientist and a sex addict.

Tie Me Up! Tie Me Down! (*Átame!*; 1990, Spain) Comedy-Romance ΨΨΨ
A Pedro Almodóvar film about a former mental patient, kidnapping, masochism, and sex roles. Many critics have maintained that the film trivializes the problem of sexual violence and denigrates women.

Torch Song Trilogy (1988) Drama ΨΨΨ
Anne Bancroft and Matthew Broderick in a film adaptation Harvey Fierstein's play about a homosexual drag queen and his lovers, enemies, and mother.

Towelhead (2007) Drama ΨΨΨ
A naïve, 13-year-old, Arab American girl moves from Syracuse to Houston and encounters several challenges associated with her emerging sexuality, including being the victim of ephebophilia.

Venus (2006) Drama ΨΨΨ
Peter O'Toole plays an aging actor with prostate cancer who falls in love with a teenage girl.

Viridiana (1961, Spain) Drama ΨΨΨΨ
This complex Luis Buñuel film tells the story of a young woman who returns home to visit her uncle just before taking vows as a nun. She resembles her dead aunt, and her uncle drugs her while she is wearing her aunt's wedding dress. He plans to rape her but is unable to commit the act. He commits suicide; she inherits his estate and devotes her life to serving the poor.

Visiting Desire (1996) Documentary ΨΨ
Twelve strangers are brought together to act out their sexual fantasies.

Voyeur Confessions (2001) Drama ΨΨ
This film captures the pain associated with the life of the voyeur. The movie touches on the etiology of voyeurism, and helps serious students better understand paraphilias.

"Stealing images from life is my life."

A voyeur describes himself, in *Voyeur Confessions* (2001)

Weiner (2016) Documentary ΨΨΨ
A disgraced Congressman resigns after confessing to sexting, then tries to make a political comeback in a campaign for mayor of New York City. He fails, loses his marriage, and is eventually sent to prison for sending obscene material to a minor.

Wild Orchid 2: Two Shades of Blue (1991) Drama Ψ
Disappointing film about the daughter of a heroin addict who becomes a prostitute to support her father's habit while maintaining a double identity.

Woodsman, The (2004) Drama ΨΨΨ
Kevin Bacon plays a pedophile recently released from prison struggling to establish a satisfying sexual relationship with a mature coworker.

World's Greatest Dad (2009) Black Comedy ΨΨΨ
An unhappy high school English teacher (Robin Williams) discovers his son has died from autoerotic asphyxiation. To save his son from being humiliated, the teacher hangs his son in his closet and attaches a poetic suicide note. The father eventually distributes a journal that he claims his son wrote, and the writing achieves the notoriety that the father could never achieve on his own. Eventually the father confesses to his duplicity.

Andrew: "You know what's strange about the book?"
Lance Clayton: "What?"
Andrew: "Kyle never talks about vaginas, anal sex, fisting, felching, or rimjobs."
Lance Clayton: "Yeah, it is a little light in the felching area, you're right. But I think it's there, Andrew, in its own way."

High school boys question their friend's literary ability, in *World's Greatest Dad*

Violence, Physical and Sexual Abuse

2LDK (2002) Drama-Action ΨΨ
A little-known but striking independent film about two girls rooming together temporarily as they compete in an acting audition. A simple argument turns into a violent battle between the two roommates. The methods of violence are unique and extraordinary, despite being contained in one apartment.

3-Iron (2004, South Korea) ΨΨΨ
A man breaks into houses when people are away for vacation and engages in mundane activities while living there temporarily. He encounters a mute woman who is the victim of domestic violence, and they continue his activities together.

5 x 2 (2004, France) Drama ΨΨΨ
Five stages of a couple's romance are portrayed backwards from their divorce; the film depicts conflict, rape, emotional stonewalling, poor decisions, and neglect of their relationship.

8 Mile (2002) Drama ΨΨ
Director Curtis Hanson depicts the struggles, racism, and abuse of rapper, Eminem. "8 mile" is a road in Detroit that represents several cinematic themes: it is the borderline and boundary between Blacks and Whites, city and suburbia, and the authentic and nonauthentic.

300 (2006) Action-History ΨΨΨ
Leonidas, the fearless leader of Sparta, leads 300 men against the vast Persian army of well over 100,000 in the infamous 480 BC Battle of Thermopylae.

Accused, The (1988) Drama ΨΨΨΨ
Jodie Foster won an Academy Award for Best Actress for her role as a woman who is gang raped in a bar. Her character chooses to prosecute for rape rather than aggravated assault; and the film examines the legal relevance of lifestyle (alcohol, drugs, and promiscuity) to the event and the complicity of bystanders. Based on a true story.

Aileen: Life and Death of a Serial Killer ΨΨΨ
(2003) Documentary
Nick Broomfield directed this documentary about serial killer Aileen Carol Wuornos, a highway prostitute who was executed in Florida in 2002 for killing seven men. The film includes the filmmaker's testimony at Wuornos' trial. (See also *Monster.*)

Air I Breathe, The (2007) Crime-Drama ΨΨ
Violent, action-filled gangster movie that explores interesting themes – happiness, pleasure, sorrow, and love – yet falls short of delivering something meaningful.

Alphabet Killer, The (2008) Drama Ψ
A detective is determined to arrest the alphabet killer, a man who is both a serial rapist and murderer; however, her work is set back when she is diagnosed with paranoid schizophrenia.

American History X (1998) Drama-Suspense ΨΨΨ
Edward Norton plays a former skinhead who has decided to leave gang life but must also convince his younger brother.

American Psycho (1999) Drama-Suspense ΨΨΨ
Christian Bale plays Patrick Bateman, a narcissistic Wall Street executive, who emphasizes excess and style over substance in everything from business cards and facial

cleansers to restaurant selection and conversation. He is depicted as a serial killer who saves the victim's heads in his refrigerator. However, there is cinematic evidence to suggest that there were no murders at all, and everything in the film simply reflects the fantasies of an antisocial mind.

Amores Perros (2000, Mexico) ΨΨΨ
Action-Suspense
Mexican film with a nonlinear plot with various hit men, murderers, and other perpetrators of highly graphic violence. Abuse and senseless killing of humans and animals are depicted. Also marketed under the title *Love's a Bitch.*

Anatomy of a Murder (1959) Drama ΨΨΨΨ
Classic courtroom drama in which Jimmy Stewart plays a prosecuting attorney in a case involving rape and promiscuity. The film presents an interesting analysis of the "irresistible impulse" defense.

Antonia's Line (1995) Comedy ΨΨΨΨ
Remarkable film about the resiliency of the human spirit, the power of love, and the importance of families. It is included here because of its treatment of a rapist, but also because of its treatment of people with an intellectual disability, the suicide of a major character, the film's open acceptance of sexual differences, and the characters' healthy attitudes about aging and death.

Apocalypse Now (1979) War ΨΨΨΨΨ
Francis Ford Coppola produced and directed this classic war film, which stars Marlon Brando, Robert Duvall, and Martin Sheen. The film is loosely based on Joseph Conrad's *Heart of Darkness* and was designed to drive home the madness and folly of war. Perhaps the best-known line in the film is "I love the smell of Napalm in the morning."

"Every man has got a breaking point. You and I have. Walter Kurtz has reached his. And, very obviously, he has gone insane."

An army general speaking of Colonel Kurtz in *Apocalypse Now* (1979), trying to describe his aberrant behavior

---

Apocalypto (2006) Thriller-Drama ΨΨ
Exceedingly violent Mel Gibson film depicting the collapse of the Mayan civilization.

Babel (2006) Drama ΨΨΨΨ
Stories from a variety of cultures (Morocco, Mexico, Japan) interweave around themes of communication and the tragic consequences of violence and miscommunication.

Badlands (1973) Crime-Drama ΨΨΨ
Film based on a true story about a sociopathic young man who takes up with a 15-year-old girl and goes on a killing spree. The film effectively portrays the lack of guilt and remorse that in part defines the antisocial personality.

Bad Lieutenant (1992) Drama ΨΨΨ
Cocaine-addicted, alcoholic police officer who abuses his position and his family reexamines his life and values after investigating the case of a nun who refuses to identify the man who has raped her.

Ballast (2008) Drama ΨΨ
A man's suicide profoundly affects three lonely people living in the Mississippi Delta.

Beyond Right And Wrong: Stories of Justice And Forgiveness (2012) Documentary ΨΨΨΨ
This sensitive film examines survivors of atrocities around the globe and emphasized the healing that can come through forgiveness.

Blood Diamond (2006) Action-Drama ΨΨΨΨ
Leonardo DiCaprio portrays a rough, mercenary, diamond smuggler who grapples with an American journalist (Jennifer Connelly) and must decide between money and assisting a fisherman (Djimon Hounsou) whose child has been kidnapped and turned into a terrorist. The film is a wake-up call on the topic of conflict diamonds.

Blue Velvet (1986) Mystery ΨΨΨΨ
A powerful and engrossing film about drugs, sexual violence, and sadomasochism. Dennis Hopper plays Frank Booth, a sociopathic and sadistic drug addict who appears to be evil personified. Watch for a young Laura Dern.

"He kidnapped them to control her, to make her do things. Then she wanted to commit suicide, so he started cutting off ears as a warning to her to stay alive. I'm not kidding. Frank loved blue. Blue velvet."

***Blue Velvet* (1986)**

Bonnie and Clyde (1967) Crime ΨΨΨΨΨ
Perhaps the best of its genre, this landmark film examines the lives of two of the most fascinating characters in the history of crime.

> **"I ain't much of a lover boy. But that don't mean nothin' personal about you. I never saw no percentage in it. Ain't nothin' wrong with me. I don't like boys...."**
>
> **Clyde Barrow to Bonnie Parker, in *Bonnie and Clyde* (1967)**

Boston Strangler, The (1968) Crime ΨΨ
Tony Curtis, George Kennedy, and Henry Fonda in a film that attempts to portray the inner life of a serial killer.

Bridge on the River Kwai, The (1957) Drama ΨΨΨΨ
Alec Guinness plays an Academy Award–winning role as a British colonel who becomes so obsessed with building a bridge that he loses sight of his loyalty and allegiance to the allied forces.

> **"Do not speak to me of rules. This is war. This is not a game of cricket. He's mad, your Colonel. Quite mad."**
>
> ***The Bridge on the River Kwai* (1957)**

Boy, A (2007, UK) Drama ΨΨΨ
Two young boys commit murder and are sent away; when Jack is eventually released, he attempts to establish a new life, but Jack's past catches up with him and makes renewal impossible. There is a sympathetic portrayal of a rehabilitation counselor in the film.

Cape Fear (1991) Thriller ΨΨΨΨ
Interesting Scorsese remake of a 1962 classic. This version includes Nick Nolte playing a sleazy attorney and Robert De Niro is a sociopathic ex-con out to get revenge by hurting Nolte and his family and seducing his teenage daughter.

Casualties of War (1989) Drama ΨΨΨ
Sean Penn leads a group of five soldiers who kidnap and rape a Vietnamese girl and subsequently kill her. Michael J. Fox subsequently shows the moral courage necessary to confront the four rapists and murderers. Based on a true story.

Celebration, The (1998, Denmark/Sweden) Drama ΨΨΨ
A man confronts his sexually abusive father during a family gathering celebrating his father's 60th birthday. The film presents a realistic approach to abuse confrontation and documents its effect on a family.

City of God (2003, Brazil) Drama-Foreign ΨΨΨΨ
Painfully sobering and graphic look at violence associated with child and adolescent gang life, drug trafficking, and poverty in a section of Rio de Janeiro, Brazil. Depiction of young children and adolescents walking around with no fear, carrying guns, with only revenge on their minds.

Clockwork Orange, A (1971) Science Fiction ΨΨΨΨΨ
Stanley Kubrick's masterpiece about "ultra-violence," stereotypes, Beethoven, pathological youth, the future of society, the evils of aversion therapy, good versus evil, the rehabilitation of prisoners, and free will versus determinism. It is regarded by many as one of the greatest films ever made.

> **"There was me, that is Alex, and my three droogs, that is Pete, Georgie, and Dim, and we sat in the Korova Milkbar trying to make up our rassoodocks what to do with the evening. The Korova milkbar sold milk-plus, milk plus vellocet or synthemesc or drencrom, which is what we were drinking. This would sharpen you up and make you ready for a bit of the old ultraviolence."**
>
> **Opening lines in *A Clockwork Orange* (1971)**

Cold Mountain (2003) Drama-Romance ΨΨ
Amidst a dramatic love story (between characters played by Jude Law and Nicole Kidman), there is a lot of antisocial behavior, violence, immoral behavior, attempted rape, and senseless tortures and killings.

Compulsion (1959) Crime ΨΨΨ
Two homosexual law students kidnap and kill a young boy. Based on the Leopold-Loeb case, the film examines the morality of capital punishment and features Orson Welles in the role played by Clarence Darrow in the actual case.

Cook, the Thief, His Wife & Her Lover, The (1989) Drama ΨΨΨΨ
Peter Greenaway film far too complex to capture in a sentence or two. Full of psychopathology, the film deals with passion, deceit, gluttony, murder, cannibalism, and man's inhumanity to man.

Crash (2004) Drama ΨΨΨΨΨ
Director Paul Haggis blends several stories in this eclectic mix of races and ethnicities in Los Angele that examines racism, discrimination, corruption, and the possibility of redemption.

Das Experiment (2001) Drama-Suspense ΨΨΨ
Depiction of psychological research experiment in a prison setting where subjects are divided into prisoners who waive their civil rights and guards who are expected to maintain peace and order. While this film bears some initial structural similarity to the famous Zimbardo Prison Experiment, it in no way portrays it accurately, as the film's violence goes well beyond actual events.

Dead Man Walking (1995) Drama ΨΨΨΨ
Susan Sarandon and Sean Penn star in this dramatic examination of a nun's need to understand and help a man sentenced to die for the rape and murder of two teenagers. The film skillfully examines the death penalty, family dynamics, themes of redemption, and the mitigating role of drugs, without ever providing easy answers. Sarandon won an Academy Award for her performance in this film.

> **"They got me on a greased rail to the Death House here."**
>
> ***Dead Man Walking* (1995)**

Deliberate Stranger, The (1986) Drama Ψ
Made-for-TV movie about serial killer Ted Bundy.

Deliverance (1972) Adventure ΨΨΨΨ
Jon Voight, Ned Beatty, and Burt Reynolds on a whitewater rafting trip in Appalachia. Beatty winds up being sodomized, and Reynolds kills the rapist, using a bow and arrow. Based on a James Dickey novel, the film raises interesting questions about personal responsibility and social justice.

> **"Lewis, don't play games with these people."**
>
> ***Deliverance* (1972)**

Dentist, The (1996) Horror Ψ
A successful Beverly Hills dentist goes mad when he discovers his wife having oral sex with the boy who cleans their pool.

Disclosure (1994) Drama ΨΨ
A less-than-illuminating film about reverse sexual discrimination. Stars include Demi Moore and Michael Douglas; the film is based on a novel by Michael Crichton.

Disco Pigs (2001, Ireland) Drama ΨΨ
A boy and a girl born seconds apart become inseparable until the age of 17 when sexual tension complicates their lives.

Dog Day Afternoon (1975) Crime ΨΨΨ
Al Pacino holds up a bank to get enough money to fund a sex-change operation for his homosexual lover. Good illustration of a basically good person caught up in a stressful situation.

Domino (2005) Action Ψ
A tough, rebellious, female bounty hunter tries to fight fair.

Don't Tell (2005, Italy/UK/France/Spain) ΨΨΨΨ
Drama
A young adult woman realizes she has repressed nearly all her childhood, and following the death of her parents, begins to have nightmares of her father sexually abusing her as a young girl. She consults with her brother to put the pieces together.

Down and Dirty (1976) Drama ΨΨ
An interesting examination of the effects of poverty, squalor, and alcoholism on an Italian family.

Dressed to Kill (1980) Thriller Ψ
The film confuses transsexualism and schizophrenia but offers good suspense. Mimics Hitchcock.

Eastern Promises (2007) Thriller-Drama ΨΨΨ
David Cronenberg film about Russian gangsters. The film features an unforgettable, intense fight scene in a steam room.

Elephant (2003) Drama ΨΨΨΨΨ
Well-crafted, foreboding, and eerie Gus Van Sant film that attempts to explain a tragic school shooting. Powerful parallels with Columbine. Winner of the Palm awards at Cannes for Best Picture and Director.

End of Violence, The (1997) Drama-Suspense ΨΨΨ
Bill Pullman plays an action-violence film director who is almost murdered, so he hides out from society and starts a new life. While his character both promotes and greatly fears violence, a secret government worker tries to prevent violence by watching over the city with thousands of cameras.

Executioner's Song, The (1982) ΨΨ
Made for TV Drama
Tommy Lee Jones plays serial killer Gary Gilmore. Based on the story by Norman Mailer.

Extremities (1986) Drama Ψ
Farrah Fawcett plays a victimized woman who gets revenge on the man who raped her.

Fallout, The (2021) Drama ΨΨΨΨΨ
Megan Park directed this film about two teen girls trying to cope with a school shooting. The film differs from others in the genre by focusing on the aftermath of the shooting rather than the event itself.

Fight Club (1999) Drama-Suspense ΨΨΨΨ
A disillusioned insomniac (Edward Norton) meets a dangerous, malcontent part of himself in the character of Brad Pitt. Norton then establishes "fight clubs" where men can violently release their aggressions by fighting one another.

> **"The first rule of Fight Club is: you do not talk about Fight Club. The second rule of Fight Club is: you DO NOT talk about Fight Club! Third rule of Fight Club: someone yells "stop!", goes limp, taps out, the fight is over. Fourth rule: only two guys to a fight. Fifth rule: one fight at a time, fellas. Sixth rule: No shirts, no shoes. Seventh rule: fights will go on as long as they have to. And the eighth and final rule: if this is your first time at Fight Club, you have to fight."**
>
> The rules for *Fight Club* (1999)

Freedomland (2006) Mystery-Drama Ψ
Julianne Moore portrays a neglectful mother; her character stands in marked contrast to Samuel L. Jackson's character who is attempting to redeem himself by caring for his adult son who is in prison.

Funny Games (1997, Austria; Remake 2007) ΨΨΨ
Drama-Horror
Two sadistic, psychopathic killers ask to borrow eggs from, and then go on to capture, torture, and kill, a vacationing family.

Gangs of New York (2002) Crime-Drama ΨΨΨ
Martin Scorsese film about the revenge perpetrated upon a gang kingpin named Bill "the Butcher" Cutting (Daniel Day-Lewis).

Godfather, The (1972), **The Godfather, Part II** (1974), and **The Godfather, Part III** (1990) Drama ΨΨΨΨΨ
The three-part gangster trilogy, directed by Francis Ford Coppola, examines violence, corruption, and crime in America.

> **"We'll make him an offer he can't refuse."**
>
> *The Godfather* (1972)

Gone Baby Gone (2007) Crime-Drama ΨΨΨΨ
An interesting and complex film, and Ben Affleck's directorial debut. The film is about a young girl who has been neglected by her drug-dependent mother and has gone missing. The movie raises fascinating questions about parental responsibility and the role of society.

Good Son, The (1993) Drama ΨΨ
A 12-year-old boy goes to stay with his uncle, aunt, and cousin, only to discover that the cousin is a psychopath and a killer. The boy's aunt eventually discovers the truth about her son and must make a difficult decision that pits the love of her son against her sense of right and justice.

Grindhouse: Death Proof (2007) and **Grindhouse: Planet Terror** (2007) Thrillers ΨΨΨ
Two feature lengths films often shown together that pay homage to gory exploitation films. Both feature significant violence – the first involves a gang of women who face off with a murderous racecar driver, and the second features an army of flesh-eating zombies. Not surprisingly, the Tarantino-directed film (the first one) is more engaging and interesting.

Halloween (1978; and its sequels: 1981, 1982, 1988, 1998, 2002, 2006, 2007, 2009) Horror Ψ
Infamous mass murderer depicted as an escaped mental patient and a deranged toy maker. These films have contributed significantly to negative stereotypes of mental illness and the belief that psychiatric patients are homicidal maniacs.

Hand That Rocks the Cradle, The (1992) Ψ
Thriller-Drama
Sociopathic woman seeks revenge for the suicide of her husband by moving in and taking over the family of the woman she holds responsible for her husband's death. Predictable performances, but still an interesting film.

Heavenly Creatures (1994) Drama ΨΨΨΨ
A New Zealand film directed by Peter Jackson and based on the true story of two adolescent girls who grow up sharing a fantasy world. When the mother of one of the girls decides to separate the children, they murder her. One of the girls, Ann Perry, served five years in prison, but now lives in England and writes mystery novels.

Henry: Portrait of a Serial Killer (1990) ΨΨΨΨ
Crime-Horror
A violent, controversial film about mass murderer and sociopath Henry Lee Lucas. A scene in which Lucas and his roommate videotape one of their murders is especially unnerving.

> **"She'd make me watch it... She'd beat me when I wouldn't watch her... She'd make me wear a dress and they would laugh."**
>
> **Henry Lee Lucas describing abuse by his mother, a prostitute, in *Henry: Portrait of a Serial Killer* (1990)**

History of Violence, A (2005) Drama-Mystery ΨΨΨΨ
David Cronenberg film about a quiet, unassuming family man who springs to action when the workers and customers of his café are threatened by thugs. His fighting prowess causes his family to question his past and who he really is.

Honeymoon Killers, The (1970) Crime Ψ
A very realistic black-and-white film based on the true story of a couple who lured, exploited, and then killed lonely women. Both the man and the woman were executed in Sing-Sing Prison.

Hotel Rwanda (2004) Drama-Documentary ΨΨΨΨΨ
Depicts the genocide of the Hutus upon the Tutsis in Rwanda and the courageous efforts of Paul Rusesabagina, the owner of the Hôtel des Mille Collines in the Rwandan capital of Kigali, who saved over 1,200 refugees. The film illustrates courage and persistence; it also shows how one ordinary man can be extraordinary and triumph over evil.

House of 1000 Corpses (2003) Horror Ψ
Musician Rob Zombie directed this film about a family of eerie serial killers that contains some comic relief.

Hunger Games, The (2012) Drama ΨΨΨ
Children between the ages of 12–18 are selected to compete to the death in televised games, the rules of which allow only one couple to survive.

Hunger Games, The: Catching Fire (2013) Drama ΨΨ
An engaging sequel in which the winners of the Hunger Games are required to compete once again.

In Cold Blood (1967) Biography-Crime ΨΨΨ
This film is based on a Truman Capote biographical novel about two sociopaths who kill a Kansas family. The film explores the family dynamics that in part lead to the senseless murders.

I Spit on Your Grave (1978) Horror Ψ
A terrible film in which a woman systematically gets revenge on the four men who raped her. The original was awful, and none of the sequels are any better.

> **"They all felt physically inferior or sexually inadequate. Their childhood was violent.... They couldn't distinguish between fantasy and reality. They didn't hate their victims; they didn't even know them."**
>
> **A doctor describes serial killers, in *In Cold Blood* (1967)**

Interrupters, The (2011) Documentary ΨΨΨ
Former gang members in Chicago work to curb street violence.

Invisible Man, The (2020) Drama, Horror, Mystery, Science Fiction ΨΨ
Elisabeth Moss stars as a woman in a violent relationship with a man she cannot see. The suspense is palpable, but the film doesn't teach the viewer much about mental illness. The film is a good illustration though of gaslighting.

Kill Bill: Vol. 1 (2003) Action-Suspense ΨΨΨΨΨ
Dynamic Tarantino story of a samurai bride (Uma Thurman) betrayed by her ex-lover and boss. This first film sets up the mythology and the world of the characters. It has more extensive graphic violence than Vol. 2 and an "eastern" martial arts emphasis.

> **"I've kept you alive for two reasons. First reason is information... But I am gonna ask you questions and every time you don't give me answers, I'm gonna cut something off. And I promise you they will be things you will miss!"**
>
> **The Bride in *Kill Bill: Vol. 1* (2003)**

Kill Bill: Vol. 2 (2004) Action-Suspense ΨΨΨΨΨ
Tarantino's conclusion to the revenge story of The Bride. This part emphasizes the unfolding of the stories and further deepening of characters in a more "western" style.

> **"I'm a killer. I'm a murdering bastard and there are consequences for breaking the heart of a murdering bastard."**
>
> **Bill in *Kill Bill: Vol. 2* (2004)**

Killing Fields, The (1984) Drama ΨΨΨΨ
Gripping film about the horrors of war and the particularly gruesome and cruel practices of the Khmer Rouge in Cambodia following the evacuation of American soldiers from Vietnam in 1975.

Killing of a Sacred Deer (2017) ΨΨΨΨ
Mystery-Horror
Nicole Kidman plays the wife of an affluent suburban cardiologist (Colin Farrell) who develops an unlikely and unhealthy relationship with fawning young man whose father had died in surgery that Farrell's character had performed years ago. The ending of the film is surprising and unforgettable. The title comes from a Greek myth retold by Euripides and Ovid.

Lilya 4-Ever (2002) Drama ΨΨΨ
A powerful depiction of cruelty and violence. An adolescent girl experiences neglect, abandonment, rejection, physical and sexual abuse, gang rape, exploitation, and forced prostitution, all by the age of 16.

Looking for Mr. Goodbar (1977) Drama ΨΨ
Diane Keaton plays a special education teacher with a compulsive need to pick up men in bars and engage in sadomasochistic sex. There are numerous examples of family pathology in the film, and it is interesting to remember how casually we treated sex in a time before AIDS.

Lovely Bones, The (2009): Drama-Suspense ΨΨΨ
Peter Jackson film about a young teenage girl who is raped and murdered by a pedophile in her neighborhood. The focus in the film is on the perpetrator's acts of violence; his subsequent cover-up behaviors; his craving, obsession, intent, and plan to kill again; and the impact of the death on the girl's family.

Luckiest Girl Alive (2022) Drama ΨΨ
A disappointing film that deals with double trauma (rape and a school shooting) in a young woman who appears to have everything going for her.

M (1931, Germany) Crime-Drama-Horror ΨΨ
A must-see Fritz Lang film (his first "talkie") starring Peter Lorre as a sexual psychopath who molests and murders little girls. When tried by a vigilante jury, he claims to have irresistible impulses, but the jury is not impressed.

Magdalene Sisters, The (2002) Docudrama ΨΨΨ
Troubled adolescent girls are sent to a dehumanizing boarding home where they are treated by the nuns who run the home, with abuse, neglect, and humiliation. The film follows four girls as they experience and respond differently to the highly abusive situation.

Mad Max: Fury Road (2015) Action-Adventure ΨΨ
The fourth of a series of *Mad Max* films, and possibly the best. The films portray an apocalyptic world in which violence is rampant. I enjoyed the film – I just didn't learn much about mental illness.

Mass (2021) Drama ΨΨΨΨ
A powerful film about two sets of grieving parents: One set are the parents of a child murdered in a school shooting years earlier; the other set, the parents of the teenage boy who did the shooting.

Metallica: Some Kind of Monster (2004) ΨΨΨ
Documentary
Inside look at the heavy metal band, Metallica, and their personal and interpersonal struggles. The handling of anger is a key theme in the film. The honest expression of emotions by these rock stars is likely to have a positive impact on many fans.

Midnight Express (1978) Biography ΨΨΨ
True story about an American college student who is busted for trying to smuggle 2 kg of hashish out of Turkey and is treated brutally in Turkish prisons before eventually escaping.

Midsommar (2019, Sweden) Drama-Horror ΨΨΨΨ
A long, violent, and unforgettable film about young American students who travel to Sweden to study a cult. The film is violent, but the violence is critical to the storyline.

Monster (2003) Drama ΨΨΨΨ
A powerful film based on the life of Aileen Carol Wuornos, a highway prostitute who was executed for killing seven men in Florida during the 1980s. (Also see *Aileen: Life and Death of a Serial Killer*, in this section of Appendix 6.)

Murder in the First (1995) Drama ΨΨ
A man imprisoned in Alcatraz for petty theft in the 1930s is put in solitary confinement for 3 years, becomes deranged, and then kills a guard. The film suggests the system is to blame for the crime. Based on a true story.

Mysterious Skin (2004) Drama ΨΨΨ
A coach sexually molests two boys, and their lives go in completely different directions. Intense, realistic portrayal of the ways sexual abuse affects children when they become adolescents and adults.

Natural Born Killers (1994) Crime-Drama ΨΨΨΨΨ
A violent Oliver Stone film based on a story written by Quentin Tarantino and starring Woody Harrelson and Juliette Lewis. The film depicts a couple who celebrate their roles as mass murderers and find their new status as cult figures a welcome reprieve from the dreariness of the life they left behind.

"Insane, no. Psychotic, yes. A menace to living creatures, yes. But to suggest that they're insane gives the impression that they don't know right from wrong. Mickey and Mallory know the difference between right and wrong. They just don't give a damn."

A psychiatric opinion in *Natural Born Killers* (1994)

Night Porter, The (1974) Drama–War ΨΨ
A former Nazi officer who sexually abused a 14-year-old girl in a concentration camp has the tables turned on him when she shows up at the hotel in which he works. This is one of several films linking Nazi practices with sadomasochistic sex.

No Man's Land (2001) Drama–Suspense ΨΨΨΨ
A Bosnian escapes a battle field and finds himself in no man's land between enemy lines. A Serb goes to ensure there were no survivors and finds himself in a standoff with the Bosnian. Another Bosnian survivor, barely alive, awakes on top of a land mine that will explode if he rises. Heated debates, murder attempts, threats, desperation, and hopelessness characterize the responses of each of the three men.

North Country (2005) Drama ΨΨΨΨ
Charlize Theron transforms herself again (following up her role as a serial killer in *Monster*), this time to play a woman who goes to great lengths to support her children by working in a blue-collar mine where she experiences significant sexual harassment.

Old Man (2022) Mystery ΨΨ
This is a difficult film to categorize; the ending is extremely violent, but the old man at the center of the film is clearly a paranoid personality. He lives alone with his dog until a stranger shows up, and then it turns out that the stranger is a younger version of himself. I found the film chaotic and confusing, and it has little to teach us about mental illness.

"It's the same old story. I've got to learn to keep my mouth shut."

Beth blaming herself for the beating she has received from her husband, in *Once Were Warriors* (1994)

Once Were Warriors (1994) Drama ΨΨΨΨ
Important New Zealand film about substance abuse and domestic violence among urban Māori tribal people. The film will help you understand a different culture, as well as the ways in which alcoholism interacts with spousal and child abuse in almost every society.

Osama (2003, Afghanistan) Drama ΨΨΨΨ
Based on a true story of the heavy discrimination, abuse, and oppression of women under Taliban rule.

Paper Tiger (2020) Drama ΨΨΨΨ
Based on a true story, this film depicts a teenage boy diagnosed with schizophrenia. He is isolated and a loner, fascinated with Adolph Hitler, violent videogames, and school shootings. His widowed mother, afraid that he is planning a shooting himself, buys a gun, checks into a hotel with her son, and then murders her son.

Parasite (2019) Drama ΨΨΨΨΨ
A remarkable film by Korean director Bong Joon Ho contrasting two families, one very rich and one very poor. The film's complex plot involves ongoing tension and deception between the two families and underscores the harsh cruelty of wealth inequality. The ending of the film is especially violent, but the violence never seems gratuitous. This movie won the prestigious Palme d'Or at Cannes, as well as Academy Awards for Best Motion Picture, Best Achievement in Directing, Best Original Screenplay, and Best Achievement in Production Design.

Passion of the Christ, The (2004) Drama–Biography ΨΨΨΨ
Mel Gibson film depicting the violent torture and suffering of the final hours of Jesus Christ. This highly controversial film is intensely graphic and visual in its portrayal of violence. It is interesting to note that it is Mel Gibson's hand that nails Jesus to the cross.

Personal Velocity (2002) Drama ΨΨΨ
Independent film about three strong women divided into three segments. One segment addresses issues of domestic violence.

"She imagined going back to him like she had done so many times before but this time her body wouldn't follow."

Narration on the escape from an abusive husband, in *Personal Velocity* (2002)

Play Misty for Me (1971) Thriller ΨΨΨ
The first film directed by Clint Eastwood. A California disc jockey becomes involved with a listener who is clinging, dependent, fanatical, and ultimately homicidal. Interesting portrayal of sexual obsession.

Precious (2009) Drama ΨΨΨΨ
Gabourey Sidibe gives a riveting performance as Claireece "Precious" Jones, an illiterate, obese, Black 16-year-old, who is pregnant for the second time by her father. Living in Harlem with her abusive mother, Precious struggles to cope with constant degradation and abuse through fantasies and dissociation. She gradually builds self-esteem through the help of a teacher at an alternative school.

Prick Up Your Ears (1987) Biography ΨΨΨΨ
A film showing the homosexual relationship and eventual murder-suicide of playwright Joe Orton and his lover.

Princess Aurora (2005, Korea) Drama ΨΨ
A saleswoman goes on a killing spree and leaves a cartoon sticker of Princess Aurora at the scene of each crime.

Promising Young Woman (2020) Drama ΨΨΨ
An attractive medical school dropout spends her days working in a coffee shop and her evenings pretending to be drunk and picking up sexual predators as a way of avenging the rape of a former classmate. The films ending is both surprising and dramatic.

Prophet, A (*Un Prophète;* 2009, France) Drama ΨΨΨΨ
A19-year-old boy is sent to prison for 6 years where he confronts racial tension and extreme violence.

Rampage (1992) Drama-Thriller ΨΨΨ
This movie, directed by William Friedkin, challenges many of the assumptions educated people are likely to hold about the insanity defense.

Rashomon (1950) Drama ΨΨΨΨΨ
Classic Akira Kurosawa film in which a rape-murder is described from four different perspectives by the four people involved. The film makes the point that reality is subjective and that truth, like beauty, is truly in the eye of the beholder.

Rendition (2007) Drama-Thriller ΨΨΨ
An Egyptian man traveling in South Africa at a conference is detained without due process. The film addresses extraordinary rendition – detaining suspected terrorists and interrogating them on foreign soil without judicial process – and depicts torture (e.g., waterboarding), brainwashing-training of suicide bombers, and the various realities politicians face.

Reservoir Dogs (1992) Drama ΨΨΨΨΨ
Extremely violent but powerful Tarantino film with a graphic and realistic torture scene in which a sociopathic sadist derives great pleasure from using a razor to slowly torment a bound and gagged undercover police officer.

"Now I'm not gonna bullshit you. I don't really care about what you know or don't know. I'm gonna torture you for a while regardless. Not to get information, but because torturing a cop amuses me. There's nothing you can say, there's nothing you can do. Except pray for death."

The sadistic Mr. Blonde in *Reservoir Dogs* (1992)

River's Edge (1986) Drama ΨΨΨΨ
A riveting film based on a true-life incident in which a young man kills his girlfriend and then shows the decomposing body to a series of friends. It takes days before one of his friends finally notifies authorities about the murder.

Rope (1948) ΨΨΨΨ
Experimental Hitchcock film about two young homosexual men who kill a friend for sport and then hide the body in a room in which they are hosting a cocktail party. Based on the Leopold-Loeb case, the film stars James Stewart.

Santa Sangre (1989) Horror-Thriller ΨΨ
A controversial but unquestionably powerful Jodorowsky film about a boy growing up in bizarre circumstances. There are strong themes of violence and incest. Roger Ebert called this film "a collision between Freud and Fellini."

Saving Private Ryan (1998) War-Action ΨΨΨΨΨ
Steven Spielberg World War II film regarded by some as the most realistic and powerful war film ever made.

Series 7: The Contenders (2001) ΨΨ
Suspense-Comedy
Highly violent, tongue-in-cheek film about a reality television show where the contestants must seek out and kill one another.

Se7en (1995) Drama ΨΨΨ
Morgan Freeman and Brad Pitt star in this engrossing film about a serial killer (Kevin Spacey) who is obsessed with the seven deadly sins (pride, envy, gluttony, lust, anger, covetousness, and sloth) and who kills his victims accordingly (e.g., a man who is gluttonous is forced to eat until he dies from overeating).

Seven Beauties (1976) Comedy-Drama ΨΨΨ
Lina Wertmuller film in which the protagonist (the brother of the seven sisters alluded to in the title) must perform degrading sexual acts for the female commandant of a German prison camp to survive the war.

Shelter Island (2003) Drama-Suspense Ψ
A lesbian couple goes away to an island house to relax. A stranger (Stephen Baldwin) appears on their doorstep during a storm, and things are not what they seem. Simplistic psychology that is not well-applied or developed.

She Said (2022) Drama ΨΨΨ
Two New York Times reporters break a story that led to the arrest and imprisonment of Harvey Weinstein and the beginning of the #MeToo movement. The film may give you some insight into the mind of a sexual predator and the sense of privilege that allowed Weinstein get away with so much for so long.

Sin City (2005) Action-Noir ΨΨΨ
Stylized graphic violence tempered by computerized graphics, based on Frank Miller's comic books, with an all-star cast.

Single White Female (1992) Drama-Horror ΨΨ
A woman breaks up with her boyfriend and takes in a roommate who admires and emulates her - and later tries to kill her.

Sleepers (1996) Drama ΨΨΨ
Guards at a reform school physically and sexually abuse young boys. After the boys grow up, they avenge their abuse and attempt to manipulate the courts to avoid sentencing. The film has a stellar cast including Robert De Niro, Dustin Hoffman, Brad Pitt, and Kevin Bacon.

Slumdog Millionaire (2008) Drama ΨΨΨΨΨ
An Academy Award-winning rags-to-riches story about a young man's destiny that intersperses his performance on *Who Wants to Be a Millionaire* with flashbacks showing significant life experiences that include poverty, abuse, and torture. The film is a classic underdog story with poignant themes of persistence, integrity/honesty, and self-confidence.

Snowtown Murders, The (2011, Australia) ΨΨΨΨ
Drama
A difficult to watch but engrossing movie based on a true story of John Butting who is now serving consecutive life sentences for 11 murders, disposing of the bodies in barrels in an abandoned bank vault. Butting holds a place in history as Australia's worst serial killer.

"It's not fuckin' mean if you kick the shit out of some diseased prick. He fuckin' deserves it. It's an Australian fuckin' tradition, anyway. Eh?"

John Bunting,
in *The Snowtown Murders* (2011)

South Central (1992) Action-Suspense ΨΨ
A man is released from prison and tries to lead an upright, gang-free life.

Stone Boy, The (1984) Drama ΨΨ
Robert Duvall and Glenn Close star in this slow-moving but intelligent film about a young man who accidentally shoots his brother. The film depicts the effect the shooting has on the entire family.

Straw Dogs (1971) Crime ΨΨΨ
Provocative and violent Sam Peckinpah film, with Dustin Hoffman as a peace-loving mathematician who resorts to violence after his wife is raped.

Sweeney Todd: The Demon Barber of Fleet Street (2007) Musical-Thriller ΨΨΨ
Extensive violence tuned to music and dance in Tim Burton's story of revenge starring Johnny Depp and Helena Bonham Carter.

Take My Eyes (*Te Doy Mis Ojos;* 2003, Spain) ΨΨΨΨ
Drama
A compelling film about domestic violence. The abusive husband is treated by a psychologist but continues to abuse his wife.

Tattoo (1981) Drama Ψ
Mentally ill tattoo artist kidnaps a model and uses her body as a canvas for his art. This is a movie that perpetuates stigma and prejudice about mental illness.

Terribly Happy (*Frygtelig Lykkelig;* 2008, Denmark) Drama ΨΨ
A policeman from Copenhagen has a nervous breakdown and is transferred to a small Danish town where he discovers both secrets and violence.

Louise: "We'll be drinking margaritas by the sea, mamacita."
Thelma: "Hey, we could change our names."
Louise: "We could live in a hacienda."
Thelma: "I'm gonna get a job. I'm gonna work at Club Med."

***Thelma and Louise* plan their future**

Thelma & Louise (1991) Drama–Comedy ΨΨΨ
Two women friends on the road for a weekend lark wind up fleeing from the law and end their lives in a defiant suicidal act. This is a powerful feminist film that stars Susan Sarandon, Geena Davis, Harvey Keitel, and a young Brad Pitt.

They Shall Not Grow Old (2018) ΨΨΨΨ
War–Documentary
Director Peter Jackson used computer restoration technology to colorize and restore World War I film footage. The film personalizes and accurately captures the horrors of war and the kind of stress soldiers experience on the battlefield.

Till (2022) Drama–Biography ΨΨΨΨΨ
Moving story about a mother's heroism following the murder of her son, Emmett Till, who was abducted, tortured, and murdered in Mississippi on a trip to visit his cousins. Till was accused of offending a White woman, and his killers were found not guilty; later, they went on to confess and sell their story to Look magazine for $4,000, protected by laws against double jeopardy.

Time to Kill, A (1996) Drama ΨΨΨ
Samuel Jackson plays an angry father who murders two White men who have raped his daughter. The film explores themes of racial and social injustice, temporary insanity, and justifiable homicide.

Triumph of the Spirit (1989) Biography ΨΨΨ
Story of Auschwitz concentration camp during World War II. Good introduction to the horrors and stress of concentration camp life.

Twist of Faith (2004) Documentary ΨΨ
A firefighter faces the trauma of childhood sexual abuse by a priest, speaking to the shame, horror, anger, and dissociation that occurs. He discusses the significant impact of abuse on his life.

Two Women (1960, Italy) War–Drama ΨΨΨ
This Vittorio De Sica film starring Sophia Loren examines war, rape, coming of age, and mother–daughter relations. Loren won an Academy Award for Best Actress for this film.

Virgin Spring, The (1959) Drama ΨΨΨ
An Ingmar Bergman film examining the rape and murder of a young girl by three bandits.

Vulgar (2002) Drama ΨΨ
A man working as a clown for children decides he can make more money working as a clown at bachelor parties. He is tortured, gang raped, and blackmailed by a psychopath and his two sons. The film graphically depicts trauma and violence, but there are also comic moments.

Waitress (2007) Comedy–Drama ΨΨΨΨΨ
Inspirational story of a young, pregnant waitress (Keri Russell) who is not enthusiastic about her pregnancy because the child's father is her psychologically abusive and controlling husband (Jeremy Sisko). Sadly, the film's director, Adrienne Shelly, was murdered before the film was widely released to critical acclaim. Shelly's young daughter appears in the final scene.

War of the Roses, The (1989) Drama–Thriller ΨΨ
Marital conflict slowly progresses into an incredibly destructive battle between Oliver and Barbara Rose (Michael Douglas and Kathleen Turner).

Warrior, The (2001, UK/France/Germany) ΨΨΨ
Drama–Adventure
A warrior, working for a cruel lord as an executioner in feudal India, takes up the practice of nonviolence. His vows becomes particularly challenging when his son is kidnapped and killed in front of him.

We Need To Talk About Kevin (2011) Drama ΨΨΨΨ
A successful woman puts her career on hold to have two children, one of whom is distant, withdrawn, and hostile. The angry child eventually commits mass murder at his high school after killing his father and sister. He spares his mother, wanting to maximize the grief and suffering she will have to endure.

White Ribbon, The (2009, Germany) Drama ΨΨΨ
Strange things happen in a small German village in the months leading up to World War I. These include a wire being strung across a road that almost kills the local doctor when he is thrown from his horse, cabbages beheaded in a field, the suicide of a farmer, and a handicapped child who is bound to a tree and tortured.

Whore's Glory (2011) Documentary ΨΨΨ
A fascinating and nonjudgmental examination of prostitutes and the lives they lead in Thailand, Bangladesh, and Mexico.

Zodiac (2007) Crime–Biography ΨΨ
Jake Gyllenhaal portrays an amateur detective in San Francisco who becomes obsessed with tracking down a serial killer, in this David Fincher film.

Treatment

Antwone Fisher (2003) Drama–Biography ΨΨΨ
A troubled and angry sailor gets in fights and is referred to a psychiatrist (Denzel Washington). Their relationship develops, and Antwone becomes comfortable sharing his history of childhood abuse and trauma; he makes amends for his past, and healing begins. Fair and balanced portrayal of a psychiatrist, although the film includes clear boundary violations (e.g., sharing a Thanksgiving dinner with the psychiatrist's family).

Article 99 (1992) Comedy Ψ
Unsuccessful M*A*S*H*-like attempt to ridicule the quality of care provided in Veterans Administration medical centers.

Bad Timing: A Sensual Obsession (1980) Drama ΨΨ
Interesting and provocative film in which a psychiatrist becomes sexually involved with a troubled and self-destructive woman.

Beautiful Dreamers (1992) Drama–Biography ΨΨΨΨ
True story about poet Walt Whitman's visit to an asylum in London, Ontario. Whitman is shocked by what he sees and persuades the hospital director to offer humane treatment. Eventually, the patients wind up playing the townspeople in a game of cricket.

Beautiful Mind, A (2001) Drama ΨΨΨΨΨ
Based on Sylvia Nasar's biography with the same name. Russell Crowe portrays John Forbes Nash, a mathematical genius and Nobel Prize laureate in Economics who battles schizophrenia and is treated with antipsychotics and insulin-shock therapy.

"Without treatment, John, the fantasies may take over entirely."

Dr. Rosen attempting to educate John Nash on the importance of continuing his treatment regimen, in *A Beautiful Mind* (2001)

Beyond Therapy (1987) Comedy Ψ
Disappointing Robert Altman film about New York yuppies and their psychiatrists.

Butcher's Wife, The (1991) Romance–Fantasy ΨΨ
Greenwich Village psychiatrist Jeff Daniels finds Demi Moore, the butcher's wife, is giving advice at least as good as his own.

Cabinet of Dr. Caligari, The (1920) Horror ΨΨΨΨΨ
German expressionistic film about hypnosis and the power of a hypnotist to induce others to do his bidding. One of the earliest stereotypic presentations of a madman who runs a psychiatric hospital.

Captain Newman, M.D. (1963) ΨΨΨ
Comedy–Drama
Sympathetic story about an Army psychiatrist (Gregory Peck) taking on the military bureaucracy to provide effective treatment for Bobby Darin. Darin is clearly manic and ultimately commits suicide.

Carefree (1938) Musical–Dance ΨΨ
Fred Astaire is a psychiatrist who was talked out of being a dancer. Ginger Rogers is referred to him for treatment (hypnosis) so she can learn to love one of Astaire's friends; he complies with her request, but predictably falls in love with her himself.

Caretakers, The (1963) Drama Ψ
Second-rate film that documents life in a West Coast psychiatric hospital and portrays some of the problems associated with introducing innovations in hospital settings.

Changeling (2008) Drama ΨΨΨ
Angelina Jolie portrays a desperate but persistent mother whose son is kidnapped by a serial child murderer. She battles with a corrupt Los Angeles police force and a manipulative psychiatrist who twists her words, attempts to blackmail her, uses ECT to punish his patients, and holds innocent women captive in the hospital to protect the police department. Based on a true story.

Chattahoochee (1990) Drama ΨΨΨ
Korean war veteran with PTSD is hospitalized and treated. Dennis Hopper has a major role as a fellow patient.

Clockwork Orange, A (1971) Science Fiction ΨΨΨΨΨ
Fascinating interpretation of Anthony Burgess's novel. The portrayal of aversion therapy is somewhat heavy-handed but raises legitimate questions about the appropriate limits of behavior modification.

Color of Night (1994) Drama Ψ
Bruce Willis plays a disillusioned psychologist who gives up his practice after a patient commits suicide. Willis's character discovers he is no longer able to perceive the color red. Much of the plot revolves around a patient with multiple personalities who is simultaneously a group therapy patient and, unknown to Willis, his lover as a woman (in a core personality named Rose).

Couch Trip, The (1988) Comedy Ψ
Dan Aykroyd plays a psychiatric patient who escapes from an institution and then passes himself off as a Beverly Hills psychiatrist. The film reinforces the notion that psychiatry is mainly pretentious language, social manipulation, and "the purchase of friendship."

Dangerous Method, A (2011, UK) ΨΨΨ
Biography–Drama
A David Cronenberg film documenting the early days of psychoanalysis and some of the interactions between Freud and Jung. In the film, Jung has erotic and sadomasochistic sex with his patient, Sabina.

Dark Past, The (1948) Crime ΨΨ
A psychologist who is taken prisoner tries to use his training to help his captor. Remake of the film *Blind Alley*.

David and Lisa (1962) Drama ΨΨΨΨ
A dated but still sensitive portrayal of life in a psychiatric institution. Perpetuates the myth that love will conquer mental illness, but gives a strong and balanced portrayal of a compassionate psychiatrist.

Dead Man Out (1989) Drama ΨΨ
Superior and timely made-for-TV movie about a psychiatrist treating a convict so the man will be sane enough to be executed. The firm raises meaningful questions about ethical issues and the appropriate limits of professional practice.

Dream Team, The (1989) Comedy ΨΨ
Four psychiatric patients are being taken to a game in Yankee Stadium when their doctor–escort is knocked unconscious and hospitalized. The entire film appears to be based on the well-known (and better done) shipboard outing by Jack Nicholson and his friends in *One Flew Over the Cuckoo's Nest*.

Jack McDermott: "What about dinner? Who's gonna get us our dinner?"
Billy: "Aren't you the same guy who changed water into wine? Huh? J.C.? Ain't the son of God good for a burger in his town? You get us something!"

***The Dream Team* (1989)**

Elephant Song (2014, Canada) Drama ΨΨΨ
A psychiatrist and a nurse both commit numerous ethical violations as they treat a disturbed and dangerous young man who has murdered his mother and perhaps another ward psychiatrist.

Face to Face (*Ansikte Mot Ansikte;* 1976, Sweden) Drama ΨΨΨΨ
Liv Ullmann plays a psychiatrist whose life is falling apart. She attempts suicide by taking an overdose and winds up in a coma. Interesting dream sequences with Bergman's usual presumption of childhood trauma as the trigger for adult unhappiness.

Fear Strikes Out (1957) Biography–Sports ΨΨΨ
Anthony Perkins as baseball player Jimmy Piersall, who suffers a mental breakdown because of his inability to please a domineering, demanding father. Piersall was successfully treated with psychotherapy and ECT and eventually staged a comeback.

Final Analysis (1992) Thriller–Drama ΨΨ
A complex film that pays homage to Hitchcock; interesting issues of childhood sexual abuse, repressed memories, professional responsibility, and the doctor–patient relationship.

"Just repeat the last two words they say and phrase it like a question."

A psychiatrist joking about his profession, in *Final Analysis* (1992)

Fine Madness, A (1966) Drama ΨΨΨ
Sean Connery plays Samson Shillitoe, an eccentric and unconventional poet who is hospitalized and lobotomized because of his sexual peccadilloes and the fact that he can't conform to societal expectations. The film was ahead of its time in raising important issues about the rights of people with mental illness.

Flame Within, The (1935) Drama Ψ
Dated and insipid film about a psychiatrist who falls in love with a patient.

Frances (1982) Biography ΨΨΨΨΨ
A vivid portrayal of the life of actress Frances Farmer, including her institutionalization, lobotomy, and alcoholism.

Good Will Hunting (1997) Drama ΨΨΨΨ
Robin Williams won an Academy Award for Best Supporting Actor for his role as a counseling psychologist teaching at a community college and treating a troubled young man (Matt Damon) who is extraordinarily gifted mathematically.

High Anxiety (1977) Comedy ΨΨ
Mel Brooks spoofs Hitchcock films and introduces The Psycho-Neurotic Institute for the Very, Very Nervous.

House of Fools (2002) Drama ΨΨΨΨ
Based on a true story: the chief psychiatrist and treatment staff of a mental institution flee due to conflicts in Chechnya, leaving the patients to fend for themselves. Soon soldiers occupy the hospital, and the viewer is left with various questions about war, politics, mental health treatment and which is crazier – the mentally ill or the politics of war. The film is loaded with examples of psychopathology.

I Heart Huckabees (2005) Comedy-Mystery ΨΨΨ
Dustin Hoffman and Lilly Tomlin play existential psychologists in this quirky, offbeat comedy. Although there is no formal therapy, there are plenty of therapeutic moments.

Inside/Out (1997) Drama ΨΨΨ
A Rob Tregenza film about life in a psychiatric hospital that was well received at the 1998 Sundance Film Festival. The film documents that both patients and staff find it hard to cope with the difficult demands of life.

Intimate Strangers (*Confidences Trop Intimes;* 2004, France) Drama ΨΨΨΨ
A woman mistakenly receives psychotherapy from an accountant in this thoughtful film.

Invisible Class, The (2019) Documentary ΨΨΨΨΨ
A powerful documentary that documents the myriad problems associated with homelessness in the United States. Some of the filming was done in San Francisco's tenderloin district, and many of the individuals interviewed are addicted to substances or mentally ill.

It's Kind of a Funny Story (2010) Comedy-Drama ΨΨΨ
A suicidal 16-year-old high school student checks himself into a psychiatric hospital where he is mentored by an older and more experienced patient played by Zach Galifianakis.

King of Hearts (1966) Comedy-Drama-War ΨΨΨΨ
In World War I, a Scotsman (Alan Bates) is assigned to enter a town and investigate a report that the retreating Germans have left a bomb, and finds that the town has been abandoned by all except the inmates of the local insane asylum. This is a must-see film for anyone interested in public attitudes about mental illness.

Ladybird, Ladybird (1993) Drama ΨΨΨΨ
Dramatic presentation of the clash between the rights of a parent and society's need to protect children.

Lilith (1964) Drama ΨΨ
Strong cast (Peter Fonda, Gene Hackman, Warren Beatty, and Kim Hunter) supports a weak script about a psychiatric inpatient who seduces a neophyte therapist.

Lost Angels (1989) Drama ΨΨ
Donald Sutherland plays a psychiatrist treating a Los Angeles adolescent who is angry and troubled but probably not mentally ill.

> **"When insurance paid for a year in a place like this, we said it took a year to help a kid. Now insurance pays for three months, and, presto, it takes three months to turn a kid around."**
>
> **Dr. Charles Loftis complaining about the system, in *Lost Angels* (1989)**

Ludwig (1973) Biography Ψ
Long and somewhat tedious film about the mad King Ludwig of Bavaria. Good costumes and scenery, but the film teaches us little about mental illness or Ludwig himself.

Man Facing Southeast (*Hombre Mirando Al Sudeste;* 1986, Argentina) Drama ΨΨΨΨ
Fascinating Argentine film about a man without identity who shows up at a psychiatric hospital claiming to be from another planet. It seems that this is not just another patient, and neither the hospital staff nor the film's audience ever figures out exactly what is happening. Compare with *K-Pax* (2001).

Manic (2001) Drama ΨΨΨ
A psychologist played by Don Cheadle tries to help an angry adolescent. Interesting group therapy sessions and inpatient hospital scenes with adolescents who have bipolar disorder, intermittent explosive disorder, major depression, self-injurious behavior, and night terrors.

Man Who Loved Women, The (1983) Comedy Ψ
A remake of the François Truffaut film of the same name. This film involves long sequences in which Burt Reynolds unburdens himself to his psychiatrist.

Marat/Sade (1966) Drama ΨΨΨΨ
In the early 1800s, the inmates of a French asylum put on a play directed by the Marquis de Sade (a patient)

based on the bathtub assassination of Jean Paul Marat. The play incites the patients to riot.

Mine Own Executioner (1947) Drama ΨΨ
Confused and troubled psychoanalyst tries to help a schizophrenic veteran.

Mr. Deeds Goes to Town (1936) Comedy ΨΨΨ
Frank Capra film in which a character played by Gary Cooper inherits 20 million dollars and is judged insane when he decides to give it all away to needy farmers.

Mr. Jones (1993) Drama-Comedy ΨΨΨ
Richard Gere portrays a bipolar patient treated by a psychiatrist who falls in love with him. This film raises interesting and important questions about the therapeutic relationship and boundary issues in psychotherapy.

Mumford (1999) Drama ΨΨΨ
A man named Mumford pretending to be a psychologist sets up shop in a small town (also named Mumford) and begins to help the townspeople.

Nobody's Child (1986) Biography ΨΨ
Marlo Thomas won an Emmy for her role as a woman who experiences tremendous personal and professional success when she is released after spending 20 years in a mental hospital.

No Time for Sergeants (1958) Comedy Ψ
Andy Griffith stars; Don Knotts plays an Army psychiatrist.

No Way Out (1950) Drama ΨΨΨ
This was Sidney Poitier's first film. Poitier plays a black physician treating two racist hoodlums. When one dies, his brother (Richard Widmark) incites a race riot. The film was one of the earliest serious examinations of racism in postwar America.

Now, Voyager (1942) Drama ΨΨΨ
Her psychiatrist and inpatient treatment both help sexually repressed Bette Davis find meaning and purpose in her life by serving as a surrogate mother for the daughter of a man she loves. The title comes from Walt Whitman's *Leaves of Grass* ("The untold want by life and land ne'er granted/Now voyager sail thou forth to seek and find.")

> **"Oh Jerry, don't let's ask for the moon. We have the stars."**
>
> **Charlotte Vale addressing her married lover, in *Now, Voyager* (1942)**

Nuts (1987) Drama ΨΨΨ
Barbra Streisand plays a prostitute who has killed a patron. She is resisting an insanity defense, and through flashbacks we learn that she was sexually abused as a child. Interesting examination of civil liberties and forensic psychiatry.

Office Space (1999) Comedy Ψ
A hypnotherapist induces a trance in a patient but suffers a heart attack before the patient comes out of the trance.

One Flew Over the Cuckoo's Nest (1975) ΨΨΨΨΨ
Drama
Classic film with Jack Nicholson as Randle P. McMurphy, who takes on Nurse Ratched and the psychiatric establishment. The film offers good insight into life on an inpatient ward, although the portrayal of ECT is stereotyped and inaccurate; in addition, the suicide of Billy seems to be simplistically linked to his domineering mother. This film took all five of the top Oscars in 1975: Best Picture, Best Actor, Best Actress, Best Director, and Best Screenplay.

> **"They was giving me ten thousand watts a day, you know, and I'm hot to trot! The next woman takes me on is gonna light up like a pinball machine and pay off in silver dollars!"**
>
> **Randle P. McMurphy commenting on ECT, in *One Flew Over the Cuckoo's Nest* (1975)**

Passion of Joan of Arc, The (1928) Historical ΨΨΨ
Historically important silent film that portrays the burning of Joan of Arc as a heretic. The mental status of Joan of Arc remains a controversial subject for historians interested in psychopathology, with many scholars believing the voices she heard and the visions she saw were manifestations of schizophrenia.

President's Analyst, The (1967) Spy-Comedy ΨΨ
James Coburn plays a psychoanalyst working for the president of the United States.

Pressure Point (1962) Drama ΨΨΨ
A black psychiatrist (Sidney Poitier) treats a racist patient (Bobby Darin). Based on a case from Robert Linder's book *The Fifty-Minute Hour*.

Prime (2005) Drama ΨΨ
A therapist discovers that her patient is having an affair with the therapist's son and has failed to disclose this dual relationship. I use this film when teaching medical ethics, and it has led to fascinating class discussions.

Prince of Tides, The (1991) Drama–Romance ΨΨΨ
Barbra Streisand plays a psychiatrist who becomes sexually involved with Nick Nolte's character, the brother of one of her patients. Nolte's character is married to someone else. The film raises interesting questions about the proper limits of the doctor–patient relationship.

Quills (2000) Drama ΨΨΨ
Geoffrey Rush stars in this Philip Kaufman film about the notorious French author who is responsible for the word "sadism." The film depicts the abuses that occurred in the 18th century in the Charenton Insane Asylum, a mental hospital located in the suburbs of Paris. The Marquis de Sade died at Charenton in 1814.

"I write of the great, eternal truths that bind together all mankind. The whole world over, we eat, we shit, we fuck, we kill, and we die."

The Marquis de Sade describes his views on literature, in *Quills* (2000)

Rachel Getting Married (2008) Drama ΨΨΨ
Kym has been in a rehabilitation center for 9 months, but she gets a few days off to attend her sister's wedding. Predictable tensions result, most of which result from Kym's role in the death of her younger brother when Kym, who was drunk at the time, lost control of her car and drove off a bridge. The film highlights the links between substance abuse and depression and the ways in which family dramas serve as triggers for relapse in recovering alcoholics and drug addicts. Rachel also meets DSM-5 criteria for narcissistic personality disorder.

Rampage (1992) Drama–Thriller ΨΨΨ
William Friedkin film about a sociopath who is arrested and tried for murder. The film raises important questions about capital punishment, the not guilty by reason of insanity (NGRI) plea, and the role of the expert witness in the courtroom.

Saving Grace B. Jones (2009) Drama Ψ
A disappointing story about how life is affected when a woman is discharged from a psychiatric hospital and comes to live with her brother and sister-in-law in a small Missouri town.

See You in the Morning (1989) Drama ΨΨ
A film about a Manhattan psychiatrist with multiple problems, including a failed first marriage. Interesting group therapy sequences and lots of speculation about motivation and purpose.

Shock Corridor (1963) Drama ΨΨ
Samuel Fuller film in which a journalist has himself admitted to an insane asylum to get an inside story on a murder but soon becomes psychotic himself. The film is better than it sounds.

Shrink (2009) Drama ΨΨ
Kevin Spacey plays a burned-out therapist who writes popular self-help books and provides therapy for movie stars; however, he is depressed after his wife's suicide and increasingly believes that his profession and his life are futile and pointless.

Spellbound (1945) Thriller ΨΨΨΨΨ
Ingrid Bergman plays a psychiatrist treating Gregory Peck's amnesia. Salvador Dali helped lay out the film's dream sequence. Producer David Selznick wanted the film to be based on his own experiences with psychotherapy, and he used his own analyst as a technical advisor. Watch for the Hitchcock cameo.

"Good night and sweet dreams ... which we'll analyze in the morning."

***Spellbound* (1945)**

Still of the Night (1982) Thriller Ψ
A psychiatrist becomes romantically involved with a woman who may have murdered one of his patients.

Stutz (2022) Biography–Documentary ΨΨΨΨΨ
Jonah Hill interviews his therapist, iconoclastic psychiatrist Phil Stutz, and the two men review the "tools" that Hill claims turned his life around. Therapists are likely to find the film especially engaging.

Teresa (1951) Drama Ψ
Notable only because it stars Rod Steiger in his first role. Steiger plays a psychiatrist in the film.

Through a Glass Darkly (1962) Drama ΨΨΨΨΨ
Classic Bergman film that follows the life of a mentally ill woman after she is treated with ECT and released from a mental hospital.

Tin Cup (1996) Comedy ΨΨ
A promiscuous Texas real estate salesperson becomes a psychologist and trades psychotherapy for golf lessons, eventually winding up in bed with the golf pro (Kevin Costner).

"From the moment I first saw you, I knew I was through with bar girls and... strippers and motorcycle chicks, and... when we first started talking, I was smitten with you, and I'm smitten with you more every day I think about you, and the fact that you know I'm full of crapola only makes you more attractive to me."

Kevin Costner's character hits on his therapist, Dr. Molly Griswold, in *Tin Cup*

Touched (1983) Romance ψ
Two patients on a psychiatric ward fall in love and try to set up a life together after they escape.

Twelve Monkeys (1995) ψψψ
Mystery–Science Fiction
Terry Gilliam film in which Bruce Willis's character travels back in time to stop a plague and winds up in a psychiatric hospital.

Unit of Difficult Patients: What Future for the Criminally Insane? (2017, France) ψψψ
Documentary
A documentary documenting the day-to-day life of 90 male patients committed to a French hospital for the criminally insane. The film has English subtitles and will give students a sense for what it is like to work with patients who are severely mentally ill. Note the frequency of OCD diagnoses; these would be far less common is a similar institution in the United States.

What About Bob? (1991) Comedy ψψ
Bill Murray plays Bob Wiley, a patient who becomes overly dependent on his therapist, Leo Marvin, played by Richard Dreyfuss. The film is very funny, and it raises interesting questions about transference and countertransference. Note the inane discussion of potential psychotropic medications.

"I'm not a shmuck, Bob, and I'm not going to let you breeze into town and steal my family away just because you're crazy enough to be fun."

Dr. Leo Marvin to patient Bob Wiley, in *What About Bob?* (1991)

Whispers in the Dark (1992) Thriller–Drama ψψ
This murder mystery revolves around a psychiatrist who becomes overly involved in the lives of her patients. Mainly useful as a vehicle for discussion of professional issues and lessons on how *not* to behave in therapy.

Film Index

Notes on Supplementary Materials

Materials for your book can be downloaded free of charge once you register on the Hogrefe website.

In addition to Appendices 1–6 the downloadable file includes one or more of the following exploration aids for each chapter:

Questions to Consider While Watching Suggested Movies

Patient Evaluation Sheets Based on Movie Characters

Discussion Questions For Suggested Movies

Critical Thinking Questions on the Disorders/Topics Discussed in the Book

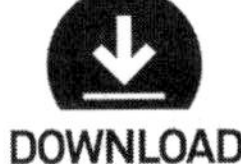

How to proceed:

1. Go to www.hgf.io/media and create a user account. If you already have one, please log in.
2. Go to **My supplementary materials** in your account dashboard and enter the code below. You will automatically be redirected to the download area, where you can access and download the supplementary materials.

Code: B-U2PBTT

To make sure you have permanent direct access to all the materials, we recommend that you download them and save them on your device.

Praise for the Book

"*Movies and Mental Illness* is a great book. No, I should really say that it's two great books in one. First, the book is about movies and thus chock-full of insights that should delight any cinephile. In fact, its cinematic scope is impressive, from classics to contemporary and from Hollywood to international. Second, the book is about mental illness in all its diverse manifestations. Indeed, the coverage goes beyond the strict DSM-5 categories. At the same time, these two books are intricately interwoven into a coherent treatment. That successful integration should not surprise us. The author, Danny Wedding, has already demonstrated his distinctive expertise in prior editions of this work. The current 5th edition just brings everything up to date. Plus, the volume's instructional value remains superlative."

Dean Keith Simonton, PhD, author of *Great flicks: Scientific Studies of Cinematic Creativity and Aesthetics* and co-editor of *The Social Science of Cinema*

"Danny Wedding has outdone himself in this 5th edition. A gifted clinician, he possesses that unique ability to actively engage the reader within the lives of film characters they may have seen, while at the same time lifting them up to appreciate broader underlying themes, both within the mental health field, as well as society. Not only are the latest movies covered, frequently placed within their historical context, the same can be said for changes occurring within mental health - including persisting myths and evolving treatments. What a wonderful way to expose the audience to creative artists within both the film and mental health fields."

Pat DeLeon, PhD, MPH, JD, Past President of the American Psychological Association

"Psychology in one way or another is at the heart of most movies, this book shows how and why. Insightful, creative, enjoyable, this 5th edition takes film criticism and psychology to a new level."

Frank Farley, PhD, Past President, American Psychological Association; Society for the Psychology of Aesthetics, Creativity and the Arts; Society for Media Psychology and Technology

"Two Thumbs Up! The 5th edition of *Movies and Mental Illness* is a masterwork trifecta of scholarly value, valiancy, and vitality and is a must-have guide for educators, practitioners, and film aficionados alike. Dr. Wedding's abilities to explore established diagnoses, to so comprehensively illustrate how their depictions in movies impact, inform, and influence our mental health beliefs and behaviors, and to interweave how these films can be used as both teaching and healing tools are nothing short of brilliant."

Don Grant, PhD, Past President, APA Division 46: Society for Media Psychology and Technology; Fellow, The American Psychological Association